Moving Forward to New Trends in Pulmonary Diseases

Moving Forward to New Trends in Pulmonary Diseases

Guest Editors

Ramona Cioboata
Costin Teodor Streba

MDPI

Basel • Beijing • Wuhan • Barcelona • Belgrade • Novi Sad • Cluj • Manchester

Guest Editors
Ramona Cioboata
Department of Internal Medicine-Pneumology
University of Medicine and Pharmacy
Craiova
Romania

Costin Teodor Streba
Department of Internal Medicine-Pneumology
University of Medicine and Pharmacy of Craiova
Craiova
Romania

Editorial Office
MDPI AG
Grosspeteranlage 5
4052 Basel, Switzerland

This is a reprint of the Special Issue, published open access by the journal *Journal of Clinical Medicine* (ISSN 2077-0383), freely accessible at: https://www.mdpi.com/journal/jcm/special_issues/41E5JFZLDQ.

For citation purposes, cite each article independently as indicated on the article page online and as indicated below:

Lastname, A.A.; Lastname, B.B. Article Title. *Journal Name* **Year**, *Volume Number*, Page Range.

ISBN 978-3-7258-8275-5 (Hbk)
ISBN 978-3-7258-8276-2 (PDF)
https://doi.org/10.3390/books978-3-7258-8276-2

Contents

About the Editors

Ramona Cioboata

Ramona Cioboata is a Lecturer of Pulmonology, a primary physician in Pulmonology and Head of Pulmonology Department at "Victor Babes" Clinical Hospital of Pulmonology and Infectious Disease, which is the reference centre for Tuberculosis and Infectious Disease in the Dolj County. The hospital is affiliated with the University and has an ongoing partnership for research and training of resident physicians, 4th year medical students.

As a pulmonologist, I have experience in diagnosing and treating respiratory conditions, including tuberculosis and other infectious disease. My role as Head of the Pulmonology Department involves not only patient care but also overseeing research initiatives and implementing innovative treatment protocols. I am committed to advancing the field of pulmonology through continuous learning and collaboration with colleagues both locally and internationally. I am actively engaged in multiple clinical trials, with a primary focus on respiratory disorders. These trials contribute to the broader field of respiratory medicine and aim to advance our understanding of lung-related conditions and their management.

Tuberculosis has been the central focus of my ongoing research efforts. This dedication to studying pulmonary tuberculosis has yielded important advancements in our comprehension of how the disease spreads and can be treated. I have led investigative projects focusing on the relationship between COVID-19 and tuberculosis. These studies aimed to elucidate the potential synergistic or antagonistic effects between these two respiratory infections as well as to assess the pandemic's influence on tuberculosis diagnosis, treatment, and patient outcomes. I have over 60 published papers Hirsch Index of 15.

Costin Teodor Streba

Costin Teodor Streba is currently serving as Research Director at the University of medicine and Pharmacy of Craiova, after a four-year mandate as the Pro-Dean with Research at the Faculty of Medicine within the same University. I am a PhD advisor in Pulmonology, also serving as a member of the Doctoral School Council since 2021. I am a Professor of Pulmonology, a primary physician in Pulmonology and a specialist physician in Gastroenterology. I am the founder of the Research Center for AI Applications in Medicine at the University. I have recently coordinated the creation of the Center for Technology Transfer in Medicine, the first of its kind in the South-West Oltenia region of Romania. My ongoing research has always focused on the development of novel, innovative technologies that use computer technology, artificial intelligence, and advanced imaging analysis techniques for the diagnosis of various pathologies. My teams and I received the prestigious "Professor Dr. Gheorghe Badea" award granted by the Romanian Society of Ultrasound in Medicine and Biology in 2023. I was involved in managing data collection from the largest cohort of COVID-19 patients from the South Western region of Romania during the pandemic heights. The influence of large-scale medical emergencies on pre-existing widespread pathologies such as tuberculosis was one of the main focuses of the 2020-2022 period, when we successfully predicted the re-emergence of tuberculosis as a high-risk transmissible threat (a 10% increase in incidence between 2023 and 2020, as well as a raise from 70 to 78 cases per 100,000 inhabitants in our county). Results were successfully communicated, and the national prevention strategy was correctly adjusted to meet the increasing demand for available treatment and hospital beds in dedicated facilities. I have over 100 published papers Hirsch Index of 20, three international books as Editor and participated as author in six reference volumes in national publishing houses.

Preface

Pulmonary diseases remain a major challenge for clinicians, researchers, and health systems because they include heterogeneous conditions with diverse mechanisms, clinical courses, and therapeutic needs. This Reprint was prepared to bring together recent evidence on emerging topics in respiratory medicine and to emphasize the need for earlier diagnosis, better risk assessment, and individualized management. Its scope includes chronic obstructive pulmonary disease, asthma, sleep apnea, lung cancer, COVID-19-related respiratory impairment, rehabilitation, environmental risk factors, and innovations in diagnostic and therapeutic strategies.

The contributions collected here reflect the multidisciplinary nature of modern pulmonary care. They examine biological and clinical markers, new approaches to functional assessment, applications of artificial intelligence, advances in oncologic classification and treatment, the role of bronchoscopy in staging, and the importance of coordinated rehabilitation. Together, these works show how progress in respiratory medicine depends on collaboration among pneumologists, oncologists, radiologists, rehabilitation specialists, laboratory scientists, and other professionals involved in patient care.

This Reprint is addressed to clinicians, researchers, trainees, and healthcare professionals seeking an updated view of pulmonary diseases and their management. We hope that it will support clinical reflection, stimulate further investigation, and contribute to more precise, integrated, and patient-centered care for individuals affected by respiratory disorders.

Ramona Cioboata and Costin Teodor Streba
Guest Editors

Journal of
Clinical Medicine

MDPI

Article

One-Minute Sit-to-Stand Test Versus Six-Minute-Walk Test in Post-COVID-19 Patients: A Cross-Sectional Observational Study

Marta Duarte-Silva [1,2,*], Pedro Fiúza [1,3], Neuza Reis [1] and Miguel Toscano-Rico [1,3]

1 Clínica de Atendimento Post-COVID, ULS São José, 1169-024 Lisboa, Portugal; neuza.reis@ulssjose.min-saude.pt (N.R.); miguel.rico@ulssjose.min-saude.pt (M.T.-R.)
2 Department of Respiratory Medicine, Santa Marta Hospital, ULS São José, 1169-024 Lisboa, Portugal
3 Department of Internal Medicine, Santa Marta Hospital, ULS São José, 1169-024 Lisboa, Portugal
* Correspondence: maria.silva42@ulssjose.min-saude.pt

Abstract

Background: Simplified field tests have gained increasing interest for the assessment of functional capacity in patients with post-COVID-19 condition; however, direct comparisons of functional performance and physiological responses between the 1-minute sit-to-stand test (1MSTST) and the 6-minute walk test (6MWT) remain limited. This study aimed to examine the associations between the two tests by evaluating functional performance, cardiopulmonary responses, oxygen desaturation, perceived exertion, and peripheral muscle strength. Furthermore, we explored whether the 1MSTST can be used as a complementary assessment, particularly within telerehabilitation pathways and in contexts where resource-intensive testing is not feasible. **Methods:** We conducted a cross-sectional observational study of adults recovering from moderate to severe COVID-19 between May and July 2021. Participants performed both the 1MSTST and 6MWT on the same day. Functional performance, peak heart rate, nadir peripheral oxygen saturation (SpO_2), perceived exertion, and handgrip dynamometry were recorded. Associations between test performances were assessed using correlation and partial correlation analyses, including adjustment for peripheral muscle strength. **Results:** Fifty-four patients were included. A moderate correlation was observed between 1MSTST repetitions and 6MWT distance (Spearman's $\rho = 0.47$, $p < 0.001$), which was attenuated after adjustment for muscle strength and demographic variables. Peak heart rate and nadir SpO_2 responses were strongly correlated between tests ($r = 0.75$ and $\rho = 0.83$, respectively; both $p < 0.001$), with no significant differences in magnitude. Exercise-induced oxygen desaturation ($\geq$4% SpO_2 drop) occurred at similar frequencies during both tests. Perceived exertion increased similarly following the 1MSTST and the 6MWT. **Conclusions:** In post-COVID-19 patients, the 1 min sit-to-stand test shows moderate concordance with the 6 min walk test for functional performance and strong agreement in cardiopulmonary responses. These findings suggest that the two tests assess overlapping but distinct aspects of functional capacity. This supports the use of the 1MSTST as a pragmatic complementary assessment when standard walking tests are not feasible, particularly within telerehabilitation pathways, primary care, and resource-limited settings.

Keywords: COVID-19; 1MSTST; 6MWT

1. Introduction

The coronavirus disease 2019 (COVID-19) pandemic has resulted in a growing population of individuals experiencing persistent symptoms and functional limitations long after recovery from the acute infection. A substantial proportion of survivors develop post-acute sequelae of SARS-CoV-2 infection (PASC), commonly referred to as long COVID, characterized by ongoing fatigue, exertional dyspnoea, reduced exercise tolerance, and impaired quality of life [1].

Growing longitudinal evidence indicates that traditional resting assessments alone may be insufficient to capture post-COVID-19 impairment. Several prospective studies have shown that pulmonary function parameters such as forced vital capacity and diffusion capacity may remain stable over time despite persistent symptoms. In a large prospective cohort study with structured follow-up at 3 and 6 months after acute COVID-19, Freund et al. demonstrated that routine pulmonary function measures did not consistently change over time and were poorly correlated with radiological improvement, highlighting the limited sensitivity of standard evaluations and the need for additional functional testing in selected patient populations [2]. Consistent with these findings, systematic reviews and longitudinal cohorts have reported persistent reductions in exercise capacity and physical performance months after COVID-19, even when resting lung function appears normal. Objective functional tests are therefore increasingly recognized as important components of post-COVID-19 follow-up and rehabilitation strategies [3,4].

The 6-minute walk test (6MWT) is widely regarded as a standard field test for the evaluation of functional exercise capacity and exertional oxygen desaturation in patients with cardiopulmonary disease. It is a simple, inexpensive, and well-standardized test with established reference equations and broad use in clinical practice [5]. The primary outcome of the test is the total distance walked over 6 minutes (6MWD), which provides clinically relevant information on submaximal exercise capacity and gas-exchange abnormalities. However, the execution of the 6MWT requires a corridor of 20–30 m and strict methodological standardization, which may limit its feasibility in outpatient, primary care, or resource-limited settings.

In the context of COVID-19, the 6MWT is recommended as a screening tool in the British Thoracic Society guidance for respiratory follow-up, particularly in patients with persistent respiratory symptoms and/or incomplete radiographic resolution [6]. Several studies have demonstrated reduced 6MWT performance in post-COVID-19 patients months after hospital discharge, particularly in those with greater comorbidity burden, prior intensive care admission, or residual pulmonary abnormalities on chest imaging [5,7]. Exercise-induced desaturation during the 6MWT has also been associated with poorer pulmonary function and greater structural lung involvement, reinforcing its role as a tool to identify patients with more pronounced functional impairment [8].

The sit-to-stand test (STST) represents a complementary field test designed to assess physical performance in individuals for whom walking-based assessments may be impractical. The STST requires participants to repeatedly stand up from and sit down on a chair for a defined period and exists in several formats, including the five-repetition, 30 s, and 1-min versions. Among these, the 1-min sit-to-stand test (1-min STST) has demonstrated the strongest association with walking-based functional tests, including the 6MWT, in chronic respiratory diseases such as chronic obstructive pulmonary disease, interstitial lung diseases, and pulmonary hypertension [9–11]. Although the 1 min STST places greater mechanical demand on the lower limbs and may stress muscular endurance to a greater extent, it provides valuable information on overall physical capacity and exercise-induced desaturation while requiring minimal space, equipment, and time [5].

In post-COVID-19 populations, the 1 min STST has been shown to be feasible, safe, have excellent test–retest reliability and sensitivity to functional impairment, with a substantial proportion of patients demonstrating reduced performance relative to reference values and clinically relevant oxygen desaturation during the test [5,12]. Importantly,

https://doi.org/10.3390/jcm15072479

the 1 min STST exhibits minimal learning effect and can be performed as a single trial, making it particularly suitable for outpatient assessment, rehabilitation planning, and telehealth-based monitoring [13].

Despite growing interest in simplified field tests for the assessment of functional capacity, direct comparisons of functional performance and physiological responses between the 1 min sit-to-stand test (1MSTST) and the 6 min walk test (6MWT) in adults recovering from acute COVID-19 remain limited. The present study aimed to examine the relationship between the 1MSTST and the 6MWT in post-COVID-19 patients by evaluating associations with test performance, cardiopulmonary responses, oxygen desaturation, perceived exertion, and peripheral muscle strength. Specifically, we sought to determine whether the 1MSTST elicits physiological and perceptual responses comparable to those of the 6MWT, thereby supporting its use as a complementary, pragmatic assessment particularly within telerehabilitation pathways and when logistical constraints limit the feasibility of standard testing, notably in primary care and resource-limited environments.

2. Materials and Methods

We conducted a cross-sectional observational study in adult patients with post-COVID-19 condition who had experienced moderate to severe acute SARS-CoV-2 infection and were referred for follow-up to the Post-COVID Outpatient Clinic (CAP-COVID) of Unidade Local de Saúde (ULS) de São José, Lisbon, Portugal. CAP-COVID is a multidisciplinary clinic dedicated to the integrated management of patients with acute sequelae and long COVID, involving specialists from internal medicine, pulmonology, physical and rehabilitation medicine, neurology, psychiatry, and nutrition. At the time of the study, follow-up assessments were coordinated through the Department of Internal Medicine. Participants were recruited between May and July 2021. Upon admission to the clinic, written informed consent was obtained, and patients underwent standardized clinical evaluation.

The severity of the acute SARS-CoV-2 infection was classified according to the Portuguese Directorate-General of Health (DGS) guideline (Norma n° 004/2020) [14]. To assess recovery after SARS-CoV-2 infection (including changes in lifestyle, sports, and social activities), the post-COVID-19 Functional Status (PCFS) scale was used. This is a validated ordinal scale developed to quantify functional limitations following COVID-19 infection, ranging from 0 (no functional limitations) to 4 (severe functional limitations) [15,16]. Functional exercise capacity was evaluated using both the 1 min sit-to-stand test (1MSTST) and the 6 min walk test (6MWT). Both tests were performed on the same day, separated by a 1-h rest interval, and tested by the same trained examiner. Participants received standardized instructions prior to each test, without verbal encouragement during performance.

The 1MSTST was conducted using a standardized chair (seat height 46 cm) without armrests. Participants were instructed to stand up and sit down as many times as possible within 1 min, and the total number of completed repetitions was recorded. The 6MWT was performed in accordance with American Thoracic Society guidelines, using a flat, straight 30 m indoor corridor [16]. The total distance walked over 6 min was recorded. For both tests, systolic and diastolic blood pressure were measured immediately before and after exercise. Heart rate and peripheral oxygen saturation (SpO_2) were continuously monitored from 2 min before to 3 min after test completion. Perceived exertion was assessed using the Modified Borg scale immediately before and after each test. Handgrip strength was measured as an index of peripheral muscle strength using a Jamar® hydraulic hand dynamometer, following standardized procedures.

A total of 54 patients completed both the 1MSTST and the 6MWT and were included in the final analysis. Participant inclusion was contingent on the availability of hospital

https://doi.org/10.3390/jcm15072479

staff to administer both tests on the same day. Exclusion criteria are detailed in Table 1. The study was conducted in accordance with the Declaration of Helsinki and was approved by the Ethics Committee of ULS São José, Lisbon, Portugal (approval no. 1209/2022). Patient recruitment and data collection were performed under the institutional framework established for COVID-19 research during the pandemic, regulated by an institutional circular on personal data protection and consent procedures (Circular Informativa No. 160/2020). This framework allowed the collection and processing of personal and clinical data for observational COVID-19–related research, provided that participants gave informed consent and that data protection procedures were respected.

Table 1. Exclusion criteria for this study.

Exclusion Criteria
Patients with a history of orthostatic hypotension
Patients with osteoarticular or neuromuscular diseases that affect standing or walking
Patients with unstable angina, myocardial infarction during the previous month, or arrhythmia
Patients with mental illness or cognitive impairment that prevents them from performing the examination safely and accurately
5. Who meet any of the following conditions
5-1. Pulse rate at rest ≤40/min or ≥120/min
5-2. Systolic blood pressure at rest ≤70 mmHg or ≥180 mmHg
5-3. Diastolic blood pressure at rest ≥100 mmHg
5-4. Complaining of palpitations, shortness of breath, chest pain at rest
5-5. Complaining of dizziness, cold sweat, or nausea in a sitting position at rest
6. Patients who are judged to be ineligible for 6MWT

Statistical Analysis

Sample size determination was based on the detection of a 0.45 correlation coefficient between both tests with a power of 90% and an alpha level of 0.05. The number of participants required for the study was determined to be 47. Continuous variables were expressed as mean ± standard deviation (SD) when normally distributed and as median (interquartile range, IQR) when non-normally distributed. Categorical variables were summarized as frequencies and percentages. Normality was assessed using the Shapiro–Wilk test.

The association between functional performance in the 1 min sit-to-stand test (1MSTST; repetitions) and the 6 min walk test (6MWT; distance in meters) was evaluated using Spearman's rank correlation coefficient. Peak heart rate (HR) responses during the two tests were compared using a paired-samples *t*-test, and their association was assessed using Pearson's correlation coefficient. Nadir peripheral oxygen saturation (SpO_2) values were compared using the Wilcoxon signed-rank test, and associations between SpO_2 values across tests were evaluated using Spearman's rank correlation. Exercise-related oxygen desaturation was defined as a ≥4% decrease in SpO_2 from resting values. The proportion of participants meeting this criterion during each test was calculated, and paired comparisons were performed using McNemar's test. Perceived dyspnoea (Modified Borg scale) changes from rest to post-test were analyzed separately for each test using Wilcoxon signed-rank tests. Modified Borg scale scores obtained after the 1MSTST and 6MWT were compared using a Wilcoxon signed-rank test, and their association was assessed using Spearman's rank correlation coefficient. For non-parametric paired comparisons, effect

https://doi.org/10.3390/jcm15072479

size was calculated as $r = Z/\sqrt{N}$ and interpreted as small ($r \approx 0.1$), moderate ($r \approx 0.3$), or large ($r \geq 0.5$). Partial correlation analyses were conducted to explore the influence of peripheral muscle strength (handgrip dynamometry) on the association between functional test outcomes. Additional exploratory analyses controlling for age, sex, and post-COVID-19 functional status (PCFS) were performed to assess the robustness of observed associations.

All tests were two-tailed, and a p-value < 0.05 was considered statistically significant. Statistical analyses were performed using IBM SPSS Statistics (version 31.0.0.0 (117)).

3. Results

A total of 54 patients completed both the 1 min sit-to-stand test (1MSTST) and the 6 min walk test (6MWT) and were included in the analysis. The mean age of the cohort was 57.9 ± 12.5 years, and 29 participants (54%) were male. Most patients had experienced a moderate SARS-CoV-2 infection (n = 32, 59%). The most frequently observed post-COVID-19 functional status category was PCFS 2 (slight functional limitation), accounting for 42.6% of participants. The mean time from acute infection to evaluation was 3.0 ± 2.4 months. The mean number of repetitions achieved during the 1MSTST was 20.5 ± 6.1, and the mean distance walked during the 6MWT was 412 ± 90 m (Table 2).

Table 2. Baseline characteristics of study population.

Characteristic	Participants (n = 54)
Age (years), mean ± SD	57.9 ± 12.5
Male sex, n (%)	29 (54%)
Time from acute COVID-19 to assessment (months), mean ± SD	3.0 ± 2.4
Acute COVID-19 severity, n (%)	
• Moderate	32 (59%)
• Severe	22 (41%)
Post-COVID-19 Functional Status (PCFS), n (%)	
• Grade 0	9 (16.7%)
• Grade 1	16 (29.6%)
• Grade 2	23 (42.6%)
• Grade 3	6 (11.1%)
• Grade 4	0 (0%)
Handgrip strength (kg), mean ± SD	18.6 ± 9.2
1 min sit-to-stand test (repetitions), mean ± SD	20.5 ± 6.1
6 min walk test distance (m), mean ± SD	412 ± 90

Values are presented as mean ± standard deviation or number (percentage), as appropriate.

A moderate positive association was observed between the number of repetitions achieved during the 1MSTST and the distance walked during the 6MWT (Spearman's $\rho = 0.47$, $p < 0.001$; Figure 1). Peripheral muscle strength assessed by hand grip dynamometry was positively correlated with performance in both the 1MSTST ($\rho = 0.49$, $p < 0.001$) and the 6MWT ($\rho = 0.41$, $p = 0.003$). When controlling for peripheral muscle strength, the association between 1MSTST repetitions and 6MWT distance was attenuated but remained statistically significant (partial $r = 0.35$, $p = 0.012$), although the magnitude of the association was smaller than that assumed for sample size estimation. Further adjustment for age, sex, and post-COVID-19 functional status resulted in additional attenuation of the association, which was no longer statistically significant (partial $r = 0.26$, $p = 0.070$) (Table 3).

https://doi.org/10.3390/jcm15072479

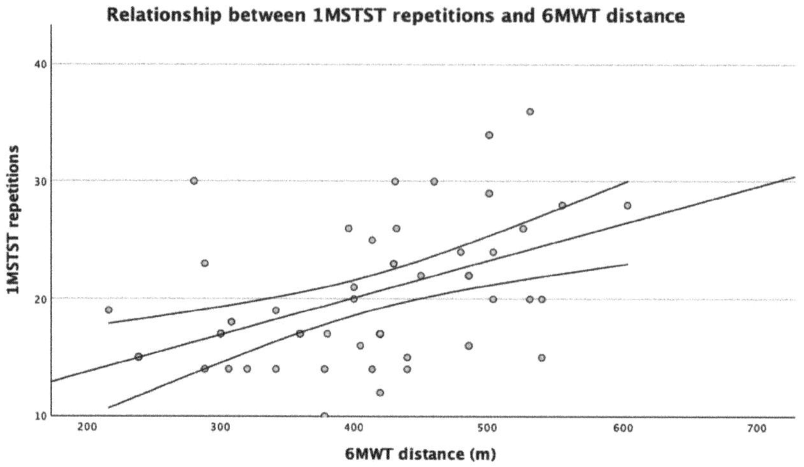

Figure 1. Relationship between 1MSTST repetitions and 6MWT distance. Each point represents an individual participant. The solid line indicates the fitted linear trend, and the outer lines represent the 95% confidence interval of the mean predicted value. A moderate association was observed between 1MSTST repetitions and 6MWT distance (Spearman's $\rho = 0.47$, $p < 0.001$).

Table 3. Associations between functional performance measures before and after adjustment.

Analysis	Correlation Coefficient	*p*-Value
1MSTST repetitions vs. 6MWT distance	ρ = 0.47	<0.001
Hand grip dynamometry vs. 1MSTST repetitions	ρ = 0.49	<0.001
Hand grip dynamometry vs. 6MWT distance	ρ = 0.41	0.003
1MSTST vs. 6MWT (adjusted for peripheral muscle strength)	r = 0.35	0.012
1MSTST vs. 6MWT (adjusted for peripheral muscle strength, age, sex, PCFS)	r = 0.26	0.070

Spearman's rank correlation coefficients (ρ) were used for unadjusted analyses. Partial correlation coefficients (r) were used for adjusted analyses.

Peak heart rate responses during the 1MSTST and the 6MWT did not differ significantly (paired *t*-test, $p = 0.160$), while a strong positive correlation was observed between peak heart rate values achieved during the two tests (Pearson's $r = 0.75$, $p < 0.001$; Figure 2a). Nadir SpO_2 values did not differ significantly between the 1MSTST and the 6MWT (Wilcoxon signed-rank test, $p = 0.919$). A very strong positive correlation was observed between nadir SpO_2 values obtained during the two tests (Spearman's $\rho = 0.83$, $p < 0.001$; Figure 2b). Exercise-related oxygen desaturation (defined as a $\geq$4% drop from resting SpO_2) occurred in 11 participants (20.4%) during the 1MSTST and 12 participants (22.2%) during the 6MWT. The proportion of participants meeting this criterion did not differ between tests (McNemar's test, $p = 1.00$). Perceived dyspnoea increased significantly from rest following both the 1MSTST and the 6MWT (both $p < 0.001$). Modified Borg scale scores obtained after the two tests were strongly correlated (Spearman's $\rho = 0.76$, $p < 0.001$). No statistically significant difference was observed between Modified Borg scale scores following the 1MSTST and the 6MWT (Wilcoxon signed-rank test, $p = 0.058$). The associated effect size was small ($r = 0.26$) (Table 4).

https://doi.org/10.3390/jcm15072479

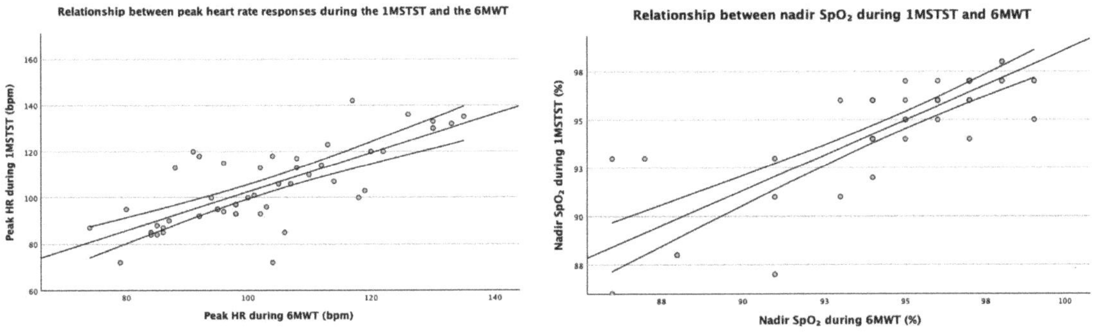

(a) (b)

Figure 2. (**a**,**b**) Relationship between peak heart rate responses and SpO_2 nadir values during the 1 min sit-to-stand test (1MSTST) and the 6 min walk test (6MWT). Each point represents an individual participant. The solid line represents the fitted linear trend; outer lines indicate the 95% confidence interval of the mean predicted value. Peak heart rate responses were strongly correlated between tests (Pearson's r = 0.75, $p < 0.001$). Nadir SpO_2 values were also strongly correlated between tests (Spearman's $\rho = 0.83$, $p < 0.001$).

Table 4. Cardiopulmonary and perceived exertion responses during the 1MSTST and the 6MWT.

Variable	1MSTST	6MWT	*p*-Value
Peak heart rate (bpm), mean ± SD	104.6 ± 16.8	102.4 ± 14.9	0.160
Nadir SpO_2 (%), median (IQR)	96 (3)	96 (3)	0.919
≥4% SpO_2 drop, n (%)	11 (20.4)	12 (22.2)	1.00
Perceived dyspnoea (Modified Borg scale, post-test), median (IQR)	5 (3)	4.5 (4)	0.058

Values are presented as mean ± standard deviation or median (interquartile range), as appropriate. Paired comparisons were performed using paired *t*-tests, Wilcoxon signed-rank tests, or exact McNemar tests, as appropriate.

No adverse events occurred during testing. All participants completed both tests without interruptions.

4. Discussion

In this study of adults recovering from moderate to severe COVID-19, we found that performance in the 1 min sit-to-stand test (1MSTST) was moderately associated with distance walked during the 6 min walk test (6MWT), while cardiopulmonary responses—including peak heart rate and nadir SpO_2—were strongly correlated between tests. Perceived exertion also showed substantial agreement. Together, these findings contribute to a growing body of evidence indicating that simplified field tests such as the 1MSTST capture overlapping aspects of functional capacity assessed by longer, standardized tests, while reflecting important physiological distinctions [17,18].

Although direct comparisons between the 1MSTST and the 6MWT in post-COVID-19 populations remain scarce, moderate to strong correlations between 1MSTST performance and 6MWT distance have been reported by available studies [19,20], supporting the concept that these tests assess related functional domains. Our findings extend existing literature by accounting for peripheral muscle strength and demographic and functional confounders.

The attenuation of the association between 1MSTST and 6MWT performance after adjustment for peripheral muscle strength highlights the distinct physiological determinants underlying each test. Sit-to-stand performance is strongly influenced by muscle

https://doi.org/10.3390/jcm15072479

strength and power, whereas walking-based tests depend more heavily on aerobic capacity, endurance, and cardiopulmonary integration [5]. Additional adjustment for age, sex, and post-COVID-19 functional status resulted in further attenuation and was no longer statistically significant, suggesting that shared patient characteristics rather than test equivalence accounted for much of the observed relationship.

Despite differing mechanical and temporal demands, the 1MSTST and the 6MWT elicited comparable cardiopulmonary responses, as reflected by similar mean peak heart rate and median nadir spO2 values and strong correlations in individual heart rate and oxygen saturation responses. Similar observations have been reported in patients with other chronic respiratory diseases, where shorter functional tests produced cardiovascular stress comparable to longer walking tests [9–11]. These findings support the physiological validity of the 1MSTST as a meaningful stimulus for cardiopulmonary assessment.

Most participants exhibited normal resting oxygen saturation and did not meet conventional criteria for exercise-induced hypoxemia. Nevertheless, neither the magnitude nor the frequency of clinically relevant oxygen desaturation ($\geq$4% drop from rest) differed between the two tests. This pattern suggests that exertional desaturation primarily reflects individual physiological susceptibility—likely related to persistent pulmonary, vascular, or gas-exchange abnormalities after COVID-19—rather than a test-specific effect. The strong within-subject concordance in SpO_2 responses supports the use of the 1MSTST for screening exertional desaturation when the 6MWT is not feasible.

Perceived exertion increased similarly following both tests, with strong correlations between post-test Borg scores. The small effect size observed for differences in Borg ratings suggests that both tests impose a comparable subjective burden, despite emphasizing different physiological components. This finding is consistent with previous reports comparing perceived exertion across functional field tests of differing duration and movement patterns [21].

Taken together, these findings align with existing recommendations emphasizing the value of simple, low-resource functional assessments in clinical practice, particularly in settings where space, time, or staffing constraints limit the feasibility of standardized walking tests. Beyond face-to-face evaluation, the 1MSTST has emerged as a particularly relevant tool for telerehabilitation in post-COVID-19 care. Its simplicity, minimal equipment requirements, absence of a clinically relevant learning effect, and short duration make it well suited for remote monitoring of functional status and therapeutic response [13].

Despite these contributions, the two tests should not be considered interchangeable. While the 6MWT remains the reference standard for detailed assessment of walking endurance and global functional capacity, the strong concordance observed in cardiopulmonary responses in the present study supports the role of the 1MSTST as a pragmatic complementary assessment, particularly within telerehabilitation pathways and in contexts where resource-intensive testing is not feasible.

Several limitations should be noted. First, convenience-based recruitment may have introduced selection bias toward individuals with better functional capacity and greater willingness to participate. Second, comorbidity data were not systematically collected in the original study database, which may limit adjustment for potential clinical confounders, nor did it include long-term follow-up to assess responsiveness or prognostic value. Third, our cohort reflects patients recovering in the early pandemic period, and findings may not generalize to later SARS-CoV-2 variants or to patients with milder disease phenotypes. Fourth, while handgrip dynamometry is a validated surrogate of overall muscle strength, the absence of direct lower-limb strength assessment may limit its ability to fully reflect the specific muscular demands of sit-to-stand performance. Fifth, the relatively preserved resting SpO_2 in our sample may reduce sensitivity to detect exercise-induced desaturation in

https://doi.org/10.3390/jcm15072479

more severely desaturating populations. Finally, the single-center design and convenience sampling may limit external validity.

5. Conclusions

In adults recovering from moderate to severe COVID-19, the 1MSTST demonstrates moderate concordance with the 6MWT in functional performance and strong agreement in cardiopulmonary responses. These findings indicate that the two tests assess overlapping but distinct aspects of functional capacity. The 1MSTST may therefore serve as a practical, complementary assessment—particularly within telerehabilitation pathways and in primary care or resource-limited settings—when standard walking tests cannot be routinely implemented. Although the COVID-19 pandemic is now largely under control, the experience gained from functional exercise assessment in post-COVID-19 patients may provide a useful framework for evaluating recovery after other viral infections with respiratory tropism, a hypothesis that should be explored in future studies.

Author Contributions: Conceptualization, M.D.-S., N.R. and M.T.-R.; Methodology, N.R. and M.T.-R.; Validation, P.F., N.R. and M.T.-R.; Formal analysis, M.D.-S.; Investigation, M.D.-S., N.R. and M.T.-R.; Resources, N.R. and M.T.-R.; Data curation, M.D.-S. and N.R.; Writing—original draft, M.D.-S.; Writing—review & editing, M.D.-S., N.R. and M.T.-R.; Supervision, M.T.-R. All authors have read and agreed to the published version of the manuscript.

Funding: This research received no external funding. The Article Processing Charge (APC) was supported by BIAL.

Institutional Review Board Statement: The study was conducted in accordance with the Declaration of Helsinki and approved by the Ethics Committee of Centro Hospitalar Universitário de Lisboa Central (approval number 1209/2022, dated 18 March 2022).

Informed Consent Statement: Informed consent was obtained from all subjects involved in the study.

Data Availability Statement: The data presented in this study are available on request from the corresponding author due to ethical reasons.

Acknowledgments: During the preparation of this manuscript, the authors used Grammarly (https://www.grammarly.com/) and ChatGPT (OpenAI, GPT-5 series) for the purposes of language enhancement or proofreading. The authors have reviewed and edited the output and take full responsibility for the content of this publication.

Conflicts of Interest: The authors declare no conflicts of interest. BIAL provided support for the APC only and had no role in the design, execution, interpretation, or writing of the study.

Abbreviations

The following abbreviations are used in this manuscript:

6MWT	6-minute walk test
1MSTS	1-minute sit-to-stand test
SpO2	Peripheral oxygen saturation
HR	Heart rate
PCFS	Post-COVID Functional Status
COVID-19	Coronavirus disease 2019
SD	Standard deviation
IQR	Interquartile range

https://doi.org/10.3390/jcm15072479

References

1. World Health Organization. *A Clinical Case Definition of Post COVID-19 Condition;* World Health Organization: Geneva, Switzerland, 2021.
2. Freund, O.; Breslavsky, A.; Givoli-Vilensky, R.; Zacks, N.; Gershman, E.; Melloul, A.; Wand, O.; Bilenko, N.; Bar-Shai, A. Assessment of a close respiratory follow-up schedule at 3 and 6 months after acute COVID-19 and its related investigations. *Respir. Med.* **2023**, *217*, 107367. [CrossRef] [PubMed]
3. Zheng, C.; Chen, J.J.; Dai, Z.H.; Wan, K.W.; Sun, F.H.; Huang, J.H.; Chen, X.K. Physical exercise-related manifestations of long COVID: A systematic review and meta-analysis. *J. Exerc. Sci. Fit.* **2024**, *22*, 341–349. [CrossRef] [PubMed]
4. Müller, K.; Ottiger, M.; Poppele, I.; Wastlhuber, A.; Stegbauer, M.; Schlesinger, T. Physical Health in Patients with Post-COVID-19 6 and 12 Months after an Inpatient Rehabilitation: An Observational Study. *J. Clin. Med.* **2024**, *13*, 3988. [CrossRef] [PubMed]
5. Torres-Castro, R.; Núñez-Cortés, R.; Larrateguy, S.; Alsina-Restoy, X.; Barberà, J.A.; Gimeno-Santos, E.; García, A.R.; Sibila, O.; Blanco, I. Assessment of Exercise Capacity in Post-COVID-19 Patients: How Is the Appropriate Test Chosen? *Life* **2023**, *13*, 621. [CrossRef] [PubMed]
6. BTS Guidance on Respiratory Follow Up of Patients with a Clinico-Radiological Diagnosis of COVID-19 Pneumonia v1.2 11 5 2020 Final Checked 4 2021. Available online: https://www.brit-thoracic.org.uk/document-library/quality-improvement/covid-19/resp-follow-up-guidance-post-covid-pneumonia/ (accessed on 1 January 2021).
7. Cortés-Telles, A.; López-Romero, S.; Figueroa-Hurtado, E.; Pou-Aguilar, Y.N.; Wong, A.W.; Milne, K.M.; Ryerson, C.J.; Guenette, J.A. Pulmonary function and functional capacity in COVID-19 survivors with persistent dyspnoea. *Respir. Physiol. Neurobiol.* **2021**, *288*, 103644. [CrossRef] [PubMed]
8. González, J.; Benítez, I.D.; Carmona, P.; Santisteve, S.; Monge, A.; Moncusí-Moix, A.; Gort-Paniello, C.; Pinilla, L.; Carratalá, A.; Zuil, M.; et al. Pulmonary Function and Radiologic Features in Survivors of Critical COVID-19 A 3-Month Prospective Cohort. Available online: https://repositoriosaludmadrid.es/server/api/core/bitstreams/7300cf41-ea6e-419f-b9f7-083d47fd22d1/content (accessed on 1 May 2023).
9. Ozalevlia, S.; Ozden, A.; Itilb, O.; Akkoclub, A. Comparison of the Sit-to-Stand Test with 6 min walk test in patients with chronic obstructive pulmonary disease. *Respir. Med.* **2007**, *101*, 286–293. [CrossRef] [PubMed]
10. Briand, J.; Behal, H.; Chenivesse, C.; Wémeau-Stervinou, L.; Wallaert, B. The 1-minute sit-to-stand test to detect exercise-induced oxygen desaturation in patients with interstitial lung disease. *Ther. Adv. Respir. Dis.* **2018**, *12*, 1753466618793028. [CrossRef] [PubMed]
11. Takeda, K.; Shigeta, A.; Inagaki, T.; Hayama, N.; Kawame, C.; Naraki, Y.; Naito, A.; Sekine, A.; Suda, R.; Sugiura, T.; et al. The utility and safety of one-minute sit-to-stand test in pulmonary hypertension: A prospective study. *Respir. Investig.* **2024**, *63*, 61–66. [CrossRef] [PubMed]
12. Amput, P.; Tapanya, W.; Wongphon, S.; Naravejsakul, K.; Sritiyot, T. Test–Retest Reliability and Minimal Detectable Change of the 6-Minute Step Test and 1-Minute Sit-to-Stand Test in Post-COVID-19 Patients. *Adv. Respir. Med.* **2025**, *93*, 33. [CrossRef] [PubMed]
13. Sevillano-Castaño, A.; Peroy-Badal, R.; Torres-Castro, R.; Gimeno-Santos, E.; García Fernández, P.; Garcia Vila, C.; Ariza Alfaro, A.; De Dios Álvarez, R.; Vilaró, J.; Blanco, I. Is there a learning effect on 1-min sit-to-stand test in post-COVID-19 patients? *ERJ Open Res.* **2022**, *8*, 00189–2022. [CrossRef] [PubMed]
14. Sáude, D.G.d. Abordagem das Pessoas com Suspeita ou Confirmação de COVID-19. 23 March 2020. Available online: https://www.ordemenfermeiros.pt/media/26675/norma-004-2020-covid-19-abordagem-das-pessoas-com-suspeita-ou-confirma%C3%A7%C3%A3o-de-covid-19-atualizada-a-06072022.pdf (accessed on 1 January 2021).
15. Klok, F.A.; Boon, G.J.; Barco, S.; Endres, M.; Geelhoed, J.M.; Knauss, S.; Rezek, S.A.; Spruit, M.A.; Vehreschild, J.; Siegerink, B. The Post-COVID-19 Functional Status scale: A tool to measure functional status over time after COVID-19. *Eur. Respir. J.* **2020**, *56*, 2001494. [CrossRef] [PubMed]
16. ATS Committee on Proficiency Standards for Clinical Pulmonary Function Laboratories. ATS statement: Guidelines for the six-minute walk test. *Am. J. Respir. Crit. Care Med.* **2002**, *166*, 111–117; Erratum in *Am. J. Respir. Crit. Care Med.* **2016**, *193*, 1185. [CrossRef] [PubMed]
17. Crook, S.; Büsching, G.; Schultz, K.; Lehbert, N.; Jelusic, D.; Keusch, S.; Wittmann, M.; Schuler, M.; Radtke, T.; Frey, M.; et al. A multicentre validation of the 1-min sit-to-stand test in patients with COPD. *Eur. Respir. J.* **2017**, *49*, 1601871. [CrossRef] [PubMed]
18. Bohannon, R.W.; Crouch, R. 1-Minute Sit-to-Stand Test. *J. Cardiopulm. Rehabil. Prev.* **2018**, *39*, 2–8. [CrossRef] [PubMed]
19. Srithawong, A.; Poncumhak, P.; Promsrisuk, T.; Amput, P. Cut-off values of one-minute sit-to-stand test for determining physical performance in mild-post-COVID-19 individuals. *Can. J. Respir. Ther.* **2024**, *60*, 143–151. [CrossRef] [PubMed]

https://doi.org/10.3390/jcm15072479

20. Honpode, S.L.; Rajam, R.S.; Mhatre, B.S.; Sawant, S.S.; Wagh, V.M.; Iyer, S. Relationship between 6-minute walk test and 1-minute sit to stand test in patients with COVID-19: A retrospective analysis. *World J. Adv. Res. Rev.* **2021**, *12*, 470–477. [CrossRef]
21. Peroy-Badal, R.; Sevillano-Castaño, A.; Torres-Castro, R.; García-Fernández, P.; Maté-Muñoz, J.; Dumitrana, C.; Rodriguez, E.S.; De Frutos Lobo, M.; Vilaró, J. Comparison of different field tests to assess the physical capacity of post-COVID-19. *Pulmonology* **2022**, *30*, 17–23. [CrossRef] [PubMed]

https://doi.org/10.3390/jcm15072479

Journal of
Clinical Medicine

MDPI

Review

Non-Small-Cell Lung Cancer: From Histopathological Classification to Precision Oncology—A Narrative Review

Simona-Maria Roșu [1,*,†], Viorel Biciușcă [2,*], Sorina-Ionelia Stan [2], Denisa Maria Mitroi [1], Beatrice Mahler [3,4,†], Diana-Maria Trașcă [2], Mihaela Popescu [5], Marian-Marius Pădureanu [1], Ana-Ștefania Stoica [1], Tania-Ioana Pencea [1,3], Ionela-Alina Croitoru [3,4] and Mara Amalia Bălteanu [3,6]

1 Doctoral School, University of Medicine and Pharmacy of Craiova, 200349 Craiova, Romania; denisa_maria2@yahoo.com (D.M.M.); marius.padureanu98@yahoo.com (M.-M.P.); stoicaanastefania@gmail.com (A.-Ș.S.); taniagoncea@yahoo.com (T.-I.P.)
2 Department of Internal Medicine, Faculty of Medicine, University of Medicine and Pharmacy of Craiova, 200349 Craiova, Romania; sorina_stan@icloud.com (S.-I.S.); diana.trasca@umfcv.ro (D.-M.T.)
3 Department of Pneumology, "Marius Nasta" Institute for Pneumology, 050159 Bucharest, Romania; beatrice.mahler@umfcd.ro (B.M.); alinahaulinca@umfcd.ro (I.-A.C.); mara.balteanu@prof.utm.ro (M.A.B.)
4 Department of Pneumology, Faculty of Medicine, University of Medicine and Pharmacy Carol Davila of Bucharest, 020021 Bucharest, Romania
5 Department of Endocrinology, Faculty of Medicine, University of Medicine and Pharmacy of Craiova, 200349 Craiova, Romania; mihaela.popescu.e@umfcv.ro
6 Department of Pneumology, Faculty of Medicine, "Titu Maiorescu" University, 040051 Bucharest, Romania
* Correspondence: simona.vulpe1995@gmail.com (S.-M.R.); biciuscaviorel@gmail.com (V.B.)
† These authors contributed equally to this work.

Abstract

Non-Small-Cell Lung Cancer (NSCLC) represents the most prevalent form of lung cancer and remains one of the leading causes of cancer-related morbidity and mortality worldwide. This disease has evolved far beyond traditional histopathological classification. While histology remains foundational, it is no longer sufficient to guide optimal patient management in the era of precision oncology. This review uniquely integrates the full spectrum of NSCLC evaluation, from underlying pathophysiological mechanisms to histological, immunohistochemical, and molecular analyses, culminating in individualized therapeutic planning. We highlight actionable genetic alterations—including EGFR, ALK, ROS1, BRAF, and KRAS—and their roles in guiding targeted therapies, alongside the transformative impact of immune checkpoint inhibitors in selected patients. By emphasizing the interplay between tumor biology, diagnostic workflows, and treatment selection, this review underscores the necessity of comprehensive molecular testing and data integration. Finally, we discuss emerging biomarkers and rational combination strategies that promise to further refine patient stratification and improve outcomes.

Keywords: non-small-cell lung cancer; histological subtypes; actionable oncogenic drivers; treatment; multidisciplinary management

1. Introduction

NSCLC represents the most common form of lung cancer and exhibits significant histological, molecular, and clinical heterogeneity. Historically, NSCLC classification relied primarily on morphological assessment of tumor tissue, distinguishing major subtypes such as adenocarcinoma, squamous cell carcinoma, and large cell carcinoma. While these histopathological distinctions provided a foundation for prognosis and therapeutic decision-making, they were insufficient to guide personalized treatment in the era of precision oncology. Over the past decade, advances in molecular biology and immunohistochemistry have transformed the diagnostic and therapeutic landscape of NSCLC [1]. The identification of actionable oncogenic drivers—including EGFR mutations, ALK and ROS1 rearrangements, BRAF alterations, and KRAS mutations—has enabled targeted therapies that achieve superior response rates and improved survival [2]. Simultaneously, the assessment of PD-L1 expression and other immune biomarkers has facilitated patient selection for immunotherapy, providing durable responses in selected populations [3]. These developments have shifted the focus from morphology alone to an integrated approach in which histology, immunohistochemistry, and molecular profiling collectively inform treatment strategies [4]. This review aims to provide a contemporary perspective on NSCLC by emphasizing how traditional histopathological classification has evolved in the context of modern precision medicine. We discuss which histological distinctions remain clinically meaningful, how immunohistochemical markers complement morphological evaluation, and how comprehensive genomic profiling guides targeted and immunotherapeutic interventions. By framing NSCLC management within this integrated paradigm, the review highlights the convergence of morphology and molecular biology in current clinical practice, illustrating the transition from descriptive classification to biomarker-driven precision oncology.

2. Epidemiology

2.1. General Data

NSCLC is the most common subtype of lung cancer globally and remains a major contributor to cancer deaths. Despite advances in screening and prevention programs, its incidence continues to be elevated in both high- and low-income regions. In countries that have implemented strong smoking control strategies, a slow but steady decline in overall lung cancer rates has been observed. Even so, this positive trend is tempered by the increasing proportion of adenocarcinoma cases. In particular, the increasing incidence of adenocarcinoma among women and non-smokers underscores changing risk patterns and highlights the increasingly complex epidemiology of this lung cancer subtype. NSCLC accounts for approximately 85% of all reported cases, and the burden of the disease is not evenly distributed worldwide [5]. The highest incidence rates are consistently documented in regions such as Central and Eastern Europe, East Asia, and North America. In addition, several areas in Africa appear to have lower reported rates, a pattern that is often attributed to limited access to diagnostic tools and underdiagnosis of the disease in clinical practice. Socioeconomic conditions also play a critical role in shaping the prevalence of NSCLC [6]. Communities that experience economic hardship tend to be more exposed to major risk factors—including higher rates of smoking, unsafe occupational environments, and high levels of environmental pollutants (Figure 1). This underscores the importance of both public health interventions and improved access to medical infrastructure [7].

2.2. Risk Factors

Smoking continues to be the dominant risk factor for NSCLC, with most cases caused by active smoking, as well as prolonged exposure to tobacco smoke—passive smoking [7]. Several environmental and occupational factors also significantly increase the likelihood of developing NSCLC. Prolonged exposure to radon, asbestos fibers, heavy metals, and polycyclic aromatic hydrocarbons plays an important role in lung carcinogenesis, particularly among people working in industries such as mining, construction, and metallurgy [8]. Air pollution has emerged as a critical factor contributing to the risk of lung cancer. Fine particles, particularly PM2.5, have been strongly associated with an increased incidence of NSCLC in heavily industrialized or densely populated urban areas [9]. Although NSCLC

https://doi.org/10.3390/jcm15083042

is primarily an acquired disease, genetic factors may influence individual susceptibility. A positive family history may indicate an inherited predisposition, and even though true hereditary mutations are uncommon, certain germline genetic variants may alter the body's response to carcinogens and therefore increase overall risk [10]. Additionally, certain pulmonary diseases may act as risk factors for lung cancer. A history of pulmonary tuberculosis may increase this risk through persistent infection with Mycobacterium tuberculosis, which promotes chronic inflammation, fibrosis, and parenchymal scarring, creating a microenvironment that may favor neoplastic development [11]. This chronic inflammatory process is also characteristic of chronic obstructive pulmonary disease, which likewise represents an important risk factor for the development of lung cancer [12].

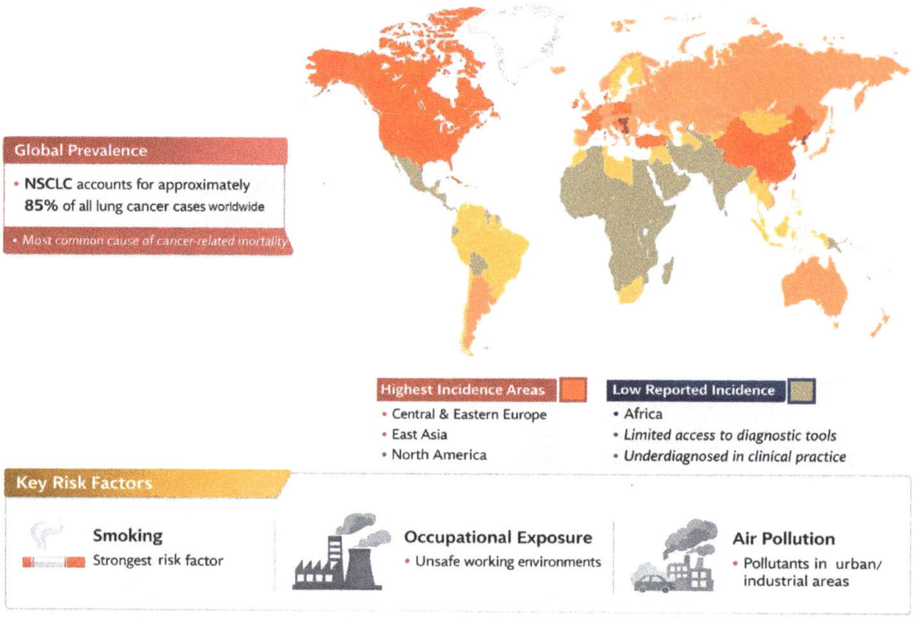

Figure 1. Epidemiology of Non-Small-Cell Lung Cancer.

2.3. Sex and Age Distribution

Epidemiological data show a steady increase in the number of cases among women, although NSCLC is still more common in men. This trend is associated both with the increase in the incidence of smoking among women in recent decades and with specific biological characteristics that influence individual susceptibility to the disease [13]. Adenocarcinoma is considered particularly common in women and in people who have never smoked [14]. The incidence of NSCLC increases considerably after the age of 50 and reaches its highest levels in the sixth and seventh decades of life. However, in recent years, an increasing number of cases have been reported in younger patients. Although less common, these manifestations are frequently linked to well-defined oncogenic mutations, such as alterations in the EGFR, ALK, or ROS1 genes, which can influence both tumor behavior and response to targeted therapies [15].

3. Pathogenesis

The development of NSCLC is driven by a complex interplay between genetic predisposition, epigenetic modifications, and environmental exposures. All these factors lead to

https://doi.org/10.3390/jcm15083042

the gradual transformation of healthy respiratory epithelial cells into malignant tissue [16]. The process unfolds over time as key molecular abnormalities accumulate, disrupting normal regulatory pathways that govern cell division, differentiation, and programmed cell death [17].

3.1. General Mechanisms

NSCLC develops through the gradual transformation of normal respiratory epithelial cells into malignant tissue, driven by the interplay of genetic predisposition, epigenetic changes, and environmental exposures. Key molecular abnormalities disrupt cell cycle regulation, apoptosis, and immune surveillance, enabling sustained proliferation and survival of abnormal cells. Chronic irritation from tobacco smoke or air pollutants promotes inflammation and oxidative stress, further damaging DNA and fostering genomic instability [18,19]. Aberrant activation of signaling pathways, such as PI3K/AKT, RAS/RAF/MEK, and JAK/STAT, enhances tumor growth, angiogenesis, and invasiveness, laying the foundation for NSCLC progression and metastasis [20].

3.2. Specific Genetic Alterations

Each histological subtype of NSCLC displays a unique molecular signature that influences both tumor behavior and therapeutic response. Adenocarcinoma is frequently associated with activating mutations in EGFR, rearrangements in ALK and ROS1, and mutations in KRAS and BRAF. These alterations result in abnormal activation of signaling pathways such as tyrosine kinase receptors or G-protein-coupled cascades, promoting sustained proliferation, evasion of apoptosis, and enhanced survival [21]. Squamous cell carcinoma is commonly linked to TP53 mutations, impairing DNA damage repair, and FGFR1 amplifications, which promote tumor growth and survival [22]. Large cell carcinoma is molecularly heterogeneous, with no single predominant driver mutation, and is often a diagnosis of exclusion after other NSCLC subtypes are ruled out [23]. Importantly, these molecular alterations are not only involved in tumorigenesis but also represent clinically actionable targets. The identification of EGFR mutations, ALK or ROS1 rearrangements, and BRAF and KRAS alterations enables the use of targeted therapies, such as tyrosine kinase inhibitors and BRAF/MEK inhibitors, which have demonstrated superior response rates, improved survival, and effective control of both systemic and intracranial disease. This therapeutic relevance underscores the necessity of comprehensive molecular profiling in modern NSCLC management, bridging traditional histopathology with precision oncology [24].

3.3. Mechanisms of Tumor Progression and Metastasis

Profound remodeling of the tumor microenvironment through the gradual accumulation of genetic alterations leads to NSCLC progression, allowing tumor cells to grow abnormally, resist apoptosis, and acquire invasive properties. Epithelial–mesenchymal transition is the mechanism by which tumor cells become mesenchymal and can invade surrounding tissues and disseminate distantly. The release of vascular endothelial growth factor leads to angiogenesis and neovascularization at the tumor level, which provides essential nutrients and oxygen to support tumor growth and constitutes an access route for cancer cells to enter the circulation [25]. Once in the blood or lymphatic system, tumor cells disseminate and can form secondary tumors in the brain, bones, liver, adrenal glands, and the contralateral lung. Secondary cardiac metastases in NSCLC are frequently underdiagnosed despite their significant clinical impact. They can arise via direct invasion, hematogenous spread, or lymphatic dissemination, affecting the pericardium, myocardium, and endocardium, and are often overlooked by clinicians because symptoms—such as dyspnea, palpitations, arrhythmias, chest pain, or signs of heart failure—are nonspecific

https://doi.org/10.3390/jcm15083042

and may be attributed to systemic tumor progression or pre-existing cardiovascular comorbidities. Early detection is crucial, as cardiac involvement has direct implications for treatment planning and prognosis: the presence of cardiac lesions may influence decisions regarding chemotherapy, radiotherapy, or targeted therapies and may necessitate closer cardiac monitoring [26]. Together, all these mechanisms underscore the aggressive and adaptive nature of NSCLC, highlighting the challenges in controlling tumor progression and preventing metastasis [27].

4. Pathological Features

The pathological features of NSCLC constitute a fundamental component of diagnostic evaluation and play a decisive role in prognosis and therapeutic planning. A thorough pathological evaluation integrates macroscopic appearance, detailed microscopic examination, immunohistochemical profiling, and molecular characterization. These features allow for the precise determination of tumor subtype, biological behavior, and characteristics that predict recurrence, progression, or metastatic spread [28].

4.1. General Macroscopic and Microscopic Characteristics

From a macroscopic perspective, NSCLC demonstrates considerable heterogeneity, influenced primarily by tumor histology and anatomical site of origin. Centrally located tumors usually arise from the larger bronchi and may obstruct the airway, while peripheral lesions typically develop within the distal lung parenchyma, sometimes in association with areas of fibrosis or chronic inflammatory remodeling [29]. Adenocarcinoma, the most prevalent subtype, frequently presents as a peripheral nodule. These tumors may appear solid, partially solid, or with regions of parenchymal consolidation. Some lesions exhibit a desmoplastic reaction or are associated with pre-existing interstitial scarring, reflecting their origin from alveolar epithelial cells [30]. Squamous cell carcinoma commonly develops in the central airways. Macroscopically, it often forms bulky, firm masses capable of invading and distorting the bronchial lumen. Areas of necrosis and cavitation are frequent due to impaired vascular supply within the tumor core [31]. Large cell carcinoma usually manifests as a well-circumscribed mass with a soft, friable texture. Pronounced necrosis is a typical finding, consistent with its high-grade, poorly differentiated nature [32]. Microscopically, adenocarcinomas display a spectrum of architectural patterns—lepidic, acinar, papillary, micropapillary, and solid. These patterns are not merely descriptive but carry prognostic weight: for example, micropapillary and solid components are associated with increased aggressiveness and poorer clinical outcomes [33]. Squamous cell carcinomas are characterized by unequivocal squamous differentiation, evidenced by keratinization, formation of keratin pearls, and identifiable intercellular bridges. These features help distinguish them from other epithelial malignancies [34]. Large cell carcinoma is diagnosed largely by exclusion [35]. These tumors lack glandular or squamous differentiation, both morphologically and immunohistochemically and represent a poorly differentiated, high-grade neoplasm.

4.2. Invasion Patterns and Pathological Staging Criteria (TNM)

Assessment of tumor invasion into adjacent anatomical structures is a central component of the pathological evaluation of NSCLC. As the tumor grows, it may infiltrate the bronchial tree, compromise the pulmonary vasculature, or penetrate the visceral and parietal pleura. More advanced lesions may extend beyond the lung into the chest wall, diaphragm, pericardium, or mediastinum, and such local invasion is associated with an advanced stage and a poor prognosis [36]. Lung cancer staging is based on the internationally standardized Tumor-Node-Metastasis (TNM) staging system, the 9th version of which was last published in 2025. The T category refers to the maximum size of the primary lesion, its

https://doi.org/10.3390/jcm15083042

extent, and the presence of pleural, vascular, or airway invasion. The N category assesses regional lymph node involvement. The number, size, and anatomical location of involved nodes—especially spread to mediastinal or subcarinal sites—have major prognostic implications and frequently influence the therapeutic strategy. The M category documents the presence of distant spread, either to the contralateral lung, pleura, or to the bone, liver, brain, or other organs [37]. Accurate staging requires meticulous examination of resected specimens, including systematic lymph node dissection or sampling, careful assessment of surgical margins, and detailed histological evaluation of the routes of invasion. This approach ensures appropriate classification, facilitates individualized treatment planning, and ultimately contributes to improved prognostic accuracy.

4.3. Predictive and Prognostic Factors

In addition to the parameters defined by the TNM classification, multiple additional pathological features significantly influence the course of NSCLC. Thus, blood and lymphatic vessel invasion stands out as one of the strongest predictors of an unfavorable prognosis, as this fact reflects an increased capacity for systemic dissemination and is associated with both early recurrence and distant metastasis [38]. The degree of cellular differentiation also provides important prognostic information. Well-differentiated tumors generally show slower growth and a more favorable course, compared with poorly differentiated or undifferentiated neoplasms that tend to have rapid progression, increased invasive potential, and a higher probability of resistance to treatment. Tumor necrosis, which often reflects hypoxia in rapidly proliferating lesions, is frequently associated with aggressive behavior. The density and composition of inflammatory infiltrates—including lymphocytes, macrophages, and stromal cells—may indicate an altered immune microenvironment that supports tumor progression [39]. Additionally, predictive factors in NSCLC have increasingly shifted from purely morphological criteria toward molecularly defined subgroups. Driver mutations (EGFR, ALK, ROS1, BRAF, KRAS) and PD-L1 expression not only influence prognosis but are critical for therapeutic decision-making, guiding the selection of tyrosine kinase inhibitors, immune checkpoint inhibitors, and combination therapies. In current practice, histopathological classification alone is insufficient for optimal patient management. Accurate subtyping is achieved through a combination of histology, immunohistochemical markers, and comprehensive molecular profiling, ensuring that each patient is matched with the most effective targeted or immunotherapeutic approach. This integrative strategy bridges traditional morphology with precision oncology, enabling both prognostic assessment and predictive therapeutic selection.

5. Clinical Manifestations

The clinical presentation of NSCLC includes multiple signs and symptoms, depending on the location, size, growth rate, and local or distant spread of the tumor. In the early stages, it does not produce obvious symptoms, allowing the disease to progress silently. Therefore, a significant percentage of cases are identified incidentally during routine imaging evaluations, such as preoperative imaging or cardiovascular investigations. When symptoms occur, they usually correlate with disruption of normal lung structure and function. Tumors located centrally in the main bronchi or proximal airways are more likely to cause early respiratory symptoms. Symptoms may include persistent cough, dyspnea, wheezing, or hemoptysis due to airway obstruction, mucosal irritation, or erosion of vascular structures. Peripheral tumors, on the other hand, may remain clinically silent until they reach a considerable size or invade the pleura, at which point patients may develop chest pain or signs of pleural effusion [40]. Systemic manifestations usually accompany more advanced disease and are often the result of tumor-induced metabolic derangements,

https://doi.org/10.3390/jcm15083042

chronic inflammation, or cytokine release, and include fatigue, anorexia, weight loss, and generalized decline in functional status. Some patients may present with manifestations of paraneoplastic syndromes that signify ectopic hormone secretion or immune-mediated processes occurring in association with the tumor [41]. All of this highlights the heterogeneous nature of NSCLC and emphasizes the importance of correlating clinical manifestations with imaging and pathological studies for timely diagnosis and effective management of the disease.

5.1. Respiratory Symptoms

Respiratory manifestations are the most common clinical features of NSCLC and are often the initial reason for patient presentation. Cough is the dominant symptom and may present in various forms—persistent, dry, or productive—depending on the degree of bronchial irritation and airflow obstruction. In central tumors, cough usually occurs early because the lesion involves large airways, stimulating cough receptors or causing partial narrowing of the bronchi. Hemoptysis, although uncommon, usually reflects erosion of the bronchial vasculature, friability of the tumor surface, or bleeding from necrotic intratumoral tissue. Even minor hemoptysis requires careful evaluation because it may indicate aggressive local invasion [42]. Dyspnea develops either from segmental or lobar bronchial obstruction, which can lead to distal atelectasis, impairing ventilation, or from tumor-induced pleural effusion or compression of the lung parenchyma, which reduces the effective respiratory surface area, resulting in respiratory distress. In advanced stages, tumor expansion or post-obstructive changes may further compromise pulmonary reserve [43]. Recurrent or persistent respiratory infections are another important manifestation, especially when a tumor obstructs the bronchial lumen. Impaired airflow promotes mucus retention, reduces mucociliary clearance, and creates an environment conducive to bacterial growth. These infections—which usually present as repeated episodes of pneumonia or chronic bronchitis—may have a limited response to standard antibiotic therapy. In some patients, such infectious episodes serve as the earliest clue suggesting an underlying endobronchial malignancy [44].

5.2. General Symptoms

In addition to respiratory manifestations, patients with NSCLC also present with general, nonspecific symptoms. Among these, unintentional weight loss is notable, serving as a clinical indicator of active metabolism and tumor progression. This weight loss often coincides with anorexia, alterations in nutrient absorption and utilization, and the development of cachexia, a complex metabolic syndrome characterized by muscle atrophy, fat depletion, and systemic inflammation [45]. Persistent fatigue is another common feature and may result from multiple overlapping mechanisms. Chronic inflammation induced by tumor-secreted cytokines, anemia secondary to bone marrow suppression or chronic disease, and the direct metabolic demands of tumor growth contribute to the depletion of energy reserves. Functional impairment caused by respiratory compromise, pain, or reduced exercise tolerance further exacerbates the feeling of fatigue. Although these general symptoms are nonspecific and can be attributed to a wide range of chronic conditions, their presence in combination—or in the context of progressive respiratory disease—may signal an underlying neoplastic process. Over time, these systemic manifestations contribute to the overall deterioration of health, often prompting patients to seek medical evaluation and requiring further diagnostic investigations. Therefore, awareness of these subtle but impactful signs is essential for early detection and comprehensive management of NSCLC [46].

https://doi.org/10.3390/jcm15083042

5.3. Paraneoplastic Syndromes

Paraneoplastic syndromes are systemic disorders that arise from the ectopic production of hormones, cytokines, or growth factors by tumor cells. These syndromes, although relatively rare, can serve as early diagnostic indicators of NSCLC [47]. Hypercalcemia occurs primarily in association with squamous cell carcinoma, and tumor cells may produce parathyroid hormone-related protein, leading to elevated serum calcium levels. Clinically, it may present with nausea, vomiting, polyuria, dehydration, confusion, and, in severe cases, cardiac arrhythmias or neurological manifestations, occasionally representing a medical emergency requiring rapid intervention [48]. Although ectopic hormone secretion, such as ACTH production, is more commonly associated with small-cell lung cancer, it can occasionally occur in NSCLC. In these rare cases, patients may develop paraneoplastic manifestations, including features of Cushing's syndrome and hyperpigmentation, reflecting the systemic impact of aberrant hormone production. While uncommon, recognition of these phenomena in NSCLC underscores the importance of comprehensive clinical evaluation and may influence both diagnostic workup and management strategies [49]. Another notable paraneoplastic phenomenon is hypertrophic osteoarthropathy, characterized by periostitis of the digits and joint pain. This syndrome is more commonly associated with adenocarcinoma, and although its precise pathophysiological mechanisms remain incompletely elucidated, it is hypothesized to involve circulating growth factors or vascular endothelial mediators that stimulate the formation of new bone and soft tissue [50]. In addition, there is the syndrome of inappropriate antidiuretic hormone secretion, which causes hyponatremia, skin hyperpigmentation such as acanthosis nigricans, and paraneoplastic coagulopathy characterized by blood hypercoagulability and the development of thrombosis. Early recognition of these syndromes not only facilitates timely diagnostic investigations but may also improve the likelihood of identifying NSCLC at a stage that may be amenable to curative or disease-modifying treatment.

6. Paraclinical Evaluation

Paraclinical assessment of NSCLC is an essential element in diagnosis, influencing both staging and selection of appropriate therapeutic strategies. This evaluation involves advanced imaging modalities, targeted invasive procedures for tissue acquisition, and increasingly modern molecular analyses. Imaging methods provide critical information about tumor location, size, local invasion, and the presence of nodal or distant metastases. Posterior–anterior chest radiography, computed tomography (CT), and magnetic resonance imaging (MRI) allow for detailed anatomical mapping, while positron emission tomography (PET) and PET/CT fusion imaging provide functional information, such as metabolic activity, that can improve the detection of occult metastatic disease and guide biopsy targeting. Tissue sampling remains the key to definitive histopathological diagnosis. Techniques range from minimally invasive procedures—such as flexible bronchoscopy with biopsy, ultrasound-guided endobronchial fine-needle aspiration (EBUS-FNA), and CT-guided transthoracic biopsy—to surgical approaches, including mediastinoscopy or video-assisted thoracoscopic surgery (VATS) for more extensive sampling. These methods enable precise classification of tumor subtypes and assessment of histological features critical for prognosis. Advances in molecular and genomic profiling have transformed the clinical landscape. Analysis of driver mutations, genetic rearrangements, and predictive biomarkers informs the use of targeted therapies and immunotherapeutic agents, enabling a shift from generalized to personalized oncology management. Techniques such as next-generation sequencing (NGS) and circulating tumor DNA (ctDNA) assays further refine the diagnostic process by detecting actionable alterations and monitoring minimal residual disease [51].

https://doi.org/10.3390/jcm15083042

6.1. Imaging

Chest radiography remains one of the oldest and most widely used diagnostic tools in the evaluation of patients with suspected pulmonary disease, including those ultimately diagnosed with NSCLC. Although its diagnostic performance is limited compared with more advanced imaging modalities, it continues to serve as a practical and widely available initial evaluation technique, particularly in symptomatic individuals or in situations where rapid triage is required. Although it has relatively low sensitivity, chest radiography can reveal many abnormalities that require further investigation. These findings may include pulmonary nodules or masses, areas of lobar or segmental atelectasis, pleural effusions, or mediastinal widening, each of which may raise suspicion of an underlying neoplastic process [52]. Radiographs are particularly useful for detecting large peripheral tumors or secondary changes, such as atelectasis caused by endobronchial obstruction. However, the value of chest radiography is limited by several disadvantages. Small lesions, especially those <1 cm, often escape detection, and centrally located tumors may be obscured by overlapping anatomical structures, such as the heart or major vessels. Dense and overlapping thoracic structures may further mask early-stage disease, reducing the sensitivity of radiographs for detecting subtle or early malignancies [52]. Despite these shortcomings, chest radiography remains clinically relevant. It provides a rapid, inexpensive, and widely available means of identifying macroscopic abnormalities and guiding the selection of more sensitive imaging modalities, such as chest CT or PET-CT. Contrast-enhanced computed tomography of the chest is widely considered the cornerstone imaging modality in the diagnosis of NSCLC. Its high spatial resolution and ability to precisely delineate thoracic anatomy make it indispensable for the characterization of both primary tumors and associated structural involvement. By administering intravenous contrast, chest CT enhances visualization of vascular, mediastinal, and pleural structures, allowing for a more precise assessment of tumor size, contour, and internal features. This level of detail facilitates the assessment of contact with adjacent anatomical structures, such as invasion of pulmonary arteries, veins, bronchi, and the chest wall [53]. In addition, it reliably identifies pleural infiltration, satellite lesions, and mediastinal or hilar lymphadenopathy, all of which have significant staging implications. Beyond its role in tumor characterization, chest CT is fundamental in differential diagnosis, helping to distinguish malignant lesions from benign entities such as infections, granulomatous disease, or vascular abnormalities. It is also essential in planning invasive procedures, including percutaneous biopsies and endobronchial sampling, guiding physicians to the most accessible and diagnostically significant ones. In the context of staging, it helps determine tumor extension and regional lymph node involvement within the TNM classification system, and it also directly informs therapeutic decision-making, influencing eligibility for surgical resection, radiotherapy planning, and selection of systemic treatments [53]. PET-CT, most often performed with fluorodeoxyglucose, has become the standard imaging technique for assessing the metabolic activity of tissues suspected of malignancy. It is particularly valuable in detecting regional lymph node involvement and distant metastatic spread, areas in which it consistently demonstrates greater sensitivity than standard chest CT [54]. The increased glucose uptake characteristic of most malignant cells allows it to highlight metastatic deposits that may be morphologically incongruent or occult on structural imaging. PET-CT can also reveal synchronous primary tumors, atypically localized metastatic disease, or early recurrences, thus influencing treatment planning and monitoring strategies [54]. Magnetic resonance imaging (MRI) of the brain plays a critical role in the evaluation of patients with non-small-cell lung cancer when there is clinical suspicion of brain involvement. Due to its superior soft tissue contrast and high sensitivity, brain MRI remains the most accurate modality for identifying brain metastases, especially small lesions or those located in anatomically

https://doi.org/10.3390/jcm15083042

complex regions that may be missed by computed tomography. Brain MRI is strongly recommended for symptomatic individuals, for example, those presenting with headache, neurological deficits, seizures, or cognitive impairment, as well as for patients with advanced disease, in whom the likelihood of occult brain metastases is increased [55]. In certain histologic subtypes, particularly adenocarcinoma, brain MRI may be warranted even in the absence of neurological symptoms, as brain metastases are common in this histologic subtype. Identification of intracranial metastases can modify systemic treatment plans, determine eligibility for targeted therapies or immunotherapy, and guide the selection between stereotactic radiotherapy and whole-brain radiotherapy [55]. Cardiac magnetic resonance imaging (CMR) has proven to be the most sensitive and specific method for detecting cardiac metastases, providing precise information on lesion location, size, extent, and involvement of adjacent structures. Compared with CT or echocardiography, CMR offers high-resolution, multiplanar assessment and tissue characterization, making it the gold standard for identifying these metastases. Integrating CMR into the diagnostic workflow for advanced NSCLC can help explain unexplained systemic symptoms and guide personalized therapeutic strategies, thereby improving prognosis for patients with metastatic disease [56].

6.2. Histological and Cytological Diagnosis

Diagnostic certainty in NSCLC is based on histological or cytological confirmation, which remains the gold standard for identifying the specific tumor subtype. Obtaining a sufficient volume of high-quality biological material is essential—not only for accurate morphological evaluation but also to allow immunohistochemistry, which has become indispensable for guiding personalized therapeutic strategies in modern oncology. The choice of sampling technique depends on the location of the tumor, the patient's characteristics, and the need for auxiliary methods. Flexible bronchoscopy is the first-line diagnostic procedure for centrally located tumors, due to its ability to provide direct endoscopic visualization of the tracheobronchial tree. This technique facilitates targeted biopsy of endobronchial lesions while allowing for bronchial aspirate collection, brush cytology, and transbronchial biopsy of adjacent parenchymal regions, when necessary. Its main advantage lies in the minimally invasive access to the central airways and the possibility of obtaining multiple tissue fragments, thus increasing diagnostic accuracy [57]. A diagnostic method that also contributes to the staging of lung cancer is ultrasound-guided transbronchial fine-needle aspiration (EBUS-TBNA). This technique is used especially in cases where the tumor is not accessible by fiberoptic bronchoscopy or does not show endobronchial expression, and there is tumor infiltration in the mediastinal nodes or, in the case of inconclusive biopsies, is performed directly from the endobronchial lesion [57]. For peripheral pulmonary nodules or masses that cannot be reached endoscopically, CT-guided transthoracic needle biopsy is considered the procedure of choice. This method ensures a high diagnostic yield due to its precise imaging-based guidance, which enables accurate targeting of even small or deep-seated lesions. Despite its effectiveness, the procedure carries a recognized risk of complications, most commonly pneumothorax, necessitating careful patient selection and performance in centers with substantial experience. Specimens obtained through transthoracic biopsy are typically suitable for comprehensive histologic examination and molecular testing, including mutation analysis and immunohistochemical profiling [58]. When less invasive diagnostic approaches fail to provide conclusive results, video-assisted thoracoscopic surgery (VATS) represents an advanced alternative that allows direct visualization and sampling of pulmonary nodules, pleural lesions, or mediastinal lymph nodes. VATS provides access to high-quality tissue samples, improving the likelihood of establishing an accurate diagnosis. In addition, surgical specimens obtained by lobectomy, segmentectomy, or other forms of lung resection constitute the most complete material for histopathological evaluation, immunohistochemistry, and molecular analyses [59]. These samples play a crucial role in accurate pathological staging, which is essential for determining prognosis and selecting the optimal therapeutic course.

6.3. Molecular and Immunohistochemical Analyses

The integration of molecular and IHC analyses has become the cornerstone of contemporary NSCLC management, moving beyond morphology-based classification to a precision oncology framework. Histopathological evaluation, while essential, is now complemented by IHC markers and comprehensive genomic profiling to guide diagnostic confirmation, prognostic stratification, and therapeutic selection. Molecular testing is considered mandatory in adenocarcinoma and strongly recommended in poorly differentiated or non-squamous NSCLC, given the high probability of identifying oncogenic factors with therapeutic implications [60]. A comprehensive genomic profile is essential to guide precision therapy in adenocarcinoma and in subtypes of NSCLC that do not show clear squamous differentiation. Adenocarcinomas arise from epithelial cells in the terminal respiratory unit and have variable morphological appearances, being of several acinar, lepidic, and papillary types, usually expressing thyroid transcription factor 1 (TTF1), Napsin A and cytokeratin 7 (CK7) [61]. There is some data in the literature suggesting that in Caucasian patients, the lack of TTF1 expression by tumor cells has a strong negative predictive value for activating EGFR mutations in adenocarcinomas, although this is less clear for ALK/ROS1. On the other hand, squamous carcinomas arise from basal bronchial epithelial cells, and morphologically, these lesions usually show keratinization and intercellular bridges with concomitant expression of p40, p63 and cytokeratin 5/6. In this context, testing for EGFR mutations, ALK and ROS1 rearrangements, and other key genomic alterations such as KRAS, BRAF, or MET mutations has become standard practice. In large cell lung cancer, key IHC markers are synaptophysin or chromogranin A, and in this context, multiple actionable genetic alterations like EGFR, ALK, KRAS, and ROS1 are tested. In the case of adenocarcinomas in "non-smokers", they present a significantly higher frequency of mutations in EGFR, ALK, and ROS, while smokers present a high frequency of KRAS mutations, suggesting potentially different pathogenetic mechanisms of tumor development in smokers and non-smokers. The detection of these molecular abnormalities enables the use of tyrosine kinase inhibitors (TKIs) and other targeted agents, which have demonstrated superior response rates, improved quality of life, and significantly reduced systemic toxicity compared with traditional cytotoxic chemotherapy. As a result, molecular stratification transforms the therapeutic landscape, offering individualized treatment pathways tailored to the tumor's specific genetic profile [62]. Assessment of PD-L1 expression through immunohistochemistry has emerged as a cornerstone of immunotherapy selection in NSCLC. PD-L1 levels are reported as the tumor proportion score (TPS), reflecting the percentage of tumor cells exhibiting membranous staining. This quantitative evaluation guides the decision to initiate immune checkpoint inhibitor therapy, either as monotherapy in cases with high PD-L1 expression or in combination with chemotherapy when moderate or heterogeneous expression patterns are observed. Although PD-L1 is not an ideal biomarker—owing to intratumoral heterogeneity, variability in testing platforms, and limited predictive accuracy—it remains the most widely implemented tool for determining eligibility for immunotherapy and for estimating the likelihood of therapeutic response [63]. Molecular alterations are not merely academic; they are clinically actionable. Identification of targetable mutations directly informs the use of tyrosine kinase inhibitors, BRAF/MEK inhibitors, and immune checkpoint inhibitors, providing superior response rates, improved survival, and effective

https://doi.org/10.3390/jcm15083042

systemic and intracranial disease control. Consequently, comprehensive molecular and IHC profiling is now considered mandatory for all newly diagnosed advanced NSCLC cases, representing a shift from morphology-centric to biomarker-driven decision-making. Beyond guiding treatment, integrated analyses refine prognostic assessment. Certain histologic patterns combined with specific molecular alterations can predict disease aggressiveness, recurrence risk, and likelihood of response to immunotherapy, enabling truly individualized patient management.

7. Treatment

The treatment of NSCLC results from the integration of clinical, imaging, histological, and molecular information in a multidisciplinary context involving a pulmonologist, an oncologist, a pathologist, and a thoracic surgeon. Treatment selection is no longer stage-based alone, but is critically dependent on molecular and immunohistochemical profiling. (Figure 2) [64]. In localized stages, curative treatment is pursued, while in advanced stages, the goals are to prolong survival and improve quality of life. Stages I–II are generally managed with curative intent by surgery or stereotactic radiotherapy, while stage III involves sequential or concomitant combinations of surgery, radiotherapy, and chemotherapy [65,66]. Stage IV is managed mainly by systemic therapy, guided by molecular and immunological profiling [67]. Evaluation of biomarkers such as EGFR, ALK, ROS1, BRAF, KRAS, or PD-L1 expression is indispensable before initiating treatment in most cases of advanced disease [68].

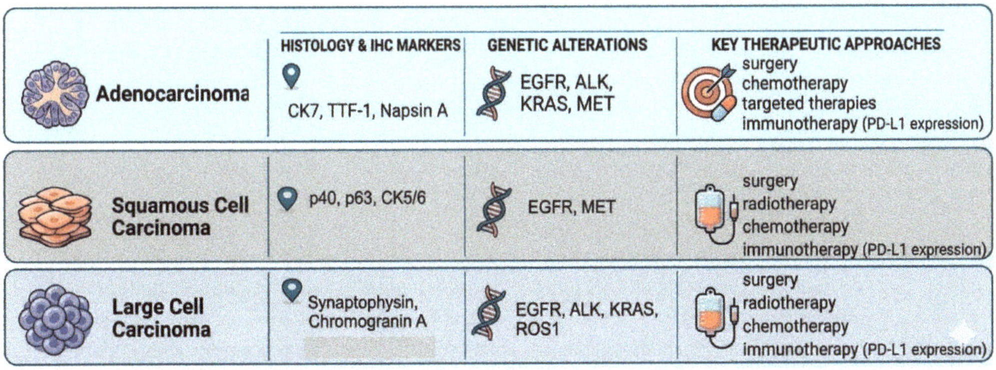

Figure 2. From Histopathological Classification to Precision Oncology.

7.1. Surgical Treatment

Surgical resection remains the standard treatment with curative intent for early-stage (I–II) and selected stage IIIA NSCLC with limited and resectable nodal involvement. The primary goal is complete excision of the tumor with negative margins while preserving as much functional lung parenchyma as possible. Lobectomy is considered the gold standard, providing an optimal balance between oncological control and preservation of lung function. Sublobar resections, such as anatomical segmentectomy, may be indicated for small peripheral tumors (<2 cm) or in patients with significant comorbidities. Pneumonectomy is reserved for cases in which limited resections cannot achieve complete tumor clearance, due to its higher morbidity [66]. Adjuvant chemotherapy is recommended in the presence of nodal involvement or other high-risk features. Furthermore, in patients with EGFR sensitizing mutations, adjuvant therapy with EGFR tyrosine kinase inhibitors—particularly osimertinib—significantly reduces the risk of recurrence and improves disease-free survival [69].

https://doi.org/10.3390/jcm15083042

7.2. Radiotherapy

Radiotherapy plays a key role in the management of NSCLC as a curative, definitive or palliative treatment modality, depending on the stage of the disease, the characteristics of the tumor, and the operability of the patient. By minimizing radiation-induced toxicity to surrounding normal tissues, various radiation techniques have distinguished and evolved. In the case of patients with early-stage NSCLC who are medically inoperable or refuse surgery, stereotactic body radiotherapy has become the treatment of choice. It offers the possibility of administering high doses of radiation in a limited number of fractions with maximum precision, resulting in excellent local control rates, comparable to those obtained with surgical resection. This approach is very effective for small peripheral tumors, with a diameter of less than 3 cm, where the risk of toxicity to critical thoracic structures is relatively low. For patients with locally advanced disease, radiotherapy is most often administered in combination with systemic chemotherapy [70]. Concurrent chemoradiotherapy is the standard of care for inoperable stage III NSCLC and has demonstrated superior survival outcomes compared with sequential treatment approaches. The cumulative effect of chemotherapy increases radiosensitivity, thereby improving local tumor control, although it is associated with an increased risk of acute and late toxicities, requiring careful patient selection and monitoring [71]. Technological innovations in radiotherapy have further optimized the precision and safety of treatment. Techniques such as intensity-modulated radiotherapy and image-guided radiotherapy allow for increased tumor dose while sparing adjacent organs at risk, including the lungs, heart, and esophagus. This has reduced treatment-related morbidity and improved patient tolerance to treatment. In addition to its curative and definitive applications, radiotherapy remains an essential component of palliative care in NSCLC, being effective in alleviating tumor-related symptoms such as pain, hemoptysis, dyspnea, and complications arising from mediastinal compression, thus improving the quality of life in patients with advanced or metastatic disease [70].

7.3. Chemotherapy

Chemotherapy continues to be a fundamental component of the therapeutic strategy for NSCLC, especially in patients with advanced disease and as adjuvant or neoadjuvant treatment in early stages, and remains indispensable in multiple clinical settings. Platinum-based doublet chemotherapy constitutes the basis of systemic treatment for NSCLC. Standard regimens usually combine cisplatin or carboplatin with a third-generation cytotoxic agent such as vinorelbine, gemcitabine, paclitaxel, or pemetrexed. Chemotherapeutic agents are chosen according to the patient's general condition, comorbidities, and histological subtype. Pemetrexed has demonstrated superior efficacy and a more favorable toxicity profile, especially in adenocarcinoma, and is therefore preferentially recommended in this subgroup, while its use is contraindicated in squamous cell carcinoma due to inferior results [72]. In inoperable stage III NSCLC, concurrent chemoradiotherapy is the standard of care, providing improved survival compared with sequential therapeutic approaches. In addition, consolidation therapy with the anti-PD-L1 monoclonal antibody durvalumab, after definitive chemoradiotherapy, has been shown to significantly improve progression-free survival and overall survival, establishing a new therapeutic paradigm in this setting [73]. In metastatic disease (stage IV), chemotherapy is used either alone or in combination with immunotherapy, depending on tumor PD-L1 expression. In the absence of actionable oncogenic driver mutations, chemoimmunotherapy combinations have demonstrated superior clinical outcomes compared with chemotherapy alone [74]. Conversely, in patients with high PD-L1 expression, immunotherapy-based therapeutic

https://doi.org/10.3390/jcm1508304

regimens may be preferred, with chemotherapy reserved for cases of disease progression or contraindications to immunotherapy [74].

7.4. Targeted Therapy

Targeted therapy represents one of the most significant advances in the management of NSCLC, reflecting a paradigm shift toward precision oncology based on the identification of oncogenic driver alterations. By selectively inhibiting molecular pathways essential for tumor growth and survival, targeted agents have demonstrated superior efficacy and improved tolerability compared with conventional chemotherapy in appropriately selected patient populations [75]. Among the most extensively studied targets in NSCLC are activating mutations of the epidermal growth factor receptor (EGFR), which are predominantly observed in adenocarcinoma histology. First-, second-, and third-generation EGFR tyrosine kinase inhibitors (TKIs), including erlotinib, gefitinib, afatinib, and osimertinib, have shown substantial clinical benefit in tumors harboring sensitizing EGFR mutations, particularly exon 19 deletions and the L858R point mutation. Osimertinib is currently the recommended first-line treatment because it works better, has fewer side effects, and can better penetrate the central nervous system. This leads to better control of the disease throughout the body and in the brain [76]. Another specific group of non-small-cell lung cancer (NSCLC) is defined by changes in the anaplastic lymphoma kinase (ALK) gene. ALK inhibitors, such as alectinib, brigatinib, and lorlatinib, have shown high response rates and lasting disease control in tumors with ALK mutations. These drugs are particularly effective at preventing and treating brain metastases, which are common in this group of patients [77]. Tumors harboring ROS1 gene fusions may be effectively treated with TKIs such as crizotinib and entrectinib, both of which have shown meaningful systemic and intracranial activity [78]. In patients with BRAF V600E mutations, combined inhibition of BRAF and MEK using dabrafenib in conjunction with trametinib has emerged as the standard targeted approach, yielding significant clinical responses [79]. More recently, the development of KRAS G12C inhibitors, including sotorasib and adagrasib, has addressed one of the most common cancer-causing factors in NSCLC, which was previously considered impossible to treat with drugs [80]. These treatments have shown promising results in patients with advanced disease who have not responded to previous systemic therapies, thus expanding the treatment options for this common molecular subtype. Accurate identification of targetable molecular changes is crucial for the best use of targeted therapy. Therefore, comprehensive molecular profiling using next-generation sequencing (NGS) is strongly recommended whenever possible, as it allows for the simultaneous detection of multiple genomic alterations and supports personalized treatment choices [75].

7.5. Immunotherapy

Immunotherapy is notable for providing significant and sustained improvements in survival outcomes with immune checkpoint inhibitors. These agents inhibit key immune checkpoint pathways that tumors use to evade immune surveillance, and the most widely used inhibitors target programmed cell death protein 1 (PD-1) and its ligand PD-L1. Monoclonal antibodies directed against PD-1, such as pembrolizumab and nivolumab, as well as PD-L1 inhibitors, including atezolizumab and durvalumab, have demonstrated robust clinical efficacy across multiple disease stages. These agents stimulate T-cell activation and proliferation, thereby promoting immune-mediated tumor cell killing by blocking the PD-1/PD-L1 interaction. Pembrolizumab monotherapy is recommended for patients whose tumors have high PD-L1 expression (tumor proportion score $\geq 50\%$) in the absence of actionable molecular alterations and in the first-line treatment of metastatic NSCLC. In this subgroup, immunotherapy alone has been shown to significantly improve overall

https://doi.org/10.3390/jcm15083042

survival and quality of life compared with platinum-based chemotherapy [81]. For patients with low or absent PD-L1 expression, immune checkpoint inhibitors are most commonly administered in combination with chemotherapy. Chemoimmunotherapy regimens have demonstrated significant survival benefits regardless of PD-L1 status and have therefore become the standard of care in this clinical setting [82]. In unresectable stage III NSCLC, consolidation immunotherapy with durvalumab after definitive concurrent chemoradiotherapy is the current standard of care. This strategy has been associated with durable improvements in progression-free survival and overall survival, marking a major advance in the management of locally advanced disease [83]. A defining feature of immunotherapy is the potential for durable and long-lasting responses. A subgroup of patients achieves prolonged disease control or complete remission, highlighting the ability of immune checkpoint inhibition to induce sustained antitumor immunity and fundamentally alter the natural history of advanced NSCLC.

7.6. Palliative Treatment

In patients with advanced NSCLC or those with limited functional reserve who are not candidates for curative intent therapies, the main goals of treatment include symptom control, optimization of quality of life, and psychosocial support. Therefore, palliative care is an essential component of the complex management of NSCLC and should be individualized according to the severity of symptoms and patient preferences. Effective pain management through appropriate analgesic therapy with opioid and non-opioid medications is fundamental to improving patient comfort. Dyspnea, one of the most common and distressing symptoms, can be managed primarily by supplemental oxygen therapy when indicated and by non-pharmacological interventions [84]. Recurrent malignant pleural effusions can be addressed by therapeutic thoracentesis, indwelling pleural catheters, or pleurodesis, depending on the context. In addition, prompt treatment of infectious complications and provision of adequate nutritional support are crucial in maintaining functional status and reducing symptom burden [84]. Palliative radiotherapy can provide rapid and effective relief of bone pain, refractory cough, hemoptysis, and symptoms related to compression of mediastinal or neural structures, thereby contributing significantly to symptom relief and overall well-being [85]. Importantly, early integration of palliative care alongside disease-directed treatment has demonstrated substantial benefits in patients with metastatic NSCLC. Early palliative involvement is associated with improved symptom control, increased quality of life, better patient and carer satisfaction, and, in some studies, prolonged survival. This integrated approach emphasizes the importance of incorporating palliative principles throughout the disease trajectory, rather than reserving them exclusively for end-of-life care [84].

8. Prognosis

The prognosis of this type of cancer is influenced by clinical, histological, molecular, and therapeutic factors, with the stage of the disease at diagnosis remaining the most important determinant of prognosis. Overall survival is significantly superior in early stages of the disease, where complete surgical resection with curative intent is feasible, compared with advanced stages, where regional lymph node involvement or distant metastases preclude definitive local treatment [86]. Histological subtype also plays a significant role in prognostic stratification, with adenocarcinoma being the most common histological variant of NSCLC and generally associated with a poor prognosis. However, outcomes have improved substantially due to the availability of targeted therapies and immunotherapy in molecularly tested patients. Squamous cell carcinoma, on the other hand, often presents a more aggressive clinical course and is associated with a more limited

https://doi.org/10.3390/jcm15083042

spectrum of actionable molecular alterations, which may restrict therapeutic options. Large cell carcinoma, due to its biological heterogeneity and predisposition to early dissemination, is usually associated with a poor prognosis and high metastatic potential [87]. The presence of actionable oncogenic factors, such as activating mutations of EGFR or rearrangements of the ALK and ROS1 genes, allows the use of targeted therapies that are associated with higher response rates, prolonged progression-free survival, and improved overall survival. Similarly, increased PD-L1 expression has been correlated with increased responsiveness to immune checkpoint inhibitors [88]. In contrast, molecular alterations, such as TP53 mutations or complex genomic profiles, are frequently associated with more aggressive tumor behavior, resistance to therapy, and poorer clinical outcomes [89]. Survival outcomes vary considerably depending on the stage of the disease. In patients with stage I NSCLC, five-year survival rates can exceed 60–70%, reflecting the effectiveness of surgical treatment in early-stage disease. In stage II, five-year survival rates drop to approximately 40–50%, while in stage III disease, long-term survival is observed in only 20–30% of patients, despite multimodal therapeutic approaches [90]. In metastatic stage IV NSCLC, median overall survival typically ranges from 12 to 30 months, depending on tumor biology, molecular profile, and access to contemporary systemic therapies, including targeted agents and immunotherapy [91]. Ultimately, response to treatment, durability of disease control, and the ability to tailor therapy to individual tumor characteristics remain essential for improving the prognosis of patients with NSCLC. Continued advances in molecular diagnostics and therapeutic innovation are expected to further refine prognostic assessment and improve survival outcomes in the future.

9. Conclusions

The landscape of NSCLC has evolved far beyond traditional histopathological classification. While histology remains a fundamental component of diagnosis, it is no longer sufficient to guide optimal patient management in the era of precision oncology. Comprehensive molecular profiling has become the standard of care, enabling the identification of clinically actionable alterations and guiding targeted therapeutic strategies. The integration of histological, immunohistochemical, and genomic data is essential for accurate diagnosis, prognostic assessment, and individualized treatment planning. Looking ahead, the future of NSCLC management lies in combining innovative targeted therapies with immunotherapies and incorporating emerging biomarkers to further refine patient selection and improve outcomes, underscoring the necessity of a holistic, data-driven approach that bridges morphology with molecular precision.

Author Contributions: Conceptualization: S.-M.R., M.A.B. and V.B.; validation: M.A.B., V.B., B.M., D.-M.T., M.P., S.-I.S. and I.-A.C.; writing—original draft preparation: S.-M.R., M.-M.P., A.-Ș.S., T.-I.P. and D.M.M.; writing—review and editing: V.B.; data curation: S.-M.R. All authors have read and agreed to the published version of the manuscript.

Funding: The Article Processing Charges were funded by the University of Medicine and Pharmacy of Craiova.

Institutional Review Board Statement: Not applicable.

Informed Consent Statement: Not applicable.

Data Availability Statement: The data presented in this study are available on request from the corresponding authors.

Conflicts of Interest: The authors declare no conflicts of interest.

https://doi.org/10.3390/jcm15083042

Abbreviations

The following abbreviations are used in this manuscript:

NSCLC	Non-small-cell lung cancer
SCLC	Small-cell lung cancer
EGFR	Epidermal growth factor receptor
ALK	Anaplastic lymphoma kinase
ROS1	Proto-oncogene tyrosine-protein kinase ROS
KRAS	Kristen rat sarcoma viral oncogene homolog
PD-1	Programmed cell death protein
PD-L1	Programmed death-ligand 1
PM2.5	Fine particles with diameters less than 2.5 μm
DNA	Deoxyribonucleic acid
PI3K/AKT	Phosphatidylinositol 3-kinase/protein kinase B
JAK/STAT	Janus kinases/signal transducer and activator of transcription proteins
FGFR1	Fibroblast growth factor receptor 1
TNM	Tumor-node-metastasis
ACTH	Adrenocorticotropic hormone
MRI	Magnetic resonance imaging
CT	Computed tomography
PET	Positron emission tomography
EBUS-TBNA	Endobronchial ultrasound-guided transbronchial needle aspiration
VATS	Video-assisted thoracoscopic surgery
NGS	Next-generation sequencing
ctDNA	Circulating tumor DNA
TTF1	Thyroid transcription factor 1
TKIs	Tyrosine kinase inhibitors
TP53	Tumor protein 53
TPS	Tumor proportion score

References

1. Chen, Z.; Fillmore, C.M.; Hammerman, P.S.; Kim, C.F.; Wong, K.-K. Non-Small-Cell Lung Cancers: A Heterogeneous Set o Diseases. *Nat. Rev. Cancer* **2014**, *14*, 535–546. [CrossRef] [PubMed]
2. Zappa, C.; Mousa, S.A. Non-Small Cell Lung Cancer: Current Treatment and Future Advances. *Transl. Lung Cancer Res.* **201** *5*, 288–300. [CrossRef]
3. Aguiar, P.N.; De Mello, R.A.; Hall, P.; Tadokoro, H.; de Lima Lopes, G. PD-L1 Expression as a Predictive Biomarker in Advance Non-Small-Cell Lung Cancer: Updated Survival Data. *Immunotherapy* **2017**, *9*, 499–506. [CrossRef]
4. Ramos, R.; Moura, C.S.; Costa, M.; Lamas, N.J.; Correia, R.; Garcez, D.; Pereira, J.M.; Lindahl, T.; Sousa, C.; Vale, N. Lung Cance Therapy: The Role of Personalized Medicine. *Cancers* **2025**, *17*, 725. [CrossRef]
5. Cheng, T.-Y.D.; Cramb, S.M.; Baade, P.D.; Youlden, D.R.; Nwogu, C.; Reid, M.E. The International Epidemiology of Lung Cance Latest Trends, Disparities, and Tumor Characteristics. *J. Thorac. Oncol.* **2016**, *11*, 1653–1671. [CrossRef]
6. Onwuka, J.U.; Zahed, H.; Feng, X.; Alcala, K.; Erhunmwunsee, L.; Williams, R.M.; Aldrich, M.C.; Ahluwalia, J.S.; Albanes, D Arslan, A.A.; et al. Association between Socioeconomic Position and Lung Cancer Incidence in 16 Countries: A Prospectiv Cohort Consortium Study. *eClinicalMedicine* **2025**, *82*, 103152. [CrossRef]
7. Bade, B.C.; Dela Cruz, C.S. Lung Cancer 2020. *Clin. Chest Med.* **2020**, *41*, 1–24. [CrossRef] [PubMed]
8. Olsson, A.; Bouaoun, L.; Schüz, J.; Vermeulen, R.; Behrens, T.; Ge, C.; Kromhout, H.; Siemiatycki, J.; Gustavsson, P.; Boffett P.; et al. Lung Cancer Risks Associated with Occupational Exposure to Pairs of Five Lung Carcinogens: Results from a Poole Analysis of Case-Control Studies (SYNERGY). *Environ. Health Perspect.* **2024**, *132*, 17005. [CrossRef] [PubMed]
9. Wang, M.; Kim, R.Y.; Kohonen-Corish, M.R.J.; Chen, H.; Donovan, C.; Oliver, B.G. Particulate Matter Air Pollution as a Cause o Lung Cancer: Epidemiological and Experimental Evidence. *Br. J. Cancer* **2025**, *132*, 986–996. [CrossRef] [PubMed]
10. Citarella, F.; Takada, K.; Cascetta, P.; Crucitti, P.; Petti, R.; Vincenzi, B.; Tonini, G.; Venanzi, F.M.; Bulotta, A.; Oresti, S.; et a Clinical Implications of the Family History in Patients with Lung Cancer: A Systematic Review of the Literature and a Nev Cross-Sectional/Prospective Study Design (FAHIC: Lung). *J. Transl. Med.* **2024**, *22*, 714. [CrossRef]

https://doi.org/10.3390/jcm1508304

1. Mitroi, D.M.; Balteanu, M.A.; Cioboata, R.; Vlasceanu, S.G.; Zlatian, O.M.; Catana, O.M.; Mirea, A.A.; Mogos, G.F.R.; Rotaru, I.; Biciusca, V. Hypercoagulability in Tuberculosis: Pathophysiological Mechanisms, Associated Risks, and Advances in Management—A Narrative Review. *J. Clin. Med.* **2025**, *14*, 762. [CrossRef] [PubMed]
2. Cioboata, R.; Balteanu, M.A.; Mitroi, D.M.; Vrabie, S.C.; Vlasceanu, S.G.; Andrei, G.M.; Riza, A.L.; Streata, I.; Zlatian, O.M.; Olteanu, M. Beyond Smoking: Emerging Drivers of COPD and Their Clinical Implications in Low- and Middle-Income Countries: A Narrative Review. *J. Clin. Med.* **2025**, *14*, 4633. [CrossRef] [PubMed]
3. Ratnakaram, K.; Yendamuri, S.; Groman, A.; Kalvapudi, S. Sex-Based Differences in Lung Cancer Incidence: A Retrospective Analysis of Two Large US-Based Cancer Databases. *Cancers* **2024**, *16*, 3244. [CrossRef]
4. Huang, C.; Qu, X.; Du, J. Proportion of Lung Adenocarcinoma in Female Never-Smokers Has Increased Dramatically over the Past 28 Years. *J. Thorac. Dis.* **2019**, *11*, 2685–2688. [CrossRef]
5. Hughes, D.J.; Kapiris, M.; Podvez Nevajda, A.; McGrath, H.; Stavraka, C.; Ahmad, S.; Taylor, B.; Cook, G.J.R.; Ghosh, S.; Josephs, D.; et al. Non-Small Cell Lung Cancer (NSCLC) in Young Adults, Age < 50, Is Associated with Late Stage at Presentation and a Very Poor Prognosis in Patients That Do Not Have a Targeted Therapy Option: A Real-World Study. *Cancers* **2022**, *14*, 6056. [CrossRef]
6. Yang, M.; Hu, X.; Tang, B.; Deng, F. Exploring the Interplay between Methylation Patterns and Non-Coding RNAs in Non-Small Cell Lung Cancer: Implications for Pathogenesis and Therapeutic Targets. *Heliyon* **2024**, *10*, e24811. [CrossRef]
7. Skoulidis, F.; Heymach, J.V. Co-Occurring Genomic Alterations in Non-Small-Cell Lung Cancer Biology and Therapy. *Nat. Rev. Cancer* **2019**, *19*, 495–509. [CrossRef]
8. Gu, Q.; Chen, F.; Chen, N.; Wang, J.; Li, Z.; Deng, X. Effect of EGCG on Bronchial Epithelial Cell Premalignant Lesions Induced by Cigarette Smoke and on Its CYP1A1 Expression. *Int. J. Mol. Med.* **2021**, *48*, 220. [CrossRef]
9. Wen, Y.; Zhu, Y.; Zhang, C.; Yang, X.; Gao, Y.; Li, M.; Yang, H.; Liu, T.; Tang, H. Chronic Inflammation, Cancer Development and Immunotherapy. *Front. Pharmacol.* **2022**, *13*, 1040163. [CrossRef] [PubMed]
0. Li, Q.; Li, Z.; Luo, T.; Shi, H. Targeting the PI3K/AKT/MTOR and RAF/MEK/ERK Pathways for Cancer Therapy. *Mol. Biomed.* **2022**, *3*, 47. [CrossRef] [PubMed]
1. Preobrazhenskaya, E.V.; Mulkidjan, R.S.; Zagrebin, F.A.; Romanko, A.A.; Saitova, E.S.; Korzun, P.R.; Binnatova, J.O.; Tiurin, V.I.; Bizin, I.V.; Imyanitov, E.N. Novel Kinase-Activating Genetic Events in Non-Small Cell Lung Carcinomas. *Explor. Target. Anti-Tumor Ther.* **2025**, *6*, 1002330. [CrossRef]
2. Vynnychenko, O.; Moskalenko, Y.; Moskalenko, R. The Role of TP53 Gene Mutation in the Survival of Non-Small Cell Lung Cancer Patients. *East. Ukr. Med. J.* **2025**, *13*, 245–256. [CrossRef]
3. Simbolo, M.; Centonze, G.; Gkountakos, A.; Monti, V.; Maisonneuve, P.; Golovco, S.; Sabella, G.; Del Gobbo, A.; Gobbo, S.; Ferrero, S.; et al. Characterization of Two Transcriptomic Subtypes of Marker-Null Large Cell Carcinoma of the Lung Suggests Different Origin and Potential New Therapeutic Perspectives. *Virchows Arch.* **2024**, *484*, 777–788. [CrossRef] [PubMed]
4. Rothschild, S. Targeted Therapies in Non-Small Cell Lung Cancer—Beyond EGFR and ALK. *Cancers* **2015**, *7*, 930–949. [CrossRef]
5. Huang, Y.; Hong, W.; Wei, X. The Molecular Mechanisms and Therapeutic Strategies of EMT in Tumor Progression and Metastasis. *J. Hematol. Oncol.* **2022**, *15*, 129. [CrossRef]
6. Jin, T.; Jiang, Y.; Song, Y. Asymptomatic Lung Adenocarcinoma with Cardiac Metastasis at Initial Diagnosis: A Case Report. *Am. J. Case Rep.* **2025**, *26*, e951223. [CrossRef]
7. Zhu, T.; Bao, X.; Chen, M.; Lin, R.; Zhuyan, J.; Zhen, T.; Xing, K.; Zhou, W.; Zhu, S. Mechanisms and Future of Non-Small Cell Lung Cancer Metastasis. *Front. Oncol.* **2020**, *10*, 585284. [CrossRef]
8. Suster, D.I.; Mino-Kenudson, M. Molecular Pathology of Primary Non-Small Cell Lung Cancer. *Arch. Med. Res.* **2020**, *51*, 784–798. [CrossRef] [PubMed]
9. Tsubokawa, N.; Mimae, T.; Miyata, Y.; Kanno, C.; Kudo, Y.; Nagashima, T.; Ito, H.; Ikeda, N.; Okada, M. Comparative Oncological Features of Centrally and Peripherally Located Small-Sized Radiologically Solid-Dominant Non-Small-Cell Lung Cancer. *Eur. J. Cardio-Thorac. Surg.* **2025**, *67*, ezaf072. [CrossRef]
0. Li, Q.; He, X.-Q.; Fan, X.; Luo, T.-Y.; Huo, J.-W.; Huang, X.-T. Computed Tomography Morphological Classification of Lung Adenocarcinoma and Its Correlation with Epidermal Growth Factor Receptor Mutation Status: A Report of 1075 Cases. *Int. J. Gen. Med.* **2021**, *14*, 3687–3698. [CrossRef] [PubMed]
1. Matache, R.S.; Stanciu-Gavan, C.; Pantile, D.; Iordache, A.M.; Bejgăneanu, A.O.; Șerboiu, C.S.; Nemes, A.F. Clinical and Paraclinical Characteristics of Endobronchial Pulmonary Squamous Cell Carcinoma—A Brief Review. *Diagnostics* **2023**, *13*, 3318. [CrossRef]
2. Ghosh, S. Large-Cell Carcinoma. In *Handbook of Imaging in Pulmonary Disease*; Springer International Publishing: Cham, Switzerland, 2021; pp. 13–14.
3. He, B.; Song, Y.; Wang, L.; Wang, T.; She, Y.; Hou, L.; Zhang, L.; Wu, C.; Babu, B.A.; Bagci, U.; et al. A Machine Learning-Based Prediction of the Micropapillary/Solid Growth Pattern in Invasive Lung Adenocarcinoma with Radiomics. *Transl. Lung Cancer Res.* **2021**, *10*, 955–964. [CrossRef] [PubMed]

34. Berezowska, S.; Maillard, M.; Keyter, M.; Bisig, B. Pulmonary Squamous Cell Carcinoma and Lymphoepithelial Carcinoma Morphology, Molecular Characteristics and Differential Diagnosis. *Histopathology* **2024**, *84*, 32–49. [CrossRef]
35. Rekhtman, N.; Tafe, L.J.; Chaft, J.E.; Wang, L.; Arcila, M.E.; Colanta, A.; Moreira, A.L.; Zakowski, M.F.; Travis, W.D.; Sima, C.S. et al. Distinct Profile of Driver Mutations and Clinical Features in Immunomarker-Defined Subsets of Pulmonary Large-Cell Carcinoma. *Mod. Pathol.* **2013**, *26*, 511–522. [CrossRef] [PubMed]
36. Uota, F.; Iwano, S.; Kamiya, S.; Ito, R.; Nakamura, S.; Chen-Yoshikawa, T.F.; Naganawa, S. Diagnostic Utility of Chest Wall Vessel Involvement Sign on Ultra-High-Resolution CT for Primary Lung Cancer Infiltrating the Chest Wall. *Eur. Radiol.* **2025** *35*, 4824–4833. [CrossRef]
37. Kifjak, D.; Mura, R.; Khenkina, N.; Pochepnia, S.; Heidinger, B.H.; Milos, R.-I.; Beer, L.; Prosch, H. Something Old Something New—Introduction to the Ninth Edition TNM Classification of Lung Cancer. *Br. J. Radiol.* **2025**, *98*, 1543–1555. [CrossRef] [PubMed]
38. Wang, J.; Wang, B.; Zhao, W.; Guo, Y.; Chen, H.; Chu, H.; Liang, X.; Bi, J. Clinical Significance and Role of Lymphatic Vessel Invasion as a Major Prognostic Implication in Non-Small Cell Lung Cancer: A Meta-Analysis. *PLoS ONE* **2012**, *7*, e52704 [CrossRef]
39. Swinson, D.E.; Jones, J.L.; Richardson, D.; Cox, G.; Edwards, J.G.; O'Byrne, K.J. Tumour Necrosis Is an Independent Prognostic Marker in Non-Small Cell Lung Cancer: Correlation with Biological Variables. *Lung Cancer* **2002**, *37*, 235–240. [CrossRef]
40. Anupozu, R.; Vanamala, M. Non-Small Cell Lung Cancer (NSCLC)—A Comprehensive Review. *Int. J. Pharma Sci. Res.* **2020** *11*, 215–223. [CrossRef]
41. Garrana, S.H.; Dagogo-Jack, I.; Cobb, R.; Kuo, A.H.; Mendoza, D.P.; Zhang, E.W.; Heeger, A.; Sequist, L.V.; Digumarthy, S.R Clinical and Imaging Features of Non–Small-Cell Lung Cancer in Young Patients. *Clin. Lung Cancer* **2021**, *22*, 23–31. [CrossRef]
42. Harle, A.; Molassiotis, A.; Buffin, O.; Burnham, J.; Smith, J.; Yorke, J.; Blackhall, F.H. A Cross Sectional Study to Determine the Prevalence of Cough and Its Impact in Patients with Lung Cancer: A Patient Unmet Need. *BMC Cancer* **2020**, *20*, 9. [CrossRef] [PubMed]
43. Hui, D.; Bohlke, K.; Bao, T.; Campbell, T.C.; Coyne, P.J.; Currow, D.C.; Gupta, A.; Leiser, A.L.; Mori, M.; Nava, S.; et al. Management of Dyspnea in Advanced Cancer: ASCO Guideline. *J. Clin. Oncol.* **2021**, *39*, 1389–1411. [CrossRef]
44. Saad Melegy, A.S.; Madkour, A.M.; Elhady Elkady, M.A.; Mahmood Ali Ibraheem, Y.M. Bronchial Bacterial Colonization in Patients with Lung Cancer. *QJM Int. J. Med.* **2024**, *117*, hcae175.159. [CrossRef]
45. Argilés, J.M.; López-Soriano, F.J.; Stemmler, B.; Busquets, S. Cancer-Associated Cachexia—Understanding the Tumour Macroenvironment and Microenvironment to Improve Management. *Nat. Rev. Clin. Oncol.* **2023**, *20*, 250–264. [CrossRef]
46. Sawant Dessai, A.; Chakrabarty, J.; Sulochana, B. The Relationship between Fatigue, Quality of Life, and Performance Status among Cancer Patients with Anemia. *Clin. Epidemiol. Glob. Health* **2025**, *31*, 101899. [CrossRef]
47. Miret, M.; Horváth-Puhó, E.; Déruaz-Luyet, A.; Sørensen, H.T.; Ehrenstein, V. Potential Paraneoplastic Syndromes and Selected Autoimmune Conditions in Patients with Non-Small Cell Lung Cancer and Small Cell Lung Cancer: A Population-Based Cohort Study. *PLoS ONE* **2017**, *12*, e0181564. [CrossRef]
48. Ogawa, T.; Miyata, J.; Fukunaga, K.; Kawana, A.; Inoue, T. Successful Treatment for Hypercalcemia Due to Cosecretion of Parathyroid Hormone-Related Protein and 1,25-Dihydroxyvitamin D_3 in Non-Small-Cell Lung Cancer: A Case Report and Literature Review. *Case Rep. Pulmonol.* **2020**, *2020*, 2475725. [CrossRef] [PubMed]
49. Morar, A.; Ghemigian, A.; Tupea, C.; Petrova, E.; Popescu, M.; Carsote, M.; Dumitru, N.; Valea, A. Twist of Endocrine Scenario Approach of Ectopic Cushing Syndrome (Review). *Rom. J. Med. Pract.* **2020**, *15*, 405–409. [CrossRef]
50. Condé, K.; Guelngar, C.O.; Mohamed, A.; Kadidjatou, I.; Daouya, D.G.; Barry, M.C.; Diallo, M.H.; Diawara, K.; Mamady, K Moriba, T.; et al. Secondary Hypertrophic Osteoarthropathy or Pierre-Marie Syndrome Bamberger: Clinical Case and Literature Review. *Open J. Rheumatol. Autoimmune Dis.* **2021**, *11*, 73–78. [CrossRef]
51. Popat, S.; Navani, N.; Kerr, K.M.; Smit, E.F.; Batchelor, T.J.P.; Van Schil, P.; Senan, S.; McDonald, F. Navigating Diagnostic and Treatment Decisions in Non-Small Cell Lung Cancer: Expert Commentary on the Multidisciplinary Team Approach. *Oncologist* **2021**, *26*, e306–e315. [CrossRef] [PubMed]
52. Panunzio, A.; Sartori, P. Lung Cancer and Radiological Imaging. *Curr. Radiopharm.* **2020**, *13*, 238–242. [CrossRef]
53. Larici, A.R.; Franchi, P.; del Ciello, A.; Sica, G.; Coviello, D.; De Waure, C.; Cicchetti, G.; Rovere, G.; Storto, M.L.; Farchione, A. et al. Role of Delayed Phase Contrast-Enhanced CT in the Intra-Thoracic Staging of Non-Small Cell Lung Cancer (NSCLC): What Does It Add? *Eur. J. Radiol.* **2021**, *144*, 109983. [CrossRef] [PubMed]
54. Owens, C.; Hindocha, S.; Lee, R.; Millard, T.; Sharma, B. The Lung Cancers: Staging and Response, CT, 18F-FDG PET/CT, MRI DWI: Review and New Perspectives. *Br. J. Radiol.* **2023**, *96*, 20220339. [CrossRef] [PubMed]
55. Mayer, N.; Boschetti, L.; Scarci, M.; Cioffi, U.; De Simone, M.; Schnider, M.; Kestenholz, P.; Minervini, F. Brain Imaging in Patients with Non-Small Cell Lung Cancer—A Systematic Review. *J. Clin. Med.* **2025**, *14*, 708. [CrossRef]

https://doi.org/10.3390/jcm15083042

Paolisso, P.; Bergamaschi, L.; Angeli, F.; Belmonte, M.; Foà, A.; Canton, L.; Fedele, D.; Armillotta, M.; Sansonetti, A.; Bodega, F.; et al. Cardiac Magnetic Resonance to Predict Cardiac Mass Malignancy: The CMR Mass Score. *Circ. Cardiovasc. Imaging* **2024**, *17*, e016115. [CrossRef]

Roșu, S.-M.; Mitroi, D.M.; Catană, O.M.; Biciușcă, V.; Stan, S.I.; Mahler, B.; Parliteanu, O.-A.; Mirea, A.A.; Bălteanu, M.A. Flexible Bronchoscopy and Non-Small-Cell Lung Cancer Staging: A Narrative Review of Modern Techniques for Optimized Clinical Decision-Making. *J. Clin. Med.* **2025**, *14*, 5773. [CrossRef]

Balasubramanian, P.; Abia-Trujillo, D.; Barrios-Ruiz, A.; Garza-Salas, A.; Koratala, A.; Chandra, N.C.; Yu Lee-Mateus, A.; Labarca, G.; Fernandez-Bussy, S. Diagnostic Yield and Safety of Diagnostic Techniques for Pulmonary Lesions: Systematic Review, Meta-Analysis and Network Meta-Analysis. *Eur. Respir. Rev.* **2024**, *33*, 240046. [CrossRef]

Nath, T.S.; Mohamed, N.; Gill, P.K.; Khan, S. A Comparative Analysis of Video-Assisted Thoracoscopic Surgery and Thoracotomy in Non-Small-Cell Lung Cancer in Terms of Their Oncological Efficacy in Resection: A Systematic Review. *Cureus* **2022**, *14*, e25443. [CrossRef]

Penault-Llorca, F.; Socinski, M.A. Emerging Molecular Testing Paradigms in Non-Small Cell Lung Cancer Management—Current Perspectives and Recommendations. *Oncologist* **2025**, *30*, oyae357. [CrossRef]

Lamberti, G.; Andrini, E.; Sisi, M.; Rizzo, A.; Parisi, C.; Di Federico, A.; Gelsomino, F.; Ardizzoni, A. Beyond EGFR, ALK and ROS1: Current Evidence and Future Perspectives on Newly Targetable Oncogenic Drivers in Lung Adenocarcinoma. *Crit. Rev. Oncol. Hematol.* **2020**, *156*, 103119. [CrossRef] [PubMed]

Dorward, D.A.; Walsh, K.; Oniscu, A.; Wallace, W.A. Molecular Pathology of Non-Small Cell Lung Cancer. *Diagn. Histopathol.* **2017**, *23*, 450–457. [CrossRef]

Doroshow, D.B.; Bhalla, S.; Beasley, M.B.; Sholl, L.M.; Kerr, K.M.; Gnjatic, S.; Wistuba, I.I.; Rimm, D.L.; Tsao, M.S.; Hirsch, F.R. PD-L1 as a Biomarker of Response to Immune-Checkpoint Inhibitors. *Nat. Rev. Clin. Oncol.* **2021**, *18*, 345–362. [CrossRef] [PubMed]

Jeon, H.; Wang, S.; Song, J.; Gill, H.; Cheng, H. Update 2025: Management of Non-Small-Cell Lung Cancer. *Lung* **2025**, *203*, 53. [CrossRef] [PubMed]

Sigel, K.; Yin Kong, C.; Leiter, A.; Kale, M.; Mhango, G.; Huang, B.; Gould, M.K.; Wisnivesky, J. Assessment of Treatment Strategies for Stage I Non-Small Cell Lung Cancer in Patients with Comorbidities. *Lung Cancer* **2022**, *170*, 34–40. [CrossRef]

Howington, J.; Souter, L.H.; Arenberg, D.; Blasberg, J.; Detterbeck, F.; Farjah, F.; Lanuti, M.; Leighl, N.; Videtic, G.M.; Murthy, S. Management of Patients with Early-Stage Non-Small Cell Lung Cancer. *Chest* **2025**, *168*, 810–827. [CrossRef] [PubMed]

Alexander, M.; Kim, S.Y.; Cheng, H. Update 2020: Management of Non-Small Cell Lung Cancer. *Lung* **2020**, *198*, 897–907. [CrossRef]

Hirsch, F.R.; Kim, C. The Importance of Biomarker Testing in the Treatment of Advanced Non-Small Cell Lung Cancer: A Podcast. *Oncol. Ther.* **2024**, *12*, 223–231. [CrossRef]

Chen, R.-L.; Sun, L.-L.; Cao, Y.; Chen, H.-R.; Zhou, J.-X.; Gu, C.-Y.; Zhang, Y.; Wang, S.-Y.; Hou, W.; Lin, L.-Z. Adjuvant EGFR-TKIs for Patients With Resected EGFR-Mutant Non-Small Cell Lung Cancer: A Meta-Analysis of 1283 Patients. *Front. Oncol.* **2021**, *11*, 629394. [CrossRef]

Prezzano, K.M.; Ma, S.J.; Hermann, G.M.; Rivers, C.I.; Gomez-Suescun, J.A.; Singh, A.K. Stereotactic Body Radiation Therapy for Non-Small Cell Lung Cancer: A Review. *World J. Clin. Oncol.* **2019**, *10*, 14–27. [CrossRef]

Conibear, J. Rationale for Concurrent Chemoradiotherapy for Patients with Stage III Non-Small-Cell Lung Cancer. *Br. J. Cancer* **2020**, *123*, 10–17. [CrossRef]

Stinchcombe, T.E. Flashback Foreword: Cisplatin/Pemetrexed in Non–Small-Cell Lung Cancer. *J. Clin. Oncol.* **2023**, *41*, 2455–2456. [CrossRef] [PubMed]

Antonia, S.J.; Villegas, A.; Daniel, D.; Vicente, D.; Murakami, S.; Hui, R.; Yokoi, T.; Chiappori, A.; Lee, K.H.; de Wit, M.; et al. Durvalumab after Chemoradiotherapy in Stage III Non–Small-Cell Lung Cancer. *N. Engl. J. Med.* **2017**, *377*, 1919–1929. [CrossRef] [PubMed]

Pérol, M.; Felip, E.; Dafni, U.; Polito, L.; Pal, N.; Tsourti, Z.; Ton, T.G.N.; Merritt, D.; Morris, S.; Stahel, R.; et al. Effectiveness of PD-(L)1 Inhibitors Alone or in Combination with Platinum-Doublet Chemotherapy in First-Line (1L) Non-Squamous Non-Small-Cell Lung Cancer (Nsq-NSCLC) with PD-L1-High Expression Using Real-World Data. *Ann. Oncol.* **2022**, *33*, 511–521. [CrossRef]

Mosele, M.F.; Westphalen, C.B.; Stenzinger, A.; Barlesi, F.; Bayle, A.; Bièche, I.; Bonastre, J.; Castro, E.; Dienstmann, R.; Krämer, A.; et al. Recommendations for the Use of Next-Generation Sequencing (NGS) for Patients with Advanced Cancer in 2024: A Report from the ESMO Precision Medicine Working Group. *Ann. Oncol.* **2024**, *35*, 588–606. [CrossRef] [PubMed]

Zhang, M.; Sun, L. First-Line Treatment for Advanced or Metastatic EGFR Mutation-Positive Non-Squamous Non-Small Cell Lung Cancer: A Network Meta-Analysis. *Front. Oncol.* **2025**, *14*, 1498518. [CrossRef]

Damuzzo, V.; Gasperoni, L.; Del Bono, L.; Ossato, A.; Inno, A.; Messori, A. Treatment of Metastatic ALK-Positive Non-Small Cell Lung Cancer: Indirect Comparison of Different ALK Inhibitors Using Reconstructed Patient Data. *Front. Oncol.* **2025**, *15*, 1566816. [CrossRef]

https://doi.org/10.3390/jcm15083042

78. D'Angelo, A.; Sobhani, N.; Chapman, R.; Bagby, S.; Bortoletti, C.; Traversini, M.; Ferrari, K.; Voltolini, L.; Darlow, J.; Roviello, C Focus on ROS1-Positive Non-Small Cell Lung Cancer (NSCLC): Crizotinib, Resistance Mechanisms and the Newer Generation c Targeted Therapies. *Cancers* **2020**, *12*, 3293. [CrossRef]
79. Planchard, D.; Besse, B.; Groen, H.J.M.; Hashemi, S.M.S.; Mazieres, J.; Kim, T.M.; Quoix, E.; Souquet, P.-J.; Barlesi, F.; Baik, C.; et a Phase 2 Study of Dabrafenib Plus Trametinib in Patients with BRAF V600E-Mutant Metastatic NSCLC: Updated 5-Year Surviva Rates and Genomic Analysis. *J. Thorac. Oncol.* **2022**, *17*, 103–115. [CrossRef]
80. O'Sullivan, É.; Keogh, A.; Henderson, B.; Finn, S.P.; Gray, S.G.; Gately, K. Treatment Strategies for KRAS-Mutated Non-Small-Ce Lung Cancer. *Cancers* **2023**, *15*, 1635. [CrossRef]
81. Majem, M.; Cobo, M.; Isla, D.; Marquez-Medina, D.; Rodriguez-Abreu, D.; Casal-Rubio, J.; Moran-Bueno, T.; Bernabé-Caro, R Pérez-Parente, D.; Ruiz-Gracia, P.; et al. PD-(L)1 Inhibitors as Monotherapy for the First-Line Treatment of Non-Small-Cell Lun Cancer Patients with High PD-L1 Expression: A Network Meta-Analysis. *J. Clin. Med.* **2021**, *10*, 1365. [CrossRef]
82. Chai, Y.; Wu, X.; Zou, Y.; Zhang, X.; Bai, H.; Dong, M.; Duan, J. Immunotherapy Combined with Chemotherapy versu Chemotherapy Alone as the First-line Treatment of PD-L1-negative and Driver-gene-negative Advanced Nonsquamous Nor small-cell Lung Cancer: An Updated Systematic Review and Meta-analysis. *Thorac. Cancer* **2022**, *13*, 3124–3132. [CrossRef]
83. Garassino, M.C.; Khalifa, J.; Reck, M.; Chouaid, C.; Bischoff, H.; Reinmuth, N.; Cove-Smith, L.; Mansy, T.; Cortinovis, D.L Migliorino, M.R.; et al. Durvalumab after Sequential Chemoradiotherapy in Unresectable Stage III Non-Small-Cell Lun Cancer—Final Analysis from the Phase II PACIFIC-6 Trial. *ESMO Open* **2025**, *10*, 105071. [CrossRef] [PubMed]
84. Gonçalves, F.; Gaudêncio, M.; Rocha, A.; Paiva, I.; Rego, F.; Nunes, R. A Review on the Management of Symptoms in Patient with Incurable Cancer. *Curr. Oncol.* **2025**, *32*, 433. [CrossRef] [PubMed]
85. Allende, S.; Turcott, J.G.; Verástegui, E.; Rodríguez-Mayoral, O.; Flores-Estrada, D.; Pérez Camargo, D.A.; Ramos-Ramírez, M Martínez-Hernández, J.-N.; Oñate-Ocaña, L.F.; Pina, P.S.; et al. Early Incorporation to Palliative Care (EPC) in Patients wit Advanced Non-Small Cell Lung Cancer: The PACO Randomized Clinical Trial. *Oncologist* **2024**, *29*, e1373–e1385. [CrossRe [PubMed]
86. Torrente, M.; Sousa, P.A.; Guerreiro, G.R.; Franco, F.; Hernández, R.; Parejo, C.; Sousa, A.; Campo-Cañaveral, J.L.; Pimentão, Provencio, M. Clinical Factors Influencing Long-Term Survival in a Real-Life Cohort of Early Stage Non-Small-Cell Lung Cance Patients in Spain. *Front. Oncol.* **2023**, *13*, 1074337. [CrossRef]
87. Shen, Y.; Chen, J.-Q.; Li, X.-P. Differences between Lung Adenocarcinoma and Lung Squamous Cell Carcinoma: Driver Gene Therapeutic Targets, and Clinical Efficacy. *Genes Dis.* **2025**, *12*, 101374. [CrossRef]
88. Restrepo, J.C.; Martínez Guevara, D.; Pareja López, A.; Montenegro Palacios, J.F.; Liscano, Y. Identification and Application o Emerging Biomarkers in Treatment of Non-Small-Cell Lung Cancer: Systematic Review. *Cancers* **2024**, *16*, 2338. [CrossRef]
89. Canale, M.; Andrikou, K.; Priano, I.; Cravero, P.; Pasini, L.; Urbini, M.; Delmonte, A.; Crinò, L.; Bronte, G.; Ulivi, P. The Role c TP53 Mutations in EGFR-Mutated Non-Small-Cell Lung Cancer: Clinical Significance and Implications for Therapy. *Cancers* **202** *14*, 1143. [CrossRef]
90. Rajaram, R.; Huang, Q.; Li, R.Z.; Chandran, U.; Zhang, Y.; Amos, T.B.; Wright, G.W.J.; Ferko, N.C.; Kalsekar, I. Recurrence-Fre Survival in Patients with Surgically Resected Non-Small Cell Lung Cancer. *Chest* **2024**, *165*, 1260–1270. [CrossRef]
91. Satoh, H.; Okuma, Y.; Shinno, Y.; Masuda, K.; Matsumoto, Y.; Yoshida, T.; Goto, Y.; Horinouchi, H.; Yamamoto, N.; Ohe, Evolving Treatments and Prognosis in Stage IV Non-Small Cell Lung Cancer: 20 Years of Progress of Novel Therapies. *Lun Cancer* **2025**, *202*, 108453. [CrossRef]

Journal of
Clinical Medicine

MDPI

eview

Artificial Intelligence in Asthma and COPD: Current Status and Future Potential

ederica Marrelli [1], Chiara Lupia [1], Saverio Nucera [1], Daniela Pastore [1], Paolo Zaffino [2], Carolina Muscoli [1], irolamo Pelaia [1] and Corrado Pelaia [3,*]

1 Department of Health Sciences, "Magna Graecia" University—Catanzaro, 88100 Catanzaro, Italy; federicamarrelli1@gmail.com (F.M.); c.lupia@unicz.it (C.L.); saverio.nucera@unicz.it (S.N.); danielapastore11@gmail.com (D.P.); muscoli@unicz.it (C.M.); pelaia@unicz.it (G.P.)
2 Department of Experimental and Clinical Medicine, "Magna Graecia" University—Catanzaro, 88100 Catanzaro, Italy; p.zaffino@unicz.it
3 Department of Medical and Surgical Sciences, "Magna Graecia" University—Catanzaro, Viale Europa—Località Germaneto, 88100 Catanzaro, Italy
* Correspondence: pelaia.corrado@unicz.it; Tel.: +39-0961-3647007; Fax: +39-0961-3647193

Abstract

Interest in artificial intelligence (AI) is rapidly growing. In healthcare, especially through machine learning and deep learning, AI is emerging as a promising tool to support the diagnosis, management, and prevention of lung diseases and to advance personalized care, although it requires large, well-structured datasets. Clinicians must learn how to integrate AI into routine practice for conditions such as asthma and chronic obstructive pulmonary disease (COPD), while ensuring patient safety and building trust in these tools. Chronic respiratory diseases are major global causes of morbidity and mortality and place a substantial burden on healthcare systems; among them, asthma and COPD are chronic disorders characterized by airway obstruction and inflammation. This review highlights the rapid advancement of AI, and it aims to explore the literature's evidence of its applicability in controlling chronic respiratory disorders, particularly in asthma and COPD. We conducted a narrative literature review by searching ScienceDirect, PubMed, and Google Scholar for English-language studies on artificial intelligence applications in asthma and COPD and by screening the references of relevant articles. The reviewed literature suggests that AI-based approaches are being applied across the asthma–COPD spectrum to support diagnosis and phenotyping, improve risk stratification and prediction of clinically relevant outcomes, and enable more continuous monitoring using heterogeneous data sources (e.g., clinical records, imaging, and digital health data). AI-based tools are poised to support clinicians in asthma and COPD across diagnosis, phenotyping, and monitoring; however, their safe implementation in routine care will require robust validation, transparency, and governance to ensure reliability and patient safety.

Keywords: asthma; COPD; machine learning; deep learning; artificial intelligence

1. Introduction

Artificial intelligence (AI) has gained widespread clinical utilization and opens new opportunities for prevention, early diagnosis, and prompt and appropriate therapeutic intervention. Research in chronic respiratory diseases (CRDs) is gradually adopting AI techniques, following the overall trend of implementation in healthcare-related studies. The term AI refers to the simulation of human intelligence by computer systems, or the use of a computer to mimic intelligent behavior with minimal human interaction; it encompasses functions such as reasoning, learning, language processing, and the display of knowledge or information. When combined with vast volumes of well-characterized data, AI can provide models that are expected to enhance clinical practice and lead to improved care delivery, particularly in the management of chronic diseases [1]. Over the last decade, the application of AI has garnered substantial interest in the field of lung diseases [2]. In the domain of CRD care, there is a growing necessity for early identification, accurate staging, and effective management strategies. AI can improve the efficiency and accessibility of high-quality healthcare. Consequently, AI has attracted considerable interest, especially for early detection of asthma, monitoring COPD progression in at-risk groups, and enhancing diagnoses [3]. AI and machine learning (ML) models are heavily reliant on accessible data, and the healthcare sector generates vast amounts of data that must be mined for underlying insights. Large and complex datasets containing multiple sources of data can be examined appropriately using modern AI/ML approaches [1]. AI may be able to reduce the global burden of asthma and COPD, as well as the morbidity and mortality rates associated with them.

2. Data Source and Study Selection

In this narrative review, we performed a structured literature search to identify studies investigating the application of artificial intelligence (AI) to the diagnosis, classification/phenotyping, monitoring, prognostication, and management of asthma and chronic obstructive pulmonary disease (COPD). We searched PubMed, ScienceDirect, and Google Scholar from database inception to 20 December 2025 using combinations of keywords related to the following: (i) respiratory diseases ("asthma", "COPD", "chronic respiratory disease", "lung disease"); (ii) AI methods ("artificial intelligence", "machine learning", "deep learning", "neural network", "natural language processing", "NLP"); and (iii) clinical tasks ("diagnosis", "management", "treatment", "prognosis", "monitor", "prediction", "exacerbation", "stratification", "phenotype"). Boolean operators and alternative spellings were used to broaden retrieval where appropriate. The search retrieved n = 142 records (plus n = 10 from reference screening); after de-duplication (n = 29), n = 123 titles/abstracts were screened and n = 35 full texts were assessed, yielding n = 27 included studies.

We included peer-reviewed articles that reported the development, validation, or clinical evaluation of AI/ML/DL/NLP approaches applied to asthma and/or COPD using clinical data (e.g., electronic health records), pulmonary function tests, imaging (e.g., CT/HRCT), wearable/sensor data, or non-invasive biomarkers. We excluded studies not focused on asthma/COPD (or not clearly related to chronic respiratory diseases), studies without a clear AI component, purely technical papers without clinical data or outcomes, animal-only studies, conference abstracts without full-text availability, and editorials/commentaries. When multiple papers reported overlapping cohorts or models, the most complete and up-to-date report was prioritized.

Titles and abstracts were screened for relevance, followed by full-text assessment of potentially eligible articles. Reference lists of included papers and relevant reviews were also screened to identify additional eligible studies. For each included study, we extracted key methodological and clinical features (study design and setting, population, sample size, data modality, AI technique, target outcome, validation strategy, including internal vs. external validation when available, main performance metrics, and reported limitations). Findings were synthesized qualitatively and organized by application domain to highlight current evidence, methodological gaps, and future directions.

Table 1 summarizes the key characteristics of the representative included studies.

https://doi.org/10.3390/jcm1506244

Table 1. Summary of representative included studies: overview of study designs, sample sizes, and validation strategies.

Author, Year, Reference	Country	Study Design	Sample Size	Validation Strategies
Srivastava et al., 2021. [4]	India	Retrospective observational study	126 patients	Internal validation of the deep learning model
Spathis et al., 2019. [5]	Greece	Retrospective observational study	132 patients	Train/Test Split, Cross-Validation (5-fold and 10-fold) and standard performance metrics
Zein et al., 2021. [6]	USA	Retrospective observational cohort study	60,302 patients	Train/test split, 5-fold cross-validation and standard performance metrics such as AUC, precision and F1 score
Altan et al., 2020. [7]	Turkey	Retrospective observational study	41 patients	Training set/test set, k-fold cross-validation, accuracy, precision, F1 score, compared with clinical standard.
Yang et al., 2022. [8]	China	Retrospective observational study	468 patients	Training/test split, internal cross-validation and ROC metrics
Kaur et al., 2018. [9]	USA	Cross-sectional study nested in a birth cohort study	427 patients	Manual review of medical records, separate training/test sets, and standard diagnostic metrics to evaluate the accuracy of the NLP model
Ross et al., 2018. [10]	USA	Retrospective observational cohort study	1688 patients	Training/test sets, internal cross-validation, standard predictive metrics, and comparison with traditional methods
Karabulut et al., 2015. [11]	Turkey	Retrospective observational study	93 patients	Training/test split, cross-validation and comparison with clinical assessments

3. Artificial Intelligence Techniques in Lung Disease Management

In this review, we use "AI" as an umbrella term that includes (i) machine learning (ML), which learns predictive relationships from structured data (e.g., logistic regression, random forest, gradient boosting) and is commonly applied to EHR-based risk prediction such as exacerbation forecasting in asthma; (ii) deep learning (DL), a subset of ML that uses multi-layer neural networks and excels in high-dimensional inputs such as CT imaging (e.g., CNN- or transformer-based models for emphysema quantification and COPD severity assessment); (iii) natural language processing (NLP), which extracts structured variables from free-text clinical notes (e.g., automated chart review for asthma prediction indices); and (iv) large language models (LLMs), a newer class of NLP models that can generate or summarize text and may support tasks such as clinical documentation assistance or structured extraction from unstructured records, although clinical deployment requires careful validation, governance, and bias monitoring.

AI techniques that simulate human-like intelligence, including DL, ML and NLP, demonstrate their effectiveness in enhancing diagnostic accuracy and prognostic capabilities across lung diseases [2]. Figure 1 illustrates the relationship between AI, ML and DL.

https://doi.org/10.3390/jcm15062445

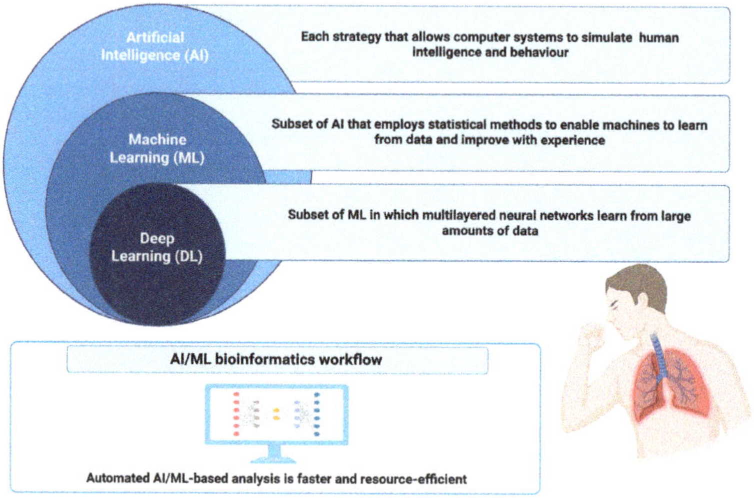

Figure 1. Relationship between Artificial Intelligence (AI), Machine Learning (ML), and Deep Learning (DL), as well as their role in data-driven clinical and bioinformatics workflows for faster and more efficient automated analyses. Created in BioRender. Marrelli, F. (2026) https://BioRender.com/ya9xdr9.

ML and DL, sub-domains of AI, provide different features and applications in medical imaging. ML models generate predictions using algorithms that learn from data and often use structured datasets from medical imaging to discover trends and support diagnosis. ML includes supervised learning, in which models learn from labelled data to assist in tasks such as disease subtype classification and treatment response prediction; unsupervised learning, where patterns are identified without labelled data, which helps segment similar regions in CT images [12–14]. DL, an advanced subset of ML, employs multilayered neural networks. DL can learn from vast amounts of data, identifying intricate patterns and subtle changes that conventional image processing methods or expert humans could overlook [14,15]. Convolutional neural network (CNN) designs have significantly advanced DL and are utilized in various computer vision applications, including image classification, object detection, and semantic segmentation. The CNN identifies characteristics that vary from fundamental edges to intricate patterns [15,16]. Every design has unique characteristics and trade-offs regarding accuracy, computational complexity, and memory demands.

Understanding the design principles and performance attributes of these architectures is crucial for selecting the most suitable model for a specific task. Creating new CNN architectures is essential for choosing suitable models for specific tasks and for designing innovative CNN models tailored to domain-specific requirements, such as medical image analysis for characterizing and identifying COPD using CT scans [4,15,17–19]. Factors facilitating the rise of DL in imaging include massive, labelled datasets, advanced network architectures, and increasing computing capabilities. Both ML and DL offer advantages in medical imaging; however, the choice between the two depends on the specific requirements of the work. AI provides notable advancements in the field of radiology. Its integration not only improves diagnostic precision but also indicates a more patient-centered methodology, whereby personalized therapies and heightened safety become the norm. Generating high-quality images from lower-dose scans using AI techniques achieves a balance between patient safety and image clarity [20]. Moreover, predictive modelling is enabled by AI's capacity to merge imaging data with electronic clinical information. This

https://doi.org/10.3390/jcm1506244

facilitates individualized patient management by providing insights into potential disease trajectories, therapeutic responses, or even complications [12]. As the volume of imaging performed in medicine continues to increase rapidly, AI will play an increasingly crucial role in image interpretation.

Accordingly, we organize the evidence below by clinical task (differential diagnosis, phenotyping, outcome prediction, imaging-based characterization, and remote monitoring), specifying the AI method and the data modality used in each study.

4. Asthma and COPD

4.1. Disease Burden and Artificial Intelligence Applications

Asthma and COPD are chronic respiratory disorders characterized by airflow limitation and inflammation and represent a major global burden. Asthma is a heterogeneous condition with variable respiratory symptoms and expiratory airflow obstruction that may resolve spontaneously or with treatment [21]. COPD is characterized by persistent respiratory symptoms (e.g., dyspnea, cough, sputum) and progressive airflow limitation related to airway and/or alveolar abnormalities. Globally, asthma and COPD account for a substantial share of chronic respiratory disease morbidity and mortality, as also highlighted by Global Burden of Disease estimates [22–25].

Asthma and COPD are recognized as heterogeneous conditions with distinct prognoses and treatment options, and making a clear distinction between them can be challenging in some patients due to overlapping clinical traits [21,24]. Pulmonary function tests remain central to diagnosis and severity assessment, requiring interpretation of ventilatory patterns and grading of airflow limitation according to international guidance [21,24]. In recent years, CT has become increasingly available in research and clinical practice, improving characterization of structural abnormalities, phenotypes, severity, and outcomes in asthma and COPD [21,24].

Because routine clinical data and spirometry are widely available, AI/ML models can support discrimination between asthma and COPD even with limited clinical variables [19]. For example, a decision support system using clinical factors (e.g., age, sex, sputum production, chest pain, smoking history) combined with spirometry has been proposed to detect and differentiate asthma and COPD [5]. These approaches are clinically relevant given that early stages may be managed in outpatient settings, whereas advanced disease and clinical worsening often require inpatient care [26,27]. Optimizing outpatient evaluation can contribute to early diagnosis, reducing avoidable hospitalizations and improving prognostic assessment [28–31].

In asthma, ML models (e.g., logistic regression, boosting, random forest) have been used to predict exacerbations using variables such as systemic steroid use, short-acting β_2-agonist use, emergency department visits, age, and exacerbation history [6,32,33]. In parallel, wearable technologies coupled with AI have been explored to monitor physiologic signals and generate predictive alarms for impending asthma attacks, supporting earlier interventions [34]. In COPD, AI has also been applied to accessible modalities such as lung sounds (including DL-based approaches for disease detection/classification), supporting potential use in resource-limited settings [7,35–37]. In imaging-based assessment, radiomics combined with ML (e.g., SVM models) has been investigated to classify and stage COPD severity from chest CT features [8,38–40], and DL systems using CT imaging have shown potential for identification and staging while predicting clinically relevant outcomes (e.g., exacerbation risk, emphysema severity, spirometric obstruction, mortality) [12,41,42].

Figure 2 summarizes key domains in which AI has been applied along the clinical pathway in asthma and COPD, ranging from identification and severity stratification to targeted management and remote monitoring.

https://doi.org/10.3390/jcm15062445

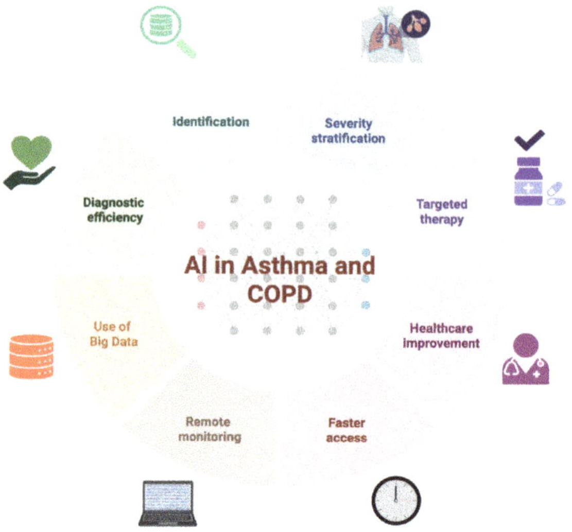

Figure 2. The use of AI in asthma and COPD, mapped to clinical tasks including differential diagnosis, severity stratification, phenotyping, outcome prediction (e.g., exacerbations/hospitalizations), and remote monitoring. Created in BioRender. Marrelli, F. (2026) https://BioRender.com/m3v3veq.

4.2. Role of Artificial Intelligence Techniques for Asthma Phenotyping

Asthma is a heterogeneous condition, and phenotyping/endotyping aims to identify clinically meaningful subgroups based on symptom patterns, lung-function impairment, and inflammatory traits to guide personalized therapy [43,44]. There is considerable promise in using AI to identify individuals at higher risk of developing asthma by integrating large-scale genetic data with routinely collected clinical information; similarly, ML can analyze medication histories and digital medical records to detect early signals that may be missed by clinicians [33]. AI and ML approaches are increasingly employed to classify patients according to disease severity and phenotype and to support monitoring strategies [1]. Clinical information, including medical history, symptom patterns, pulmonary function tests, and auscultated lung sounds, represents a major data source for asthma diagnosis, screening, and phenotype-related assessment [9].

In this context, respiratory sounds represent a scalable phenotype-related signal that can be captured outside the clinic. The primary aim of Oletic and Bilas's wearable sensor was to identify wheeze by recording breathing sound signals and transmitting them to a smartphone after specific signal alterations. The accuracy, sensitivity, and specificity of the final model were 94.91%, 89.34%, and 96.28%, respectively [45].

The forced oscillation technique (FOT) provides effort-independent measurements of respiratory mechanics and can capture airway obstruction traits relevant to asthma phenotyping, particularly in children or in patients unable to perform reliable spirometry. Amaral et al. evaluated multiple ML approaches using FOT-derived parameters as input to detect airway obstruction in asthma, supporting the feasibility of oscillometry features as phenotype-relevant signals for ML-based assessment [46]. Unlike conventional lung function tests, FOT is non-invasive and has the advantage of not requiring forced breathing maneuvers, enabling repeated measurements and potential longitudinal monitoring [46].

https://doi.org/10.3390/jcm15062445

Beyond respiratory sounds, physiology-based signals can further support phenotype-oriented assessment by capturing airway mechanics and ventilation dynamics that may not be fully reflected by symptoms alone.

Capnography yields a continuous CO_2 waveform (capnogram) that reflects ventilation dynamics and expiratory flow characteristics. Singh et al. performed automatic quantitative analysis of the respired CO_2 waveform and used a support vector machine classifier to differentiate asthma from non-asthma subjects, demonstrating the potential of capnogram-derived features as ML inputs for asthma-related classification [47]. However, the limited dataset and lack of broad external validation in this work prevent an adequate assessment of the proposed modality for routine phenotype-oriented assessment or monitoring [47].

The exhaled breath condensate (EBC) of 89 asthmatic patients and 20 healthy controls was examined, and a random forest classifier was developed to differentiate between the two groups. The final classifier exhibited 80% sensitivity and 75% specificity. Looking for non-invasive asthma biomarkers, the EBC could be another potential target. However, this technology requires better standardization before it can be implemented in broader clinical settings [48,49].

Regarding asthma classification and phenotypes, several scientists have developed an ML technique for identifying pediatric asthma phenotypes based on patients' responses to controller drugs. Bronchodilator response and blood eosinophils have been identified as the strongest predictive indicators of asthma management in the pediatric group under study [10]. Asthma exacerbations are crucial to the disease's progression and management, resulting in significant direct and indirect expenditures. Asthma models have been created to assess attack risk in real time, utilizing sensors that collect physiological and environmental information. The information obtained is sent to a smartphone and analyzed by a random forest classifier, which recognizes asthma attacks with an overall accuracy of 80.1% [34]. Determining whether hospitalization is necessary during an asthma attack is a crucial decision. The suggested gradient-boosting machine-based approach measures total risk and determines whether hospitalization is needed [50].

Overall, current asthma phenotyping work using AI falls into several reproducible patterns: treatment-response phenotypes, such as pediatric subgrouping based on response to controller medications [10]; biomarker-/omics-informed approaches, including exhaled breath condensate-based classifiers and breath biomarker frameworks that support non-invasive phenotype discovery, while highlighting the need for standardization [48,49]; and digital phenotyping, where respiratory sounds or wearable-derived signals provide measurable traits (e.g., wheeze detection) outside the clinic [45], complemented by physiology-based traits captured by oscillometry and capnography-derived waveform analysis [46,47]. In parallel, ML models have been developed for actionable decisions during exacerbations, such as estimating the need for hospitalization at emergency department triage [50]. Despite promising results, many studies remain limited by sample size, single-center design, and inconsistent external validation, which may affect generalizability and clinical reliability [1].

4.3. Role of Artificial Intelligence Techniques for COPD Classification

Radiology and CT are central to COPD characterization because they enable quantitative assessment of emphysema, airway remodeling, and extrapulmonary features that are clinically linked to outcomes. In this context, AI methods have been applied to automate CT-derived quantification and to support COPD diagnosis and severity stratification ("staging"), often by integrating imaging information with clinical variables such as spirometry to improve classification performance [8,12,38–40]. High-resolution CT (HRCT) provides detailed views of airway and parenchymal structure, and AI-driven analysis can reduce inter-reader variability and scale interpretation across large datasets [51,52].

CT can also capture clinically relevant COPD comorbidities and overlapping conditions. For example, bronchiectasis is detectable on CT in a substantial proportion of COPD patients and is associated with exacerbations and mortality [53]. In addition, CT-derived measures such as coronary artery calcium, pulmonary artery enlargement, bone density, and muscle mass provide prognostic information and are independently associated with all-cause mortality [54,55].

HRCT generates high-dimensional data, and radiomics can extract quantitative descriptors associated with COPD presence and severity [8,38]. These features can then be exploited by ML models to classify COPD from CT and to support severity stratification [39]. Notably, adding radiomic descriptors to an SVM classifier has been reported to reliably categorize COPD stages and to outperform prior approaches, supporting radiomics+ML as a viable pathway for CT-based COPD staging [40]. More broadly, AI methods can automate and optimize CT analysis once trained on appropriate datasets, improving consistency and throughput [51–53].

Beyond parenchymal radiomics, airway-structure features such as branching patterns, lengths, and wall thickness can further improve CT-based COPD characterization and may enhance ML performance when combined with original CT image features [56,57]. Examining the bronchial tree's branching, lengths, and wall thicknesses may provide useful data [56]. It is possible to generate a full representation of the lung using representations of 3D airway trees and lung fields, for COPD diagnosis and combining these characteristics with the original CT image features, improving the performance of ML models in COPD [12,57].

Additionally, DL algorithms are used to identify and stage COPD: a specific DL system may recognize notable regional image characteristics from high-resolution CT scans of COPD patients, revealing strong predictive capabilities for exacerbation risk, emphysema severity, spirometric obstruction, and mortality, which may improve both research and clinical practice [12,41].

AI impacts emphysema diagnosis, subtyping, and phenotypes. Emphysema is defined as the irreversible destruction of the alveoli and it is typically classified into three subtypes based on CT scans distribution: centrilobular emphysema (CLE), prevalent in smokers; panlobular emphysema (PLE), often linked to α1-antitrypsin deficiency; and paraseptal emphysema (PSE). CT can assess the severity of emphysema using densitometric analysis, which quantifies the lung's mean attenuation and the proportion of lung volume with low attenuation [12,58].

AI algorithms can assess the degree of emphysema by automatically estimating the compromised lung capacity, offering a more objective and consistent classification than human densitometry [59]. AI has improved the diagnosis of emphysema in several ways: enhanced sensitivity through ML and traditional features; utilizing DL to extract features automatically; convolutional neural networks demonstrate promising accuracy levels while reducing processing time, automatically identifying and isolating emphysematous regions without the need for manual feature engineering, and discriminating between subtypes of emphysema in high-resolution CT lung images [11,60]. Large patches clipped from CT images are employed for embedding and classification in a vision transformer (ViT) model for categorizing emphysema subtypes. The ViT model holds potential for additional medical applications and accurately classifies emphysema subtypes [61].

Automated CT algorithms could enhance COPD severity staging and provide prognostic insights by measuring emphysema and air trapping in CT images using a DL-based method [62]. CT also aids in the decision-making process for lung volume reduction

https://doi.org/10.3390/jcm1506244

surgery (LVRS) or endobronchial valve insertion. However, there is a growing inclination towards quantitative analysis of emphysema position, size, and fissure integrity to facilitate decision-making for endobronchial valve treatment. Emphysema is associated with an accelerated drop in forced expiratory volume in one second (FEV_1), an elevated mortality risk, and an increased probability of lung cancer development [24].

Dosovitskiy et al. use the Transformer architecture for image categorization in the ViT model, which is useful for identifying different types of emphysema and may increase the precision and effectiveness of COPD assessment. The model uses data augmentation and transfer learning on a labelled dataset of CT scans with annotated emphysema subtypes to improve performance and generalizability [12,63].

Pang et al. suggested the Generative Adversarial Network (GAN) technique for producing contrast-enhanced or non-contrast CT images. A discriminator and a generator make up the network architecture of the suggested synthesizer. The generator can learn to create realistic contrast-enhanced (CE) or non-contrast (NC) CT scans, by using the discriminator to distinguish between real and fake images. In order to create a probability map, the NC CT and real CE CT are also combined and fed into the discriminator [64,65].

MIL is particularly relevant for COPD because CT labels are often available at the patient level (COPD vs. non-COPD, or severity groups), while disease patterns are regionally heterogeneous within the lung; MIL can therefore learn from weak labels by aggregating patch-level information [57,66]. Using CT scans, Multiple Instance Learning (MIL) can detect COPD. With the support of labelled bags and a large number of examples, the MIL paradigm facilitates learning of COPD patterns from weakly labelled data, such as the overall COPD status of each CT scan. A CT scan is represented by a bag, and the examples inside the bag stand in for different areas or patches of the picture. MIL can control the disease's heterogeneity because it can detect COPD through local patterns or anomalies in particular areas of the CT scan. Patch extraction, feature extraction, attention-guided instance-level prediction, and bag-level aggregation are the steps needed to set up MIL-based COPD identification [57,66].

CNN aims to identify unique characteristics that represent regional variations and patterns linked to COPD in the feature extraction process. Airway thickness, the presence of mucus plugs, emphysema, and other anatomical changes in the lungs that signify disease can all be recognized by training Convolutional Neural Networks (CNNs). The degree of these alterations, which reflects the severity of the illness, can also be measured using CNNs [12,56,57]. The risk level of the population may be measured with the help of CNN analysis. A multilayer CNN was able to predict episodes of acute respiratory illness, smoker mortality, and accurately diagnose and stage COPD using only CT imaging data [42]. Events in attention-guided instance-level prediction are assigned varying weights according to their significance for COPD prediction. The attention process ignores the less significant portions while identifying and prioritizing the most instructive. Each instance is given an attention rating, which is then used to modify the instance-level predictions. Either adding attention layers to the MIL design or using a separate attention network, can produce an attention score. A bag-level evaluation that reflects the overall COPD state of the CT image is produced by combining the instance-level predictions. Max pooling, average pooling, and attention-based mechanisms are examples of common aggregation strategies [57,66].

The MIL framework has a number of advantages, including adaptability and the ability to be used with different aggregation algorithms and DL architectures to improve the precision and resilience of COPD detection [57,66]. In order to create a highly precise automatic algorithm for the severity of COPD, Ying et al. used a deep belief network,

https://doi.org/10.3390/jcm15062445

proving that it is a useful tool for determining the risk of exacerbations in patients with COPD [67].

Both pulmonary and extrapulmonary vascular alterations are associated with the pathophysiology of COPD. Submillimeter vascular changes can be detected by AI tools, improving our knowledge of vessel dynamics [68]. Various methods are employed, including transformer-based networks, CNN, and generative adversarial networks [69,70].

Overall, current work on AI in CT-based COPD classification spans radiomics-driven staging, DL-based identification and outcome prediction, the use of weakly supervised frameworks such as MIL to capture regional heterogeneity, and vessel-focused models to quantify pulmonary and extrapulmonary alterations [8,12,38–41,57,66–70].

Table 2 summarizes the main AI-driven applications investigated in asthma and COPD, reporting for each area the typical algorithms, input data sources, and the corresponding clinical purpose.

Table 2. Current Applications of Artificial Intelligence in the Diagnosis and Characterization of Asthma and COPD.

Application Domain	AI/ML Technique Used	Purpose/ Function	Input Data	Key Results/ Performance	Limitations
Diagnosis and Differential Diagnosis	Logistic Regression, Random Forest, Boosting [1,6,19].	Differentiate asthma from COPD and predict exacerbations.	Clinical data (age, smoking history, symptoms) and spirometry [5,6,19].	Identification of key predictors for exacerbations (e.g., steroid use) [1,6].	Risk of inaccurate diagnosis; misclassify asthma vs. COPD; reducing reliability and reproducibility [1,5,6,19].
Asthma Phenotyping	Random Forest [10].	Identify pediatric phenotypes and classify patients based on treatment response.	Response to controller medications, blood eosinophils, bronchodilator test [10].	Identification of predictive biomarkers for personalized therapy [10,43,44].	Heterogeneous or incomplete data; small or unrepresentative cohorts; reduced interpretability; challenging to apply clinically.
COPD Classification from Imaging	Support Vector Machine (SVM) with Radiomics [40].	Stage COPD severity.	Radiomic features extracted from chest CT scans [8,38,40].	Accurate classification of COPD stages, outperforming existing methods [40].	Limits generalisability; affects model consistency; risk of overfitting; reduced interpretability of models.
Wheezing and Respiratory Sound Detection	Deep Learning Algorithms [4,7,45].	Detect wheezing and classify COPD severity from lung sounds.	Respiratory sound recordings (12-channel auscultation or wearable sensors) [7,45].	Accuracy > 94% in wheezing detection [45] and COPD classification (AUC 0.965) [7].	Reduced generalizability and interpretability; sensitivity to environmental noise and microphone quality; difficulty distinguishing wheezing from other respiratory sounds.

https://doi.org/10.3390/jcm15062445

Table 2. *Cont.*

Application Domain	AI/ML Technique Used	Purpose/ Function	Input Data	Key Results/ Performance	Limitations
Lung Structure Analysis (Emphysema)	Convolutional Neural Network (CNN), Vision Transformer (ViT) [11,12,42,61].	Quantify, segment, and classify emphysema subtypes.	High-resolution CT (HRCT) scans [12,58].	Automation of quantification and accurate classification of emphysema subtypes (CLE, PLE, PSE) [11,59,61].	Limited generalisability and external validation; reduced interpretability; indirect clinical correlation.

4.4. Future Perspectives of Artificial Intelligence in Asthma and COPD

The reviewed literature indicates that AI can support asthma and COPD across diagnosis, phenotyping/severity stratification, quantitative imaging, and outcome prediction, with particular strengths in processing high-dimensional data such as CT and longitudinal digital health streams [12,65,71–73]. However, the clinical usefulness of many proposed tools remains contingent on robust validation and demonstration of added value within real-world workflows. Key benefits, current challenges/limitations, and future perspectives of AI applications in asthma and COPD are summarized in Figure 3.

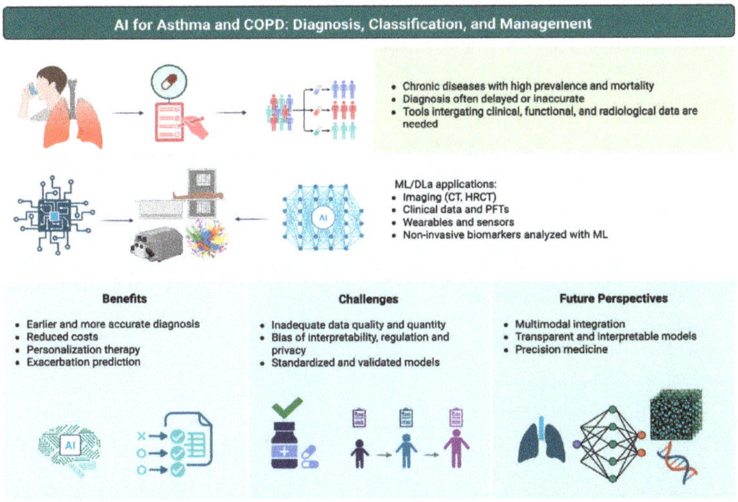

Figure 3. Conceptual overview of AI in asthma and COPD management: benefits, challenges/limitations, and future perspectives. Created in BioRender. Pelaia, C. (2026) https://BioRender.com/qy3blub.

In COPD, AI-enabled CT analysis has shown promise for quantitative emphysema assessment, region segmentation, and severity stratification, while also enabling prediction of clinically meaningful outcomes (e.g., exacerbations and mortality) [12,41,42]. In parallel, lightweight approaches for COPD screening in primary care (e.g., simplified spirometry + mobile-enabled workflows) may improve early identification in underserved settings [65]. For asthma, integrating sensor data and sequential models (e.g., LSTM-based pipelines) may improve real-time risk prediction and proactive management [33,34].

Across both diseases, barriers to adoption include data quality and dataset shift, limited external validation, interpretability constraints, and privacy/regulatory requirements [2,12,33,74]. Under-representation of specific demographic or clinical subgroups may

https://doi.org/10.3390/jcm15062445

distort predictions and exacerbate bias, underscoring the need for diverse training cohorts and continuous monitoring after deployment [33]. Clear data regulations and governance frameworks are also necessary to ensure patient data ownership, access, sharing, and secure monitoring [74].

Improving clinical trust requires interpretable models and transparent reporting of model rationale (e.g., attention maps or clinically meaningful feature importance), together with integration into existing clinical pathways [2,12,57,71].

Table 3 summarizes future perspectives and key development priorities for AI in asthma and COPD management.

Table 3. Future Perspectives on and the Development Potential of Artificial Intelligence in the Management of Asthma and COPD.

Future Development Area	Potential Application	Related Technologies/ Challenges	Expected Impact
Integrated Precision Medicine	Combine imaging (CT), genomic, proteomic, and environmental sensor data for holistic predictive models [12,33,73].	Data integration challenges, interoperability, governance, and privacy [2,74].	Identification of endotypes, prediction of treatment response, and discovery of new drug targets [12,43,44].
Dynamic and Real-Time Predictive Models	Develop 4D models to visualize airway dynamics and predict exacerbations in real time [12,33,34].	Integration with wearable sensor data (IoT), sequential AI models (e.g., LSTM) [33,34].	Timely preventive interventions, reduction in hospitalizations, and proactive disease management [1,33].
Interpretability (XAI) and Clinical Reliability	Develop "Explainable AI" (XAI) models to clarify the rationale behind AI decisions [12,71].	Development of algorithms for attention maps and clinically relevant feature importance [12,57].	Increased clinician trust, easier implementation into routine clinical practice [2,12,71].
Early Screening and Primary Care Diagnostics	Implement lightweight algorithms for COPD screening in primary care settings [65].	Development of mobile apps, analysis of basic clinical data and simplified spirometry [65].	Early diagnosis, reduced underutilization of resources, and access to care in underserved populations [37,65].
Clinical Trial Optimization	Identify and enroll patients for clinical trials by screening electronic databases [9].	Natural Language Processing (NLP) for medical records, identification of digital phenotypes [9].	Accelerated recruitment, more efficient trials, and development of more targeted therapies [72].

5. Conclusions

AI is expected to remain a prominent research hotspot in the coming years for the diagnosis and treatment of CRDs. Advanced algorithms expedite diagnosis, facilitating more efficient and tailored therapies. AI/ML methods are particularly beneficial when analyzing large, complex datasets that include information from various sources. Since asthma and COPD are chronic conditions that require monitoring over several years and whose symptoms can be identified at the cellular, organ, and organismal levels, they are ideal candidates for the application of AI/ML. Large-scale data must be analyzed in tandem, as environmental factors are crucial to the pathophysiology and natural history of asthma and COPD. To frame all potential CRD effects across scale and time, a theoretical study should ideally collect genomic, metabolomic, clinical, and environmental data from vast and heterogeneous patient cohorts across successive time slices. Asthma and COPD are

https://doi.org/10.3390/jcm1506244

common and treatable diseases, yet extensive underdiagnosis and misdiagnosis result in patients receiving no treatment or inappropriate treatment. Additionally, while they share similarities and comparable symptoms, these conditions also exhibit significant differences that should impact clinical decision-making. The ability of AI to create personalized health plans is evident, as it can offer customized solutions based on the patient's history and current condition. This review provides an integrative synthesis of AI applications for asthma and COPD in outpatient care, highlighting potential clinical and economic benefits, the main implementation challenges (e.g., misdiagnosis risk, bias, data quality, interpretability, regulation and privacy), and the most relevant future development priorities to support safe translation into practice. Furthermore, AI's transformative potential in clinical trials—particularly to enable decentralized participation and remote monitoring—holds significant promise. However, safe implementation requires addressing key challenges such as misdiagnosis risk, systematic errors, spurious associations, limitations in differential diagnostic criteria, and security and privacy vulnerabilities. Future investigations on AI for CRD management should concentrate on the following main goals: standardizing AI models and algorithms to guarantee consistent outcomes and facilitate broad clinical adoption; developing interpretable AI systems to bolster clinicians' comprehension and confidence in AI-generated predictions; tackling data privacy concerns with stringent protocols to foster trust among patients and healthcare providers; and augmenting diverse datasets to enhance AI model robustness, thereby improving generalization and accuracy in diagnosing lung diseases. These collaborative efforts will strengthen effectiveness, transparency, and trust within healthcare environments. Despite the challenges posed by the complex 'black box' nature of some AI approaches and the need for rigorous training and validation, the future appears promising.

Author Contributions: Conceptualization, F.M., C.L. and C.P.; methodology, F.M., C.L., S.N., D.P., P.Z., C.M., G.P. and C.P.; writing—original draft preparation, F.M., C.L. and S.N.; writing—review and editing, F.M., C.L., S.N., D.P., P.Z., C.M., G.P. and C.P. All authors have read and agreed to the published version of the manuscript.

Funding: This research received no external funding.

Institutional Review Board Statement: Not applicable.

Informed Consent Statement: Not applicable.

Data Availability Statement: No new data were created or analyzed in this study.

Conflicts of Interest: The authors have no relevant affiliations or financial involvement with any organization or entity with a financial interest in or financial conflict with the subject matter or materials discussed in the manuscript.

Abbreviations

AI	Artificial Intelligence
CNN	Convolutional Neural Network
COPD	Chronic Obstructive Pulmonary Disease
CRDs	Chronic Respiratory Diseases
CT	Computed Tomography
DL	Deep Learning
EBC	Exhaled Breath Condensate
FOT	Forced Oscillation Technique
GAN	Generative Adversarial Network
LVRS	Lung Volume Reduction Surgery
MIL	Multiple Instance Learning

https://doi.org/10.3390/jcm15062445

ML	Machine Learning
NLP	Natural Language Processing
SVM	Support Vector Machine
HRCT	High-Resolution Computed Tomography
PFT	Pulmonary Function Test
FEV_1	Forced Expiratory Volume in 1 s
AUC	Area Under the Curve
ViT	Vision Transformer
CLE/PLE/PSE	Centrilobular/Panlobular/Paraseptal Emphysema
IoT	Internet of Things
LSTM	Long Short-Term Memory networks

References

1. Exarchos, K.P.; Beltsiou, M.; Votti, C.A.; Kostikas, K. Artificial intelligence techniques in asthma: A systematic review and critica appraisal of the existing literature. *Eur. Respir. J.* **2020**, *56*, 2000521. [CrossRef] [PubMed]
2. Hussain, A.; Marlowe, S.; Ali, M.; Uy, E.; Bhopalwala, H.; Gullapalli, D.; Vangara, A.; Haroon, M.; Akbar, A.; Piercy, J. A Systemati Review of Artificial Intelligence Applications in the Management of Lung Disorders. *Cureus* **2024**, *16*, e51581. [CrossRef] [PubMed
3. Zhang, B.; Wang, J.; Chen, J.; Ling, Z.; Ren, Y.; Xiong, D.; Guo, L. Machine learning in chronic obstructive pulmonary diseas *Chin. Med. J.* **2023**, *136*, 536–538. [CrossRef]
4. Srivastava, A.; Jain, S.; Miranda, R.; Patil, S.; Pandya, S.; Kotecha, K. Deep learning based respiratory sound analysis for detectio of chronic obstructive pulmonary disease. *PeerJ Comput. Sci.* **2021**, *7*, e369. [CrossRef]
5. Spathis, D.; Vlamos, P. Diagnosing asthma and chronic obstructive pulmonary disease with machine learning. *Health Inform.* **2019**, *25*, 811–827. [CrossRef]
6. Zein, J.G.; Wu, C.P.; Attaway, A.H.; Zhang, P.; Nazha, A. Novel Machine Learning Can Predict Acute Asthma Exacerbation. *Ches* **2021**, *159*, 1747–1757. [CrossRef]
7. Altan, G.; Kutlu, Y.; Gokçen, A. Chronic obstructive pulmonary disease severity analysis using deep learning on multi-channe lung sounds. *Turk. J. Electr. Eng. Comput. Sci.* **2020**, *28*, 2979–2996. [CrossRef]
8. Yang, Y.; Li, W.; Guo, Y.; Zeng, N.; Wang, S.; Chen, Z.; Liu, Y.; Chen, H.; Duan, W.; Li, X.; et al. Lung radiomics features fo characterizing and classifying COPD stage based on feature combination strategy and multi-layer perceptron classifier. *Math Biosci. Eng.* **2022**, *19*, 7826–7855. [CrossRef]
9. Kaur, H.; Sohn, S.; Wi, C.I.; Ryu, E.; Park, M.A.; Bachman, K.; Kita, H.; Croghan, I.; Castro-Rodriguez, J.A.; Voge, G.A.; et a Automated chart review utilizing natural language processing algorithm for asthma predictive index. *BMC Pulm. Med.* **2018**, *1* 34. [CrossRef]
10. Ross, M.K.; Yoon, J.; van der Schaar, A.; van der Schaar, M. Discovering Pediatric Asthma Phenotypes on the Basis of Response t Controller Medication Using Machine Learning. *Ann. Am. Thorac. Soc.* **2018**, *15*, 49–58. [CrossRef] [PubMed]
11. Karabulut, E.M.; Ibrikci, T. Emphysema discrimination from raw HRCT images by convolutional neural networks. In *Proceeding of the 2015 9th International Conference on Electrical and Electronics Engineering (ELECO), Bursa, Turkey, 26–28 November 2015*; IEEE Piscataway, NJ, USA, 2015; pp. 705–708.
12. Wu, Y.; Xia, S.; Liang, Z.; Chen, R.; Qi, S. Artificial intelligence in COPD CT images: Identification, staging, and quantitatior *Respir. Res.* **2024**, *25*, 319. [CrossRef] [PubMed]
13. Xu, M.; Qi, S.; Yue, Y.; Teng, Y.; Xu, L.; Yao, Y.; Qian, W. Segmentation of lung parenchyma in CT images using CNN trained wit a clustering algorithm-generated dataset. *Biomed. Eng. Online* **2019**, *18*, 2. [CrossRef]
14. Kaplan, A.; Cao, H.; FitzGerald, J.M.; Iannotti, N.; Yang, E.; Kocks, J.W.H.; Kostikas, K.; Price, D.; Reddel, H.K.; Tsiligianni, I.; et a Artificial Intelligence/Machine Learning in Respiratory Medicine and Potential Role in Asthma and COPD Diagnosis. *J. Allerg Clin. Immunol. Pract.* **2021**, *9*, 2255–2261. [CrossRef]
15. Sathiya, S.; Priyanka, G.; Jeyanthi, S. Detection of chronic obstructive pulmonary disease in computer-aided diagnosis syster with CNN classification. *Int. J. Pure Appl. Math.* **2018**, *119*, 13815–13821.
16. LeCun, Y.; Bengio, Y.; Hinton, G. Deep learning. *Nature* **2015**, *521*, 436–444. [CrossRef] [PubMed]
17. Wu, Y.; Du, R.; Feng, J.; Qi, S.; Pang, H.; Xia, S.; Qian, W. Deep CNN for COPD identification by Multi-View snapshot integratior of 3D airway tree and lung field. *Biomed. Signal Process. Control* **2023**, *79*, 104162.
18. Sun, J.; Liao, X.; Yan, Y.; Zhang, X.; Sun, J.; Tan, W.; Liu, B.; Wu, J.; Guo, Q.; Gao, S.; et al. Detection and staging of chroni obstructive pulmonary disease using a computed tomography-based weakly supervised deep learning approach. *Eur. Radio* **2022**, *32*, 5319–5329. [CrossRef]

https://doi.org/10.3390/jcm150624

Joumaa, H.; Sigogne, R.; Maravic, M.; Perray, L.; Bourdin, A.; Roche, N. Artificial intelligence to differentiate asthma from COPD in medico-administrative databases. *BMC Pulm. Med.* **2022**, *22*, 357. [CrossRef]

Greffier, J.; Hamard, A.; Pereira, F.; Barrau, C.; Pasquier, H.; Beregi, J.P.; Frandon, J. Image quality and dose reduction opportunity of deep learning image reconstruction algorithm for CT: A phantom study. *Eur. Radiol.* **2020**, *30*, 3951–3959. [CrossRef]

Global Initiative for Asthma (GINA) Report: Global Strategy for Asthma Management and Prevention. Available online: https://ginasthma.org/2025-gina-strategy-report/ (accessed on 7 May 2025).

Global Asthma Network. Global Asthma Report 2025. Available online: https://www.globalasthmanetwork.org (accessed on 7 May 2025).

Miligkos, M.; Oh, J.; Kwon, R.; Konstantinou, G.N.; Kim, S.; Yon, D.K.; Papadopoulos, N.G. Epidemiology of asthma across the ages. *Ann. Allergy Asthma Immunol.* **2025**, *134*, 376–384.e13. [CrossRef] [PubMed]

Global Strategy for Diagnosis, Management and Prevention of COPD (2025 Report). Available online: https://www.goldcopd.org (accessed on 7 May 2025).

Viegi, G.; Maio, S.; Fasola, S.; Baldacci, S. Global Burden of Chronic Respiratory Diseases. *J. Aerosol Med. Pulm. Drug Deliv.* **2020**, *33*, 171–177. [CrossRef]

Bellocq, A.; Gaspard, W.; Couffignal, C.; Vigan, M.; Guerder, A.; Ambard, J.; Caruana, S.; Similowski, T.; Garcia, G.; Taillé, C. Outpatient pulmonary rehabilitation for severe asthma with fixed airway obstruction: Comparison with COPD. *J. Asthma* **2019**, *56*, 1325–1333. [CrossRef]

Sutherland, E.R. Outpatient treatment of chronic obstructive pulmonary disease: Comparisons with asthma. *J. Allergy Clin. Immunol.* **2004**, *114*, 715–725. [CrossRef]

Riley, C.M.; Sciurba, F.C. Diagnosis and Outpatient Management of Chronic Obstructive Pulmonary Disease: A Review. *JAMA* **2019**, *321*, 786–797. [CrossRef]

Al-Zahrani, J.M.; Ahmad, A.; Al-Harbi, A.; Khan, A.M.; Al-Bader, B.; Baharoon, S.; Shememeri, A.A.; Al-Jahdali, H. Factors associated with poor asthma control in the outpatient clinic setting. *Ann. Thorac. Med.* **2015**, *10*, 100–104. [CrossRef]

Ali, Z.; Dirks, C.G.; Ulrik, C.S. Long-term mortality among adults with asthma: A 25-year follow-up of 1075 outpatients with asthma. *Chest* **2013**, *143*, 1649–1655. [CrossRef]

Gutiérrez, F.J.Á.; Galván, M.F.; Gallardo, J.F.M.; Mancera, M.B.; Romero, B.R.; Falcón, A.R. Predictive factors for moderate or severe exacerbations in asthma patients receiving outpatient care. *BMC Pulm. Med.* **2017**, *17*, 77. [CrossRef] [PubMed]

Feng, Y.; Teh, H.S.; Cai, Y. Deep learning for chest radiology: A review. *Curr. Radiol. Rep.* **2019**, *7*, 25. [CrossRef]

Al Meslamani, A.Z. How AI is advancing asthma management? Insights into economic and clinical aspects. *J. Med. Econ.* **2023**, *26*, 1489–1494. [CrossRef] [PubMed]

Hosseini, A.; Buonocore, C.M.; Hashemzadeh, S.; Hojaiji, H.; Kalantarian, H.; Sideris, C.; Bui, A.A.T.; King, C.E.; Sarrafzadeh, M. Feasibility of a Secure Wireless Sensing Smartwatch Application for the Self-Management of Pediatric Asthma. *Sensors* **2017**, *17*, 1780. [CrossRef] [PubMed]

Nikolaou, V.; Massaro, S.; Fakhimi, M.; Stergioulas, L.; Price, D. COPD phenotypes and machine learning cluster analysis: A systematic review and future research agenda. *Respir. Med.* **2020**, *171*, 106093. [CrossRef] [PubMed]

Estépar, R.S.J. Artificial Intelligence in COPD: New Venues to Study a Complex Disease. *Barc. Respir. Netw. Rev.* **2020**, *6*, 144–160. [CrossRef]

Bian, H.; Zhu, S.; Zhang, Y.; Fei, Q.; Peng, X.; Jin, Z.; Zhou, T.; Zhao, H. Artificial Intelligence in Chronic Obstructive Pulmonary Disease: Research Status, Trends, and Future Directions—A Bibliometric Analysis from 2009 to 2023. *Int. J. Chron. Obstruct. Pulmon. Dis.* **2024**, *19*, 1849–1864. [CrossRef]

Yang, K.; Yang, Y.; Kang, Y.; Liang, Z.; Wang, F.; Li, Q.; Xu, J.; Tang, G.; Chen, R. The value of radiomic features in chronic obstructive pulmonary disease assessment: A prospective study. *Clin. Radiol.* **2022**, *77*, e466–e472. [CrossRef]

Cheplygina, V.; Pena, I.P.; Pedersen, J.H.; Lynch, D.A.; Sorensen, L.; de Bruijne, M. Transfer Learning for Multicenter Classification of Chronic Obstructive Pulmonary Disease. *IEEE J. Biomed. Health Inform.* **2018**, *22*, 1486–1496. [CrossRef]

Li, Z.; Liu, L.; Zhang, Z.; Yang, X.; Li, X.; Gao, Y.; Huang, K. A Novel CT-Based Radiomics Features Analysis for Identification and Severity Staging of COPD. *Acad. Radiol.* **2022**, *29*, 663–673. [CrossRef] [PubMed]

Singla, S.; Gong, M.; Riley, C.; Sciurba, F.; Batmanghelich, K. Improving clinical disease subtyping and future events prediction through a chest CT-based deep learning approach. *Med. Phys.* **2021**, *48*, 1168–1181. [CrossRef] [PubMed]

González, G.; Ash, S.Y.; Vegas-Sánchez-Ferrero, G.; Onieva Onieva, J.; Rahaghi, F.N.; Ross, J.C.; Díaz, A.; San José Estépar, R.; Washko, G.R.; COPDGene and ECLIPSE Investigators. Disease Staging and Prognosis in Smokers Using Deep Learning in Chest Computed Tomography. *Am. J. Respir. Crit. Care Med.* **2018**, *197*, 193–203. [CrossRef]

Howard, R.; Rattray, M.; Prosperi, M.; Custovic, A. Distinguishing Asthma Phenotypes Using Machine Learning Approaches. *Curr. Allergy Asthma Rep.* **2015**, *15*, 38. [CrossRef]

Ray, A.; Das, J.; Wenzel, S.E. Determining asthma endotypes and outcomes: Complementing existing clinical practice with modern machine learning. *Cell Rep. Med.* **2022**, *3*, 100857. [CrossRef] [PubMed]

https://doi.org/10.3390/jcm15062445

45. Oletic, D.; Bilas, V. Asthmatic Wheeze Detection From Compressively Sensed Respiratory Sound Spectra. *IEEE J. Biomed. Healt Inform.* **2018**, *22*, 1406–1414. [CrossRef]
46. Amaral, J.L.M.; Lopes, A.J.; Veiga, J.; Faria, A.C.D.; Melo, P.L. High-accuracy detection of airway obstruction in asthma usin machine learning algorithms and forced oscillation measurements. *Comput. Methods Programs Biomed.* **2017**, *144*, 113–12 [CrossRef]
47. Singh, O.P.; Palaniappan, R.; Malarvili, M. Automatic quantitative analysis of human respired carbon dioxide waveform fo asthma and non-asthma classification using support vector machine. *IEEE Access* **2018**, *6*, 55245–55256. [CrossRef]
48. Sinha, A.; Desiraju, K.; Aggarwal, K.; Kutum, R.; Roy, S.; Lodha, R.; Kabra, S.K.; Ghosh, B.; Sethi, T.; Agrawal, A. Exhaled breat condensate metabolome clusters for endotype discovery in asthma. *J. Transl. Med.* **2017**, *15*, 262. [CrossRef]
49. Horváth, I.; Barnes, P.J.; Loukides, S.; Sterk, P.J.; Högman, M.; Olin, A.C.; Amann, A.; Antus, B.; Baraldi, E.; Bikov, A.; et al. European Respiratory Society technical standard: Exhaled biomarkers in lung disease. *Eur. Respir. J.* **2017**, *49*, 1600965. [CrossRe [PubMed]
50. Patel, S.J.; Chamberlain, D.B.; Chamberlain, J.M. A Machine Learning Approach to Predicting Need for Hospitalization fo Pediatric Asthma Exacerbation at the Time of Emergency Department Triage. *Acad. Emerg. Med.* **2018**, *25*, 1463–1470. [CrossRef [PubMed]
51. Williams, L.H.; Drew, T. What do we know about volumetric medical image interpretation?: A review of the basic science an medical image perception literatures. *Cogn. Res. Princ. Implic.* **2019**, *4*, 21. [CrossRef] [PubMed]
52. Kumar, R.; Wang, W.; Kumar, J.; Yang, T.; Khan, A.; Ali, W.; Ali, I. An Integration of blockchain and AI for secure data sharin and detection of CT images for the hospitals. *Comput. Med. Imaging Graph.* **2021**, *87*, 101812. [CrossRef]
53. Castiglioni, I.; Rundo, L.; Codari, M.; Di Leo, G.; Salvatore, C.; Interlenghi, M.; Gallivanone, F.; Cozzi, A.; D'Amico, N.C Sardanelli, F. AI applications to medical images: From machine learning to deep learning. *Phys. Med.* **2021**, *83*, 9–24. [CrossRef
54. Martínez-García, M.Á.; de la Rosa-Carrillo, D.; Soler-Cataluña, J.J.; Catalan-Serra, P.; Ballester, M.; Roca Vanaclocha, Y.; Agramun M.; Ballestin, J.; Garcia-Ortega, A.; Oscullo, G.; et al. Bronchial Infection and Temporal Evolution of Bronchiectasis in Patient With Chronic Obstructive Pulmonary Disease. *Clin. Infect. Dis.* **2021**, *72*, 403–410. [CrossRef]
55. Ezponda, A.; Casanova, C.; Divo, M.; Marín-Oto, M.; Cabrera, C.; Marín, J.M.; Bastarrika, G.; Pinto-Plata, V.; Martin-Palmer Á.; Polverino, F.; et al. Chest CT-assessed comorbidities and all-cause mortality risk in COPD patients in the BODE coho *Respirology* **2022**, *27*, 286–293. [CrossRef] [PubMed]
56. Zhang, L.; Jiang, B.; Wisselink, H.J.; Vliegenthart, R.; Xie, X. COPD identification and grading based on deep learning of lun parenchyma and bronchial wall in chest CT images. *Br. J. Radiol.* **2022**, *95*, 20210637. [CrossRef]
57. Wu, Y.; Qi, S.; Feng, J.; Chang, R.; Pang, H.; Hou, J.; Li, M.; Wang, Y.; Xia, S.; Qian, W. Attention-guided multiple instance learnin for COPD identification: To combine the intensity and morphology. *Biocybern. Biomed. Eng.* **2023**, *43*, 568–585. [CrossRef]
58. Martini, K.; Frauenfelder, T. Advances in imaging for lung emphysema. *Ann. Transl. Med.* **2020**, *8*, 1467. [CrossRef]
59. Bermejo-Peláez, D.; San José Estépar, R.; Ledesma-Carbayo, M.J. Emphysema classification using a multi-view convolutiona network. *Proc. IEEE Int. Symp. Biomed Imaging* **2018**, *2018*, 519–522. [CrossRef]
60. Peng, L.; Lin, L.; Hu, H.; Zhang, Y.; Li, H.; Iwamoto, Y.; Han, X.H.; Chen, Y.W. Semi-Supervised Learning for Semanti Segmentation of Emphysema with Partial Annotations. *IEEE J. Biomed. Health Inform.* **2020**, *24*, 2327–2336. [CrossRef]
61. Wu, Y.; Qi, S.; Sun, Y.; Xia, S.; Yao, Y.; Qian, W. A vision transformer for emphysema classification using CT images. *Phys. Me Biol.* **2021**, *66*, 245016. [CrossRef] [PubMed]
62. Hasenstab, K.A.; Yuan, N.; Retson, T.; Conrad, D.J.; Kligerman, S.; Lynch, D.A.; Hsiao, A.; COPDGene Investigators. Automate CT Staging of Chronic Obstructive Pulmonary Disease Severity for Predicting Disease Progression and Mortality with a Dee Learning Convolutional Neural Network. *Radiol. Cardiothorac. Imaging* **2021**, *3*, e200477. [CrossRef] [PubMed]
63. Dosovitskiy, A.; Beyer, L.; Kolesnikov, A.; Weissenborn, D.; Zhai, X.; Unterthiner, T.; Dehghani, M.; Minderer, M Heigold, G.; Gelly, S.; et al. An image is worth 16x16 words: Transformers for image recognition at scale. In Proceed ings of the International Conference on Learning Representations (ICLR), Vienna, Austria, 4 May 2021; Available onlin https://openreview.net/forum?id=YicbFdNTTy (accessed on 7 May 2025).
64. Pang, H.; Qi, S.; Wu, Y.; Wang, M.; Li, C.; Sun, Y.; Qian, W.; Tang, G.; Xu, J.; Liang, Z.; et al. NCCT-CECT image synthesizers an their application to pulmonary vessel segmentation. *Comput. Methods Programs Biomed.* **2023**, *231*, 107389. [CrossRef]
65. Yang, X. Application and Prospects of Artificial Intelligence Technology in Early Screening of Chronic Obstructive Pulmonar Disease at Primary Healthcare Institutions in China. *Int. J. Chronic Obstr. Pulm. Dis.* **2024**, *19*, 1061–1067. [CrossRef]
66. Chen, L.; Feng, Q.; Yin, X.; Min, X.; Shi, L.; Yang, D.; Chen, Y.W.; Zhang, D.; Zhu, W. A Graph Convolutional Multiple Instanc Learning on a Hypersphere Manifold Approach for Diagnosing Chronic Obstructive Pulmonary Disease in CT Images. *IEEE Biomed. Health Inform.* **2022**, *26*, 6058–6069. [CrossRef]
67. Ying, J.; Dutta, J.; Guo, N.; Xia, L.; Sitek, A.; Li, Q. Gold classification of COPDGene cohort based on deep learning. In *Proceeding of the IEEE International Conference on Acoustics, Speech and Signal Processing (ICASSP), Shanghai, China, 20–25 March 2016*; IEEE Piscataway, NJ, USA, 2016; pp. 2474–2478.

8. Lin, A.; Kolossváry, M.; Motwani, M.; Išgum, I.; Maurovich-Horvat, P.; Slomka, P.J.; Dey, D. Artificial intelligence in cardiovascular CT: Current status and future implications. *J. Cardiovasc. Comput. Tomogr.* **2021**, *15*, 462–469. [CrossRef]
9. Nardelli, P.; Jimenez-Carretero, D.; Bermejo-Pelaez, D.; Washko, G.R.; Rahaghi, F.N.; Ledesma-Carbayo, M.J.; San Jose Estepar, R. Pulmonary Artery-Vein Classification in CT Images Using Deep Learning. *IEEE Trans. Med. Imaging* **2018**, *37*, 2428–2440. [CrossRef]
0. Tan, W.; Zhou, L.; Li, X.; Yang, X.; Chen, Y.; Yang, J. Automated vessel segmentation in lung CT and CTA images via deep neural networks. *J. X-Ray Sci. Technol.* **2021**, *29*, 1123–1137. [CrossRef] [PubMed]
1. Akduman, S.; Yilmaz, K. Examining the effectiveness of artificial intelligence applications in asthma and COPD outpatient support in terms of patient health and public cost: SWOT analysis. *Medicine* **2024**, *103*, e38998. [CrossRef] [PubMed]
2. Gogali, A.; Kyriakopoulos, C.; Potonos, D.; Ladias, A.; Tatsis, K.; Kostikas, K. Artificial Intelligence in Asthma: Current Status, Opportunities, and Pitfalls. *J. Allergy Clin. Immunol. Pract.* **2025**, *13*, 2891–2901. [CrossRef] [PubMed]
3. Feng, Y.; Wang, Y.; Zeng, C.; Mao, H. Artificial Intelligence and Machine Learning in Chronic Airway Diseases: Focus on Asthma and Chronic Obstructive Pulmonary Disease. *Int. J. Med. Sci.* **2021**, *18*, 2871–2889. [CrossRef]
4. Martin, C.; DeStefano, K.; Haran, H.; Zink, S.; Dai, J.; Ahmed, D.; Razzak, A.; Lin, K.; Kogler, A.; Waller, J.; et al. The ethical considerations including inclusion and biases, data protection, and proper implementation among AI in radiology and potential implications. *Intell.-Based Med.* **2022**, *6*, 100073. [CrossRef]

https://doi.org/10.3390/jcm15062445

Journal of
Clinical Medicine

MDPI

Review

Update on the Treatment of Non-Small Cell Lung Carcinoma (NSCLC)

Yousif A. Kariri

Department of Clinical Laboratory Sciences, Collage of Applied Medical Sciences, Shaqra University, Shaqra 11961, Saudi Arabia; ykuriri@su.edu.sa

Abstract

Non-small cell lung carcinoma (NSCLC) is a prominent type, with an 85–90% incidence in all lung cancer cases. The evidence for a particular therapy strategy for people with NSCLC is still inadequate. This review evaluates NSCLC therapies that have passed phase IV trials, emphasizing their efficiency and adverse effects. Crucial therapeutic approaches, including dacomitinib, lorlatinib, durvalumab, osimertinib, and rivaroxban, are discussed, highlighting their mechanisms of action, uses, and adverse effects. Immune checkpoint medications are recommended because of their specific activity and minimal adverse reactions. The review also investigates cooperation therapies, such as targeting immune checkpoint inhibitors and hemostasis, alongside chemotherapy, as they offer potential for future therapies. However, further research is needed to improve the safety and efficacy of current treatments, and to explore novel ways to achieve better long-term outcomes.

Keywords: non-small lung carcinoma; adverse effects; efficacy; tyrosine kinase inhibitors; epithelial growth factor receptor; clinical trials; phase IV

1. Introduction

Lung cancer is one of the most common leading cancers, resulting in high mortality and morbidity around the globe [1]. In 2022, lung cancer accounted for 1.57 million new cases in males, making it the most frequent cancer diagnosed globally, according to GLOBOCAN, lung cancer was the first most diagnosed cancer in males and the second most in females, with approximately 910,000 new cases [2]. Recently, lung cancer was demonstrated to have only a 25% probability of 5-year survival, one of the lowest survival rates of all cancers in 2024 [3]. Despite recent developments in lung cancer screening, diagnosis, prevention, and therapy, the significant connection between incidence and mortality indicates that the disease is still generally fatal.

The occurrence of lung cancer cases by gender and population is anticipated to be mainly determined by cigarette smoking. Although lung cancer has been generally more common among males who smoked more frequently in the past few decades, recent studies reveal an increasing incidence of lung cancer cases in women, especially among younger age groups, and a drop in lung cancer instances in men [4]. A study conducted in the United States reported that the incidence of lung cancer was higher in young women compared to young men [5], and it certainly indicates that this development does not just hinge on changing patterns in cigarette smoking [4]. Exposure to asbestos, as the main risk factor for the development of malignant mesothelioma, secondhand smoking, mineral and metal dusts, and radon are other recognized risk factors for lung cancer [6]. The United States' lung cancer mortality rate has recently dropped by 59% for men, from its peak in men in

1990, and 36% for women, from its peak in women in 2002, due to the implementation of screening guidelines and an overall decrease in tobacco usage [3].

Based on cancer cells' histology, lung cancer can be divided into two distinct groups: NSCLC and small cell lung carcinoma (SCLC). NSCLC is the dominant lung cancer type with 85–90% incidence in all lung cancer cases. Remarkably, NSCLC is a very severe disease characterized by high rates of metastasis and recurrence, and composed of several histological subtypes, including large-cell carcinoma, lung squamous carcinoma, and lung adenocarcinoma [7]. Another histological subclassification classified NSCLC according to cell types into squamous NSCLC (constituting up to 30% of NSCLC cases), and non-squamous carcinoma NSCLC, which may be further classified into adenocarcinoma (constituting up to around 40% of NSCLCs), big cell carcinoma, and other cell types [8].

The stage of NSCLC at diagnosis impacts significantly on treatment options and prognoses. To illustrate, in the early stages, surgery is a highly effective therapeutic option, whereas it is not recommended once metastasis occurs. Moreover, NSCLC treatment is often multimodal, including surgery, radiotherapy, and chemotherapy; for stage 4, systemic treatment is the current standard of care, but radiotherapy and surgery may also have a role (i.e., palliative treatment) [9,10]. Despite the utilization of conventional chemotherapeutic drugs for advanced lung carcinoma cases, some limitations reduce their effectiveness in cancer treatment, such as the development of drug resistance, non-specific targeting, and low bioavailability [11]. Hence, the most effective advance in recent years in NSCLC therapy is the focus on molecular targeted therapy. Exploring the genomic drivers is the key to identifying the etiology and understanding the pathogenesis of NSCLC. Tyrosine kinase inhibitors (TKIs) are a new group of treatments that have emerged as a result of the identification of activating mutations of epidermal growth factor receptor (EGFR) in patients with lung adenocarcinoma [12]. These therapeutic strategies open up new horizons in terms of patients' clinical management, as targeting EGFR mutations can approximately double the survival rate compared to conventional chemotherapy [13].

2. Pharmacological Approaches to NSCLC Therapy

2.1. Molecular Pharmacological Treatments

The increasing prevalence of TKI resistance has challenged the initial expectations and paved the way for the gradual development of novel medications that target multiple molecular modifications and pathways. Recently, patients diagnosed with advanced metastasis stages of NSCLC have shown mutations in several genes, including EGFR, c-ros oncogene 1 (ROS1), anaplastic lymphoma kinase (ALK), human epidermal growth factor receptor (HER2), and Kirsten rat sarcoma virus (KRAS), suggesting that mutations in these genes can be used as therapeutic targets [14–16]. Interestingly, finding a targetable mutation might assist patients in better understanding their prognosis and the progression of their medical condition, in addition to influencing clinical decision-making and therapy selection. However, to date, only medications that target EGFR or ALK mutations, as well as ROS and BRAF mutations, have been approved for clinical trials and treatments. To specify, patients with ALK modifications are recommended to be treated with brigatinib [17], or alectinib [18], whereas those with ROS1 modifications are treated with crizotinib [19]. Likewise, patients with lung adenocarcinoma harboring EFGR mutation are generally treated with osimertinib [20]. The pathways for these mutations are summarized in Figure 1. The recommendation of using these molecules, which target specific mutations, will increase in the future, driven by extensive ongoing research that aims to develop NSCLC target therapies. Furthermore, research on inhibitors with other targets is also ongoing [21]. Despite the initial effectiveness of the molecular targeted therapy approach, tumor heterogeneity and epigenetic alterations frequently lead to acquired drug resistance, which significantly reduces therapeutic efficiency in NSCLC [22,23]. Therefore, developing novel molecular targets for NSCLC is essential to improve patient outcomes.

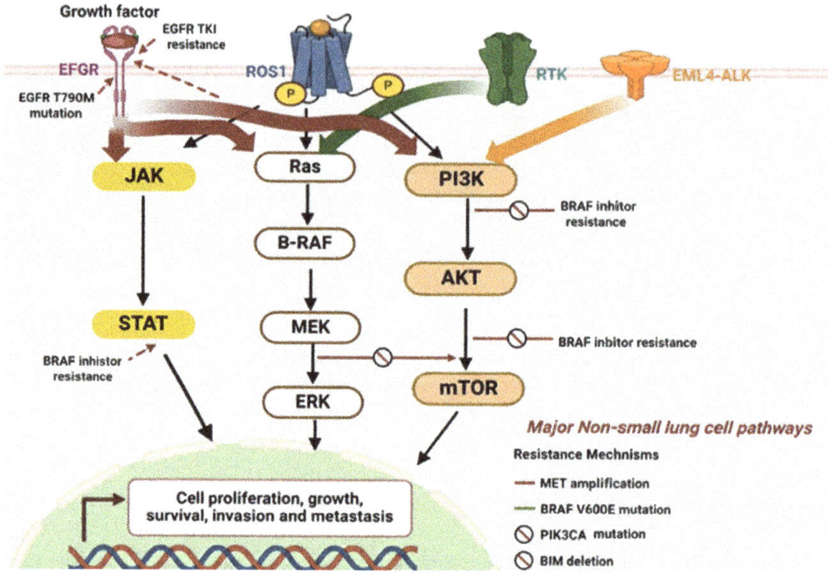

Figure 1. Summary of the major TKIs mutation pathways involved in NSCLC. JAK-STAT, RAS, and PI3K-AKT are three key signaling pathways in NSCLC. These pathways are well-known regulators of cell cycle development, growth, and apoptosis/cell survival; dysregulation is a common feature of human cancers. Modifications in essential pathways will influence DNA methylation modifications, such as elevated DNA methyltransferases (DNMTs), DNA post-translation, and reduced ten-eleven translocation methylcytosine dioxygenases (TETs), enabling amplification of mesenchymal homology box 2 (MEOX2), which has a negative association with patient survival. As a consequence, the expression of key cell cycle checkpoints and tumor suppressor biomarkers (P53, P21, and other related biomarkers) will decrease to allow cancer cell proliferation and survival. Tyrosine kinase inhibitors (TKIs) are a class of drugs specifically designed to target major genomic mutations that act as oncogenic drivers in non-small cell lung cancer (NSCLC). These mutations lead to the overactivation of key signaling pathways, which in turn drive uncontrolled cell proliferation, growth, and survival. As shown in the figure, the primary genomic mutations targeted by TKIs include the following: EGFR mutations: These are common mutations in the epidermal growth factor receptor (EGFR) gene. TKIs inhibit the signaling of the mutated EGFR protein, thereby blocking the downstream signaling pathways like RAS-RAF-MEK-ERK and PI3K-AKT-mTOR. The figure also shows the EGFR T790M mutation, a common resistance mechanism that requires a different type of TKI. ROS1 fusions: A genetic rearrangement involving the ROS1 gene that leads to a constitutively active kinase, which is targeted by specific TKIs. EML4-ALK fusions: A gene fusion that creates an oncogenic protein with constant kinase activity, which is a major target for ALK inhibitors, a type of TKI. The figure also highlights other genomic changes that can act as either primary drivers or resistance mechanisms, such as BRAF V600E mutation, MET amplification, and PIK3CA mutations, all of which can be targeted by specific inhibitors to disrupt the cancer cell's signaling.

2.2. *Immune Target Pharmacological Treatments*

Immunotherapy approaches that focus extensively on immune checkpoint inhibitors are another therapeutic option for NSCLC that is very successful and significantly safer for patients [24,25]. Immune checkpoint inhibitor-based treatments targeting PD-1 and PD-L1 are common therapies for advanced or metastatic NSCLC that lacks identifiable genetic causes [26]. Moreover, prior studies have indicated that combining immunotherapy with other medications or therapeutic modalities may be beneficial [27–29].

Although there have been significant improvements in NSCLC treatment through several options to explore the best therapeutic applications, the treatment of NSCLC is still controversial and needs improvement. This review summarizes the pharmacological effects of agents that completed phase IV clinical trials in the last 5 years for the treatment of NSCLC.

A review of recent studies on anti-PD-1 and anti-PD-L1 immune checkpoint inhibitors for non-small cell lung cancer (NSCLC) reveals nuanced differences in their efficacy and safety profiles [30]. While both classes of drugs have demonstrated a significant overall survival advantage compared to chemotherapy in second- and later-line treatments, subtle distinctions become apparent upon closer examination. A meta-analysis focusing on efficacy and safety in relapsed or refractory advanced NSCLC found that anti-PD-1 agents ranked highest for overall survival, with anti-PD-L1 agents following [31]. However, another systematic review specifically examining the safety of these inhibitors found that PD-L1 inhibitors might be a safer option regarding grade $\geq$3 treatment-related adverse events, particularly pneumonia and pneumonitis, when used alone or in combination with chemotherapy. A separate study further explored these differences, suggesting that anti-PD-1 agents may show a higher response rate and a better outcome when combined with chemotherapy for first-line treatment, especially for patients with specific PD-L1 expression levels. Conversely, the same study noted that anti-PD-L1 agents were associated with less severe immune-related adverse events [32]. These findings suggest that while both drug classes are effective, the choice between them may depend on a balance between desired efficacy and a patient's tolerance for potential side effects.

3. Completed Phase IV Clinical Trials for NSCLC Treatment

3.1. *Dacomitinib*

Dacomitinib, developed by Pfizer, is a multi-kinase receptor regulator used for NSCLC therapy with EGFR activating mutations. Dacomitinib was approved as a therapeutic agent for metastatic NSCLC by the United States Food and Drug Administration in 2018 [33].

Dacomitinib is a permanent small-molecule inhibitor that efficiently regulates the EGFR family's tyrosine kinase activity by targeting EGFR gene mutation, especially exon 19 deletions and exon 21 L858R point mutations [34,35]. Dacomitinib achieves permanent inhibition by forming covalent bonds with cysteine residues located inside the catalytic domains of HER receptors [36]. However, dacomitinib's metabolic pathway is controlled by cytochrome p450 (CYP) CYP2D6 and CYP2A4, differing from other EGFR-TKIs, which are controlled by CYP3A4. This diversity in metabolic pathways might result in variable interactions among medications and pharmacological profiles.

Around the globe, dacomitinib is used as a first-line treatment for patients diagnosed with NSCLC metastasis. A conducted study by Nishio et al. claimed that dacomitinib improves the progression of free survival in patients, with no serious adverse events [6]. This suggests the ability of dacomitinib to act as an effective and safe first-line treatment for patients with EGFR-positive advanced NSCLC. The mechanism of action of dacomitinib in NSCLC is summarized in Figure 2A.

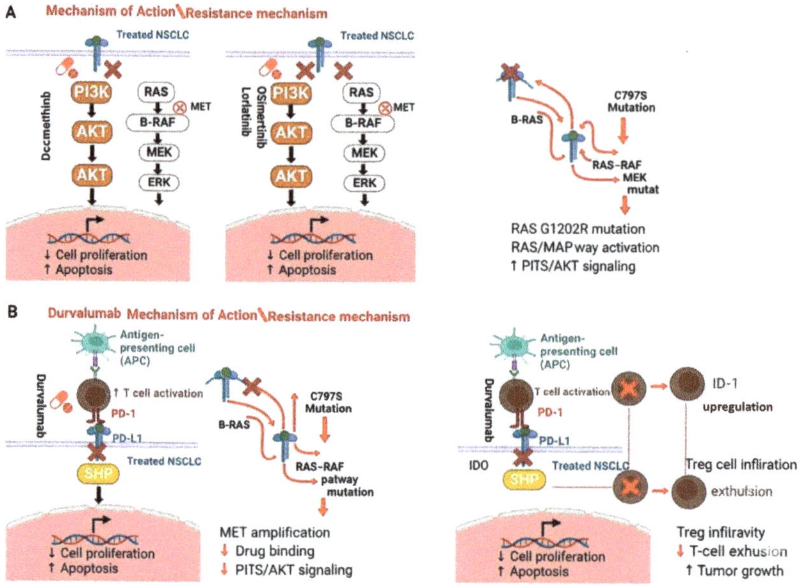

Figure 2. Mechanism of action and resistance of TKIs. PI3K-AKT, RAS, and SHP are essential TKIs drug target pathways. Human malignancies frequently exhibit deregulation of these pathways, which are prominent mediators of cell cycle development, proliferation, and apoptosis/cell survival. (**A**) Mechanism of action, dacomitinib blocks the PI3K/AKT pathway and thus promotes cell apoptosis, lorlatinib and osimertinib prevents both PI3K and RAS pathways, and hence enhances cell apoptosis. and (**B**) Durvalumab blocks the SHP pathway, and thus prevents cell survival. The resistance mechanisms are shown on the right-hand side.

Despite its proven effectiveness, dacomitinib may still have a few adverse effects, though not all of these adverse effects will necessarily occur, though they might require medical care if they do develop. These adverse effects depend on the duration of treatment, the presence of inflammations such as stomatitis and dermatitis, and the presence of other symptoms, including diarrhea, chest pain, weight loss, loss of appetite, hair loss, coughing, sleep issues, vomiting, and swollen or red eyes.

Several studies have evaluated the role of dacomitinib in phases I, II, and III. These are listed in Table 1. There is also a newly completed phase IV clinical trial (n = 115) "Dacomitinib for the Treatment of Patients in India with Metastatic Non-Small Cell Lung Cancer with EGFR Activating Mutations" (NCT04511533), conducted by Pfizer, claiming that dacomitinib is effective and safe, with no serious adverse effects.

Table 1. Overview of Dacomitinib in clinical trial phases I, II, and III.

N	Authors/Reference	Clinical Trails	Phase of the Studies	Number of Samples
1	Jung H. et al. [7]	(NCT04339829)	Phase II	30
2	Iwasaku M. et al. [8]	(jRCTs071190015)	Phase II	41
3	Tan W. et al. [9]	(NCT01858389)	Phase II	41
4	Mok T. et al. [10]	(NCT01774721)	Phase III	227
5	Pu X. et al. [11]	(NCT01774721)	Phase III	227
6	Cheng Y. et al. [12]	(NCT01774721)	Phase III	346

3.2. Lorlatinib

Larlatinib is an orally effective drug that regulates ALK and ROS1 kinases, it has been developed by Pfizer for ALK-positive NSCLC treatment [13]. Generally, ALK is a naturally occurring endogenous tyrosine kinase receptor that stimulates different kinds of neurons in the nervous system and is crucial for brain development. Larlatinib is a member of the third generation of ALK-TKI and shows extensive effectiveness against ALK-resistance mutations developed during therapies employing first-generation (crizotinib) or second-generation ALK inhibitors (alectinib, ceritinib) [14]. Moreover, lorlatinib has shown in vitro efficacy against a variety of ALK enzyme mutations, including several found in tumors where the clinical condition was worsening while using crizotinib and other ALK inhibitors [15]. Furthermore, lorlatinib penetrates the blood–brain barrier, and can also treat developing or worsening brain metastases [16]. In in vivo models, lorlatinib's overall anticancer effect seems to depend on the dose and is associated with the suppression of ALK phosphorylation [17]. The mechanism of action of lorlatinib in NSCLC is summarized in Figure 2A.

Larlatinib was first approved in Japan in September 2018, followed by the United States in November 2018, based on the findings of phase I/II studies [18]. The European Medicines Agency (EMA) later authorized larlatinib in 2019 for the treatment of a selected group of patients with advanced ALK-positive NSCLC who had already received other treatments. In 2022, the approval was further extended to cover lorlatinib as a first-line treatment option for advanced ALK-positive NSCLC [19]. A multicentric phase I/II study (NCT01970865) showed strong antitumor efficacy of lorlatinib, following the failure of prior ALK inhibitor therapy, including in patients who had been treated with either first- or second-generation ALK TKIs, or both [20,21].

Lorlatinib is highly effective in the treatment of advanced NSCLC. The adverse effects of this agent include hypertriglyceridemia, hypercholesterolemia, central nerve system effects (speech disorder, depression, cognitive disorder), peripheral neuropathy, overweight edema and gastrointestinal effects. Moreover, atrioventricular block might occur due to an excessive increase in lipase. However, there is a slim chance of long-term withdrawal based on adverse effects, though the majority of them are temporary, and therefore, lorlatinib has an exceptional safety profile compared to other ALK TKIs medications [19].

Several Phase I, II, and III clinical studies have evaluated the efficacy of larlatinib in NSCLC patients. These are summarized in Table 2. There are also two completed Phase IV clinical trials, "Lorlatinib in ALK Inhibitor Treated Unresectable Advanced/Recurrent ALK-Positive Non-Small Cell Lung Cancer Patients in India" (NCT04541706: n = 100) and "Study of Loralatinib in People with ALK-positive Non-small Cell Lung Cancer" (NCT04362072: n = 71), conducted by Pfizer, to explore the efficacy and adverse effects of lorlatinib as a therapeutic agent for NSCLC. These studies reported that lorlatinib was effective and safer for advanced NSCLC.

Table 2. Overview of Lorlatinib in clinical trial phases I, II, and III.

N	Authors/Reference	Clinical Trails	Phase of the Studies	Number of Samples
1	Goldsmith K. et al. [22]	(NCT03107988)	Phase I	65
2	Solomon B. et al. [21]	(NCT01970865)	Phase I & II	364
3	Lu S. et al. [23]	(NCT03909971)	Phase II	109
4	Felip E et al. [24]	(NCT01970865)	Phase II	139
5	Ou S. et al. [25]	(NCT01970865)	Phase I & II	364
6	Solomon B. et al. [27]	(NCT03052608)	Phase III	296

3.3. Durvalumab

Durvalumab is an immune-target therapy developed by Medimmune/AstraZeneca that produces an antitumor antibody to stimulate immune-mediated antitumor responses via activating immune cells [28]. Durvalumab is a human immunoglobulin G1 kappa (IgG1k) monoclonal antibody that exclusively inhibits the interaction of human PD-L1 with programmed cell death 1 (PD-1) and cluster differentiation (CD80) [29,37]. This stimulates anti-cancer immune responses, T-cell proliferation, and T-cell activity [29]. Furthermore, it is designed to prevent cellular cytotoxicity reactions that are dependent on antibodies. Reductions in tumor growth are linked to durvalumab-induced PD-L1 inhibition in co-engrafted human cancer and immune cell xenograft mouse models [26]. To improve the effectiveness of PD-L1 blockade, it may be combined with other chemotherapeutic agents. The mechanism of action in NSCLC is summarized in Figure 2B. Durvalumab, used alone [33] or in conjunction with chemotherapy [34], has shown antitumor effects in individuals with NSCLS during early clinical trials. Likewise, a study conducted by Rothschild et al. reported that stage III NSCLC patients who received durvalumab alongside neoadjuvant chemotherapy showed good results and manageable adverse effects [35].

In 2018, durvalumab was approved by the FDA for stage III NSCLC. Moreover, durvalumab sequential monotherapy significantly improved progression-free survival in patients with unresectable stage III NSCLC who did not progress after platinum-based chemoradiation therapy, according to a planned interim analysis of a randomized, double-blind, placebo-controlled, phase III PACIFIC trial (NCT02125461) [36]. An update on PACIFIC trials conducted by Faivre-Finn et al. demonstrated that the standard-of-care PACIFIC combination with durvalumab after chemoradiotherapy indicates sustained overall survival (OS) benefit with persistent progression-free survival (PFS), as determined by preliminary findings from PACIFIC [38].

Although durvalumab has expanded utilization as an effective therapeutic target for advanced stages of NSCLC, using durvalumab for advanced stages of NSCLC may present some limitations. These adverse effects include shortness of breath, coughing, upper respiratory tract infections, inflammation of the lungs, chest pain, and fatigue. However, these adverse effects are manageable and easy to resolve with direct healthcare, which allows a faster response to any medical adverse reaction.

Multiple studies have investigated the role of durvalumab in phase II and III clinical trials. These are summarized in Table 3. There is also a phase IV clinical trial conducted by AstraZeneca that evaluated the role of durvalumab in advanced NSCLC: "Study to Access Safety of Durvalumab in Indian Adult Patients with Locally Advanced NSCLC" (NCT04416633: n = 100).

Table 3. Overview of Durvalumab in clinical trials- phase II and III.

N	Authors/Reference	Clinical Trails	Phase of the Studies	Number of Samples
1	Besse B. et al. [39]	(NCT03334617)	Phase II	268
2	Garassino M. et al. [40]	(NCT03693300)	Phase II	117
3	Reck M. et al. [41]	(NCT05925530)	Phase II	140
4	Schoenfeld J. et al. [42]	(NCT02888743)	Phase II	90
5	Johnson M. et al. [33]	(NCT03164616)	Phase III	1013
6	Ruysscher D. et al. [43]	(NCT04026412)	Phase III	888

3.4. Osimertinib

Osimertinib (developed by AstraZeneca, UK, Cambridge) is a third-generation EFGR-TKI that particularly targets activating mutations of EGFR and the resistance of T790M mutations, a barrier mutation that enhances EGFR's tolerance of ATP in its ATP-binding domain, thus effectively inhibiting first- and second-generation TKIs from attaching to EGFR ATP-binding sites [44]. Osimertinib acts by forming a covalent bond with the C797 residue at the ATP-binding site of mutant EGFR. In contrast to both first- and second-generation EGFR-TKIs, osimertinib exhibits greater efficacy towards T790M mutants in vitro, with low off-target effects, resulting in fewer adverse outcomes generally associated with the blockage of wild-type EGFR [45]. The mechanism of action in NSCLC is summarized in Figure 2A.

Initially, osimertinib was exclusively authorized for use in individuals with EGFR T790M-positive mutations whose NSCLC was advancing after EGFR TKI treatment [46]. Subsequently, FLAURA research revealed a notable improvement in both OS and PFS with osimertinib when compared to first-generation EGFR TKI therapy [47]. Nowadays, major healthcare organizations have authorized osimertinib as the sole third-generation EGFR-TKI for the management of T790M-positive patients who have made progress with first- or second-generation EGFR-TKIs. Furthermore, osimertinib received approval in 2018 as the primary therapeutic medication for advanced EFGR-mutated NSCLC [48].

Although osimertinib is recognized as one of the primary therapies in advanced NCSCLC, patients invariably develop secondary resistance to osimertinib, despite its strong clinical efficacy. This represents a key difficulty, because there are currently limited post-osimertinib pharmacological alternatives available. Moreover, the drug may have certain adverse effects in addition to its anticipated advantages. Although not all of these adverse reactions may be seen in all patients, if they do present, medical attention is required to treat/minimize these adverse reactions. These adverse reactions include swelling or inflammation of the mouth, back pain, constipation, nausea, and skin rush.

A summary of clinical trials that have evaluated the role of osimertinib in NSCLC in phase II and III clinical trials is presented in Table 4. A recently completed Phase IV clinical trial (NCT05219162; n = 182) conducted by AstraZeneca investigated the role of osimertinib in NSCLC: "Real-World Study on Gene Profile in Patients with Advanced NSCLC Who Progressed on First-Line Osimertinib Therapy (GPS)".

Table 4. Overview of Osimertinib in clinical trials- II and III.

N	Authors/Reference	Clinical Trails	Phase of the Studies	Number of Samples
1	Okuma Y. et al. [49]	(jRCTs071200002)	Phase II	40
2	Herbst R. et al. [50]	(NCT02511106)	Phase III	682
3	Lu S. et al. [51]	(NCT03521154)	Phase III	216
4	Planchard D. et al. [52]	(NCT04035486)	Phase III	557
5	Remon J. et al. [53]	(NCT02856893)	Phase III	156

4. Antibody-Drug Conjugates in Non-Small Cell Lung Cancer

The treatment landscape for non-small cell lung cancer (NSCLC) is being reshaped by antibody-drug conjugates (ADCs), which merge the precision of monoclonal antibodies with the destructive potential of cytotoxic agents. These sophisticated molecules are engineered to selectively target tumor cells, thereby widening the therapeutic window and reducing systemic toxicity. Each ADC comprises three essential components: a monoclonal antibody designed to recognize specific tumor antigens, a chemical linker that ensures stability in circulation, and a potent cytotoxic payload. The drug-to-antibody ratio (DAR) plays a crucial role in determining both efficacy and safety profiles. A significant feature of many ADCs is the bystander effect, wherein the released payload can penetrate nearby cells, targeting heterogeneous tumor populations that may not express the antigen [54]. Significant clinical progress has been achieved with HER2-directed agents. Trastuzumab deruxtecan (T-DXd) gained regulatory approval for HER2-mutant NSCLC based on results from the DESTINY-Lung trials, which reported a 55% objective response rate and 8.2 months median progression-free survival [55]. Earlier efforts with trastuzumab emtansine (T-DM1), however, demonstrated more limited clinical activity in this setting [56].

Emerging targets beyond HER2 show considerable promise. Datopotamab deruxtecan (Dato-DXd), which targets TROP2, improved progression-free survival compared to docetaxel in the TROPION-Lung01 study, though overall survival data are still maturing [57]. Similarly, patritumab deruxtecan (HER3-DXd) achieved a 29.8% response rate in EGFR-mutant patients who had progressed on prior tyrosine kinase inhibitors and chemotherapy [58]. Telisotuzumab vedotin, targeting c-MET, has also demonstrated encouraging anti-tumor activity in selected patient subgroups. Despite these advances, several challenges require attention. Management of unique toxicities, particularly interstitial lung disease associated with T-DXd, demands careful monitoring and prompt intervention. The development of reliable predictive biomarkers beyond antigen expression levels remains a critical need for optimizing patient selection. Additionally, understanding resistance mechanisms and determining optimal sequencing strategies represent important areas for future research. ADCs have undoubtedly expanded therapeutic options for NSCLC patients. Ongoing research efforts continue to refine their clinical application, with a focus on enhancing efficacy while managing treatment-related adverse events.

5. Anti-Angiogenic Agents in the Management of Non-Small Cell Lung Cancer

Angiogenesis, the formation of new blood vessels, is a critical process for tumor growth and metastasis. Vascular endothelial growth factor (VEGF) and its receptors are key mediators of this process. Anti-angiogenic agents, such as the monoclonal antibody bevacizumab which targets VEGF-A, inhibit this pathway, thereby suppressing tumor blood supply and promoting normalization of the remaining vasculature. This normalization can reduce intratumoral pressure and improve the delivery of concurrently administered chemotherapeutic or immunotherapeutic agents. The most substantiated evidence for anti-angiogenic therapy in NSCLC comes from the IMpower150 trial [59]. This phase III study evaluated a quadruple regimen consisting of atezolizumab (an anti-PD-L1 antibody), bevacizumab (anti-VEGF), carboplatin, and paclitaxel (ABCP) compared to bevacizumab plus chemotherapy (BCP) in patients with metastatic non-squamous NSCLC without EGFR or ALK alterations. The ABCP regimen demonstrated a statistically significant improvement in overall survival (OS) compared to BCP, with a median OS of 19.5 months versus 14.7 months (HR 0.80; 95% CI, 0.67–0.95) [59]. Exploratory analyses indicated that the survival benefit was most evident in patients with high PD-L1 expression and those with liver metastases. Notably, the trial design allowed for continuous atezolizumab treatment until loss of clinical benefit, differing from the fixed-duration approach used in other immunotherapy trials. This regimen provides an important first-line option, particularly for patients with high tumor burden or aggressive disease phenotypes where rapid disease control is paramount.

The combination of an anti-angiogenic agent with immunotherapy is thought to work synergistically; bevacizumab may reverse VEGF-mediated immunosuppression in the tumor microenvironment, potentially enhancing the efficacy of immune checkpoint inhibition.

Despite its benefits, the use of bevacizumab is restricted to patients with non-squamous histology due to an elevated risk of life-threatening hemoptysis in patients with squamous cell carcinoma. Furthermore, anti-angiogenic agents are associated with a distinct toxicity profile, including hypertension, proteinuria, bleeding events, and impaired wound healing, which necessitates careful patient selection and monitoring. The IMpower150 trial also showed that the benefit was less clear in the PD-L1 negative population, highlighting that not all patients derive equal benefit from this intensive and costly combination [59]. Anti-angiogenic therapy, exemplified by bevacizumab in the IMpower150 regimen, remains a valuable component of combination therapy for a subset of patients with advanced non-squamous NSCLC. Its role has been refined rather than replaced by the advent of immunotherapy, finding a niche in synergistic quadruple regimens. Future research directions include identifying predictive biomarkers beyond histology to better select patients who will benefit most from anti-angiogenic combinations. Additionally, investigating novel anti-angiogenic agents and their combinations with newer immunotherapeutic strategies, such as bispecific antibodies or antibody-drug conjugates, may further expand the utility of this treatment modality.

6. Chimeric Antigen Receptor (CAR)-T-Cell Therapy for NSCLC

Chimeric antigen receptor (CAR)-T-cell therapy is a promising and novel strategy for the treatment of non-small-cell lung cancer (NSCLC). While anti-CD19 CAR-T cells have been approved for hematological malignancies, their application to solid tumors like NSCLC is still in development. The therapy involves genetically engineering T cells to express a CAR that specifically recognizes and binds to tumor-associated antigens (TAAs). Despite their potential, the clinical application of CAR-T cells in NSCLC faces significant challenges. These include the scarcity of truly tumor-specific antigens, an immunosuppressive tumor microenvironment, poor infiltration of CAR-T cells into tumor tissue, and the risk of tumor antigen escape. Additionally, toxicities such as cytokine release syndrome (CRS), neurological toxicity, and on-target/off-tumor effects—where CAR-T cells attack healthy tissue expressing the same antigen—remain major safety concerns [60]. Current research is focused on identifying suitable antigens to target in NSCLC. The most commonly targeted antigens in clinical trials include EGFR, mesothelin (MSLN), mucin 1 (MUC1), prostate stem cell antigen (PSCA), carcinoembryonic antigen (CEA), and programmed death-ligand 1 (PD-L1).

Several clinical trials have explored these targets. Anti-EGFR CAR-T cells have shown specific cytolytic activity against EGFR-positive tumor cells in preclinical studies. A phase I trial (NCT04153799) evaluating anti-EGFR CAR-T cells in advanced NSCLC patients reported that two out of eleven patients achieved a partial response, while five had stable disease for eight months. Anti-MSLN CAR-T cells are also being tested, and preliminary results demonstrate the rationale for their use, though some trials have been terminated due to slow patient enrollment (NCT01583686). For antigens like MUC1 and PSCA, ongoing studies are assessing the safety and efficacy of CAR-T cells for advanced solid tumors, including NSCLC (NCT02587689 and NCT03198052) [60]. A preclinical model indicated that a third-generation anti-PSCA CAR-T cell delayed tumor development. Furthermore, anti-CEA CAR-T cell therapies are in phase I trials to evaluate their safety and efficacy in lung cancer patients who are CEA-positive (NCT02349724 and NCT04348643). Researchers are also investigating anti-PD-L1 CAR-T cell therapy as a novel strategy, as PD-L1 is expressed on both tumor and stromal cells. Early phase I studies are underway to determine the safety and engraftment potential of these cells (NCT03060343, NCT03330834). Similarly, anti-ROR1 CAR-T cells are being tested for their anti-tumor effects in advanced ROR1-positive, stage IV NSCLC patients (NCT02706392). The article also notes that while a trial for anti-HER2 CAR-T cells was withdrawn due to safety considerations, this antigen remains a potential therapeutic target. While CAR-T therapy for NSCLC is still in its early stages, it has yielded promising preliminary results in both preclinical and clinical settings. Continued research is essential to overcome current challenges and realize its full therapeutic potential.

7. Bispecific Antibodies for NSCLC

Bispecific antibodies represent a transformative and highly relevant innovation in treating NSCLC. These new therapies effectively highlight a paradigm shift, moving beyond the single-target approach of conventional treatments [61]. A particular emphasis is placed on the transformative impact of amivantamab, an epidermal growth factor receptor (EGFR)/mesenchymal–epithelial transition factor (MET)-targeting antibody [62]. This therapy has revolutionized the treatment landscape for patients with EGFR exon 20 insertion mutations—a patient population that has historically shown poor response to standard tyrosine kinase inhibitors. The inclusion of other emerging agents, such as zenocutuzumab for tumors with neuregulin 1 fusions, further illustrates the expanding utility of bispecific antibodies in addressing specific, previously untreatable oncogenic drivers [62]. By synthesizing key data and recent approvals, it is clear that these agents are addressing significant unmet clinical needs and shaping future treatment strategies. Beyond the discussion of clinical efficacy, the focus is on the "real-world" aspects of integrating these novel drugs. A much-needed framework is provided for managing the unique spectrum of on-target toxicities, including dermatologic side effects and infusion-related reactions. The practical guidance offered is invaluable, ensuring that the promise of these therapies can be realized in everyday practice without compromising patient safety and well-being. Furthermore, consideration of broader patient-centered issues, such as quality-of-life outcomes and financial toxicity, sets this review apart [63]. The exploration of subcutaneous formulations as a means to improve patient adherence and convenience is a forward-thinking and crucial point for therapies that require long-term administration. This thoughtful approach ensures the content is not just a summary of clinical data, but a pragmatic tool for enhancing patient care.

The clinical application of bispecific antibodies is a significant and timely contribution to the field of thoracic oncology. It provides a balanced and thorough account of these therapies, celebrating their clinical successes while offering a realistic perspective on the challenges of their implementation. The strength of this work lies in its ability to bridge the gap between academic innovation and practical, patient-focused care. It will serve as an essential reference for clinicians as the pipeline of bispecific antibodies continues to expand and these treatments become more integrated into standard practice.

8. Alternative Medicine

While some investigations have explored the role of traditional and alternative medicine in non-small-cell lung cancer (NSCLC) management, it is crucial to maintain a cautious perspective and avoid overstating the clinical value of these approaches when used alongside established pharmacological treatments. The current evidence base, while showing some promise, requires careful interpretation.

Traditional Chinese Medicine (TCM) has been investigated for potential benefits, with some reports suggesting positive effects for chronic pain when used either alone or as a supplementary therapy [64–66]. A study by Jiang et al. indicated that patients who received TCM alone experienced effects on time to progression and overall survival that were reportedly similar to those of chemotherapy [67]. Additionally, a separate study by Li et al. suggested that prophylactic TCM might potentially help reduce the incidence of grade 3 skin toxicity [68]. There are also reports that TCM, whether as a stand-alone therapy or in combination with conventional treatments like immunotherapy, chemotherapy, radiotherapy, targeted therapy, and surgery, has been associated with improved patient outcomes for NSCLC.

These findings, however, should be viewed with a critical eye. While they hint at areas for further exploration, they do not yet definitively establish the role of TCM within the standard of care. To confirm these potential benefits, more rigorous, large-scale clinical trials are needed to validate its safety and effectiveness in improving patient outcomes [69].

9. Emerging Treatments

Fascinating novel molecules have shown potential in the ongoing fight towards NSCLC. Over many years, TKIs, which target oncogenic driver mutations, have improved in efficacy and addressed drug resistance [70]. Moreover, immune checkpoint inhibiting drugs remain vital for treating NSCLCs that lack particular identifiable genetic alterations [71]. Likewise, a study conducted by Hayashi et al. reported that a combination of liquid immune components could pinpoint individuals who are anticipated to be responsive to PD-1/PD-L1 inhibition due to terminal depletion of antitumor immunity, and therefore, this combination might be able to better predict patient response to NSCLC [72]. Another recent study reported that trophoblast cell surface antigen 2 (TROP2) expression performs a crucial role in the main resistance to PD-L1 inhibition in NSCLC, and this could help in identifying patients with NSCLC who might benefit from a combination of immunotherapy and an anti-TROP2 drug [73].

Cancer-associated thrombosis (CAT) is a significant thrombotic event in cancer patients [74]. Recent research has investigated the association between thromboembolic events and immune checkpoint inhibitor therapies in NSCLC patients, and revealed that the probability of thrombosis among NSCLC is not insignificant [75]. This detection could provide a potential insight as regards developing a novel NSCLC therapy approach, as well as its diagnostic instruments, and subsequently enhance NSCLC patient outcomes. Therefore, more investigation is warranted to explore the key mechanism factor(s) underlying the association between cancer, hemostasis, and immune response in the environment of immune checkpoint inhibitor treatments. Nevertheless, discovering predictive biomarkers to customize therapies, overcome resistance, reduce costs, and offer appropriate cancer treatment availability remains an ongoing challenge.

10. Conclusions

Effective therapy for non-small-cell lung cancer (NSCLC) remains a significant challenge, despite the pivotal role of immune checkpoint inhibitors and molecular targeted therapies. The limitations of these treatments, particularly the development of drug resistance, necessitate a focus on several key research priorities to enhance patient outcomes. A central research priority is to understand and address the mechanisms of both primary and acquired drug resistance. This requires investigating why some patients fail to respond to initial therapies and why others eventually relapse. The treatment landscape is being rapidly reshaped by novel therapeutic modalities. Antibody-drug conjugates (ADCs) have emerged as a powerful class of drugs, merging the precision of monoclonal antibodies with the potency of cytotoxic payloads to target specific tumor antigens like HER2, TROP2, and HER3, offering new options for heavily pre-treated patients. Similarly, anti-angiogenic agents continue to play a crucial role, particularly in synergistic combinations with immunotherapy and chemotherapy, as evidenced by regimens like atezolizumab–bevacizumab–carboplatin–paclitaxel, which improve survival in selected patient populations. Beyond these, cellular therapies, such as CAR-T cells targeting antigens like EGFR, MSLN, and PD-L1, represent a frontier in personalized medicine, though their application in solid tumors like NSCLC requires overcoming significant challenges related to the tumor microenvironment and toxicity. Furthermore, bispecific antibodies are demonstrating transformative potential by engaging multiple targets simultaneously; amivantamab, targeting EGFR and MET, has revolutionized care for patients with EGFR exon 20 insertion mutations, highlighting a shift towards addressing previously untreatable oncogenic drivers. Advancing personalized medicine in NSCLC depends on identifying more reliable predictive biomarkers for all these therapies. While PD-L1 expression and genetic mutations are useful indicators, they do not consistently predict treatment response. Future research should aim to discover and validate a broader range of biomarkers to allow for more precise patient selection, ensuring that individuals receive the most appropriate therapy while minimizing unnecessary exposure to ineffective treatments.

Finally, a key research priority is the seamless integration of these novel therapeutic modalities—including ADCs, anti-angiogenics, cellular therapies, and bispecific antibodies—into existing and new treatment regimens. This includes exploring their use in combination with each other and with conventional strategies like chemotherapy, radiotherapy, and surgery. By thoughtfully combining these innovative approaches, clinicians can create more comprehensive and personalized treatment plans, ultimately leading to more effective NSCLC management and improved patient outcomes.

Funding: This research received no external funding.

Acknowledgments: The author would like to thank the Deanship of Scientific Research at Shaqra University for supporting this work.

Conflicts of Interest: The authors declare no conflicts of interest.

References

1. Shirley, M. Dacomitinib: First Global Approval. *Drugs* **2018**, *78*, 1947–1953. [CrossRef] [PubMed]
2. Passaro, A.; Mok, T.; Peters, S.; Popat, S.; Ahn, M.J.; de Marinis, F. Recent Advances on the Role of EGFR Tyrosine Kinas Inhibitors in the Management of NSCLC with Uncommon, Non Exon 20 Insertions, EGFR Mutations. *J. Thorac. Oncol.* **2021**, *1* 764–773. [CrossRef]
3. Wu, S.G.; Yu, C.J.; Yang, J.C.; Shih, J.Y. The effectiveness of afatinib in patients with lung adenocarcinoma harboring comple epidermal growth factor receptor mutation. *Ther. Adv. Med. Oncol.* **2020**, *12*, 1–17. [CrossRef]
4. Niu, Z.X.; Wang, Y.T.; Lu, N.; Sun, J.F.; Nie, P.; Herdewijn, P. Advances of clinically approved small-molecule drugs for th treatment of non-small cell lung cancer. *Eur. J. Med. Chem.* **2023**, *261*, 115868. [CrossRef]
5. Shah, R.R.; Shah, D.R. Safety and Tolerability of Epidermal Growth Factor Receptor (EGFR) Tyrosine Kinase Inhibitors i Oncology. *Drug Saf.* **2019**, *42*, 181–198. [CrossRef]
6. Nishio, M.; Kato, T.; Niho, S.; Yamamoto, N.; Takahashi, T.; Nogami, N.; Kaneda, H.; Fujita, Y.; Wilner, K.; Yoshida, M.; et a Safety and efficacy of first-line dacomitinib in Japanese patients with advanced non-small cell lung cancer. *Cancer Sci.* **2020**, *11* 1724–1738. [CrossRef]
7. Jung, H.A.; Park, S.; Lee, S.H.; Ahn, J.S.; Ahn, M.J.; Sun, J.M. Dacomitinib in EGFR-mutant non-small-cell lung cancer with brai metastasis: A single-arm, phase II study. *ESMO Open* **2023**, *8*, 102068. [CrossRef]
8. Iwasaku, M.; Uchino, J.; Yamada, T.; Chihara, Y.; Shimamoto, T.; Tamiya, N.; Kaneko, Y.; Kiyomi, F.; Takayama, K. Rationale an design of a phase II study to evaluate prophylactic treatment of dacomitinib-induced dermatologic adverse events in epiderma growth factor receptor-mutated advanced non-small cell lung cancer (SPIRAL-Daco study). *Transl. Lung Cancer Res.* **2019**, *8* 519–523. [CrossRef] [PubMed]
9. Tan, W.; Giri, N.; Quinn, S.; Wilner, K.; Parivar, K. Evaluation of the potential effect of dacomitinib, an EGFR tyrosine kinas inhibitor, on ECG parameters in patients with advanced non-small cell lung cancer. *Investig. New Drugs* **2020**, *38*, 874–88 [CrossRef] [PubMed]
10. Mok, T.S.; Cheng, Y.; Zhou, X.; Lee, K.H.; Nakagawa, K.; Niho, S.; Chawla, A.; Rosell, R.; Corral, J.; Migliorino, M.R.; et a Updated Overall Survival in a Randomized Study Comparing Dacomitinib with Gefitinib as First-Line Treatment in Patient with Advanced Non-Small-Cell Lung Cancer and EGFR-Activating Mutations. *Drugs* **2021**, *81*, 257–266. [CrossRef] [PubMed]

Pu, X.; Li, J.; Zhang, B.; Zhang, J.; TS, K.M.; Nakagawa, K.; Rosell, R.; Cheng, Y.; Zhou, X.; Miglorino, M.R.; et al. Efficacy in patients with EGFR-positive non-small-cell lung cancer treated with dacomitinib who had skin adverse events: Post hoc analyses from ARCHER 1050. *Future Oncol.* **2024**, *20*, 2971–2982. [CrossRef]

Cheng, Y.; Mok, T.S.; Zhou, X.; Lu, S.; Zhou, Q.; Zhou, J.; Du, Y.; Yu, P.; Liu, X.; Hu, C.; et al. Safety and efficacy of first-line dacomitinib in Asian patients with EGFR mutation-positive non-small cell lung cancer: Results from a randomized, open-label, phase 3 trial (ARCHER 1050). *Lung Cancer* **2021**, *154*, 176–185. [CrossRef]

Choo, J.R.; Soo, R.A. Lorlatinib for the treatment of ALK-positive metastatic non-small cell lung cancer. *Expert. Rev. Anticancer. Ther.* **2020**, *20*, 233–240. [CrossRef]

Goto, Y.; Shukuya, T.; Murata, A.; Kikkawa, H.; Emir, B.; Wiltshire, R.; Miura, S. Real-world therapeutic effectiveness of lorlatinib after alectinib in Japanese patients with ALK-positive non-small-cell lung cancer. *Cancer Sci.* **2023**, *114*, 2560–2568. [CrossRef]

Solomon, B.J.; Liu, G.; Felip, E.; Mok, T.S.K.; Soo, R.A.; Mazieres, J.; Shaw, A.T.; de Marinis, F.; Goto, Y.; Wu, Y.L.; et al. Lorlatinib Versus Crizotinib in Patients with Advanced ALK-Positive Non-Small Cell Lung Cancer: 5-Year Outcomes from the Phase III CROWN Study. *J. Clin. Oncol.* **2024**, *42*, 3400–3409. [CrossRef]

Murakami, Y.; Kawashima, Y.; Chiba, S.; Hara, S.; Yamazaki, Y.; Doman, T.; Saito, S.; Odaka, T.; Ogasawara, T.; Shimizu, H.; et al. Successful application of lorlatinib in a 23-year-old patient with anaplastic lymphoma kinase (ALK)-positive lung cancer and multiple brain metastases. *Cancer Rep.* **2024**, *7*, e1981. [CrossRef]

Taniguchi, H.; Akagi, K.; Dotsu, Y.; Yamada, T.; Ono, S.; Imamura, E.; Gyotoku, H.; Takemoto, S.; Yamaguchi, H.; Sen, T.; et al. Pan-HER inhibitors overcome lorlatinib resistance caused by NRG1/HER3 activation in ALK-rearranged lung cancer. *Cancer Sci.* **2023**, *114*, 164–173. [CrossRef]

Syed, Y.Y. Lorlatinib: First Global Approval. *Drugs* **2019**, *79*, 93–98. [CrossRef]

Naik, J.; Beavers, N.; Nilsson, F.O.L.; Iadeluca, L.; Lowry, C. Cost—Effectiveness of Lorlatinib in First-Line Treatment of Adult Patients with Anaplastic Lymphoma Kinase (ALK)—Positive Non—Small—Cell Lung Cancer in Sweden. *Appl. Health Econ. Health Policy* **2023**, *21*, 661–672. [CrossRef]

Shaw, A.T.; Felip, E.; Bauer, T.M.; Besse, B.; Navarro, A.; Postel-Vinay, S.; Gainor, J.F.; Johnson, M.; Dietrich, J.; James, L.P.; et al. Lorlatinib in non-small-cell lung cancer with ALK or ROS1 rearrangement: An international, multicentre, open-label, single-arm first-in-man phase 1 trial. *Lancet Oncol.* **2017**, *18*, 1590–1599. [CrossRef]

Solomon, B.J.; Besse, B.; Bauer, T.M.; Felip, E.; Soo, R.A.; Camidge, D.R.; Chiari, R.; Bearz, A.; Lin, C.C.; Gadgeel, S.M.; et al. Lorlatinib in patients with ALK-positive non-small-cell lung cancer: Results from a global phase 2 study. *Lancet Oncol.* **2018**, *19*, 1654–1667. [CrossRef]

Goldsmith, K.C.; Park, J.R.; Kayser, K.; Malvar, J.; Chi, Y.Y.; Groshen, S.G.; Villablanca, J.G.; Krytska, K.; Lai, L.M.; Acharya, P.T.; et al. Lorlatinib with or without chemotherapy in ALK-driven refractory/relapsed neuroblastoma: Phase 1 trial results. *Nat. Med.* **2023**, *29*, 1092–1102. [CrossRef]

Lu, S.; Zhou, Q.; Liu, X.; Du, Y.; Fan, Y.; Cheng, Y.; Fang, J.; Lu, Y.; Huang, C.; Zhou, J.; et al. Lorlatinib for Previously Treated ALK-Positive Advanced NSCLC: Primary Efficacy and Safety from a Phase 2 Study in People's Republic of China. *J. Thorac. Oncol.* **2022**, *17*, 816–826. [CrossRef]

Felip, E.; Shaw, A.T.; Bearz, A.; Camidge, D.R.; Solomon, B.J.; Bauman, J.R.; Bauer, T.M.; Peters, S.; Toffalorio, F.; Abbattista, A.; et al. Intracranial and extracranial efficacy of lorlatinib in patients with ALK-positive non-small-cell lung cancer previously treated with second-generation ALK TKIs. *Ann. Oncol.* **2021**, *32*, 620–630. [CrossRef]

Ou, S.I.; Solomon, B.J.; Shaw, A.T.; Gadgeel, S.M.; Besse, B.; Soo, R.A.; Abbattista, A.; Toffalorio, F.; Wiltshire, R.; Bearz, A. Continuation of Lorlatinib in ALK-Positive NSCLC Beyond Progressive Disease. *J. Thorac. Oncol.* **2022**, *17*, 568–577. [CrossRef]

Stewart, R.; Morrow, M.; Hammond, S.A.; Mulgrew, K.; Marcus, D.; Poon, E.; Watkins, A.; Mullins, S.; Chodorge, M.; Andrews, J.; et al. Identification and Characterization of MEDI4736, an Antagonistic Anti-PD-L1 Monoclonal Antibody. *Cancer Immunol. Res.* **2015**, *3*, 1052–1062. [CrossRef]

Solomon, B.J.; Bauer, T.M.; Mok, T.S.K.; Liu, G.; Mazieres, J.; de Marinis, F.; Goto, Y.; Kim, D.W.; Wu, Y.L.; Jassem, J.; et al. Efficacy and safety of first-line lorlatinib versus crizotinib in patients with advanced, ALK-positive non-small-cell lung cancer: Updated analysis of data from the phase 3, randomised, open-label CROWN study. *Lancet Respir. Med.* **2023**, *11*, 354–366. [CrossRef]

Al-Salama, Z.T. Durvalumab: A Review in Extensive-Stage SCLC. *Target. Oncol.* **2021**, *16*, 857–864. [CrossRef]

AstraZeneca. MFINZI (Durvalumab): EU Summary of Product Characteristics. 2021. Available online: https://www.ema.europa.eu/en/documents/product-information/imfinzi-epar-product-information_en.pdf (accessed on 25 July 2025).

Banna, G.L.; Cantale, O.; Bersanelli, M.; Del Re, M.; Friedlaender, A.; Cortellini, A.; Addeo, A. Are anti-PD1 and anti-PD-L1 alike? The non-small-cell lung cancer paradigm. *Oncol. Rev.* **2020**, *14*, 490. [CrossRef]

Ando, K.; Manabe, R.; Kishino, Y.; Kusumoto, S.; Yamaoka, T.; Tanaka, A.; Ohmori, T.; Ohnishi, T.; Sagara, H. Comparative Efficacy and Safety of Anti-PD-1/PD-L1 Immune Checkpoint Inhibitors for Refractory or Relapsed Advanced Non-Small-Cell Lung Cancer—A Systematic Review and Network Meta-Analysis. *Cancers* **2020**, *13*, 52. [CrossRef]

32. Ding, J.; Liu, Z.; Ning, J.; Sun, N. Safety of PD-L1 inhibitors versus PD-1 inhibitors in the treatment of lung cancer: A systemat review and network meta-analysis. *Expert. Rev. Anticancer. Ther.* **2025**, *25*, 259–267. [CrossRef]
33. Johnson, M.L.; Cho, B.C.; Luft, A.; Alatorre-Alexander, J.; Geater, S.L.; Laktionov, K.; Kim, S.W.; Ursol, G.; Hussein, M.; Lim, F.L et al. Durvalumab with or Without Tremelimumab in Combination with Chemotherapy as First-Line Therapy for Metastati Non-Small-Cell Lung Cancer: The Phase III POSEIDON Study. *J. Clin. Oncol.* **2023**, *41*, 1213–1227. [CrossRef]
34. Heymach, J.V.; Harpole, D.; Mitsudomi, T.; Taube, J.M.; Galffy, G.; Hochmair, M.; Winder, T.; Zukov, R.; Garbaos, G.; Gao, S.; et a Perioperative Durvalumab for Resectable Non-Small-Cell Lung Cancer. *N. Engl. J. Med.* **2023**, *389*, 1672–1684. [CrossRef]
35. Rothschild, S.I.; Zippelius, A.; Eboulet, E.I.; Savic Prince, S.; Betticher, D.; Bettini, A.; Früh, M.; Joerger, M.; Lardinois, D.; Gelpk H.; et al. SAKK 16/14: Durvalumab in Addition to Neoadjuvant Chemotherapy in Patients with Stage IIIA(N2) Non-Small-Ce Lung Cancer—A Multicenter Single-Arm Phase II Trial. *J. Clin. Oncol.* **2021**, *39*, 2872–2880. [CrossRef]
36. AstraZeneca. IMFINZI™ (Durvalumab) Significantly Reduces the Risk of Disease Worsening or Death in the Phase III PACIFI Trial for Stage III Unresectable Lung Cancer. Available online: https://www.astrazeneca.com/media-centre/press-releases/201 /imfinzi-significantly-reduces-the-risk-of-disease-worsening-or-death-in-the-phase-iii-pacific-trial-for-stage-iii-unresectabl lung-cancer-12052017.html#! (accessed on 25 July 2025).
37. AstraZeneca. IMFINZI®® (Durvalumab) Injection, for Intravenous Use: US Prescribing Information. Available online: http //www.accessdata.fda.gov/drugsatfda_docs/label/2021/761069s029lbl.pdf (accessed on 25 July 2025).
38. Faivre-Finn, C.; Vicente, D.; Kurata, T.; Planchard, D.; Paz-Ares, L.; Vansteenkiste, J.F.; Spigel, D.R.; Garassino, M.C.; Reck, M Senan, S.; et al. Four-Year Survival with Durvalumab After Chemoradiotherapy in Stage III NSCLC—An Update from th PACIFIC Trial. *J. Thorac. Oncol.* **2021**, *16*, 860–867. [CrossRef]
39. Besse, B.; Pons-Tostivint, E.; Park, K.; Hartl, S.; Forde, P.M.; Hochmair, M.J.; Awad, M.M.; Thomas, M.; Goss, G.; Wheatley-Pric P.; et al. Biomarker-directed targeted therapy plus durvalumab in advanced non-small-cell lung cancer: A phase 2 umbrella tri *Nat. Med.* **2024**, *30*, 716–729. [CrossRef]
40. Garassino, M.C.; Mazieres, J.; Reck, M.; Chouaid, C.; Bischoff, H.; Reinmuth, N.; Cove-Smith, L.; Mansy, T.; Cortinovis, D Migliorino, M.R.; et al. Durvalumab After Sequential Chemoradiotherapy in Stage III, Unresectable NSCLC: The Phase PACIFIC-6 Trial. *J. Thorac. Oncol.* **2022**, *17*, 1415–1427. [CrossRef]
41. Reck, M.; Nadal, E.; Girard, N.; Filippi, A.R.; Martin, L.W.; Gay, C.M.; Petersen, C.; Gale, D.; Emeribe, U.A.; Georgoulia, N et al. MDT-BRIDGE: Neoadjuvant Durvalumab Plus Chemotherapy Followed by Either Surgery and Adjuvant Durvalumab o Chemoradiotherapy and Consolidation Durvalumab in Resectable or Borderline-resectable Stage IIB-IIIB NSCLC. *Clin. Lun Cancer* **2024**, *25*, 587–593.e583. [CrossRef]
42. Schoenfeld, J.D.; Giobbie-Hurder, A.; Ranasinghe, S.; Kao, K.Z.; Lako, A.; Tsuji, J.; Liu, Y.; Brennick, R.C.; Gentzler, R.D.; Lee, C et al. Durvalumab plus tremelimumab alone or in combination with low-dose or hypofractionated radiotherapy in metastati non-small-cell lung cancer refractory to previous PD(L)-1 therapy: An open-label, multicentre, randomised, phase 2 trial. *Lanc Oncol.* **2022**, *23*, 279–291. [CrossRef]
43. De Ruysscher, D.; Ramalingam, S.; Urbanic, J.; Gerber, D.E.; Tan, D.S.W.; Cai, J.; Li, A.; Peters, S. CheckMate 73L: A Phase Study Comparing Nivolumab Plus Concurrent Chemoradiotherapy Followed by Nivolumab with or Without Ipilimumab Versu Concurrent Chemoradiotherapy Followed by Durvalumab for Previously Untreated, Locally Advanced Stage III Non-Small-Ce Lung Cancer. *Clin. Lung Cancer* **2022**, *23*, e264–e268. [CrossRef]
44. Leonetti, A.; Sharma, S.; Minari, R.; Perego, P.; Giovannetti, E.; Tiseo, M. Resistance mechanisms to osimertinib in EGFR-mutate non-small cell lung cancer. *Br. J. Cancer* **2019**, *121*, 725–737. [CrossRef]
45. Liu, Q.; Luo, Y.; Li, Z.; Chen, C.; Fang, L. Structural modifications on indole and pyrimidine rings of osimertinib lead to hig selectivity towards L858R/T790M double mutant enzyme and potent antitumor activity. *Bioorg Med. Chem.* **2021**, *36*, 11609 [CrossRef]
46. Papadimitrakopoulou, V.A.; Mok, T.S.; Han, J.Y.; Ahn, M.J.; Delmonte, A.; Ramalingam, S.S.; Kim, S.W.; Shepherd, F.A.; Laskin, J He, Y.; et al. Osimertinib versus platinum-pemetrexed for patients with EGFR T790M advanced NSCLC and progression on prior EGFR-tyrosine kinase inhibitor: AURA3 overall survival analysis. *Ann. Oncol.* **2020**, *31*, 1536–1544. [CrossRef]
47. Ramalingam, S.S.; Vansteenkiste, J.; Planchard, D.; Cho, B.C.; Gray, J.E.; Ohe, Y.; Zhou, C.; Reungwetwattana, T.; Cheng, Y Chewaskulyong, B.; et al. Overall Survival with Osimertinib in Untreated, EGFR-Mutated Advanced NSCLC. *N. Engl. J. Me* **2020**, *382*, 41–50. [CrossRef]
48. Soria, J.C.; Ohe, Y.; Vansteenkiste, J.; Reungwetwattana, T.; Chewaskulyong, B.; Lee, K.H.; Dechaphunkul, A.; Imamura, F Nogami, N.; Kurata, T.; et al. Osimertinib in Untreated EGFR-Mutated Advanced Non-Small-Cell Lung Cancer. *N. Engl. J. Me* **2018**, *378*, 113–125. [CrossRef]
49. Okuma, Y.; Kubota, K.; Shimokawa, M.; Hashimoto, K.; Kawashima, Y.; Sakamoto, T.; Wakui, H.; Murakami, S.; Okishio, K Hayashihara, K.; et al. First-Line Osimertinib for Previously Untreated Patients with NSCLC and Uncommon EGFR Mutation The UNICORN Phase 2 Nonrandomized Clinical Trial. *JAMA Oncol.* **2024**, *10*, 43–51. [CrossRef]

Herbst, R.S.; Wu, Y.L.; John, T.; Grohe, C.; Majem, M.; Wang, J.; Kato, T.; Goldman, J.W.; Laktionov, K.; Kim, S.W.; et al. Adjuvant Osimertinib for Resected EGFR-Mutated Stage IB-IIIA Non-Small-Cell Lung Cancer: Updated Results from the Phase III Randomized ADAURA Trial. *J. Clin. Oncol.* **2023**, *41*, 1830–1840. [CrossRef]

Lu, S.; Kato, T.; Dong, X.; Ahn, M.J.; Quang, L.V.; Soparattanapaisarn, N.; Inoue, T.; Wang, C.L.; Huang, M.; Yang, J.C.; et al. Osimertinib after Chemoradiotherapy in Stage III EGFR-Mutated NSCLC. *N. Engl. J. Med.* **2024**, *391*, 585–597. [CrossRef]

Planchard, D.; Jänne, P.A.; Cheng, Y.; Yang, J.C.; Yanagitani, N.; Kim, S.W.; Sugawara, S.; Yu, Y.; Fan, Y.; Geater, S.L.; et al. Osimertinib with or without Chemotherapy in EGFR-Mutated Advanced NSCLC. *N. Engl. J. Med.* **2023**, *389*, 1935–1948. [CrossRef]

Remon, J.; Besse, B.; Aix, S.P.; Callejo, A.; Al-Rabi, K.; Bernabe, R.; Greillier, L.; Majem, M.; Reguart, N.; Monnet, I.; et al. Overall Survival from the EORTC LCG-1613 APPLE Trial of Osimertinib Versus Gefitinib Followed by Osimertinib in Advanced EGFR-Mutant Non-Small-Cell Lung Cancer. *J. Clin. Oncol.* **2024**, *42*, 1350–1356. [CrossRef]

Drago, J.Z.; Modi, S.; Chandarlapaty, S. Unlocking the potential of antibody-drug conjugates for cancer therapy. *Nat. Rev. Clin. Oncol.* **2021**, *18*, 327–344. [CrossRef]

Li, B.T.; Smit, E.F.; Goto, Y.; Nakagawa, K.; Udagawa, H.; Mazières, J.; Nagasaka, M.; Bazhenova, L.; Saltos, A.N.; Felip, E.; et al. Trastuzumab Deruxtecan in HER2-Mutant Non-Small-Cell Lung Cancer. *N. Engl. J. Med.* **2022**, *386*, 241–251. [CrossRef]

Li, B.T.; Shen, R.; Buonocore, D.; Olah, Z.T.; Ni, A.; Ginsberg, M.S.; Ulaner, G.A.; Offin, M.; Feldman, D.; Hembrough, T.; et al. Ado-Trastuzumab Emtansine for Patients with HER2-Mutant Lung Cancers: Results from a Phase II Basket Trial. *J. Clin. Oncol.* **2018**, *36*, 2532–2537. [CrossRef]

Ahn, M.J.; Tanaka, K.; Paz-Ares, L.; Cornelissen, R.; Girard, N.; Pons-Tostivint, E.; Vicente Baz, D.; Sugawara, S.; Cobo, M.; Pérol, M.; et al. Datopotamab Deruxtecan Versus Docetaxel for Previously Treated Advanced or Metastatic Non-Small Cell Lung Cancer: The Randomized, Open-Label Phase III TROPION-Lung01 Study. *J. Clin. Oncol.* **2025**, *43*, 260–272. [CrossRef]

Yu, H.A.; Goto, Y.; Hayashi, H.; Felip, E.; Chih-Hsin Yang, J.; Reck, M.; Yoh, K.; Lee, S.H.; Paz-Ares, L.; Besse, B.; et al. HERTHENA-Lung01, a Phase II Trial of Patritumab Deruxtecan (HER3-DXd) in Epidermal Growth Factor Receptor-Mutated Non-Small-Cell Lung Cancer After Epidermal Growth Factor Receptor Tyrosine Kinase Inhibitor Therapy and Platinum-Based Chemotherapy. *J. Clin. Oncol.* **2023**, *41*, 5363–5375. [CrossRef]

Socinski, M.A.; Nishio, M.; Jotte, R.M.; Cappuzzo, F.; Orlandi, F.; Stroyakovskiy, D.; Nogami, N.; Rodríguez-Abreu, D.; Moro-Sibilot, D.; Thomas, C.A.; et al. IMpower150 Final Overall Survival Analyses for Atezolizumab Plus Bevacizumab and Chemotherapy in First-Line Metastatic Nonsquamous NSCLC. *J. Thorac. Oncol.* **2021**, *16*, 1909–1924. [CrossRef]

Qu, J.; Mei, Q.; Chen, L.; Zhou, J. Chimeric antigen receptor (CAR)-T-cell therapy in non-small-cell lung cancer (NSCLC): Current status and future perspectives. *Cancer Immunol. Immunother.* **2021**, *70*, 619–631. [CrossRef]

Carlisle, J.W.; Wolner, Z.; Pannu, S.; Mitchell, C.; Hsu, M.; Aijaz, A.; Johnson, M.; Naqash, A.R. Bispecific Antibodies in Non-Small Cell Lung Cancer: From Targeted Innovation to Real-World Integration. *Am. Soc. Clin. Oncol. Educ. Book* **2025**, *45*, e472792. [CrossRef]

Frentzas, S.; Austria Mislang, A.R.; Lemech, C.; Nagrial, A.; Underhill, C.; Wang, W.; Wang, Z.M.; Li, B.; Xia, Y.; Coward, J.I.G. Phase 1a dose escalation study of ivonescimab (AK112/SMT112), an anti-PD-1/VEGF—A bispecific antibody, in patients with advanced solid tumors. *J. Immunother. Cancer* **2024**, *12*, e008037. [CrossRef]

Wang, F.; Wei, X.; Zheng, Y.; Wang, J.; Ying, J.; Chen, X.; Luo, S.; Luo, H.; Yu, X.; Chen, B.; et al. Safety, Pharmacokinetics, and Pharmacodynamics Evaluation of Ivonescimab, a Novel Bispecific Antibody Targeting PD-1 and VEGF, in Chinese Patients with Advanced Solid Tumors. *Cancer Med.* **2025**, *14*, e70653. [CrossRef]

Qian, Z.; Wang, G.Y.; Henning, M.; Chen, Y. Measurements of traditional Chinese medicine health literacy regarding chronic pain: A scoping review. *BMC Complement. Med. Ther.* **2024**, *24*, 395. [CrossRef]

Li, S.H.; Li, L.; Yang, R.N.; Liang, S.D. Compounds of traditional Chinese medicine and neuropathic pain. *Chin. J. Nat. Med.* **2020**, *18*, 28–35. [CrossRef] [PubMed]

Wei, Z.; Chen, J.; Zuo, F.; Guo, J.; Sun, X.; Liu, D.; Liu, C. Traditional Chinese Medicine has great potential as candidate drugs for lung cancer: A review. *J. Ethnopharmacol.* **2023**, *300*, 115748. [CrossRef]

Jiang, Y.; Liu, L.S.; Shen, L.P.; Han, Z.F.; Jian, H.; Liu, J.X.; Xu, L.; Li, H.G.; Tian, J.H.; Mao, Z.J. Traditional Chinese Medicine treatment as maintenance therapy in advanced non-small-cell lung cancer: A randomized controlled trial. *Complement Ther. Med.* **2016**, *24*, 55–62. [CrossRef]

Li, Z.; Feiyue, Z.; Gaofeng, L. Traditional Chinese medicine and lung cancer—From theory to practice. *Biomed Pharmacother* **2021**, *137*, 111381. [CrossRef]

Chen, H.; Zheng, M.; Zhang, W.; Long, Y.; Xu, Y.; Yuan, M. Research Status of Mouse Models for Non-Small-Cell Lung Cancer (NSCLC) and Antitumor Therapy of Traditional Chinese Medicine (TCM) in Mouse Models. *Evid. Based Complement. Altern. Med.* **2022**, *2022*, 6404853. [CrossRef]

Meyer, M.L.; Fitzgerald, B.G.; Paz-Ares, L.; Cappuzzo, F.; Jänne, P.A.; Peters, S.; Hirsch, F.R. New promises and challenges in the treatment of advanced non-small-cell lung cancer. *Lancet* **2024**, *404*, 803–822. [CrossRef]

71. Ranjan, T.; Podder, V.; Margolin, K.; Velcheti, V.; Maharaj, A.; Ahluwalia, M.S. Immune Checkpoint Inhibitors in the Managemen of Brain Metastases from Non-Small Cell Lung Cancer: A Comprehensive Review of Current Trials, Guidelines and Futur Directions. *Cancers* **2024**, *16*, 3388. [CrossRef]
72. Hayashi, H.; Chamoto, K.; Hatae, R.; Kurosaki, T.; Togashi, Y.; Fukuoka, K.; Goto, M.; Chiba, Y.; Tomida, S.; Ota, T.; et al. Solubl immune checkpoint factors reflect exhaustion of antitumor immunity and response to PD-1 blockade. *J. Clin. Investig.* **2024** *134*, e168318. [CrossRef]
73. Bessede, A.; Peyraud, F.; Besse, B.; Cousin, S.; Cabart, M.; Chomy, F.; Rey, C.; Lara, O.; Odin, O.; Nafia, I.; et al. TROP2 Is Associated with Primary Resistance to Immune Checkpoint Inhibition in Patients with Advanced Non-Small Cell Lung Cance *Clin. Cancer Res.* **2024**, *30*, 779–785. [CrossRef]
74. Freitas-Dias, C.; Gonçalves, F.; Martins, F.; Lemos, I.; Gonçalves, L.G.; Serpa, J. Interaction between NSCLC Cells, CD8$^+$ T-Cell and Immune Checkpoint Inhibitors Potentiates Coagulation and Promotes Metabolic Remodeling-New Cues on CAT-VTE. *Cell* **2024**, *13*, 305. [CrossRef] [PubMed]
75. Benariba, M.A.; Hannachi, K.; Zhu, S.; Zhang, Y.; Wang, X.; Zhou, N. A liposome-based assay for cancer biomarker detection Exploring the correlation between platelet-derived microvesicles and NSCLC-associated miRNAs. *Nanoscale* **2024**, *16*, 22037–2204 [CrossRef]

Journal of
Clinical Medicine

MDPI

view

lexible Bronchoscopy and Non-Small-Cell Lung Cancer Staging: . Narrative Review of Modern Techniques for Optimized :linical Decision-Making

mona-Maria Roşu [1,2,†], Denisa Maria Mitroi [1], Oana Maria Catană [1], Viorel Biciușcă [3,*], Sorina Ionelia Stan [3], :atrice Mahler [2,4,†], Oana-Andreea Parliteanu [5,*], Adina Andreea Mirea [6] and Mara Amalia Bălteanu [2,7]

1 Doctoral School, University of Medicine and Pharmacy, 200349 Craiova, Romania; simona.vulpe1995@gmail.com (S.-M.R.); denisa_maria2@yahoo.com (D.M.M.); oana_cattana@yahoo.com (O.M.C.)

2 Department of Pneumology, "Marius Nasta" Institute for Pneumology, 050159 Bucharest, Romania; beatrice.mahler@umfcd.ro (B.M.); mara.balteanu@prof.utm.ro (M.A.B.)

3 Department of Internal Medicine, Faculty of Medicine, University of Medicine and Pharmacy of Craiova, 200349 Craiova, Romania; sorina_stan@icloud.com

4 Department of Pneumology Faculty of Medicine, University of Medicine and Pharmacy Carol Davila of Bucharest, 020021 Bucharest, Romania

5 Department of Pathophysiology, Faculty of Medicine, "Titu Maiorescu" University, 040051 Bucharest, Romania

6 Department of Oral-Dental Prevention, University of Medicine and Pharmacy, 200349 Craiova, Romania; adinaturcu14@yahoo.com

7 Department of Pneumology, Faculty of Medicine, "Titu Maiorescu" University, 040051 Bucharest, Romania

* Correspondence: biciuscaviorel@gmail.com (V.B.); oana.parliteanu@prof.utm.ro (O.-A.P.)

† These authors contributed equally to this work.

Abstract

Non-small-cell lung cancer (NSCLC) is a widespread and aggressive form of cancer, and in cases of its occurrence, accurate diagnosis and precise staging play a crucial role in determining treatment and estimating prognosis. Flexible bronchoscopy (FB) is a minimally invasive method used to assess the local and regional extent of the disease. FB facilitates the identification of endobronchial lesions and the collection of biopsy samples for histopathological diagnosis. It also enables the evaluation of regional lymph node involvement via advanced techniques such as endobronchial ultrasound with fine-needle aspiration (EBUS-TBNA). This method has high sensitivity and specificity, reducing the need for more invasive interventions like mediastinoscopy. The integration of endobronchial ultrasound (EBUS) has revolutionized NSCLC staging by providing detailed images and guiding biopsies of suspicious lymph nodes. Additionally, FB is valuable in staging the extent of primary tumor growth, providing critical information about the invasion of adjacent structures. In conclusion, FB, supported by advanced technologies, is important for the staging of NSCLC, improving medical practice and patient prognosis.

Keywords: flexible bronchoscopy; non-small-cell lung cancer; diagnosis; staging; EBUS-TBNA

1. Introduction

In 2020, lung cancer (LC) exceeded breast cancer in cancer mortality frequency among men in Europe, and it also accounted for about 12% of all new cancer diagnoses [1]. In Romania, LC constitutes a considerable public health issue, representing approximately

20% of deaths from cancer. Tragically, only 10% of the LC Romanian patients survived after the first 5 years, primarily due to late-stage detection [2]. NSCLC, which encompasses subtypes such as adenocarcinoma, squamous cell carcinoma, and large cell carcinoma, comprises approximately 85% of LC cases. However, less than one in three NSCLC patients are identified in the early stages, when the disease is still potentially treatable [3]. Given the overwhelming financial burden of lung cancer treatment, with the U.S. spending USD 1.5 billion on care in 2019, timely and accurate diagnosis is crucial both clinically and economically [4]. FB has become an essential, minimally invasive procedure for diagnosing and assessing lung cancer, offering vital insight into the local and regional extent of the disease. One of the primary challenges of this technique is the difficulty in obtaining biopsy samples from peripheral lesions using auxiliary instruments. Once these instruments pass the bronchoscope's tip, directing them to the target area becomes problematic. Locating lesions under fluoroscopy can be difficult, leading to a preference for alternative guidance techniques such as CT-guided bronchoscopy and EBUS. EBUS-TBNA has gained increasing use as a first-line diagnostic approach for centrally located lesions that lack endobronchial visibility and/or present adenopathy. This minimally invasive technique aids in both diagnosis and disease staging, and it is now recommended when adenopathy is detected on CT scans or when lymph nodes exhibit fluorodeoxyglucose (FDG) uptake on PET-CT [5]. The purpose of this article is to emphasize the importance of bronchoscopy in clinical practice, offering evidence that supports informed clinical decisions and contributes to better patient outcomes, ultimately advancing pulmonary oncology.

2. Methodology and Search Strategy

A structured and methodologically transparent literature review was performed to identify relevant studies on the use of FB, EBUS-TBNA, and other diagnostic modalities for staging of NSCLC. The databases searched included PubMed, Scopus, and Web of Science, covering publications from 2010 to 2024, and a total of 32 articles were included in the final analysis.

The search strategy combined the following keywords and Boolean operators: ("NSCLC staging" OR "lung cancer staging") AND ("flexible bronchoscopy" OR "EBUS-TBNA" OR "BAL" OR "mediastinoscopy" OR "PET/CT" OR "AI" OR "electromagnetic navigation bronchoscopy (ENB)") AND ("diagnostic accuracy" OR "sensitivity" OR "specificity"). Inclusion criteria encompassed original research articles, meta-analyses, and systematic reviews published in English, involving human subjects, and reporting diagnostic performance metrics such as sensitivity, specificity, positive and negative predictive values, or overall diagnostic yield. Only peer-reviewed studies were considered. Case reports or case series with fewer than 10 patients, the non-peer-reviewed literature, preclinical studies, animal models, and abstracts or editorials lacking original data were excluded from our analysis.

3. Flexible Bronchoscopy and Adjunct Techniques: The Role of BAL and Bronchial Brushing in NSCLC Evaluation

FB is indispensable for identifying endobronchial lesions, staging lung cancer, and assessing invasion of the trachea, bronchi, and adjacent structures to guide treatment. It helps differentiate between resectable and unresectable tumors, thereby influencing therapeutic decisions, and it is a minimally invasive method for diagnosing LC, considered the safest and most accessible technique for obtaining biopsy material, and the gold standard in diagnosing invasive and preinvasive malignant lesions of the airways. This technique is performed using a flexible fiber-optic bronchoscope introduced through the mouth or nose, allowing for direct visualization of the tracheobronchial tree. It is primarily employed for centrally located tumors, visible lesions, or when symptoms such as hemoptysis or airway obstruction suggest endobronchial involvement. The procedure is generally performed under local anesthesia and moderate sedation. FB employs various tools depending on lesion visibility and location. Biopsy forceps are typically used to obtain tissue samples from visible endobronchial tumors and involve taking 3–5 samples to improve diagnostic accuracy. This method has become the recommended approach for all patients with suspected lung cancer, presenting a sensitivity of approximately 88% for centrally located lesions and about 78% for peripheral lesions (ranging from 36% to 88% depending on the technique used). Additionally, FB enables proper surgical planning by assessing the surface, location, tumor extent, vocal cord mobility, and lumen of the airways [6]. Patients diagnosed at an early stage of the disease have a 5-year survival rate greater than 70%, confirming that early LC detection is essential for improving the odds of survival. Given that the early detection of lung cancer, followed by prompt initiation of treatment, can improve outcomes, considerable efforts have been made to overcome the limitations of FB in white light. Innovative bronchoscopic techniques, such as autofluorescence bronchoscopy (AFB) and narrow-band imaging (NBI) bronchoscopy, have been developed to detect preinvasive malignant lesions. Wang et al. demonstrated that AFB had significantly higher sensitivity in detecting malignant and premalignant lesions compared to white light bronchoscopy (WLB). Early detection of lung cancer is indeed possible. NBI is a variant of AFB that enhances specificity for diagnosing lung cancer. A 2015 meta-analysis which encompassed eight studies found that NBI had a sensitivity of 80% and specificity of 84%. When NBI was combined with AFB, the sensitivity and specificity increased to 86% and 75%, respectively [7]. FB plays an important role in staging tumors by identifying the local extension of the primary lesion (the T component of the TNM staging system). This provides essential information regarding the invasion of the trachea, main bronchi, or adjacent structures, which is crucial for determining a patient's suitability for surgical intervention or curative radiotherapy. The ninth edition of the TNM staging system stated that T1 tumors do not involve the primary or lobar bronchi. T2 tumors include lesions that invade a main bronchus, regardless of their proximity to the carina. Tumors of any size that invade the carina are classified as T4 [8]. All of these characteristics, which highlight the degree of tissue invasion and the involvement of central airways, are essential for surgical planning; the invasion of the origin of the lobar or main bronchus may require sleeve resection or pneumonectomy. In the LC approach, it is also crucial to distinguish between resectable and unresectable lesions, given that unresectable tumors are managed with chemotherapy, immunotherapy, and/or radiotherapy only. When lesions are less well defined or localized to the peripheral airways, bronchial brushings and bronchoalveolar lavage (BAL) are more appropriate for cytological sampling. Exfoliative cytology techniques are useful for collecting cells from mucosal surfaces, providing diagnostic information about preinvasive or incipient malignant changes. These tools, when appropriately combined, increase diagnostic accuracy and support optimal clinical decision-making [9]. BAL is a minimally invasive technique used during bronchoscopy that plays an important role in the evaluation and diagnosis of patients with suspected peripheral NSCLC. Combining FB with BAL is particularly useful when lung lesions are inaccessible for direct biopsy. BAL represents a complementary method within the diagnostic algorithm of NSCLC and involves the instillation of sterile saline solution into the distal airways, followed after 10–15 min by aspiration of the fluid, which is subsequently analyzed through biochemical, cytological, and microbiological examinations [10]. BAL can contribute to the diagnosis of NSCLC by detecting malignant cells in bronchial secretions, especially in patients with visible endobronchial lesions [11]. Cytological analysis of the retrieved fluid can identify malignant cells, determine histologic subtype, and sometimes even detect actionable molecular mutations relevant for targeted therapies (e.g., EGFR, KRAS, ALK) through a polymerase chain reaction (PCR) analysis of cellular DNA collected from the BAL supernatant [12]. In addition to its diagnostic value, BAL is useful for excluding other conditions that may mimic lung cancer, such as infections or inflammatory diseases, thus supporting differential diagnosis in NSCLC. The sensitivity of BAL in detecting and analyzing neoplastic cells is variable and depends on factors such as tumor location, the degree of cellular exfoliation, and the expertise of the cytopathology laboratory [13]. Bronchial brushing is a technique in which the bronchial wall is brushed with flexible brushes guided through a fiber-optic bronchoscope under visual or radiographic control, aimed at exfoliating and collecting cells from the bronchial mucosa. It is advantageous in cases of minimal changes in the bronchial mucosa that cannot be biopsied, such as preinvasive lesions [11,12]. The histopathological subtypes of NSCLC include adenocarcinoma, squamous cell carcinoma, and large-cell carcinoma. Vishak Acharya K et al. highlighted only 11 cases out of 156 where the diagnosis was established through lavage, with a very low sensitivity of 7%. When comparing cytology by brushing with biopsy, brushing showed a sensitivity of 55.88% and a specificity of 55.56%, suggesting a better approach by combining the two techniques. Additionally, brushing had a superior yield in cases of minimally modified mucosa, with a 50% yield, increasing to 70% in infiltrative lesions. Brushing can be preferred over biopsy with forceps in patients with a high risk of bleeding. Moreover, the friable, necrotic superficial tissue obtained via biopsy is often histopathologically inconclusive [13]. Transbronchial biopsy, commonly used for tumors located peripherally, can be performed either blindly or with fluoroscopic guidance. In their study, Kumar V et al. found that for tumors not visible through bronchoscopy, the diagnostic yield was 46.15% for BAL, 76.92% for brushing, and 84.61% for transbronchial biopsy [14]. Liam CK et al. noted that for tumors visible through bronchoscopy, the diagnostic yields were 28.3% for BAL, 77.5% for endobronchial biopsy, and 53.7% for brushing [15]. Research suggests a higher rate of squamous cell carcinoma diagnosis through biopsy compared to adenocarcinoma, likely due to the central localization of squamous cell carcinoma, which makes it easier to access [16]. Kumar V et al. found that 66.22% of patients in their study were diagnosed with squamous cell carcinoma, while 26.66% were diagnosed with adenocarcinoma. Most studies conducted in India suggest a higher prevalence of squamous cell carcinoma [14]. Gupta et al. found that 42.3% of cases were squamous cell carcinoma, while only 19.9% were adenocarcinoma [17]. Thippanna et al. identified that 67.5% of patients had squamous cell carcinoma compared to 18.75% with adenocarcinoma [18]. Kashyap et al. also highlighted that 58.3% of cases were squamous cell carcinoma and 10.8% of cases were adenocarcinoma in their study group [19]. Considering the studies presented above, a preliminary conclusion is that the use of the described bronchoscopic techniques and methods results in a superior identification rate for squamous cell carcinoma (Figure 1) compared to adenocarcinoma in lung cancer can be made. Additionally, the primary methods used for sample collection required for histopathological examination, with superior diagnostic yields, are endobronchial biopsy and brushing.

Even though FB is generally considered a safe procedure, it can be associated with several complications. These are usually rare, especially when the procedure is performed by experienced medical personnel in a controlled setting. However, complications can occur, especially during blind maneuvers such as transbronchial biopsy, and must be promptly recognized and managed. One of the most common complications is iatrogenic hemorrhage, which can range from minor, self-limiting bleeding to significant episodes that require hemostatic intervention. The risk of hemorrhage increases in the presence of hypervascularized lesions, centrally located bronchial tumors with vascular invasion, or in patients with coagulation disorders [20]. Another potential complication is pneumothorax, especially after transbronchial biopsy of peripherally located lesions, where there is an increased risk of pulmonary parenchymal perforation and air leakage into the pleural space. The incidence of pneumothorax varies depending on the size and extent of the lesion but the experience of the operator is also important [21]. Post-procedural respiratory infections, although uncommon, may occur, particularly in the context of immunosuppression, pre-existing chronic lung disease, or repeated invasive exploration of the bronchial tree [22]. Other adverse reactions encountered with FB include bronchospasm, transient hypoxemia, and side effects related to sedatives or local anesthetics used during the procedure. Therefore, careful pre-procedural risk assessment and close monitoring during and after bronchoscopy are essential for the prevention and prompt treatment of these adverse events.

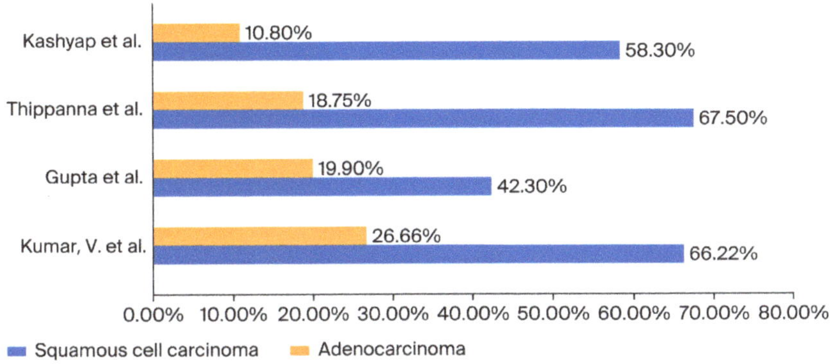

Figure 1. Hystopathological lung cancer types identified via flexible bronchoscopy in published studies. Kumar V. et al. (2017) [14], Gupta et al. (1998) [17], Thippanna et al. (1999) [18], Kashyap et al. (2003) [19].

4. Modern NSCLC Diagnostic Methodology

In contemporary practice, new technologies such as EBUS-TBNA have been introduced that feature combined imaging methods. This technique is also useful for identifying the involvement of mediastinal and hilar lymph nodes, which is necessary for staging NSCLC, along with obtaining biopsy material to confirm the histopathological diagnosis [23]. EBUS-TBNA is a procedure that combines flexible bronchoscopy with real-time ultrasound imaging and allows for the sampling of mediastinal and hilar lymph nodes. This technique constitutes a fundamental element in the staging of NSCLC, most especially for diagnosing N2 and N3 lymph node involvement. Patient preparation is performed according to institutional protocol, typically involving either conscious sedation or general anesthesia. A convex-probe bronchoscope and a 7.5 MHz ultrasound transducer are typically used. Lymph nodes are selected during the procedure for aspiration based on imaging criteria such as a size greater than 1 cm, rounded shape, absence of adipose hilum, heterogeneous echogenicity, and FDG avidity on PET-CT. Generally, a 21 G or 22 G aspiration needle is used, and for adequate tissue acquisition, a minimum of three round-trip passes of the needle per target lymph node are recommended. The application of the rapid on-site evaluation (ROSE) method, in which cytological specimens are immediately evaluated by a pathologist or trained technician, can significantly improve diagnostic accuracy and procedure yield. Doppler ultrasound is used to ensure the safety of the procedure by identifying and avoiding vascular structures before needle insertion. The puncture is generally performed at an angle of 20 to 25 degrees to the ultrasound probe, which allows for precise navigation and efficient penetration of the target node [24]. The last ten years have seen a sharp rise in the use of this minimally invasive procedure. EBUS-TBNA devices are present in about 85% of the critical care and pulmonary services that take part in different studies. Consequently, the rising use of this bronchoscopy technique for lung cancer detection and staging is becoming more and more popular. EBUS, which provides real-time pictures of mediastinal structures and enables precise navigation of the biopsy needle to suspicious lymph nodes, has transformed the staging of NSCLC by its incorporation into FB [25]. Also, EBUS-TBNA has a specificity of over 90% and a sensitivity of over 85%, which minimizes the need for more prevalent and invasive techniques like mediastinoscopy. The American Thoracic Society (ATS), European Respiratory Society (ERS), European Society of Medical Oncology (ESMO), and the American College of Chest Physicians (ACCP) have issued specific guidelines for performing invasive biopsy procedures on mediastinal adenopathy in NSCLC staging. In the latest third edition of the ACCP lung cancer guidelines, EBUS-TBNA is recommended as the first-line approach. As advanced-stage NSCLC is generally linked to a significant drop in survival rates, precise staging is very important for ensuring that patients receive the most appropriate treatment. EBUS-TBNA has also proven to be a safe technique, with minimal complications that may occur post-procedure [26]. A comprehensive systematic review including more than 1500 patients found only minor complications such as agitation, coughing, and mild bleeding at the puncture site [27]. Prospective studies have reported a complication rate of about 1%, although rare occurrences like mediastinitis, pericarditis, and even death have been noted. Despite the overall safety profile of this bronchoscopy technique, the primary risk associated with the procedure is incorrect staging [28].

In Level A staging, biopsies of every visible lymph node in all relevant stations (1, 2R, 2L, 3, 4R, 4L, and 7) are performed, requiring at least three passes through each lymph node or ROSE. Station 3A cannot be accessed through EBUS-TBNA due to the obstruction of large vessels in the mediastinum (Figure 2 [29]). Level B staging requires samples from stations 2R, 2L, 4R, 4L, and 7, using at least three passes per lymph node or ROSE. It is important to note that both Level A and Level B staging need to include samples from stations 5 and 6 if the tumor is in the left upper lobe, although these stations are generally inaccessible using EBUS-TBNA [30].

Level C staging corresponds to at least one adenopathy biopsied with fewer than three passes and no ROSE. The ability to freeze images allows for precise measurement of the evaluated nodule, ensuring accuracy in the assessment. The Doppler mode proves to be particularly valuable in evaluating vascularity within the ultrasound field, facilitating the safe insertion of the needle into the lymph node while adjusting for the 20-degree angle between the needle and transducer. Aspiration is performed by advancing the needle gently within the lymph node, with the aspirated material then transferred to glass slides for fixation and subsequent histopathological analysis. Also, material is collected for the preparation of cytoblocks or microbiological analysis, which may be essential for alternative or concurrent diagnostic evaluations [31]. Several retrospective studies have investigated the ultrasound characteristics of lymph nodes. In the most extensive study conducted by Fujiwara et al., a high negative predictive value for malignancy was observed in the absence of specific signs, including a round shape, well-defined margins, heterogeneous echogenicity, and the presence of coagulation necrosis [32]. Another study further corroborated that enlargement of the lymph node and its round or oval morphology are significant risk factors for malignancy. Increased vascularity within lymph nodes, especially beyond the main vessels leading to the center, can be an important indicator of malignant transformation. The absence of a central vessel in the lymph node during ultrasound evaluation is also recognized as a potential predictive sign of malignancy [33]. A 2008 study by Lee et al. highlighted the importance of the number of aspiration attempts on the diagnostic success rate of EBUS-TBNA. The same study found that performing three aspiration attempts resulted in a sensitivity of 95% and a specificity of 100%, which was significantly superior to the results observed with one or two aspiration attempts, where sensitivities were 69% and 83%, respectively. These findings emphasize the importance of multiple aspirations in enhancing the diagnostic accuracy of EBUS-TBNA [34]. A recent study in Toronto compared EBUS-TBNA with mediastinoscopy. All 153 eligible patients underwent EBUS-TBNA first, followed by mediastinoscopy, with both procedures showing similar results in evaluating the status of mediastinal lymph nodes. EBUS-TBNA exhibited a sensitivity of 81% and a specificity of 100%, while mediastinoscopy had a sensitivity of 79% and a specificity of 100% (Table 1).

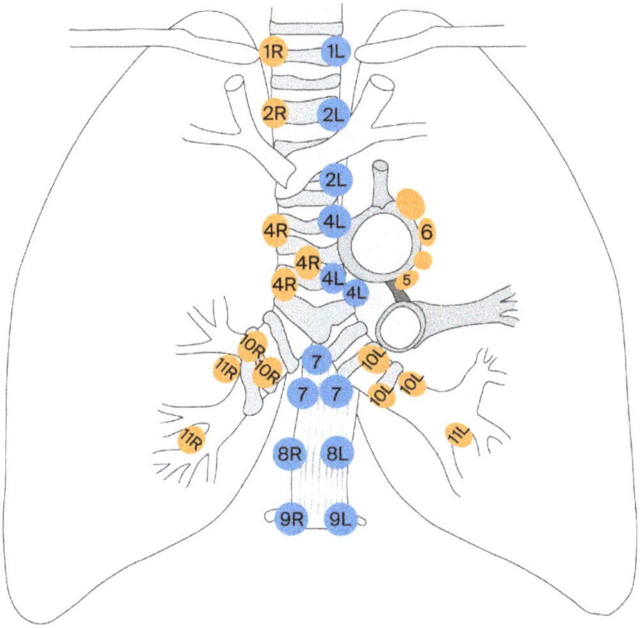

Figure 2. The different thoracic lymph node stations that can be approached by endoscopic ultrasonography. (Adapted after Kurt G. Tournoy et al. [29]).

Mediastinoscopy is an invasive surgical technique used in current practice for staging and diagnosing NSCLC. This method allows for direct visualization of mediastinal structures and biopsy of mediastinal lymph nodes, offering definitive histopathological confirmation, essential for determining the appropriate treatment strategy. While imaging methods like CT or PET-CT guide initial staging, mediastinoscopy remains the gold standard, especially in situations where non-invasive techniques such as EBUS-TBNA yield inconclusive results. Its fundamental role in identifying N2/N3 nodal involvement will have a significant impact on therapeutic decisions, being essential for establishing the optimal therapeutic regimen and improving the chances of patient survival [35]. Given the known less invasive nature of EBUS-TBNA, choosing this procedure instead of mediastinoscopy is justified, but the final decision depends on the physician's experience and the medical institution's available equipment [36].

However, certain clinical and radiological scenarios may necessitate complementary imaging methods, particularly for accurate staging, such as PET-CT. PET/CT plays an essential role in the diagnosis and staging of NSCLC and provides both anatomical information (via CT) and functional insights (via PET) [37,38]. This method is considered superior to other imaging techniques in early and accurate detection of malignant lesions, but it is not without potential confounding factors in the interpretation of the results. The use of the radiotracer 18F-FDG allows for the identification of regions with increased glucose metabolism, which is typical of tumor tissue [39]. Therefore, PET/CT is particularly useful for differentiating between benign and malignant nodules, especially in cases where conventional CT fails to offer definitive information [40]. In staging, PET/CT contributes significantly by evaluating disease extent, detecting both nodal and distant metastases—factors that critically influence therapeutic planning. Furthermore, it can help avoid unnecessary surgical interventions in patients with advanced disease. However, PET/CT has certain limitations, including false positives in cases of inflammation or infection, as well as false negatives in tumors with low metabolic activity, such as mucinous adenocarcinomas [41]. If the tomographic appearance of a patient suspected of having NSCLC is manifested as a polypoid lesion, eccentric lumen narrowing, or circumferential wall thickening, a PET-CT should be performed to confirm the absence of mediastinal lymph node involvement and distant metastases [42]. Currently, in patients with T1 tumors or peripheral T2 tumors, most guidelines do not recommend performing invasive mediastinal staging in the case of normal-sized mediastinal lymph nodes without glucose uptake on PET-CT. On the other hand, lymph nodes with pathological fluorodeoxyglucose uptake on PET-CT should be confirmed histopathologically through EBUS-TBNA, or if that is not possible, via mediastinoscopy. Therefore, invasive mediastinal staging is indicated in patients with mediastinal adenopathies larger than 1 cm or hypermetabolic on PET-CT, central tumors, or N1 lymph node staging [43]. Although imaging modalities such as PET/CT provide valuable guidance when combined with flexible bronchoscopy in staging strategies, histopathological confirmation remains the diagnostic gold standard for NSCLC.

Table 1. Lymph node station identification: EBUS vs. mediastinoscopy.

Lymph Node Station	Name/Location	Accessible via EBUS	Accessible via Mediastinoscopy
1	Lower cervical/ supraclavicular lymph nodes	yes	no (generally not accessible)
2R/2L	Upper paratracheal (right/left)	yes	yes
3A	Pre-vascular	yes (difficult)	no
3P	Retrotracheal	yes (very rare)	no
4R/4L	Lower paratracheal (right/left)	yes	yes
5	Subaortic (aorto-pulmonary)	no	yes (only via extended mediastinoscopy)
6	Para-aortic/ anterior to pulmonary artery ligament	no	no
7	Subcarinal	yes	yes
8	Lower paraesophageal	yes	no
9	Pulmonary ligament	yes (very rare)	no
10R/10L	Hilar (right/left)	yes	yes (difficult)
11R/11L	Interlobar	yes	no

5. Emerging Technologies: AI and Bronchoscopic Innovation

Recent advances in robotics and artificial intelligence (AI) are reshaping bronchoscopic practice and NSCLC staging. These techniques are formulated to improve diagnostic accuracy, increase workflow efficiency, and expand procedural coverage. Thus, AI-based systems are being developed to aid in real-time interpretation of endoscopic and ultrasound images during bronchoscopic scanning and EBUS-TBNA scanning. These platforms can detect abnormal mucosal patterns, differentiate between malignant and benign nodules, and support automated navigation to optimal biopsy sites. Convolutional neural networks, a subset of deep learning models, have demonstrated diagnostic accuracy comparable to that of expert bronchoscopists in preliminary studies. Although promising, such systems require extensive validation and clinical integration [44]. Robotic-assisted bronchoscopy platforms provide adequate stability and access to peripheral lesions. Electromagnetic navigation bronchoscopy (ENB) allows for preplanned navigation to nodules with greater precision. These methods allow access to lesions smaller than 2 cm, especially those located outside the radius of standard bronchoscopy, and have a lower risk of pneumothorax compared with transthoracic needle biopsy. The combination with real-time CT imaging further improves targeting capabilities. Despite their potential, these technologies are largely limited to clinical trials or tertiary referral centers [45].

6. Limitations

This narrative review comprises a comprehensive overview of FB and its role in the staging of NSCLC. However, several inherent limitations must be emphasized that may affect the validity and generalizability of the findings. Firstly, the narrative format does not follow a systematic methodology for a literature search, inclusion, and critical appraisal. As a result, selection bias may be introduced, with the potential omission of relevant studies or overrepresentation of certain perspectives. Secondly, the lack of quantitative synthesis prevents the assessment of pooled diagnostic performance metrics such as sensitivity, specificity, and predictive values across multiple studies. Without a meta-analytical approach, the relative efficacy of advanced FB techniques—particularly EBUS-TBNA—cannot be precisely compared to alternative staging modalities such as mediastinoscopy or PET-CT. Moreover, the review may not fully capture the variability in clinical outcomes associated with operator experience, institutional protocols, or patient-specific factors, which are crucial in real-world applications. Additionally, potential complications, limitations in access to advanced technologies, and cost-effectiveness considerations are only briefly addressed. Finally, given the rapid evolution of diagnostic tools and lung cancer management strategies, some of the included evidence may become outdated, and developing technologies like robotic bronchoscopy or artificial intelligence-assisted image analysis are not comprehensively discussed.

7. Conclusions

This review examines the evolving role of minimally invasive methods (FB and EBUS-TBNA) in NSCLC staging. By showing their clinical value, diagnostic yield, and safety profiles, this compares them to imaging techniques like PET/CT and conventional methods like mediastinoscopy. PET/CT informs staging approaches, but histopathological validation is key and EBUS-TBNA has an edge in some situations. The article also explores emerging technologies, including artificial intelligence and robotic bronchoscopy, which are expected to enhance diagnostic accuracy in the future. In summary, this review provides a structured evidence-based framework for integrating endobronchial instruments in NSCLC staging to enable personalized decision-making.

Author Contributions: Conceptualization: S.-M.R., M.A.B., and V.B.; validation: M.A.B., V.B., B.M., O.-A.P., and S.I.S.; supervision: V.B.; writing—original draft preparation: S.-M.R. and O.M.C.; writing—review and editing: V.B.; data curation: S.-M.R., A.A.M., and D.M.M. All authors have read and agreed to the published version of the manuscript.

Funding: This research received no external funding.

Institutional Review Board Statement: Not applicable.

Informed Consent Statement: Not applicable.

Data Availability Statement: The data presented in this study are available upon request from the corresponding author.

Conflicts of Interest: The authors declare no conflicts of interest.

Abbreviations

The following abbreviations are used in this manuscript:

NSCLC	Non-small-cell lung cancer
FB	Flexible bronchoscopy
EBUS-TBNA	Endobronchial ultrasound with fine-needle aspiration
PET-CT	Positron emission tomography
LC	Lung cancer
FDG	Fluorodeoxyglucose
AFB	Autofluorescence bronchoscopy
NBI	Narrow-band imaging
BAL	Bronchoalveolar lavage
WLB	White light bronchoscopy
ACCP	American College of Chest Physicians
EGFR	Epidermal growth factor
ALK	Receptor anaplastic lymphoma kinase
PD-L1	Programmed death-ligand 1
ROSE	Rapid on-site evaluation
AI	Artificial intelligence
ENB	Electromagnetic navigation bronchoscopy

References

1. Ferlay, J.; Colombet, M.; Soerjomataram, I.; Parkin, D.M.; Piñeros, M.; Znaor, A.; Bray, F. Cancer statistics for the year 2020: A overview. *Int. J. Cancer* **2021**, *5*, 33588. [CrossRef]
2. Olteanu, G.E.; Vigdorovits, A.; Barna, R.A.; Mazilu, L.; Manolache, V.; Preoteasa, V.; Curcean, S.; Roman, A.; Motas, N Dediu, M.; et al. Lung Cancer in Romania. *J. Thorac. Oncol.* **2024**, *19*, 1492–1503. [CrossRef]
3. Zappa, C.; Mousa, S.A. Non-small cell lung cancer: Current treatment and future advances. *Transl. Lung Cancer Res.* **2016**, 288–300. [CrossRef]
4. Apple, J.; DerSarkissian, M.; Shah, A.; Chang, R.; Chen, Y.; He, X.; Chun, J. Economic burden of early-stage non-small-cell lun cancer: An assessment of healthcare resource utilization and medical costs. *J. Comp. Eff. Res.* **2023**, *12*, e230107. [CrossRef] [PubMed]
5. Silvestri, G.A.; Gonzalez, A.V.; Jantz, M.A.; Margolis, M.L.; Gould, M.K.; Tanoue, L.T.; Harris, L.J.; Detterbeck, F.C. Methods fc staging non-small cell lung cancer: Diagnosis and management of lung cancer, 3rd ed: American College of Chest Physician evidence-based clinical practice guidelines. *Chest* **2013**, *143*, e211S–e250S. [CrossRef]
6. Shinagawa, N. A review of existing and new methods of bronchoscopic diagnosis of lung cancer. *Respir. Investig.* **2019**, *57*, 3– [CrossRef]
7. Iftikhar, I.H.; Musani, A.I. Narrow-Band Imaging Bronchoscopy in the Detection of Premalignant Airway Lesions: A Meta -Analysis of Diagnostic Test Accuracy. *Ther. Adv. Respir. Dis.* **2015**, *9*, 123–133. [CrossRef]
8. Argentieri, G.; Valsecchi, C.; Petrella, F.; Jungblut, L.; Frauenfelder, T.; Del Grande, F.; Rizzo, S. Implementation of the 9th TNM for lung cancer: Practical insights for radiologists. *Eur. Radiol.* **2025**, *35*, 4395–4402. [CrossRef]
9. Domagala-Kulawik, J. The relevance of bronchoalveolar lavage fluid analysis for lung cancer patients. *Expert. Rev. Respir. Me* **2020**, *14*, 329–337. [CrossRef] [PubMed]
10. Davidson, K.R.; Ha, D.M.; Schwarz, M.I.; Chan, E.D. Bronchoalveolar lavage as a diagnostic procedure: A review of know cellular and molecular findings in various lung diseases. *J. Thorac. Dis.* **2020**, *12*, 4991–5019. [CrossRef] [PubMed]
11. Zhang, H.; Deng, D.; Li, S.; Ren, J.; Huang, W.; Liu, D.; Wang, W. Bronchoalveolar lavage fluid assessment facilitates precisio medicine for lung cancer. *Cancer Biol. Med.* **2023**, *21*, 230–251. [CrossRef]
12. Kalkanis, A.; Papadopoulos, D.; Testelmans, D.; Kopitopoulou, A.; Boeykens, E.; Wauters, E. Bronchoalveolar Lavage Fluic Isolated Biomarkers for the Diagnostic and Prognostic Assessment of Lung Cancer. *Diagnostics* **2022**, *12*, 2949. [CrossRef]

Nguyen-Dang, K.; Bui-Thi, H.D.; Duong-Minh, N.; Pham-Quang, T.; Nguyen-Ho, L.; Lam-Quoc, D.; Dang-Vu, T.; Tran-Ngoc, N.; Nguyen-Thi, P.; Le-Thuong, V. The Role and Associated Factors of Liquid-Based Cytology of Bronchoalveolar Lavage Fluid in Lung Cancer Diagnosis: A Prospective Study. *Cureus* **2023**, *15*, e48483. [CrossRef]

Kumar, V.; Gupta, K.B.; Aggarwal, R. Yield of different bronchoscopic techniques in diagnosis of lung cancer. *Int. J. Res. Med. Sci.* **2017**, *5*, 4098–4103. [CrossRef]

Liam, C.K.; Pang, Y.K.; Poosparajah, S. Diagnostic yield of flexible bronchoscopic procedures in lung cancer patients according to tumour location. *Singapore Med. J.* **2007**, *48*, 625–631.

Biciuşcă, V.; Popescu, I.A.S.; Traşcă, D.M.; Olteanu, M.; Stan, I.S.; Durand, P.; Camen, G.C.; Bălteanu, M.A.; Cazacu, I.M.; Demetrian, A.D.; et al. Diagnosis of lung cancer by flexible fiberoptic bronchoscopy: A descriptive study. *Rom. J. Morphol. Embryol.* **2022**, *63*, 369–381. [CrossRef]

Gupta, R.C.; Purohit, S.D.; Sharma, M.P.; Bhardwaj, S. Primary bronchogenic carcinoma: Clinical profile of 279 cases from mid-west Rajasthan. *Indian J. Chest Dis. Allied. Sci.* **1998**, *40*, 109–116.

Thippanna, G.; Venu, K.; Gopalakrishnaiah, V.; Reddy, P.N.; Charan, B.G. A profile of lung cancer patients in Hyderabad. *J. Indian Med. Assoc.* **1999**, *97*, 357–359. [PubMed]

Kashyap, S.; Mohapatra, P.; Singh, R. Pattern of primary lung cancer among Bidi smokers in North-Western Himalayan region of India. *Lung Cancer* **2003**, *41*, S111. [CrossRef]

Bernasconi, M.; Koegelenberg, C.F.N.; Koutsokera, A.; Ogna, A.; Casutt, A.; Nicod, L.; Lovis, A. Iatrogenic bleeding during flexible bronchoscopy: Risk factors, prophylactic measures and management. *ERJ Open Res.* **2017**, *21*, 00084-2016. [CrossRef] [PubMed]

Ishak, M.; Chakraborty, D.; Kassirian, S.; Dhaliwal, I.; Mitchell, M.A. Risk of iatrogenic pneumothorax based on location of transbronchial biopsy: A retrospective cohort study. *BMC Res. Notes* **2023**, *16*, 14. [CrossRef]

Shimizu, T.; Okachi, S.; Imai, N.; Hase, T.; Morise, M.; Hashimoto, N.; Sato, M.; Hasegawa, Y. Risk factors for pulmonary infection after diagnostic bronchoscopy in patients with lung cancer. *Nagoya J. Med. Sci.* **2020**, *82*, 69–77. [CrossRef] [PubMed] [PubMed Central]

Elhidsi, M.; Zaini, J.; Rachmadi, L.; Asmarinah, A.; Kekalih, A.; Soeroso, N.; Rasmin, M. Clinical and Bronchoscopy Assessment in Diagnosing the Histopathology Type of Primary Central Lung Tumors. *Open Respir. Med. J.* **2024**, *18*, e18743064318977. [CrossRef]

Yarmus, L.B.; Akulian, J.; Lechtzin, N.; Shah, A.; Yasin, F.; Kamdar, B.; Ernst, A.; Ost, D.E. Comparison of 21-Gauge and 22-Gauge Aspiration Needle in Endobronchial Ultrasound-Guided Transbronchial Needle Aspiration: Results of the American College of Chest Physicians Quality Improvement Registry, Education, and Evaluation Registry. *Chest* **2013**, *143*, 1036–1043. [CrossRef]

Ahn, J.H. An update on the role of bronchoscopy in the diagnosis of pulmonary disease. *Yeungnam Univ. J. Med.* **2020**, *37*, 253–261. [CrossRef] [PubMed]

Detterbeck, F.C.; Lewis, S.Z.; Diekemper, R.; Addrizzo-Harris, D.; Alberts, W.M. Executive Summary: Diagnosis and Management of Lung Cancer, 3rd ed: American College of Chest Physicians evidence-based clinical practice guidelines. *Chest* **2013**, *143*, 7S–37S. [CrossRef] [PubMed]

Varela-Lema, L.; Fernández-Villar, A.; Ruano-Ravina, A. Effectiveness and safety of endobronchial ultrasound-transbronchial needle aspiration: A systematic review. *Eur. Respir. J.* **2009**, *33*, 1156–1164. [CrossRef]

Asano, F.; Aoe, M.; Ohsaki, Y.; Okada, Y.; Sasada, S.; Sato, S.; Suzuki, E.; Senba, H.; Fujino, S.; Ohmori, K. Deaths and complications associated with respiratory endoscopy: A survey by the Japan Society for Respiratory Endoscopy in 2010. *Respirology* **2012**, *17*, 478–485. [CrossRef]

Tournoy, K.G.; Annema, J.T.; Krasnik, M.; Herth, F.J.; van Meerbeeck, J.P. Endoscopic and endobronchial ultrasonography according to the proposed lymph node map definition in the seventh edition of the tumor, node, metastasis classification for lung cancer. *J. Thorac. Oncol.* **2009**, *4*, 1576–1584. [CrossRef]

Folch, E.; Santacruz, J.F.; Machuzak, M.S.; Gildea, T.R.; Majid, A. Safety and Efficacy of EBUS-Guided TBNA Through the Pulmonary Artery: A Preliminary Report. *Chest* **2011**, *140*, 600. [CrossRef]

Casal, R.F.; Staerkel, G.A.; Ost, D.; Almeida, F.A.; Uzbeck, M.H.; Eapen, G.A.; Jimenez, C.A.; Nogueras-Gonzalez, G.M.; Sarkiss, M.; Morice, R.C. Randomized clinical trial of endobronchial ultrasound needle biopsy with and without aspiration. *Chest* **2012**, *142*, 568–573. [CrossRef]

Fujiwara, T.; Yasufuku, K.; Nakajima, T.; Chiyo, M.; Yoshida, S.; Suzuki, M.; Shibuya, K.; Hiroshima, K.; Nakatani, Y.; Yoshino, I. The utility of sonographic features during endobronchial ultrasound-guided transbronchial needle aspiration for lymph node staging in patients with lung cancer: A standard endobronchial ultrasound image classification system. *Chest* **2010**, *138*, 641–647. [CrossRef] [PubMed]

Satterwhite, L.G.; Berkowitz, D.M.; Parks, C.S.; Bechara, R.I. Central intranodal vessels to predict cytology during endobronchial ultrasound transbronchial needle aspiration. *J. Bronchol. Interv. Pulmonol.* **2011**, *18*, 322–328. [CrossRef]

34. Lee, H.S.; Lee, G.K.; Lee, H.S.; Kim, M.S.; Lee, J.M.; Kim, H.Y.; Nam, B.H.; Zo, J.I.; Hwangbo, B. Real-time endobronchial ultrasound-guided transbronchial needle aspiration in mediastinal staging of non-small cell lung cancer: How many aspirations per target lymph node station? *Chest* **2008**, *134*, 368–374. [CrossRef] [PubMed]
35. Leiro-Fernández, V.; Fernández-Villar, A. Mediastinal Staging for Non-Small Cell Lung Cancer. *Transl. Lung Cancer Res.* **2021**, *10*, 496–505. [CrossRef]
36. Yasufuku, K.; Pierre, A.; Darling, G.; de Perrot, M.; Waddell, T.; Johnston, M.; da Cunha Santos, G.; Geddie, W.; Boerner, S.; Le, L.W.; et al. A prospective controlled trial of endobronchial ultrasound-guided transbronchial needle aspiration compared with mediastinoscopy for mediastinal lymph node staging of lung cancer. *J. Thorac. Cardiovasc. Surg.* **2011**, *142*, 1393–1400.e1. [CrossRef]
37. Chao, F.; Zhang, H. PET/CT in the staging of the non-small-cell lung cancer. *J. Biomed. Biotechnol.* **2012**, *2012*, 783739. [CrossRef]
38. Volpi, S.; Ali, J.M.; Tasker, A.; Peryt, A.; Aresu, G.; Coonar, A.S. The role of positron emission tomography in the diagnosis, staging and response assessment of non-small cell lung cancer. *Ann. Transl. Med.* **2018**, *6*, 95. [CrossRef]
39. Zhu, J.; Pan, F.; Cai, H.; Pan, L.; Li, Y.; Li, L.; Li, Y.; Wu, X.; Fan, H. Positron emission tomography imaging of lung cancer: An overview of alternative positron emission tomography tracers beyond F18 fluorodeoxyglucose. *Front. Med.* **2022**, *9*, 945602. [CrossRef]
40. Sun, Y.; Ge, X.; Niu, R.; Gao, J.; Shi, Y.; Shao, X.; Wang, Y.; Shao, X. PET/CT radiomics and deep learning in the diagnosis of benign and malignant pulmonary nodules: Progress and challenges. *Front. Oncol.* **2024**, *14*, 1491762. [CrossRef] [PubMed]
41. Khan, I.S.; Mashkoor, S.; Shafiq, S.; Amber, F.; Kaleemi, R.; Nausheen, S.; Kumari, P.; Hashmi, A.A. Diagnostic Accuracy of FDG PET-CT in Lymph Nodal Staging of Lung Cancer. *Cureus* **2025**, *17*, e77880. [CrossRef]
42. Matache, R.S.; Stanciu-Gavan, C.; Pantile, D.; Iordache, A.M.; Bejgăneanu, A.O.; Șerboiu, C.S.; Nemes, A.F. Clinical and Paraclinical Characteristics of Endobronchial Pulmonary Squamous Cell Carcinoma—A Brief Review. *Diagnostics* **2023**, *13*, 3318. [CrossRef] [PubMed]
43. Farsad, M. FDG PET/CT in the Staging of Lung Cancer. *Curr. Radiopharm.* **2020**, *13*, 195–203. [CrossRef] [PubMed]
44. Zhao, J.; Chen, H.; Tian, Q.; Chen, J.; Yang, B.; Liu, H. BronchoCopilot: AI in Autonomous Bronchoscopy–Reinforcement Learning Platform for Real-Time Bronchoscope Guidance. *arXiv* **2024**, arXiv:2403.01483.
45. Brownlee, A.R.; Watson, J.J.; Akhmerov, A.; Nammalwar, S.; Chen, Q.; Soukiasian, S.G.; Soukiasian, H.J. Robotic Navigational Bronchoscopy in Real-World Practice: Diagnostic Yield of 87.9%, with Low Complication Rate (5%). *J. Thorac. Dis.* **2023**, *5*, 1–6. [CrossRef]

Journal of
Clinical Medicine

MDPI

view

'hronic Obstructive Pulmonary Disease and COVID-19: The mpact of Hematological Biomarkers on Disease Severity nd Outcomes

ıbriela Mara [1,2], Gheorghe Nini [2] and Coralia Cotoraci [3,*]

[1] Multidisciplinary Doctoral School, Vasile Goldis Western University of Arad, 310414 Arad, Romania; mara.gabriela@uvvg.ro
[2] Pneumology Department, Vasile Goldis Western University of Arad, 310414 Arad, Romania; nini.gheorghe@uvvg.ro
[3] Clinical Hematology Department, Vasile Goldis Western University of Arad, 310025 Arad, Romania
* Correspondence: cotoraci.coralia@uvvg.ro

Abstract: Background/Objectives: Chronic obstructive pulmonary disease (COPD) patients are at heightened risk of severe COVID-19 due to underlying respiratory impairment, systemic inflammation, and immune dysregulation. This review explores the hematological changes that occur in COPD patients with COVID-19 and their implications for disease progression, prognosis, and clinical management. **Methods:** We conducted a comprehensive analysis of recent peer-reviewed studies from medical databases including Clarivate Analytics, PubMed, and Google Scholar. **Results:** Hematological alterations, such as lymphopenia, elevated neutrophil-to-lymphocyte ratio (NLR), increased D-dimer and fibrinogen levels, inflammatory anemia, and erythrocyte dysfunction, are commonly observed in COPD patients with COVID-19. These changes are linked to immune suppression, hyperinflammation, oxidative stress, and thromboembolic complications. **Conclusions:** Hematological biomarkers are valuable tools for early risk assessments and guiding treatment strategies in this high-risk population. The regular monitoring of D-dimer, fibrinogen, and NLR is advisable. Prophylactic anticoagulation and immunomodulatory therapies, such as corticosteroids and IL-6 and IL-1 inhibitors, may improve clinical outcomes. Further clinical studies are needed to validate personalized approaches and explore antioxidant-based interventions.

Keywords: COPD; COVID-19; hematological markers; coagulopathy; oxidative stress

1. Introduction

Chronic obstructive pulmonary disease (COPD) is a heterogeneous lung disease marked by chronic respiratory symptoms, such as dyspnea, cough, sputum production, and exacerbations, caused by airway (e.g., bronchitis and bronchiolitis) and/or alveolar (e.g., emphysema) abnormalities that lead to persistent, often progressive, airflow obstruction [1]. The disease is primarily caused by long-term exposure to harmful particles and gases, with cigarette smoking being the leading risk factor. In 2016, an estimated 251 million cases of COPD were recorded globally, according to the Global Burden of Disease (GBD) study [2]. The Burden of Obstructive Lung Disease initiative and Global Burden of Disease collaborators have led efforts to estimate global COPD burden, reporting between 212 and 384 million cases from 2010 to 2019 based on spirometry data refined through risk factor modeling [3]. Additionally, projections from the World Health Organization (WHO) suggest that by 2030, COPD will rank as the third leading cause of death worldwide [4].

The pathogenesis of COPD involves an imbalance between proteases and antiproteases, oxidative stress, and chronic inflammation, which contribute to airway remodeling, mucus hypersecretion, and lung parenchymal destruction [5]. COPD is a major global health issue, ranking as the third leading cause of death worldwide, with an increasing burden in low- and middle-income countries [2].

Patients with COPD are at a significantly higher risk of developing severe COVID-19 infections. Pre-existing respiratory impairment and chronic inflammation in COPD patients create a favorable environment for viral infections, leading to increased disease severity and complications [6]. The presence of COPD has been associated with higher rates of hospitalization, intensive care unit (ICU) admissions, and mortality in COVID-19 patients [7]. The heightened vulnerability in COPD patients is attributed to factors such as reduced mucociliary clearance, altered immune responses, and increased expression of angiotensin-converting enzyme 2 (ACE2) receptors in the lungs, which facilitate SARS-CoV-2 entry [8].

The COVID-19 pandemic, with an estimated global excess mortality of 14.9 million in 2020 and 2021 according to WHO, has had a profound impact not only on human health but also across various fields, including epidemiology, pharmaceutical innovation, behavioral sciences, and healthcare system management [9]. It possess a greater risk of severe illness and death in individuals with underlying comorbidities, such as cardiovascular disease, diabetes, and chronic respiratory conditions. These comorbidities, along with factors like advanced age, severe lymphopenia, elevated CRP, and D-dimer levels above 1 μg/L, are strongly associated with a poor prognosis and increased mortality rates [10].

Hematological alterations play a crucial role in predicting COVID-19 severity in COPD patients. Parameters such as lymphopenia, elevated neutrophil-to-lymphocyte ratio (NLR), increased levels of C-reactive protein (CRP), and thrombocytopenia have been identified as markers of disease progression and poor outcomes [11]. In COPD patients, systemic inflammation is already elevated, which may exacerbate the hyperinflammatory state induced by COVID-19, leading to cytokine storms and severe respiratory failure [12]. Understanding these hematological changes is essential for early risk stratification, timely intervention, and improved clinical management of COPD patients with COVID-19.

The aim of this review is to investigate the hematological changes that occur in patients with COPD who are infected with COVID-19 and to explore how these changes influence disease progression, clinical outcomes, and therapeutic strategies. The review seeks to highlight the pathophysiological overlap between the two conditions, particularly in terms of immune dysregulation, coagulation abnormalities, and oxidative stress, and to evaluate the clinical utility of hematological biomarkers for risk stratification and management.

2. Methodology

This review is based on a comprehensive analysis of peer-reviewed studies published between January 2020 and December 2023, which were retrieved from databases including Clarivate Analytics, PubMed, and Google Scholar. Studies were selected based on their relevance to hematological abnormalities in COPD and COVID-19, particularly those addressing markers such as lymphopenia, NLR, D-dimer, fibrinogen, and indicators of oxidative stress. Both clinical and mechanistic research was included, focusing on inflammatory and coagulopathic pathways, erythropoietic dysfunction, and prognostic implications.

3. Shared Mechanisms Between COPD and COVID-19

3.1. *Chronic Inflammation and Cytokine Storms*

Chronic inflammation is a key pathological feature of both COPD and severe COVID-19, leading to dysregulated immune responses and systemic complications (Table 1). The interplay between chronic inflammation and hematological disturbances highlights the need for targeted anti-inflammatory and anticoagulant strategies in COPD patients at risk of severe COVID-19 complications. Understanding these mechanisms can aid in the development of personalized treatment approaches to mitigate disease progression and improve patient outcomes.

Table 1. Chronic inflammation and cytokine storms in COPD and severe COVID-19.

Mechanism	Description	Relevance to COPD	Relevance to Severe COVID-19
Increased IL-6 levels	IL-6 is a key pro-inflammatory cytokine involved in immune activation.	Elevated in COPD, especially in frequent exacerbators; associated with reduced lung function.	Correlated with disease severity and cytokine storms; higher serum levels linked to poor outcomes.
Elevated TNF-α levels	Promotes macrophage activation and lung tissue damage.	Increased in COPD; contributes to alveolar destruction and exacerbations.	Associated with ARDS and lung injury; a potential target for anti-TNF therapies.
Increased IL-8 (CXCL8) expression	Recruits neutrophils and amplifies inflammation.	Associated with exacerbations and lung function decline.	Enhances neutrophil infiltration, worsening alveolar injury.
Macrophage and dendritic cell activation	Innate immune cells regulate inflammatory responses.	Overactive macrophages produce cytokines and sustain inflammation.	Excessive activation linked to cytokine storms and multiorgan failure.
NET formation and neutrophilia	Neutrophils release extracellular traps that damage tissue.	Higher levels correlate with worse symptoms and exacerbation frequency.	Associated with disease severity and increased cfDNA and mortality.
Hematological alterations and coagulopathy	Inflammation affects coagulation and increases thrombosis risk.	Advanced COPD increases VTE risk and worsens the prognosis if thrombotic events occur.	Coagulopathy may result in pulmonary embolism and stroke; associated with increased mortality.
Oxidative stress and lung damage	ROS generation exacerbates inflammation and tissue injury.	Drives COPD progression and systemic inflammation.	Contributes to endothelial injury, pulmonary fibrosis, and cytokine-mediated damage.

Table 1 summarizes the key inflammatory mediators and immune mechanisms involved in the cytokine storm observed in both COPD and severe COVID-19, highlighting their overlapping pathophysiological pathways.

3.2. Hypoxia and Oxidative Stress

COPD and severe COVID-19 are both characterized by hypoxia and oxidative stress, which contribute to systemic complications beyond lung pathology. Chronic hypoxia triggers adaptive and maladaptive responses in hematopoiesis and coagulation [13], while oxidative stress results in cellular damage and inflammation [14].

Both hypoxia and oxidative stress play a central role in the systemic complications of COPD and severe COVID-19, particularly in hematopoietic changes, immune dysregulation, and coagulation abnormalities. Understanding these mechanisms highlights the need for therapeutic strategies that target hypoxia-induced inflammation and oxidative damage, such as antioxidant therapies, oxygen supplementation, and anti-inflammatory treatments.

3.2.1. Hypoxia-Induced Hematological and Coagulation Alterations in COPD and Severe COVID-19

Chronic hypoxia plays a critical role in hematopoiesis, inflammation, and coagulation dysfunction, significantly affecting disease progression in both COPD and severe COVID-19. The body's response to persistent oxygen deprivation leads to a cascade of adaptive and maladaptive mechanisms, influencing erythropoiesis, leukocyte activity, and thrombotic risk.

Hypoxia acts as a primary stimulus for erythropoiesis, triggering the release of erythropoietin (EPO) from the kidneys to promote red blood cell (RBC) production in an effort to enhance oxygen transport, which is regulated by hypoxia-inducible factors (HIFs) [15]. In COPD, prolonged hypoxia can lead to secondary polycythemia [16], characterized by increased hematocrit levels, which may contribute to blood hyperviscosity, increased cardiovascular burden, and a higher risk of thrombotic events [17–19]. acute COPD exacerbations are linked to increased systemic inflammation, which promotes platelet activation, endothelial dysfunction, enhanced coagulation, and impaired fibrinolysis, as indicated by elevated platelet–monocyte complexes (PMCs), monocyte Mac-1 expression, Bon Willebrand factor (VWF), and thrombin generation, while prolonged clot lysis time and platelet hyperreactivity at admission are associated with a higher risk of relapse [20].

However, in severe COVID-19, erythropoiesis appears to be dysregulated, often leading to anemia instead of polycythemia [21]. In a study of 179 infected patients, 20.3% had a positive Coombs test (mainly IgG), though no cases of autoimmune hemolysis were found; Coombs-positive patients had more severe anemia, required more transfusions and intensive care, and showed an inflammatory anemia pattern with elevated hepcidin and ferritin but inappropriately low EPO and erythroferrone, with iron metabolism markers correlating with disease severity [22]. Consequently, while COPD patients frequently experience elevated RBC counts [23], COVID-19 patients may present with normocytic or microcytic anemia [24,25], contributing to worsened oxygen transport and disease severity.

In addition to altering RBC production, hypoxia significantly influences leukocyte function, leading to a state of chronic inflammation. Low oxygen availability enhances the release of pro-inflammatory cytokines, particularly IL-6, TNF-α, and IL-8, which promote neutrophil activation and immune cell recruitment [26]. This exaggerated inflammatory response contributes to the systemic inflammation observed in COPD and plays a role in the cytokine storm characteristic of severe COVID-19 [27].

A central regulator of this process is hypoxia-inducible factor 1-alpha (HIF-1α), a transcription factor that becomes stabilized under hypoxic conditions, leading to the upregulation of inflammatory pathways [28] by activating EGFR/PI3K/AKT pathway [29]. HIF-1α activation not only amplifies neutrophil-driven inflammation but also impairs immune resolution, resulting in sustained tissue damage and increased susceptibility to exacerbations in COPD and multi-organ failure in COVID-19 [30–32].

Chronic hypoxia is a well-established driver of hypercoagulability [33], predisposing patients to an increased risk of deep vein thrombosis [34,35], pulmonary embolism [36,37], and microvascular thrombosis [38,39]. This prothrombotic state is primarily mediated by

- Platelet activation and aggregation, leading to enhanced clot formation [40];
- Elevated fibrinogen levels, which contribute to increased blood viscosity [40];
- The upregulation of tissue factor (TF), a key initiator of the extrinsic coagulation cascade [41].

In COPD, chronic inflammation and endothelial dysfunction promote a hypercoagulable state, increasing the risk of cardiovascular events and stroke [42]. Similarly, in severe COVID-19, these mechanisms are further exacerbated by a viral infection, leading to the development of COVID-19-associated coagulopathy, which is strongly linked to higher mortality rates [43]. The presence of elevated D-dimer levels, along with increased fibrinogen and platelet activation, serves as a critical marker of thrombotic complications in both diseases [44].

3.2.2. Increased Production of Reactive Oxygen Species (ROS) and Their Impact on Blood Cells

Oxidative stress occurs when there is an imbalance between reactive oxygen species (ROS) production and the body's antioxidant defense, leading to cellular and tissue damage. In both COPD and severe COVID-19, excessive ROS generation plays a crucial role in disease progression, contributing to systemic inflammation, hematological alterations, and vascular dysfunction [45,46].

Several biological processes contribute to increased ROS production, further amplifying inflammation and tissue injury. Chronic hypoxia and inflammation lead to excessive mitochondrial ROS production, exacerbating oxidative stress and impairing cellular function [47]. During inflammatory responses, neutrophils generate superoxide radicals (O_2^-), hydrogen peroxide (H_2O_2), and hydroxyl radicals (OH^-), which contribute to tissue destruction and immune dysregulation [48]. ROS reduce the availability of endothelial nitric oxide (NO), leading to vasoconstriction, impaired blood flow, and increased thrombotic risk [49].

ROS directly affect blood cell function and survival, playing a key role in hematological disturbances observed in COPD and COVID-19. Oxidative stress damages RBC membranes, leading to reduced lifespan, hemolysis, and anemia, worsening oxygen transport [50–52]. ROS hyperactivate neutrophils and macrophages, intensifying inflammatory responses and immune dysregulation [53–55]. Moreover, ROS promote platelet activation and aggregation, increasing the risk of thrombosis, microvascular injury, and multi-organ dysfunction [56,57].

The pathological effects of excessive ROS production have severe consequences in both COPD and COVID-19. In COPD, chronic oxidative stress accelerates lung tissue damage, systemic inflammation, and cardiovascular complications, leading to disease progression and frequent exacerbations [58]. In severe COVID-19, heightened ROS production is strongly associated with endothelial dysfunction, hyperinflammation (cytokine storm), and increased mortality risk [55].

Both hypoxia and oxidative stress play a central role in the systemic complications of COPD and severe COVID-19, particularly in hematopoietic changes, immune dysregulation, and coagulation abnormalities (Table 2). Understanding these mechanisms highlights the need for therapeutic strategies that target hypoxia-induced inflammation and oxidative damage, such as antioxidant therapies, oxygen supplementation, and anti-inflammatory treatments.

Table 2. Biomarkers of hypoxia and oxidative stress in COPD and severe COVID-19.

Biomarker	Description	Relevance in COPD	Relevance in Severe COVID-19
Erythropoietin (EPO)	Hormone produced by the kidneys to stimulate red blood cell (RBC) production in response to hypoxia.	Increased due to chronic hypoxia, leading to secondary polycythemia [59]	Variable: May be low or normal due to inflammation-related erythropoiesis [60,61]
Hemoglobin (Hb) and Hematocrit (Hct)	Measures of oxygen-carrying capacity in blood.	Increased in some COPD patients due to chronic hypoxia [62]	Decreased in severe COVID-19, often due to anemia of inflammation [63]

Table 2. *Cont.*

Biomarker	Description	Relevance in COPD	Relevance in Severe COVID-19
Hypoxia-Inducible Factor 1-alpha (HIF-1α)	A transcription factor activated by low oxygen levels; regulates cellular responses to hypoxia.	Upregulated, promoting erythropoiesis, angiogenesis, and glycolysis [64].	Highly upregulated, contributing to immune activation, inflammation, and vascular remodeling [65].
Reactive Oxygen Species (ROS)	Free radicals produced by mitochondria and immune cells during oxidative stress.	Increased, leading to oxidative damage in lung tissue [45].	Increased, contributing to endothelial dysfunction and tissue injury [66].
Malondialdehyde (MDA)	Malondialdehyde (MDA)	Elevated, reflecting cell membrane damage due to chronic inflammation [67].	Elevated, linked to severe oxidative injury in the lung and vascular endothelium [68].
Superoxide Dismutase (SOD)	An antioxidant enzyme that neutralizes superoxide radicals.	Increased, leading to higher oxidative stress and lung injury [69].	Decreased, reducing protection against inflammation-induced ROS [70].
Glutathione (GSH)	A major intracellular antioxidant that protects against oxidative damage.	Depleted, leading to chronic lung tissue damage [71].	Depleted, impairing the immune response and increasing lung injury risk [72].
8-Hydroxy-2′-deoxyguanosine (8-OHdG)	A DNA oxidation marker, indicating oxidative DNA damage.	Increased, reflecting oxidative stress-induced genetic damage in lung cells [73].	Increased, linked to severe systemic inflammation and endothelial dysfunction [74].
Fibrinogen	An acute-phase protein involved in blood clot formation.	Elevated, contributing to hypercoagulability and increased thrombosis risk [75].	Highly elevated, associated with coagulation disorders and microthrombosis [76].
D-dimer	A fibrin degradation product and a marker of clot formation and breakdown.	Mildly elevated, especially in exacerbations or comorbid cardiovascular disease [77].	Significantly elevated, indicating high thrombotic activity and a poor prognosis [78].
Interleukin-6 (IL-6)	A pro-inflammatory cytokine involved in immune regulation and inflammation.	Increased, associated with disease severity and systemic inflammation [79].	Markedly increased, linked to cytokine storms and respiratory failure [80].
Myeloperoxidase (MPO)	An enzyme released by neutrophils and a marker of oxidative stress and inflammation.	Elevated, contributing to neutrophil-mediated lung damage [81].	Elevated, associated with endothelial dysfunction and multi-organ injury [82].

4. Hematological Changes in COPD Patients with COVID-19

Patients suffering from COPD and COVID-19 often exhibit significant hematological changes, reflecting the complex interplay between chronic inflammation, immune dysregulation, and hypercoagulability [83]. These hematological alterations contribute to disease severity, a poor prognosis, and increased risk of complications.

4.1. Lymphopenia and Impaired Immune Responses

Lymphopenia is a common hematological abnormality observed in COPD patients infected with SARS-CoV-2 [84]. This reduction in lymphocytes, particularly CD4+ and CD8+ T cells, impairs the host's ability to mount an effective antiviral immune response [85,86]. CD4+ T cells play a crucial role in orchestrating adaptive immunity by activating B cells and cytotoxic T cells, while CD8+ T cells are essential for the direct elimination of virus-infected cells [87]. The depletion of these immune cells weakens the body's defense mechanisms, allowing for uncontrolled viral replication and prolonged infection [88].

Another critical marker of immune dysfunction in COPD patients with COVID-19 is an increased NLR. A high NLR is indicative of an exaggerated inflammatory response and has been established as a reliable prognostic marker for severe disease progression and mortality [89]. The combination of lymphopenia and elevated neutrophil counts promotes systemic inflammation, tissue damage, and multi-organ failure, exacerbating the already compromised pulmonary function in COPD patients [90].

4.2. Coagulopathy and Thromboembolic Risk

Coagulopathy is a significant concern in COPD patients with COVID-19 due to the heightened inflammatory state and endothelial dysfunction associated with both conditions. Elevated levels of D-dimer, fibrinogen, and vWF have been reported in these patients, reflecting an increased propensity for thrombotic complications. D-dimer, a fibrin degradation product, serves as a biomarker of hypercoagulability and is frequently elevated in severe COVID-19 cases, correlating with a higher risk of adverse outcomes [91].

One of the most concerning thromboembolic complications in COPD patients with COVID-19 is pulmonary embolism (PE) [92]. The chronic hypoxia and systemic inflammation present in COPD contribute to a prothrombotic environment, which, when compounded by COVID-19, significantly increases the risk of PE [83]. Furthermore, the presence of disseminated intravascular coagulation has been observed in critically ill COVID-19 patients, manifesting as widespread microvascular thrombosis and the consumption of clotting factors, leading to life-threatening hemorrhagic complications [93]. These hematological alterations necessitate close monitoring and early intervention with anticoagulant therapy to mitigate thrombotic risks.

4.3. Inflammatory Anemia and Erythrocyte Dysfunction

Chronic hypoxia in COPD patients leads to compensatory erythropoiesis, often resulting in secondary polycythemia. However, in the context of COVID-19, systemic inflammation disrupts normal erythropoiesis, leading to inflammatory anemia (also known as anemia of chronic disease) [94–96]. Pro-inflammatory cytokines such as IL-6 and TNF-α interfere with iron metabolism by increasing hepcidin levels, which inhibits iron absorption and sequestration, thus impairing hemoglobin synthesis [97].

Additionally, erythrocyte dysfunction is a notable concern in COPD patients with COVID-19. Oxidative stress and systemic inflammation contribute to altered erythrocyte membrane properties, reducing their deformability and increasing their susceptibility to hemolysis [98]. This leads to impaired oxygen delivery to tissues, further exacerbating hypoxia and worsening disease outcomes [99]. The combination of chronic hypoxia, inflammation-driven iron deficiency, and erythrocyte dysfunction highlights the complex hematological challenges faced by COPD patients during COVID-19 infection [100,101].

Figure 1 highlights the hematological changes in COPD patients with COVID-19, focusing on three main aspects: lymphopenia and impaired immune response, coagulopathy and thromboembolic risk, as well as inflammatory anemia and erythrocyte dysfunction, each contributing to disease severity and patient prognosis.

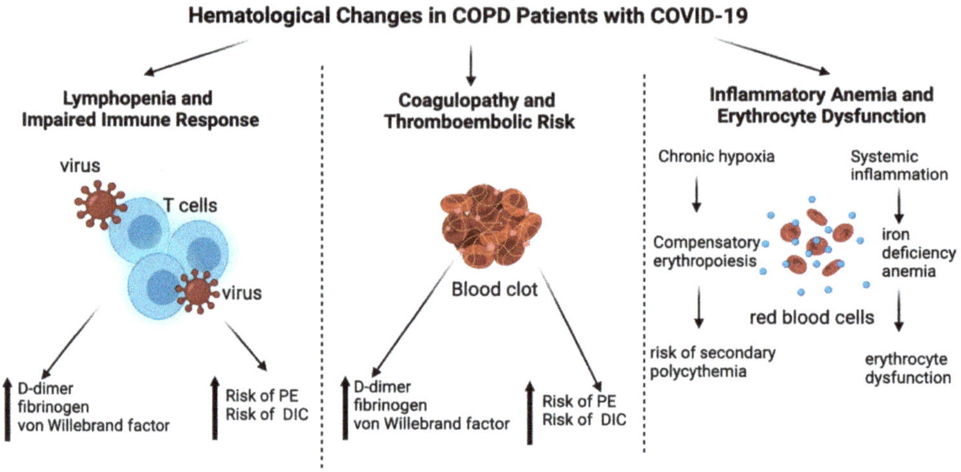

Figure 1. Hematological changes in COPD patients with COVID-19. This figure illustrates the key hematological changes observed in COPD patients with COVID-19. The three main categories included are as follows: 1. Lymphopenia and Impaired Immune Response—Characterized by a reduction in CD4+ and CD8+ T cells, leading to weakened antiviral defense, and an increased neutrophil-to-lymphocyte ratio (NLR), which serves as a prognostic marker; 2. Coagulopathy and Thromboembolic Risk—Marked by elevated D-dimer, fibrinogen, and von Willebrand factor levels, increasing the risk of pulmonary embolism (PE) and disseminated intravascular coagulation (DIC); 3. Inflammatory Anemia and Erythrocyte Dysfunction—Chronic hypoxia induces compensatory erythropoiesis, increasing the risk of secondary polycythemia, while systemic inflammation contributes to iron deficiency anemia and erythrocyte dysfunction. Arrows indicate relationships between the central concept and its specific pathological mechanisms. Created with Biorender.com.

5. Clinical Implications and Therapeutic Strategies

5.1. Monitoring Hematological Markers

The management of COPD patients infected with COVID-19 necessitates the diligent monitoring of hematological markers, which act as crucial prognostic indicators. Among these markers, D-dimer, fibrinogen, and the neutrophil-to-lymphocyte ratio (NLR) are particularly significant in assessing disease severity and predicting adverse outcomes [102].

The role of hematological markers in prognosis is significant in various medical conditions. Elevated D-dimer levels are strongly associated with an increased risk of thrombotic complications, particularly in COVID-19 patients, and can serve as an early indicator of coagulopathy [103]. High fibrinogen levels reflect an ongoing inflammatory response and a heightened risk of clot formation, both of which are crucial concerns in COPD patients with COVID-19 [104]. Additionally, a high neutrophil-to-lymphocyte ratio (NLR) is indicative of an exaggerated inflammatory response and is correlated with worse clinical outcomes in COVID-19 [105].

Given the prognostic significance of these hematological markers, screening algorithms for COPD patients with COVID-19 should incorporate routine monitoring of D-dimer, fibrinogen, and NLR. The early identification of abnormalities in these markers can help clinicians stratify patients based on risk levels and tailor interventions accordingly.

The table below outlines essential hematological monitoring strategies used in the clinical management of COPD patients with COVID-19, emphasizing their diagnostic and prognostic value, along with associated benefits and limitations (Table 3).

Table 3. Key hematological monitoring strategies in COPD patients with COVID-19.

'herapeutic ;trategy	Purpose	Advantages	Risks/Limitations	References
)-dimer monitoring	Assess thrombotic risk and predict severity	Early detection of coagulopathy and guides anticoagulation	False positives must be interpreted with other markers	[106–108]
'ibrinogen nonitoring	Evaluate inflammation and coagulation status	Helps in risk stratification	Can be elevated due to multiple factors that are not always specific to COVID-19	[109,110]
ILR assessment	Gauge severity of inflammation	Quick and cost-effective	Non-specific, influenced by other infections or stress responses	[111–113]

In clinical practice, hematological monitoring should begin at hospital admission for all COPD patients diagnosed with COVID-19. For hospitalized patients, D-dimer, fibrinogen, and NLR should be assessed on admission [114]. Suggested thresholds to consider therapeutic escalation include:

- D-dimer > 1.0 μg/mL, which is associated with increased thrombotic risk and may justify the initiation or intensification of anticoagulation;
- NLR > 7, which is predictive of severe disease progression and a poor prognosis;
- Fibrinogen > 4 g/L, which is indicative of high inflammatory burden.

These values should be interpreted along with clinical status, oxygenation levels, and imaging findings. Individualized management strategies based on dynamic changes in these markers can support timely intervention and improved outcomes.

5.2. Anticoagulation Therapy in COPD and COVID-19

Prophylactic anticoagulation plays a crucial role in preventing thromboembolic complications, particularly in patients with COPD and COVID-19, who are already prone to clot formation due to their compromised respiratory and circulatory systems. Given these risks, prophylactic anticoagulation is strongly recommended as a preventative measure to reduce morbidity and mortality in affected patients [115].

The primary benefits of prophylactic anticoagulation include the prevention of deep vein thrombosis (DVT) and pulmonary embolism (PE), which are common complications in severe COVID-19 cases, often leading to worsened respiratory function and increased mortality rates [116]. By inhibiting excessive clotting, anticoagulation significantly reduces the likelihood of these life-threatening events. Another key benefit is the reduction in mortality and morbidity. Patients receiving anticoagulation therapy show lower rates of thrombotic complications, ultimately improving their overall prognosis. By preventing clot formation, these therapies contribute to better systemic oxygenation and reduced strain on the cardiovascular system, thereby enhancing recovery outcomes.

Several anticoagulants are available for prophylactic use, each with specific advantages and considerations for patients with COPD and COVID-19.

Low-molecular-weight heparin (LMWH) is a class of anticoagulants and is often the preferred choice due to its predictable pharmacokinetics and lower risk of bleeding compared to unfractionated heparin [117]. LMWH is administered via subcutaneous injection and does not require frequent laboratory monitoring, making it a practical option for hospitalized and critically ill patients.

Direct oral anticoagulants (DOACs) are anticoagulants which offer an alternative to LMWH and are particularly useful for long-term management. However, their use requires careful dose adjustments in patients with renal impairment, which is a common comorbidity in individuals with COPD [118]. While DOACs provide convenience through oral administration, their safety profile necessitates close monitoring, especially in those with fluctuating renal function [119]. Studies have shown that direct oral anticoagulants (DOACs), such as apixaban, rivaroxaban, dabigatran, and edoxaban, offer superior efficacy and safety compared to traditional oral anticoagulant (OAC) therapies, including vitamin K antagonists (VKAs), in patients with pulmonary disease [120].

Additional clinical considerations should be given to COPD patients with coexisting COVID-19 and renal impairment. Renal dysfunction can significantly alter the pharmacokinetics of anticoagulants, particularly DOACs, increasing the risk of bleeding or subtherapeutic dosing. In this context, the regular monitoring of renal function (e.g., serum creatinine and eGFR) is essential to guide dose adjustments or the choice of anticoagulant type [121].

Although DOACs and LMWH are generally preferred, vitamin K antagonists (VKAs) such as warfarin remain in use for certain patient populations, particularly those with mechanical heart valves, antiphospholipid syndrome, or severe renal impairment, where DOACs may be contraindicated. VKAs require regular INR monitoring but may be a practical option in settings where other anticoagulants are not available or are cost-prohibitive [122].

Table 4 presents a comparative summary of anticoagulant options commonly used in COPD patients with COVID-19, detailing their mechanisms of action, clinical benefits, and associated risks to support individualized treatment decisions.

Table 4. Comparative overview of anticoagulant therapies in COPD patients with COVID-19.

Anticoagulant Type	Mechanism	Benefits	Risks/Limitations	References
LMWH	Inhibits factor Xa and prevents clot formation	Reliable dosing; fewer drug interactions	Requires injection and costlier than DOACs	[123–125]
DOACs	Directly inhibit factor Xa or thrombin	Oral administration; no need for monitoring	Bleeding risk; contraindications in renal impairment	[125–127]
VKAs (e.g., warfarin)	Inhibits vitamin K-dependent clotting factors (II, VII, IX, X)	Effective for patients with mechanical valves or antiphospholipid syndrome; cost-effective	Requires regular INR monitoring; dietary restrictions; drug interactions	[122,128]

In conclusion, prophylactic anticoagulation is a critical intervention in managing patients with COPD and COVID-19. By mitigating the risks associated with thromboembolic events, these treatments contribute significantly to improving patient outcomes, reducing complications, and ultimately enhancing survival rates in this vulnerable population. Further research and clinical guidelines will continue to refine the best practices for anticoagulation strategies, ensuring optimal care for high-risk patients.

5.3. Immunomodulators and Anti-Inflammatory Therapy

Inflammatory responses play a crucial role in the pathophysiology of COVID-19-associated respiratory deterioration, particularly in COPD patients who already have compromised pulmonary function. Immunomodulatory therapies aim to control cytokine storms and excessive inflammation [129].

Corticosteroids, such as dexamethasone, are widely used in COVID-19 management due to their ability to reduce lung inflammation and lower mortality in severe cases. Their benefits include reducing cytokine-mediated lung damage, improving oxygenation, and decreasing the need for mechanical ventilation [130]. However, they also carry certain risks, such as immune suppression, which can increase susceptibility to secondary infections and worsen COPD exacerbations [131].

Severe COVID-19 can lead to a cytokine storm, which exacerbates lung injury. Monoclonal antibodies such as Tocilizumab (IL-6 inhibitor) and Anakinra (IL-1 receptor antagonist) have been investigated for their role in mitigating excessive immune responses [132].

Another emerging strategy involves specialized pro-resolving mediators (SPMs), such as resolvins, protectins, and maresins, which actively promote the resolution phase of inflammation without inducing immunosuppression [133]. SPMs have shown potential in preclinical models for reducing cytokine-driven damage and restoring immune homeostasis [133], which could be particularly beneficial in COPD patients with COVID-19 experiencing excessive inflammatory responses.

Table 5 outlines key immunomodulatory agents used in COPD patients with COVID-19, focusing on their mechanisms of action, therapeutic benefits, and potential risks, with a particular emphasis on cytokine-targeted strategies.

Table 5. Overview of immunomodulatory therapies in the management of COPD patients with COVID-19.

Immunomodulator	Mechanism	Benefits	Risks/Limitations	References
Corticosteroids	Reduce inflammatory cytokine release	Lower mortality and improved oxygenation	Increased infection risk and hyperglycemia	[134]
Tocilizumab	An IL-6 receptor blocker; suppresses inflammation	Reduces cytokine storm severity	May cause hepatotoxicity and secondary infections	[135,136]
Anakinra	Blocks IL-1 receptor and mitigates hyperinflammation	Beneficial in severe cases	Limited evidence and high cost	[137,138]

In addition to acute management, attention must be given to the long-term consequences of SARS-CoV-2 infection in COPD patients. Recent studies have highlighted that individuals with COPD are particularly prone to developing post-COVID-19 syndrome, often characterized by persistent fatigue, dyspnea, and neuropsychiatric symptoms. In a cohort study conducted in Romania, symptoms such as fatigue (36%), cough (26%), and myalgia (23%) were observed up to six months post-infection, especially in those with pre-existing respiratory conditions and comorbidities [139]. These findings underscore the importance of integrated post-discharge care and tailored rehabilitation for COPD patients recovering from COVID-19.

6. Conclusions

Patients with chronic obstructive pulmonary disease (COPD) represent a high-risk population during the COVID-19 pandemic due to their underlying chronic inflammation, persistent hypoxia, and immune dysregulation. The presence of SARS-CoV-2 infection further exacerbates these conditions by triggering an intense systemic inflammatory response, which is closely associated with significant hematological changes.

Common hematological abnormalities in COPD patients with COVID-19, such as lymphopenia, elevated NLR, increased levels of D-dimer and fibrinogen, inflammatory anemia, and erythrocyte dysfunction, have been strongly correlated with disease severity, a poor prognosis, and a higher risk of thromboembolic complications. These alterations serve not only as reflections of disease progression but also as important prognostic markers that can guide early clinical intervention.

Chronic hypoxia and oxidative stress, which are hallmark features of both COPD and severe COVID-19, amplify inflammatory and thrombotic responses through mechanisms that involve HIFs and the excessive production of reactive oxygen species (ROS). These processes contribute to systemic damage, cellular dysfunction, and vascular complications that significantly impact patient outcomes.

From a clinical perspective, the continuous monitoring of hematological markers, particularly D-dimer, fibrinogen, and NLR, is crucial for timely risk stratification and therapeutic decision-making. Prophylactic anticoagulation-tailored anti-inflammatory therapies and immunomodulators have emerged as key strategies in managing these patients, and their use should be personalized based on individual hematological profiles and comorbid conditions.

Future research should focus on evaluating the efficacy and safety of anticoagulants and immunomodulatory treatments specifically in COPD patients with COVID-19. Additionally, clinical guidelines should emphasize personalized approaches that integrate hematological assessments as core components of care. Investigating the therapeutic potential of antioxidant strategies and targeted interventions to reduce oxidative stress may further improve clinical outcomes in this vulnerable population.

Author Contributions: Conceptualization, G.M. and C.C.; methodology, G.M.; writing—original draft preparation, G.M., G.N. and C.C.; writing—review and editing, G.M. and C.C. All authors have read and agreed to the published version of the manuscript.

Funding: This research received no external funding.

Conflicts of Interest: The authors declare no conflicts of interest.

References

1. Meng, Y.; Ji, Q.; Zhang, A.; Zhan, Y. Trends in the prevalence and incidence of chronic obstructive pulmonary disease among adults aged ≥50 years in the United States, 2000–2020. *Chronic Dis. Transl. Med.* **2024**, *10*, 302–311. [CrossRef] [PubMed]
2. Boers, E.; Barrett, M.; Su, J.G.; Benjafield, A.V.; Sinha, S.; Kaye, L.; Zar, H.J.; Vuong, V.; Tellez, D.; Gondalia, R.; et al. Global Burden of Chronic Obstructive Pulmonary Disease Through 2050. *JAMA Netw. Open* **2023**, *6*, e2346598. [CrossRef]
3. Adeloye, D.; Song, P.; Zhu, Y.; Campbell, H.; Sheikh, A.; Rudan, I.; NIHR RESPIRE Global Respiratory Health Unit. Global, regional, and national prevalence of, and risk factors for, chronic obstructive pulmonary disease (COPD) in 2019: A systematic review and modelling analysis. *Lancet Respir. Med.* **2022**, *10*, 447–458. [CrossRef]
4. Al Wachami, N.; Guennouni, M.; Iderdar, Y.; Boumendil, K.; Arraji, M.; Mourajid, Y.; Bouchachi, F.Z.; Barkaoui, M.; Louerdi, M.L.; Hilali, A.; et al. Estimating the global prevalence of chronic obstructive pulmonary disease (COPD): A systematic review and meta-analysis. *BMC Public Health* **2024**, *24*, 297. [CrossRef]
5. Vogelmeier, C.F.; Criner, G.J.; Martinez, F.J.; Anzueto, A.; Barnes, P.J.; Bourbeau, J.; Celli, B.R.; Chen, R.; Decramer, M.; Fabbri, L.M.; et al. Global Strategy for the Diagnosis, Management, and Prevention of Chronic Obstructive Lung Disease 2017 Report. GOLD Executive Summary. *Am. J. Respir. Crit. Care Med.* **2017**, *195*, 557–582. [CrossRef]
6. Lippi, G.; Henry, B.M. Chronic obstructive pulmonary disease is associated with severe coronavirus disease 2019 (COVID-19). *Respir. Med.* **2020**, *167*, 105941. [CrossRef] [PubMed]
7. Alqahtani, J.S.; Oyelade, T.; Aldhahir, A.M.; Alghamdi, S.M.; Almehmadi, M.; Alqahtani, A.S.; Quaderi, S.; Mandal, S.; Hurst, J.R. Prevalence, Severity and Mortality associated with COPD and Smoking in patients with COVID-19: A Rapid Systematic Review and Meta-Analysis. *PLoS ONE* **2020**, *15*, e0233147. [CrossRef] [PubMed]
8. Leung, M.; Alghamdi, R.; Guallart, I.; Bergamini, M.; Yu, P.; Froum, S.; Cho, S.-C. Patient-Related Risk Factors for Maxillary Sinus Augmentation Procedures: A Systematic Literature Review. *Int. J. Periodontics Restor. Dent.* **2021**, *41*, e121–e128. [CrossRef]

Ashmore, P.; Sherwood, E. An overview of COVID-19 global epidemiology and discussion of potential drivers of variable global pandemic impacts. *J. Antimicrob. Chemother.* **2023**, *78* (Suppl. S2), ii2–ii11. [CrossRef]

Marginean, C.M.; Popescu, M.; Vasile, C.M.; Cioboata, R.; Mitrut, P.; Popescu, I.A.S.; Biciusca, V.; Docea, A.O.; Mitrut, R.; Marginean, I.C.; et al. Challenges in the Differential Diagnosis of COVID-19 Pneumonia: A Pictorial Review. *Diagnostics* **2022**, *12*, 2823. [CrossRef]

Zeng, Y.; Cai, S.; Chen, Y.; Duan, J.; Zhao, Y.; Li, X.; Ma, L.; Liu, Q.; Zhu, Y.; Chen, M.; et al. Current Status of the Treatment of COPD in China: A Multicenter Prospective Observational Study. *Int. J. Chronic Obstr. Pulm. Dis.* **2020**, *15*, 3227–3237. [CrossRef] [PubMed]

Fabbri, L.M.; Luppi, F.; Beghé, B.; Rabe, K.F. Complex chronic comorbidities of COPD. *Eur. Respir. J.* **2008**, *31*, 204–212. [CrossRef]

Alvarez-Martins, I.; Remédio, L.; Matias, I.; Diogo, L.N.; Monteiro, E.C.; Dias, S. The impact of chronic intermittent hypoxia on hematopoiesis and the bone marrow microenvironment. *Pflüg. Arch.-Eur. J. Physiol.* **2016**, *468*, 919–932. [CrossRef] [PubMed]

Arunachalam, K.; Anand, K.; Palanisamy, S.; Anathy, V. Editorial: Oxidative stress related to cellular metabolism in lung health and diseases. *Front. Pharmacol.* **2022**, *13*, 1015423. [CrossRef] [PubMed]

Semenza, G.L. Regulation of Erythropoiesis by the Hypoxia-Inducible Factor Pathway: Effects of Genetic and Pharmacological Perturbations. *Annu. Rev. Med.* **2023**, *74*, 307–319. [CrossRef]

Zhang, J.; DeMeo, D.L.; Silverman, E.K.; Make, B.J.; Wade, R.C.; Wells, J.M.; Cho, M.H.; Hobbs, B.D. Secondary polycythemia in chronic obstructive pulmonary disease: Prevalence and risk factors. *BMC Pulm. Med.* **2021**, *21*, 235. [CrossRef]

Patel, A.R.; Hurst, J.R. Extrapulmonary comorbidities in chronic obstructive pulmonary disease: State of the art. *Expert Rev. Respir. Med.* **2011**, *5*, 647–662. [CrossRef]

Santos, S.; Manito, N.; Sánchez-Covisa, J.; Hernández, I.; Corregidor, C.; Escudero, L.; Rhodes, K.; Nordon, C. Risk of severe cardiovascular events following COPD exacerbations: Results from the EXACOS-CV study in Spain. *Rev. Esp. Cardiol.* **2025**, *78*, 138–150. [CrossRef]

Morgan, A.; Herrett, E.; De Stavola, B.; Smeeth, L.; Quint, J. COPD disease severity and the risk of venous thromboembolic events: A matched case-control study. *Int. J. Chronic Obstr. Pulm. Dis.* **2016**, *11*, 899. [CrossRef]

Van Der Vorm, L.N.; Li, L.; Huskens, D.; Hulstein, J.J.J.; Roest, M.; De Groot, P.G.; Ten Cate, H.; De Laat, B.; Remijn, J.A.; Simons, S.O. Acute exacerbations of COPD are associated with a prothrombotic state through platelet-monocyte complexes, endothelial activation and increased thrombin generation. *Respir. Med.* **2020**, *171*, 106094. [CrossRef]

Hanson, A.L.; Mulè, M.P.; Ruffieux, H.; Mescia, F.; Bergamaschi, L.; Pelly, V.S.; Turner, L.; Kotagiri, P.; Cambridge Institute of Therapeutic Immunology and Infectious Disease–National Institute for Health Research (CITIID–NIHR) COVID BioResource Collaboration; Göttgens, B.; et al. Iron dysregulation and inflammatory stress erythropoiesis associates with long-term outcome of COVID-19. *Nat. Immunol.* **2024**, *25*, 471–482. [CrossRef] [PubMed]

Schmitz, L.; Pirotte, M.; Lebeau, A.; Ernst, M.; Fillet, M.; Devey, A.; Schmitt, J.; Cobraiville, G.; Binsfeld, M.; Gofflot, S.; et al. Alterations of erythropoiesis in COVID-19 patients: Prevalence of positive Coombs tests and iron metabolism. *Ther. Adv. Hematol.* **2023**, *14*, 20406207231199836. [CrossRef]

Saad, E.; Maamoun, B.; Nimer, A. Increased Red Blood Cell Distribution Predicts Severity of Chronic Obstructive Pulmonary Disease Exacerbation. *J. Pers. Med.* **2023**, *13*, 843. [CrossRef]

Elemam, N.M.; Talaat, I.M.; Bayoumi, F.A.; Zein, D.; Georgy, R.; Altamimi, A.; Alkhayyal, N.; Habbal, A.; Al Ali, F.; ElKhider, A.; et al. Peripheral blood cell anomalies in COVID-19 patients in the United Arab Emirates: A single-centered study. *Front. Med.* **2022**, *9*, 1072427. [CrossRef] [PubMed]

Chandran, N.; Sigamani, K.; Khadeja Bi, A. Hematological Profile in COVID-19 Infection Among Patients in a Tertiary Care Hospital in Tamil Nadu, South India. *Cureus* **2022**, *14*, e30731. [CrossRef]

Hacievliyagil, S.S.; Gunen, H.; Mutlu, L.C.; Karabulut, A.B.; Temel, İ. Association between cytokines in induced sputum and severity of chronic obstructive pulmonary disease. *Respir. Med.* **2006**, *100*, 846–854. [CrossRef]

Merad, M.; Martin, J.C. Pathological inflammation in patients with COVID-19: A key role for monocytes and macrophages. *Nat. Rev. Immunol.* **2020**, *20*, 355–362. [CrossRef] [PubMed]

Xu, Y.-R.; Wang, A.-L.; Li, Y.-Q. Hypoxia-inducible factor 1-alpha is a driving mechanism linking chronic obstructive pulmonary disease to lung cancer. *Front. Oncol.* **2022**, *12*, 984525. [CrossRef]

Zhang, H.-X.; Yang, J.-J.; Zhang, S.-A.; Zhang, S.-M.; Wang, J.-X.; Xu, Z.-Y.; Lin, R.-Y. HIF-1α promotes inflammatory response of chronic obstructive pulmonary disease by activating EGFR/PI3K/AKT pathway. *Eur. Rev. Med. Pharmacol. Sci.* **2018**, *22*, 6077–6084.

Walmsley, S.R.; Print, C.; Farahi, N.; Peyssonnaux, C.; Johnson, R.S.; Cramer, T.; Sobolewski, A.; Condliffe, A.M.; Cowburn, A.S.; Johnson, N.; et al. Hypoxia-induced neutrophil survival is mediated by HIF-1α–dependent NF-κB activity. *J. Exp. Med.* **2005**, *201*, 105–115. [CrossRef]

Serebrovska, Z.O.; Chong, E.Y.; Serebrovska, T.V.; Tumanovska, L.V.; Xi, L. Hypoxia, HIF-1α, and COVID-19: From pathogenic factors to potential therapeutic targets. *Acta Pharmacol. Sin.* **2020**, *41*, 1539–1546. [CrossRef] [PubMed]

32. Jahani, M.; Dokaneheifard, S.; Mansouri, K. Hypoxia: A key feature of COVID-19 launching activation of HIF-1 and cytokin storm. *J. Inflamm. Lond. Engl.* **2020**, *17*, 33. [CrossRef] [PubMed]
33. Gupta, N.; Zhao, Y.-Y.; Evans, C.E. The stimulation of thrombosis by hypoxia. *Thromb. Res.* **2019**, *181*, 77–83. [CrossRef]
34. Ninivaggi, M.; de Laat, M.; Lancé, M.M.D.; Kicken, C.H.; Pelkmans, L.; Bloemen, S.; Dirks, M.L.; van Loon, L.J.C.; Gover Riemslag, J.W.P.; Lindhout, T.; et al. Hypoxia Induces a Prothrombotic State Independently of the Physical Activity. *PLoS ON* **2015**, *10*, e0141797. [CrossRef]
35. Malone, P.C.; Agutter, P.S. Deep venous thrombosis: The valve cusp hypoxia thesis and its incompatibility with modern orthodox *Med. Hypotheses* **2016**, *86*, 60–66. [CrossRef]
36. Goldhaber, S.Z.; Elliott, C.G. Acute Pulmonary Embolism: Part I: Epidemiology, Pathophysiology, and Diagnosis. *Circulatio* **2003**, *108*, 2726–2729. [CrossRef]
37. Subramanian, M.; Ramadurai, S.; Arthur, P.; Gopalan, S. Hypoxia as an independent predictor of adverse outcomes in pulmonar embolism. *Asian Cardiovasc. Thorac. Ann.* **2018**, *26*, 38–43. [CrossRef] [PubMed]
38. Matsuura, Y.; Yamashita, A.; Iwakiri, T.; Sugita, C.; Okuyama, N.; Kitamura, K.; Asada, Y. Vascular wall hypoxia promotes arteria thrombus formation via augmentation of vascular thrombogenicity. *Thromb. Haemost.* **2015**, *114*, 158–172. [CrossRef]
39. Jones, D.T.; Macdonald, J.H.; Sandoo, A.; Oliver, S.J.; Rossetti, G.M. The deleterious effects of acute hypoxia and large vesse endothelial function. *Exp. Physiol.* **2021**, *106*, 1699–1709. [CrossRef]
40. Delaney, C.; Davizon-Castillo, P.; Allawzi, A.; Posey, J.; Gandjeva, A.; Neeves, K.; Tuder, R.M.; Di Paola, J.; Stenmark, K.R.; Nozi E.S. Platelet activation contributes to hypoxia-induced inflammation. *Am. J. Physiol. Lung Cell. Mol. Physiol.* **2021**, *320*, L413–L42 [CrossRef]
41. Bhagat, S.; Biswas, I.; Ahmed, R.; Khan, G.A. Hypoxia induced up-regulation of tissue factor is mediated through extracellula RNA activated Toll-like receptor 3-activated protein 1 signalling. *Blood Cells. Mol. Dis.* **2020**, *84*, 102459. [CrossRef]
42. Ding, C.; Wang, R.; Gong, X.; Yuan, Y. Stroke risk of COPD patients and death risk of COPD patients following a stroke: systematic review and meta-analysis. *Medicine* **2023**, *102*, e35502. [CrossRef] [PubMed]
43. Conway, E.M.; Mackman, N.; Warren, R.Q.; Wolberg, A.S.; Mosnier, L.O.; Campbell, R.A.; Gralinski, L.E.; Rondina, M.T.; Van D Veerdonk, F.L.; Hoffmeister, K.M.; et al. Understanding COVID-19-associated coagulopathy. *Nat. Rev. Immunol.* **2022**, *22*, 639–64 [CrossRef] [PubMed]
44. Chandel, A.; Patolia, S.; Looby, M.; Bade, N.; Khangoora, V.; King, C.S. Association of D-dimer and Fibrinogen With Hypercoa ulability in COVID-19 Requiring Extracorporeal Membrane Oxygenation. *J. Intensive Care Med.* **2021**, *36*, 689–695. [CrossRef] [PubMed]
45. Boukhenouna, S.; Wilson, M.A.; Bahmed, K.; Kosmider, B. Reactive Oxygen Species in Chronic Obstructive Pulmonary Diseas *Oxid. Med. Cell. Longev.* **2018**, *2018*, 5730395. [CrossRef]
46. Xie, J.; Yuan, C.; Yang, S.; Ma, Z.; Li, W.; Mao, L.; Jiao, P.; Liu, W. The role of reactive oxygen species in severe acute respirator syndrome coronavirus 2 (SARS-CoV-2) infection-induced cell death. *Cell. Mol. Biol. Lett.* **2024**, *29*, 138. [CrossRef]
47. Wang, H.; Song, T.-Y.; Reyes-García, J.; Wang, Y.-X. Hypoxia-Induced Mitochondrial ROS and Function in Pulmonary Arteria Endothelial Cells. *Cells* **2024**, *13*, 1807. [CrossRef]
48. Afzal, S.; Abdul Manap, A.S.; Attiq, A.; Albokhadaim, I.; Kandeel, M.; Alhojaily, S.M. From imbalance to impairment: Th central role of reactive oxygen species in oxidative stress-induced disorders and therapeutic exploration. *Front. Pharmacol.* **202** *14*, 1269581. [CrossRef]
49. Janaszak-Jasiecka, A.; Siekierzycka, A.; Płoska, A.; Dobrucki, I.T.; Kalinowski, L. Endothelial Dysfunction Driven by Hypoxia-Th Influence of Oxygen Deficiency on NO Bioavailability. *Biomolecules* **2021**, *11*, 982. [CrossRef]
50. Yang, Q.; Chen, D.; Li, C.; Liu, R.; Wang, X. Mechanism of hypoxia-induced damage to the mechanical property in huma erythrocytes-band 3 phosphorylation and sulfhydryl oxidation of membrane proteins. *Front. Physiol.* **2024**, *15*, 1399154. [CrossRef]
51. Tariq, S.; Ismail, D.; Thapa, M.; Goriparthi, L.; Pradeep, R.; Khalid, K.; Cooper, A.C.; Jean-Charles, G. Chronic Obstructiv Pulmonary Disease and Its Effect on Red Blood Cell Indices. *Cureus* **2023**, *15*, e36100. [CrossRef] [PubMed]
52. Mullen, E.; Bergin, S.; Healy, G.; Quinn, J.; Glavey, S.; Murphy, P.T. Red blood cells from COVID-19 patients suffer from increase oxidative stress and may have increased lactate influx. *Blood Res.* **2022**, *57*, 294–296. [CrossRef] [PubMed]
53. Barnes, P.J. Oxidative Stress in Chronic Obstructive Pulmonary Disease. *Antioxidants* **2022**, *11*, 965. [CrossRef]
54. Finicelli, M.; Digilio, F.A.; Galderisi, U.; Peluso, G. The Emerging Role of Macrophages in Chronic Obstructive Pulmonary Diseas The Potential Impact of Oxidative Stress and Extracellular Vesicle on Macrophage Polarization and Function. *Antioxidants* **202** *11*, 464. [CrossRef]
55. Georgieva, E.; Ananiev, J.; Yovchev, Y.; Arabadzhiev, G.; Abrashev, H.; Abrasheva, D.; Atanasov, V.; Kostandieva, R.; Mitev, M Petkova-Parlapanska, K.; et al. COVID-19 Complications: Oxidative Stress, Inflammation, and Mitochondrial and Endothelia Dysfunction. *Int. J. Mol. Sci.* **2023**, *24*, 14876. [CrossRef] [PubMed]
56. Mallah, H.; Ball, S.; Sekhon, J.; Parmar, K.; Nugent, K. Platelets in chronic obstructive pulmonary disease: An update o pathophysiology and implications for antiplatelet therapy. *Respir. Med.* **2020**, *171*, 106098. [CrossRef]

7. Yang, M. Redox stress in COVID-19: Implications for hematologic disorders. *Best Pract. Res. Clin. Haematol.* **2022**, *35*, 101373. [CrossRef]

8. Jo, Y.S. Long-Term Outcome of Chronic Obstructive Pulmonary Disease: A Review. *Tuberc. Respir. Dis.* **2022**, *85*, 289–301. [CrossRef]

9. El-Korashy, R.I.; Amin, Y.M.; Moussa, H.A.; Badawy, I.; Bakr, S.M. Study the relationship of erythropoietin and chronic obstructive pulmonary disease. *Egypt. J. Chest Dis. Tuberc.* **2012**, *61*, 53–57. [CrossRef]

0. Soliz, J.; Schneider-Gasser, E.M.; Arias-Reyes, C.; Aliaga-Raduan, F.; Poma-Machicao, L.; Zubieta-Calleja, G.; Furuya, W.I.; Trevizan-Baú, P.; Dhingra, R.R.; Dutschmann, M. Coping with hypoxemia: Could erythropoietin (EPO) be an adjuvant treatment of COVID-19? *Respir. Physiol. Neurobiol.* **2020**, *279*, 103476. [CrossRef]

1. Ehrenreich, H.; Weissenborn, K.; Begemann, M.; Busch, M.; Vieta, E.; Miskowiak, K.W. Erythropoietin as candidate for supportive treatment of severe COVID-19. *Mol. Med.* **2020**, *26*, 58. [CrossRef]

2. Thapa, K.B.; Paudel, A.; Dhital, S.; Shrestha, A.; Ojha, L.; Shrestha, A. Polycythemia among Patients with Chronic Obstructive Pulmonary Disease Admitted to the Department of Medicine in a Tertiary Care Center: A Descriptive Cross-sectional Study. *JNMA J. Nepal Med. Assoc.* **2023**, *61*, 343–346. [CrossRef] [PubMed]

3. Ayako, R.M.; Patel, K.; Ndede, I.; Nordgren, J.; Larrson, M.; Mining, S.K. Inflammatory, Hematological, and Biochemical Biomarkers in COVID-19 Patients. *Immun. Inflamm. Dis.* **2024**, *12*, e70078. [CrossRef] [PubMed]

4. Deng, R.; Ma, X.; Zhang, H.; Chen, J.; Liu, M.; Chen, L.; Xu, H. Role of HIF-1α in hypercoagulable state of COPD in rats. *Arch. Biochem. Biophys.* **2024**, *753*, 109903. [CrossRef] [PubMed]

5. Tian, M.; Liu, W.; Li, X.; Zhao, P.; Shereen, M.A.; Zhu, C.; Huang, S.; Liu, S.; Yu, X.; Yue, M.; et al. HIF-1α promotes SARS-CoV-2 infection and aggravates inflammatory responses to COVID-19. *Signal Transduct. Target. Ther.* **2021**, *6*, 308. [CrossRef]

6. Moulaeian, M.; Ferdousmakan, S.; Banihashemi, S.; Homayounfar, S.; Pasupulla, A.P.; Malekzadegan, Y. Reactive oxygen species induced by SARS-CoV-2 infection can induce EMT in solid tumors: Potential role of COVID-19 in chemo-resistance and metastasis. *Heliyon* **2024**, *10*, e40297. [CrossRef]

7. Voskresenska, N.; Voicehovska, J.; Vojcehovska, A.; Orlikovs, G.; Skesters, A. Malondialdehyde level in chronic obstructive pulmonary disease exacerbations. In *52 Monitoring Airway Disease*; European Respiratory Society: Lausanne, Switzerland, 2015; p. OA2920.

8. Mehri, F.; Rahbar, A.H.; Ghane, E.T.; Souri, B.; Esfahani, M. Changes in oxidative markers in COVID-19 patients. *Arch. Med. Res.* **2021**, *52*, 843–849. [CrossRef]

9. Bowler, R.P.; Hokanson, J.; Taylor, M.; Levy, S.; Canaham, E.M.; Regan, E.; Wheeler, C.; Nicks, M.; Chan, E.; Crapo, J.D. Extracellular superoxide dismutase (EC-SOD) as a protective factor for risk of chronic obstructive pulmonary disease. *Eur. Respir. Rev.* **2006**, *15*, 200–201. [CrossRef]

0. Chu, J.; Hua, L.; Liu, X.; Xiong, H.; Jiang, F.; Zhou, W.; Wang, L.; Xue, G. Superoxide dismutase alterations in COVID-19: Implications for disease severity and mortality prediction in the context of omicron variant infection. *Front. Immunol.* **2024**, *15*, 1362102. [CrossRef]

1. Silvagno, F.; Vernone, A.; Pescarmona, G.P. The Role of Glutathione in Protecting against the Severe Inflammatory Response Triggered by COVID-19. *Antioxidants* **2020**, *9*, 624. [CrossRef]

2. Guloyan, V.; Oganesian, B.; Baghdasaryan, N.; Yeh, C.; Singh, M.; Guilford, F.; Ting, Y.-S.; Venketaraman, V. Glutathione Supplementation as an Adjunctive Therapy in COVID-19. *Antioxidants* **2020**, *9*, 914. [CrossRef] [PubMed]

3. Satała, J.; Woźniak, A.; Fabiś, M.; Gorzelak-Pabiś, P.; Pawlos, A.; Fabiś, J.; Broncel, M.; Woźniak, E. Severe COVID-19 classified by simple covid risk index is associated with higher levels of advanced oxidation protein products and 8-hydroxy 2 deoxyguanosine. *Epidemiol. Infect.* **2023**, *151*, e140. [CrossRef]

4. Lorente, L.; Martín, M.M.; González-Rivero, A.F.; Pérez-Cejas, A.; Cáceres, J.J.; Perez, A.; Ramos-Gómez, L.; Solé-Violán, J.; Ramos, J.A.M.Y.; Ojeda, N.; et al. DNA and RNA Oxidative Damage and Mortality of Patients With COVID-19. *Am. J. Med. Sci.* **2021**, *361*, 585–590. [CrossRef] [PubMed]

5. Ellingsen, J.; Janson, C.; Bröms, K.; Hårdstedt, M.; Högman, M.; Lisspers, K.; Palm, A.; Ställberg, B.; Malinovschi, A. CRP, Fibrinogen, White Blood Cells, and Blood Cell Indices as Prognostic Biomarkers of Future COPD Exacerbation Frequency: The TIE Cohort Study. *J. Clin. Med.* **2024**, *13*, 3855. [CrossRef]

6. Rahaghi, F.N.; Pistenmaa, C.L. Hypercoagulation in COPD: The clot thickens. *ERJ Open Res.* **2021**, *7*, 00534–02021. [CrossRef]

7. Higham, A.; Mathioudakis, A.; Vestbo, J.; Singh, D. COVID-19 and COPD: A narrative review of the basic science and clinical outcomes. *Eur. Respir. Rev. Off. J. Eur. Respir. Soc.* **2020**, *29*, 200199. [CrossRef]

8. Hilda, F.; Liana, P.; Nurtjahyo, A.; Hudari, H.; Sari, N.P.; Umar, T.P.; Amin, C.A.; Afifah, A.R. D-Dimer as a Sensitive Biomarker of Survival Rate in Patients with COVID-19. *Eurasian J. Med.* **2022**, *54*, 219–224. [CrossRef] [PubMed]

9. Hafez, W.; Nasa, P.; Khairy, A.; Jose, M.; Abdelshakour, M.; Ahmed, S.; Abdulaal, F.; Nair, N.; Ahmad, M.; Rashid, V.J.; et al. Interleukin-6 and the determinants of severe COVID-19: A retrospective cohort study. *Medicine* **2023**, *102*, e36037. [CrossRef]

80. Shekhawat, J.; Gauba, K.; Gupta, S.; Purohit, P.; Mitra, P.; Garg, M.; Misra, S.; Sharma, P.; Banerjee, M. Interleukin-6 Perpetrator of the COVID-19 Cytokine Storm. *Indian J. Clin. Biochem. IJCB* **2021**, *36*, 440–450. [CrossRef]
81. Lodge, K.M.; Vassallo, A.; Liu, B.; Long, M.; Tong, Z.; Newby, P.R.; Agha-Jaffar, D.; Paschalaki, K.; Green, C.E.; Belchamber, K.B.R. et al. Hypoxia Increases the Potential for Neutrophil-mediated Endothelial Damage in Chronic Obstructive Pulmonary Disease *Am. J. Respir. Crit. Care Med.* **2022**, *205*, 903–916. [CrossRef]
82. Teo, A.; Chan, L.L.Y.; Cheung, C.; Chia, P.Y.; Ong, S.W.X.; Fong, S.W.; Ng, L.F.P.; Renia, L.; Lye, D.C.; Young, B.E.; et al. Myeloperoxidase inhibition may protect against endothelial glycocalyx shedding induced by COVID-19 plasma. *Commun. Med.* **2023**, *3*, 62. [CrossRef] [PubMed]
83. Awatade, N.T.; Wark, P.A.B.; Chan, A.S.L.; Mamun, S.M.A.A.; Mohd Esa, N.Y.; Matsunaga, K.; Rhee, C.K.; Hansbro, P.M.; Sohal S.S.; On Behalf of The Asian Pacific Society of Respirology Apsr Copd Assembly. The Complex Association between COPD and COVID-19. *J. Clin. Med.* **2023**, *12*, 3791. [CrossRef] [PubMed]
84. Zhao, Q.; Meng, M.; Kumar, R.; Wu, Y.; Huang, J.; Deng, Y.; Weng, Z.; Yang, L. Lymphopenia is associated with severe coronavirus disease 2019 (COVID-19) infections: A systemic review and meta-analysis. *Int. J. Infect. Dis. IJID Off. Publ. Int. Soc. Infect. Dis* **2020**, *96*, 131–135. [CrossRef]
85. Guan, W.; Ni, Z.; Hu, Y.; Liang, W.; Ou, C.; He, J.; Liu, L.; Shan, H.; Lei, C.; Hui, D.S.C.; et al. Clinical Characteristics of Coronavirus Disease 2019 in China. *N. Engl. J. Med.* **2020**, *382*, 1708–1720. [CrossRef] [PubMed]
86. Pothast, C.R.; Dijkland, R.C.; Thaler, M.; Hagedoorn, R.S.; Kester, M.G.D.; Wouters, A.K.; Hiemstra, P.S.; van Hemert, M.J.; Gras S.; Falkenburg, J.H.F.; et al. SARS-CoV-2-specific CD4+ and CD8+ T cell responses can originate from cross-reactive CMV-specific T cells. *eLife* **2022**, *11*, e82050. [CrossRef]
87. Kervevan, J.; Chakrabarti, L.A. Role of CD4+ T Cells in the Control of Viral Infections: Recent Advances and Open Questions. *Int J. Mol. Sci.* **2021**, *22*, 523. [CrossRef]
88. Sun, Y.; Luo, B.; Liu, Y.; Wu, Y.; Chen, Y. Immune damage mechanisms of COVID-19 and novel strategies in prevention and control of epidemic. *Front. Immunol.* **2023**, *14*, 1130398. [CrossRef]
89. Lian, J.; Jin, C.; Hao, S.; Zhang, X.; Yang, M.; Jin, X.; Lu, Y.; Hu, J.; Zhang, S.; Zheng, L.; et al. High neutrophil-to-lymphocyte ratio associated with progression to critical illness in older patients with COVID-19: A multicenter retrospective study. *Aging* **2020** *12*, 13849–13859. [CrossRef]
90. Paliogiannis, P.; Fois, A.G.; Sotgia, S.; Mangoni, A.A.; Zinellu, E.; Pirina, P.; Negri, S.; Carru, C.; Zinellu, A. Neutrophil to lymphocyte ratio and clinical outcomes in COPD: Recent evidence and future perspectives. *Eur. Respir. Rev. Off. J. Eur. Respir. Soc* **2018**, *27*, 170113. [CrossRef]
91. Grobler, C.; Maphumulo, S.C.; Grobbelaar, L.M.; Bredenkamp, J.C.; Laubscher, G.J.; Lourens, P.J.; Steenkamp, J.; Kell, D.B. Pretorius, E. COVID-19: The Rollercoaster of Fibrin(Ogen), D-Dimer, Von Willebrand Factor, P-Selectin and Their Interactions with Endothelial Cells, Platelets and Erythrocytes. *Int. J. Mol. Sci.* **2020**, *21*, 5168. [CrossRef]
92. Singh, D.; Mathioudakis, A.G.; Higham, A. Chronic obstructive pulmonary disease and COVID-19: Interrelationships. *Curr. Opin Pulm. Med.* **2022**, *28*, 76–83. [CrossRef] [PubMed]
93. Levi, M.; Thachil, J.; Iba, T.; Levy, J.H. Coagulation abnormalities and thrombosis in patients with COVID-19. *Lancet Haematol* **2020**, *7*, e438–e440. [CrossRef] [PubMed]
94. Alisamir, M.; Ebrahimi, M.; Rahim, F. Anemia in chronic obstructive pulmonary disease: A systematic review. *Respir. Investig* **2022**, *60*, 510–521. [CrossRef]
95. Tao, Z.; Xu, J.; Chen, W.; Yang, Z.; Xu, X.; Liu, L.; Chen, R.; Xie, J.; Liu, M.; Wu, J.; et al. Anemia is associated with severe illness in COVID-19: A retrospective cohort study. *J. Med. Virol.* **2021**, *93*, 1478–1488. [CrossRef]
96. Benoit, J.L.; Benoit, S.W.; de Oliveira, M.H.S.; Lippi, G.; Henry, B.M. Anemia and COVID-19: A prospective perspective. *J. Med Virol.* **2021**, *93*, 708–711. [CrossRef] [PubMed]
97. Wessling-Resnick, M. Iron homeostasis and the inflammatory response. *Annu. Rev. Nutr.* **2010**, *30*, 105–122. [CrossRef]
98. Mendonça, M.M.; da Cruz, K.R.; Pinheiro, D.d.S.; Moraes, G.C.A.; Ferreira, P.M.; Ferreira-Neto, M.L.; da Silva, E.S.; Gonçalves R.V.; Pedrino, G.R.; Fajemiroye, J.O.; et al. Dysregulation in erythrocyte dynamics caused by SARS-CoV-2 infection: Possible role in shuffling the homeostatic puzzle during COVID-19. *Hematol. Transfus. Cell Ther.* **2022**, *44*, 235–245. [CrossRef]
99. Kent, B.D.; Mitchell, P.D.; McNicholas, W.T. Hypoxemia in patients with COPD: Cause, effects, and disease progression. *Int. J. Chronic Obstr. Pulm. Dis.* **2011**, *6*, 199–208.
100. Cavezzi, A.; Troiani, E.; Corrao, S. COVID-19: Hemoglobin, Iron, and Hypoxia beyond Inflammation. A Narrative Review. *Clin Pract.* **2020**, *10*, 1271. [CrossRef]
101. Hardang, I.M.; Søyseth, V.; Kononova, N.; Hagve, T.-A.; Einvik, G. COPD: Iron Deficiency and Clinical Characteristics in Patients With and Without Chronic Respiratory Failure. *Chronic Obstr. Pulm. Dis. J. COPD Found.* **2024**, *11*, 261–269. [CrossRef]
102. Şan, İ.; Gemcioğlu, E.; Davutoğlu, M.; Çatalbaş, R.; Karabuğa, B.; Kaptan, E.; Erden, A.; Küçükşahin, O.; Ateş, İ.; Karaahmetoğlu S.; et al. Which hematological markers have predictive value as early indicators of severe COVID-19 cases in the emergency department? *Turk. J. Med. Sci.* **2021**, *51*, 2810–2821. [CrossRef] [PubMed]

3. Al-Samkari, H.; Karp Leaf, R.S.; Dzik, W.H.; Carlson, J.C.T.; Fogerty, A.E.; Waheed, A.; Goodarzi, K.; Bendapudi, P.K.; Bornikova, L.; Gupta, S.; et al. COVID-19 and coagulation: Bleeding and thrombotic manifestations of SARS-CoV-2 infection. *Blood* **2020**, *136*, 489–500. [CrossRef] [PubMed]
4. Sui, J.; Noubouossie, D.F.; Gandotra, S.; Cao, L. Elevated Plasma Fibrinogen Is Associated With Excessive Inflammation and Disease Severity in COVID-19 Patients. *Front. Cell. Infect. Microbiol.* **2021**, *11*, 734005. [CrossRef]
5. Simadibrata, D.M.; Calvin, J.; Wijaya, A.D.; Ibrahim, N.A.A. Neutrophil-to-lymphocyte ratio on admission to predict the severity and mortality of COVID-19 patients: A meta-analysis. *Am. J. Emerg. Med.* **2021**, *42*, 60–69. [CrossRef] [PubMed]
6. Smadja, D.M.; Bory, O.M.; Diehl, J.-L.; Mareau, A.; Gendron, N.; Jannot, A.-S.; Chocron, R. Daily Monitoring of D-Dimer Allows Outcomes Prediction in COVID-19. *TH Open* **2022**, *06*, e21–e25. [CrossRef]
7. Patil, S.; Khule, S.; Toshniwal, S. Role of D-Dimer in assessing severity, monitoring, and predicating outcome in COVID-19 pneumonia: A single center study. *Glob. J. Health Sci. Res.* **2023**, *1*, 31–37. [CrossRef]
8. Beidollahkhani, S.; Fayedeh, F.; Shoja, A.; Hassan Nejad, E.; Hoseinpour, M.; Fazlpour, F.; Payandeh, A.; Pezeshki Rad, M.; Moodi Ghalibaf, A. d-dimer as a biomarker for COVID-19-associated pulmonary thromboembolism: A narrative review from molecular pathways to the imaging findings. *Egypt. J. Bronchol.* **2023**, *17*, 44. [CrossRef]
9. Kornblith, L.Z.; Sadhanandhan, B.; Arun, S.; Long, R.; Johnson, A.J.; Noll, J.; Ramchand, C.N.; Olynyk, J.K.; Farrell, D.H. γ' fibrinogen levels as a biomarker of COVID-19 respiratory disease severity. *Blood Cells. Mol. Dis.* **2023**, *101*, 102746. [CrossRef]
0. Long, W.; Yang, J.; Li, Z.; Li, J.; Chen, S.; Chen, D.; Wang, S.; Li, Q.; Hu, D.; Huang, J.; et al. Abnormal Fibrinogen Level as a Prognostic Indicator in Coronavirus Disease Patients: A Retrospective Cohort Study. *Front. Med.* **2021**, *8*, 687220. [CrossRef]
1. Toori, K.U.; Qureshi, M.A.; Chaudhry, A.; Safdar, M.F. Neutrophil to lymphocyte ratio (NLR) in COVID-19: A cheap prognostic marker in a resource constraint setting. *Pak. J. Med. Sci.* **2021**, *37*, 1435–1439. [CrossRef]
2. Ribeiro Carvalho, C.R.; Lamas, C.D.A.; Visani De Luna, L.A.; Chate, R.C.; Salge, J.M.; Yamada Sawamura, M.V.; Toufen, C.; Garcia, M.L.; Scudeller, P.G.; Nomura, C.H.; et al. Post-COVID-19 respiratory sequelae two years after hospitalization: An ambidirectional study. *Lancet Reg. Health-Am.* **2024**, *33*, 100733. [CrossRef] [PubMed]
3. Asperges, E.; Albi, G.; Zuccaro, V.; Sambo, M.; Pieri, T.C.; Calia, M.; Colaneri, M.; Maiocchi, L.; Melazzini, F.; Lasagna, A.; et al. Dynamic NLR and PLR in Predicting COVID-19 Severity: A Retrospective Cohort Study. *Infect. Dis. Ther.* **2023**, *12*, 1625–1640. [CrossRef] [PubMed]
4. Gemicioglu, B.; Uzun, H.; Borekci, S.; Karaali, R.; Kurugoglu, S.; Atukeren, P.; Sirolu, S.; Durmus, S.; Dirican, A.; Kuskucu, M.A.; et al. Focusing on Asthma and Chronic Obstructive Pulmonary Disease with COVID-19. *J. Infect. Dev. Ctries.* **2021**, *15*, 1415–1425. [CrossRef]
5. Labbé, V.; Contou, D.; Heming, N.; Megarbane, B.; Razazi, K.; Boissier, F.; Ait-Oufella, H.; Turpin, M.; Carreira, S.; Robert, A.; et al. Effects of Standard-Dose Prophylactic, High-Dose Prophylactic, and Therapeutic Anticoagulation in Patients With Hypoxemic COVID-19 Pneumonia: The ANTICOVID Randomized Clinical Trial. *JAMA Intern. Med.* **2023**, *183*, 520. [CrossRef]
6. Kaptein, F.H.J.; Stals, M.a.M.; Huisman, M.V.; Klok, F.A. Prophylaxis and treatment of COVID-19 related venous thromboembolism. *Postgrad. Med.* **2021**, *133* (Suppl. S1), 27–35. [CrossRef] [PubMed]
7. Pereyra, D.; Heber, S.; Schrottmaier, W.C.; Santol, J.; Pirabe, A.; Schmuckenschlager, A.; Kammerer, K.; Ammon, D.; Sorz, T.; Fritsch, F.; et al. Low-molecular-weight heparin use in coronavirus disease 2019 is associated with curtailed viral persistence: A retrospective multicentre observational study. *Cardiovasc. Res.* **2021**, *117*, 2807–2820. [CrossRef]
8. Roguljić, H.; Arambašić, J.; Ninčević, V.; Kuna, L.; Šesto, I.; Tabll, A.; Smolić, R.; Včev, A.; Primorac, D.; Wu, G.Y.; et al. The role of direct oral anticoagulants in the era of COVID-19: Are antiviral therapy and pharmacogenetics limiting factors? *Croat. Med. J.* **2022**, *63*, 287–294. [CrossRef]
9. Batra, G.; Modica, A.; Renlund, H.; Larsson, A.; Christersson, C.; Held, C. Oral anticoagulants, time in therapeutic range and renal function over time in real-life patients with atrial fibrillation and chronic kidney disease. *Open Heart* **2022**, *9*, e002043. [CrossRef]
0. Lai, J.; Feng, S.; Xu, S.; Liu, X. Effects of oral anticoagulant therapy in patients with pulmonary diseases. *Front. Cardiovasc. Med.* **2022**, *9*, 987652. [CrossRef]
1. Aursulesei, V.; Costache, I.I. Anticoagulation in chronic kidney disease: From guidelines to clinical practice. *Clin. Cardiol.* **2019**, *42*, 774–782. [CrossRef]
2. Ballestri, S.; Romagnoli, E.; Arioli, D.; Coluccio, V.; Marrazzo, A.; Athanasiou, A.; Di Girolamo, M.; Cappi, C.; Marietta, M.; Capitelli, M. Risk and Management of Bleeding Complications with Direct Oral Anticoagulants in Patients with Atrial Fibrillation and Venous Thromboembolism: A Narrative Review. *Adv. Ther.* **2023**, *40*, 41–66. [CrossRef] [PubMed]
3. Wei, M.Y.; Ward, S.M. The Anti-Factor Xa Range For Low Molecular Weight Heparin Thromboprophylaxis. *Hematol. Rep.* **2015**, *7*, 5844. [CrossRef]
4. Alsagaff, M.Y.; Mulia, E.P.B.; Maghfirah, I.; Azmi, Y.; Rachmi, D.A.; Yutha, A.; Andira, L.H.; Semedi, B.P. Low molecular weight heparin is associated with better outcomes than unfractionated heparin for thromboprophylaxis in hospitalized COVID-19 patients: A meta-analysis. *Eur. Heart J.-Qual. Care Clin. Outcomes* **2022**, *8*, 909–918. [CrossRef] [PubMed]

125. Wumaier, K.; Li, W.; Chen, N.; Cui, J. Direct oral anticoagulants versus low molecular weight heparins for the treatment cancer-associated thrombosis: A cost-effectiveness analysis. *Thromb. J.* **2021**, *19*, 68. [CrossRef] [PubMed]
126. Kustos, S.; Fasinu, P. Direct-Acting Oral Anticoagulants and Their Reversal Agents—An Update. *Medicines* **2019**, *6*, 103. [CrossRe
127. Lutz, J.; Jurk, K.; Schinzel, H. Direct oral anticoagulants in patients with chronic kidney disease: Patient selection and speci considerations. *Int. J. Nephrol. Renov. Dis.* **2017**, *10*, 135–143. [CrossRef]
128. Olie, R.H.; Winckers, K.; Rocca, B.; Ten Cate, H. Oral Anticoagulants Beyond Warfarin. *Annu. Rev. Pharmacol. Toxicol.* **202** *64*, 551–575. [CrossRef]
129. Kumar, A.; Sharma, A.; Tirpude, N.V.; Sharma, S.; Padwad, Y.S.; Kumar, S. Pharmaco-immunomodulatory interventions f averting cytokine storm-linked disease severity in SARS-CoV-2 infection. *Inflammopharmacology* **2022**, *30*, 23–49. [CrossRef]
130. van Paassen, J.; Vos, J.S.; Hoekstra, E.M.; Neumann, K.M.I.; Boot, P.C.; Arbous, S.M. Corticosteroid use in COVID-19 patients: systematic review and meta-analysis on clinical outcomes. *Crit. Care* **2020**, *24*, 696. [CrossRef]
131. Singanayagam, A.; Glanville, N.; Girkin, J.L.; Ching, Y.M.; Marcellini, A.; Porter, J.D.; Toussaint, M.; Walton, R.P.; Finney, L. Aniscenko, J.; et al. Corticosteroid suppression of antiviral immunity increases bacterial loads and mucus production in COP exacerbations. *Nat. Commun.* **2018**, *9*, 2229. [CrossRef]
132. Ohadian Moghadam, S. A Review on Currently Available Potential Therapeutic Options for COVID-19. *Int. J. Gen. Med.* **202** *13*, 443–467. [CrossRef] [PubMed]
133. Balta, M.G.; Papathanasiou, E.; Christopoulos, P.F. Specialized Pro-Resolving Mediators as Potential Regulators of Inflammato Macrophage Responses in COVID-19. *Front. Immunol.* **2021**, *12*, 632238. [CrossRef] [PubMed]
134. Bahsoun, A.; Fakih, Y.; Zareef, R.; Bitar, F.; Arabi, M. Corticosteroids in COVID-19: Pros and cons. *Front. Med.* **2023**, *10*, 120250 [CrossRef]
135. Abidi, E.; El Nekidy, W.S.; Alefishat, E.; Rahman, N.; Petroianu, G.A.; El-Lababidi, R.; Mallat, J. Tocilizumab and COVID-1 Timing of Administration and Efficacy. *Front. Pharmacol.* **2022**, *13*, 825749. [CrossRef]
136. Rosas, I.O.; Bräu, N.; Waters, M.; Go, R.C.; Hunter, B.D.; Bhagani, S.; Skiest, D.; Aziz, M.S.; Cooper, N.; Douglas, I.S.; et a Tocilizumab in Hospitalized Patients with Severe COVID-19 Pneumonia. *N. Engl. J. Med.* **2021**, *384*, 1503–1516. [CrossRe [PubMed]
137. Shapiro, L.; Scherger, S.; Franco-Paredes, C.; Gharamti, A.; Henao-Martinez, A.F. Anakinra authorized to treat severe coronaviru disease 2019; Sepsis breakthrough or time to reflect? *Front. Microbiol.* **2023**, *14*, 1250483. [CrossRef] [PubMed]
138. Kyriazopoulou, E.; Akinosoglou, K.; Florou, E.; Kouriannidi, E.; Bogosian, A.; Tsachouridou, O.; Syrigos, K.N.; Gatselis, N Milionis, H.; Papanikolaou, I.C.; et al. Anakinra efficacy in COVID-19 pneumonia guided by soluble urokinase plasminoge activator receptor: Association with the inflammatory burden of the host. *Int. J. Antimicrob. Agents* **2025**, *65*, 107405. [CrossRef
139. Cioboata, R.; Nicolosu, D.; Streba, C.T.; Vasile, C.M.; Olteanu, M.; Nemes, A.; Gheorghe, A.; Calarasu, C.; Turcu, A.A. Pos COVID-19 Syndrome Based on Disease Form and Associated Comorbidities. *Diagnostics* **2022**, *12*, 2502. [CrossRef]

Journal of
Clinical Medicine

MDPI

Review

Leptin and Insulin in COPD: Unveiling the Metabolic-Inflammatory Axis—A Narrative Review

Oana Maria Catana [1,†], Alexandra Floriana Nemes [2,†], Ramona Cioboata [3,*], Claudia Lucia Toma [4,*], Denisa Maria Mitroi [1], Cristina Calarasu [3] and Costin Teodor Streba [3]

1 Doctoral School, University of Medicine and Pharmacy, 200349 Craiova, Romania; oana_cattana@yahoo.com (O.M.C.); denisa_maria2@yahoo.com (D.M.M.)
2 Neonatology Department, Memorial Life Hospital Bucharest, 010719 Bucharest, Romania; alexandra-floriana.nemes@drd.umfcd.ro
3 Pneumology Department, University of Medicine and Pharmacy, 200349 Craiova, Romania; calarasu.cristina@yahoo.com (C.C.); costin.streba@umfcv.ro (C.T.S.)
4 Pneumology Department, University of Medicine Carol Davila, 020021 Bucharest, Romania
* Correspondence: ramona_cioboata@yahoo.com (R.C.); claudiatoma@yahoo.co.uk (C.L.T.)
† These authors contributed equally to this work.

Abstract: Chronic obstructive pulmonary disease (COPD) is a progressive and debilitating condition characterized by airflow limitations and systemic inflammation. The interaction between the metabolic and inflammatory pathways plays a key role in disease progression, with leptin and insulin emerging as pivotal metabolic regulators. Leptin, an adipokine that regulates energy homeostasis, and insulin, the primary regulator of glucose metabolism, are both altered in COPD patients. This narrative review provides an in-depth examination of the roles of leptin and insulin in COPD pathogenesis, focusing on the molecular mechanisms through which these metabolic regulators interact with inflammatory pathways and how their dysregulation contributes to a spectrum of extrapulmonary manifestations. These disturbances not only exacerbate COPD symptoms but also increase the risk of comorbidities such as metabolic syndrome, diabetes, cardiovascular disease, or muscle wasting. By exploring the underlying mechanisms of leptin and insulin dysregulation in COPD, this review underscores the significance of the metabolic–inflammatory axis, suggesting that restoring metabolic balance through leptin and insulin modulation could offer novel therapeutic strategies for improving clinical outcomes.

Keywords: chronic obstructive pulmonary disease; COPD; leptin; insulin; metabolic–inflammatory axis; oxidative stress

1. Introduction

Chronic obstructive pulmonary disease (COPD) ranks among the top three global causes of death and is responsible for 90% of fatalities in low- and middle-income countries [1]. The number of deaths from COPD increased by 17.5% between 2007 and 2017, accounting for 3.2 million in 2017 [2]. Moreover, in 2018, about 12.8 million adults (5% of the adult population) were diagnosed with COPD [3,4].

The prevalence of COPD is expected to rise due to higher smoking rates in low- and middle-income countries, aging populations in high-income nations, and increased biomass exposure, which may elevate the risk of non-smoking-related COPD and impact prevention and treatment strategies [5]. Current estimates suggest a 10.3% prevalence rate, with a 95% confidence interval (CI) of 8.2% to 12.8% [1,6]. Data modeled from the Global Burden of Disease database indicates that the number of global COPD cases in individuals aged 25 years and older is projected to increase by 23% between 2020 and 2050, potentially reaching 600 million cases by 2050 [7]. Furthermore, this increase is expected to be more pronounced among women and populations in low- and middle-income [1,8]. Additionally, research has demonstrated a connection between COPD and air pollution [9].

Therefore, the prevalence of COPD is typically higher than what health authorities estimate, making it an underdiagnosed condition. This underestimation can be attributed to a number of factors, such as a lack of reliable diagnostic criteria, variations in lung function tests, inconsistent terminology used for COPD, and a lack of government funding [10–12].

The recognition of significant unmet needs in the treatment of chronic obstructive pulmonary disease has led to considerable research activity in the last decade in an effort to better understand the pathophysiology behind this multifaceted disorder and enhance therapeutic options. Key concerns include the mechanisms of inflammation, metabolic dysregulation, early diagnosis, the identification of effective biomarkers, and the relationship between comorbidities and airway disease [13].

Chronic obstructive pulmonary disease is predominantly defined by airflow limitations caused by airway inflammation and remodeling, frequently linked to parenchymal destruction and the onset of emphysema [14]. Increased and progressive airway remodeling and airflow limitation contribute to a decline in exercise capacity, air trapping, and both static and dynamic hyperinflation [15]. Cigarette smoking is the leading risk factor for COPD and a significant contributor to the development of numerous chronic diseases and certain malignancies [16]. The hallmark symptom of COPD is dyspnea, and there is mounting evidence that the entirety of the symptom burden, which may also include coughing, sputum production, wheezing, and chest tightness, has a significant negative influence on quality of life and health status [17]. Currently, the international guidelines use "FEV1 (Forced expiratory volume in 1 s)/FVC (Forced vital capacity) < 70%" as the GOLD standard to diagnose COPD [18]. Although the diagnosis of COPD requires spirometric measurements, the assessment of respiratory symptoms is essential for the choice of treatment.

The clinical signs and pathological processes are not limited to airway remodeling and pulmonary inflammation. One of the main characteristics of COPD is that comorbidities have a big impact on an individual's prognosis. Cardiovascular diseases, osteoporosis, muscle weakness, metabolic and endocrinological disorders, anxiety disorders, depression, and cancer are among the most prevalent health conditions associated with these factors [19] (Figure 1).

Among the primary factors potentially contributing to the elevated occurrence of co-existing conditions, systemic inflammation is widely recognized as a key feature of the disease [20]. Besides causing inflammation of the airways and lungs, smoking also enhances systemic oxidative stress, humoral and cellular inflammation, pronounced alterations in vasomotor and endothelial function, and elevated levels of circulating procoagulant factors [21]. Along with the airway and lung abnormalities commonly seen in COPD, the systemic effects of smoking may also contribute significantly to the onset of chronic diseases, either independently or in combination with other risk factors such as obesity, hyperlipidemia, and high blood pressure [22]. Additionally, individuals with stable COPD exhibit a higher prevalence of diabetes mellitus compared to the general population (15–17%) [23].

Initially, adipose tissue was thought to be an organ solely used for energy storage. However, research conducted in recent decades has shown that this conventional understanding is no longer accurate. Adipose tissue is known to play a unique role in insulin resistance due to the production of adipokines, such as leptin and adiponectin, and the rise in circulating free-fatty acids [24]. It has also been demonstrated that non-hypoxemic COPD patients exhibit higher IR (insulin resistance) than healthy individuals. Moreover, growing evidence suggests that leptin, a protein produced by adipose tissue, may play a crucial role in enhancing the inflammatory response [25]. During acute exacerbations of COPD, serum leptin levels and the leptin/adiponectin ratio are elevated, and these increases are correlated with elevated serum levels of tumor necrosis factor alpha TNF-α and IL-6 (interleukin-6) [26].

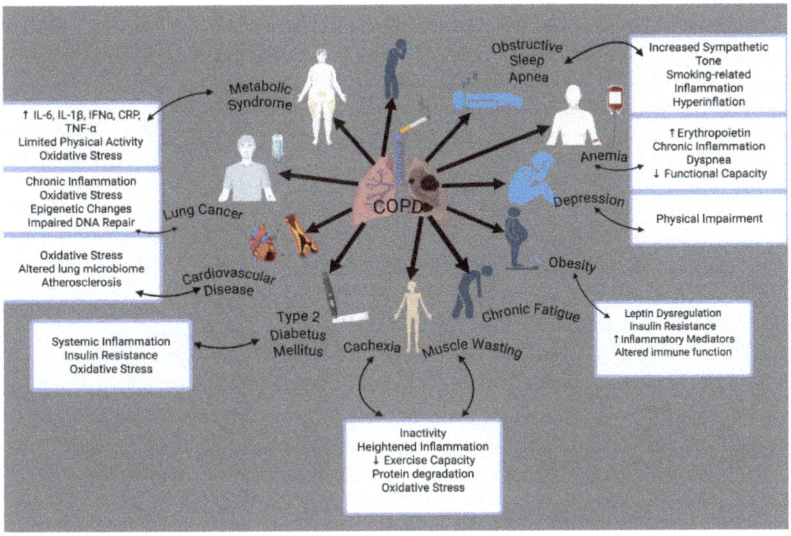

Figure 1. Comorbidities associated with COPD. Created with BioRender.com (accessed on 3 February 2025).

In spite of increasing evidence on the metabolic-inflammatory axis in COPD, the exact roles of leptin and insulin in disease progression remain incompletely understood. This narrative review aims to explore the interaction between leptin, insulin, and COPD, highlighting their impact on systemic inflammation, metabolic dysregulation, and potential therapeutic implications.

Additionally, this review discusses the clinical implications of these findings and emphasizes the need for personalized medicine approaches that consider metabolic dysfunction as a key component of COPD management, ultimately aiming to improve patient outcomes and quality of life. By achieving these objectives, insights into the complex relationship between the insulin–leptin axis and COPD will be provided, highlighting its potential as a therapeutic target for improving metabolic health and the well-being of patients with COPD in terms of life quality.

We conducted an extensive literature search using databases such as PubMed and Google Scholar, prioritizing peer-reviewed articles on COPD pathophysiology, metabolic dysregulation, and inflammatory pathways. As a narrative review, our primary objective is to offer a broad synthesis of emerging evidence on the insulin–leptin axis in COPD, underscoring the critical interplay between metabolic dysfunction and disease progression.

2. Leptin: A Metabolic and Immunological Hormone

In terms of structure, leptin is a 16 kDa non-glycosylated polypeptide that is primarily found in adipocytes, an adipokine that was first discovered to be a crucial molecule in controlling food intake and body weight [27]. In conjunction with the endocrine system and the hypothalamic–pituitary–adrenal axis, leptin plays a vital role in insulin secretion, as well as in regulating angiogenesis and energy homeostasis [28,29]. A growing amount of evidence indicates that food consumption essentially controls leptin production, and this is linked to a brief rise in ob gene (obese gene) expression, whereas fasting lowers leptin levels [30]. However, there are additional factors that can affect leptin levels; its secretion can be induced by insulin and glucocorticoids [31].

The leptin receptor (LepR) is expressed in various tissues, including adipose tissue, the heart; muscles; the lungs; the small intestine; the liver; and the central nervous system, particularly in the hypothalamus [32]. The pleiotropic effects of leptin are facilitated by the widespread expression of its receptors. Leptin is typically secreted by adipocytes into the bloodstream; it then crosses the blood–brain barrier and acts on specific areas of the brain, with particular emphasis on the hypothalamus [33]. LepR, belonging to the type I cytokine receptor family, consists of six subtypes, ranging from LepRa to LepRf [34].

Around a year after the leptin gene was discovered, it was revealed that leptin controls appetite and metabolism by inhibiting the synthesis and release of neuropeptide Y (NPY) in the arcuate nucleus (ARC) [35]. Subsequently, it was found that the dorsomedial hypothalamic nucleus (DMH), ARC, lateral hypothalamic nuclei (LH—the "hunger center"), and ventromedial hypothalamic nucleus (VMH—the "satiety center") all contain the LEP-R isoform b (LEP-Rb), which is essential for controlling body mass and energy balance [36]. Subsequent research has shown that leptin can suppress appetite by activating neural pathways targeted by anorexigenic stimulants and inhibit those activated by orexigenic stimulants. The agouti-related protein (AgRP) and NPY are two instances of orexigenic neuropeptides. Alpha-melanocyte-stimulating hormone (α-MSH), a byproduct of proopiomelanocortin (POMC), has anorexigenic properties. The central melanocortin system, which governs energy balance, consists of neurons that express AgRP, POMC, and melanocortins [37].

The interplay between leptin signaling and the primary feeding regulation is an easy-to-understand model: leptin modulates POMC transcription, prompting the release of its α-MSH product into the synapse, where it binds to the melanocortin receptor (MCR) on neurons, thereby activating them and inhibiting appetite [38]. Leptin also prevents neurons from synthesizing NPY/AgRP, which lessens the stimulatory effect of AgRP on MCR [38]. In summary, leptin controls energy homeostasis by influencing the function of NPY/AgRP and POMC neurons in the arcuate nucleus [37].

Regardless of its impact on adiposity, brain leptin signaling controls glucose homeostasis. It can be challenging to ascertain whether leptin signaling in a particular brain structure directly regulates glucose homeostasis or whether the observed effects are secondary to changes in body weight and adiposity, given that obesity is a major contributing factor to insulin resistance. When LepR is unilaterally reactivated in the arcuate nucleus of the hypothalamus of mice that are otherwise LepR-deficient, body weight and adiposity are only slightly affected, but blood glucose and hyperinsulinemia are significantly improved [39]. According to Rossi et al., the central melanocortin system regulates glucose homeostasis [40]. There is evidence that glucose homeostasis is also regulated by leptin signaling in VMH neurons. For instance, without changing body weight, selectively deactivating SOCS3 in steroidogenic factor-1 (SF1) cells improves glucose homeostasis by increasing leptin sensitivity [41].

Crucially, leptin also plays a vital part in regulating both the innate and adaptive immune system. The structural resemblance between leptin and the long-chain helical cytokine family, which comprises IL-6, IL-11, IL-12, and oncostatin M, might be the cause [42]. A reduction in plasma leptin levels usually results in compromised immune function because its immunoregulatory roles bridge nutritional health and T helper (Th)1 immune responses [43]. The involvement in the cytokine cascade, which coordinates the host defense mechanisms and innate immune response, is strongly suggested by altered leptin production during infection and inflammation [44]—its levels decrease with chronic inflammation, in contrast to the increase seen with acute inflammatory stimulation [45]. Leptin has been demonstrated to activate the Janus kinase/signal transducer and activator of transcription (JAK/STAT) pathway, just like other IL-6 family members [46]. Additionally, the suppressor-of-cytokine signaling (SOCS)-3, which suppresses STAT signaling, is expressed in response to leptin [47]. The signaling of other cytokines in the IL-6 family is also characterized by the activation of these pathways [48]. By changing the synthesis of proinflammatory and anti-inflammatory cytokines, the physiological levels of leptin can modify the body's reaction to an inflammatory challenge.

3. Insulin: Role Beyond Glucose Homeostasis

Insulin, a polypeptide hormone made up of 51 amino acids, is crucial for regulating glucose balance, promoting cell growth, and controlling metabolism. Previously, it was thought that this hormone was only produced by pancreatic β cells, but new research has revealed that some central nervous system neurons also produce it in trace amounts [49]. Food intake initiates the metabolism of glucose, leading to increased insulin production by β cells and a reduction in glucagon secretion by α cells to normalize serum glucose levels. Insulin is distributed to hepatocytes and circulates throughout the body after secretion, prompting them to store glucose as glycogen.

In addition to absorbing glucose, skeletal muscle cells, and adipocytes, other key targets of circulating insulin also contribute to lowering blood glucose levels back to baseline [50]. Insulin, through the tyrosine kinase receptor pathway, facilitates glucose uptake, skeletal muscle protein synthesis, glycogenesis, and lipogenesis, similar to other polypeptide hormones [51]. The insulin receptors (IRs) located in the plasma membrane function enzymatically to transfer phosphates from ATP to tyrosine residues on intracellular target proteins [52]. Following insulin's binding to the α subunits, the β subunits undergo phosphorylation, thereby initiating the receptor's catalytic activity [52]. Furthermore, several intracellular proteins that regulate insulin metabolism, cell division, and gene expression are phosphorylated by the activated receptor [53].

About 70% of glucose uptake is directed to skeletal muscle [54], while the liver uses the remaining amount of glucose in an insulin-dependent manner. A rise in plasma insulin levels activates glucose uptake and utilization in skeletal muscle, while postprandial hyperglycemia triggers the pancreas to release insulin [55]. Muscle cells primarily use fats and carbohydrates as energy sources to create ATP, which is necessary for muscle function [56]. Following glucose consumption, the concentration of plasma glucose influences the release of insulin by pancreatic β cells, resulting in hyperinsulinemia. This results in a decrease in lipid utilization and a drop in the concentration of plasma free fatty acids (FFA). By triggering multiple enzymes, insulin simultaneously promotes the uptake of glucose by skeletal muscle [57].

Adipose tissue is responsible for producing approximately 10% of the insulin required for glucose absorption [58]. Therefore, especially in obese people, the biological characteristics of adipose tissue from various sites may be important in the development and progression of metabolic disorders. There have been reports that insulin controls a number of aspects of the functional development and differentiation of adipose cells [59]. Adipose tissue is predominantly unaffected by glucose absorption; however, it significantly relies on the levels of FFA released into the bloodstream by insulin. This process is essential for the optimal functioning of vital organs, including the heart [58].

Endothelial dysfunction is one of the most frequently addressed issues related to endothelial function, with insulin playing a pivotal role in this context [60]. This condition is marked by the expression of pro-inflammatory and pro-thrombotic factors, a decline in nitric oxide (NO) bioavailability, heightened oxidative stress due to increased production of reactive oxygen species (ROS), and impaired vasoreactivity [60]. By controlling the production of NO, the two main signaling cascades that are triggered by the binding of insulin to endothelial insulin receptors and mediated by phosphatidylinositol 3-kinase (PI3K) and Ras–mitogen-activated protein kinase (MAPK) is subsequently implicated in these dysfunctional processes [61].

A complex and highly integrated network mediates insulin signaling and regulates multiple processes. The insulin receptor (IR) initiates the phosphorylation of insulin receptor substrate proteins (IRS proteins), which are vital for activating two key signaling pathways [62]. The Ras–mitogen-activated protein kinase pathway regulates gene expression and works in conjunction with the PI3K pathway to promote cell growth and differentiation. In contrast, the PI3K–AKT/protein kinase B (PKB) pathway primarily governs the metabolic functions of insulin [62].

The complex interaction between insulin and leptin regarding their functions is shown below. Figure 2 illustrates how both hormones play pivotal roles in regulating energy balance and metabolism. This intricate interplay is crucial for maintaining metabolic health and understanding the mechanisms behind metabolic diseases.

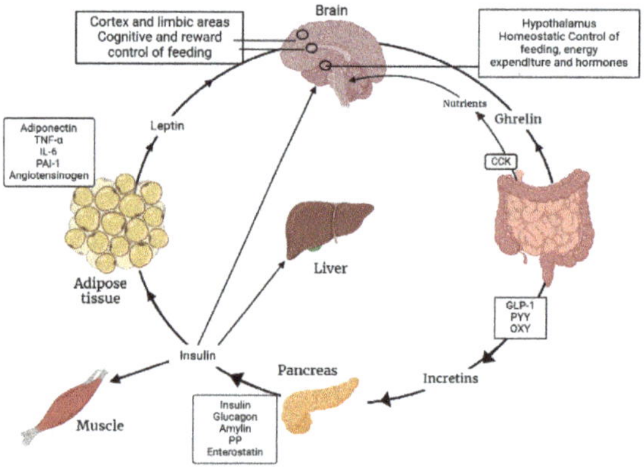

Figure 2. Synergy between insulin and leptin functions. PAI-1: Plasminogen Activator Inhibitor-1; PYY: Peptide YY; GLP-1: Glucagon-like Peptide-1; PP: Pancreatic Polypeptide; OXY: Oxytocin. Created with BioRender.com (accessed on 3 February 2025).

4. Insulin–Leptin Interplay in the Central Nervous System

In the dynamic world of hypothalamic neurons, leptin and insulin are instrumental in initiating important signaling pathways. Leptin activates the JAK–STAT3 pathway, while insulin engages the PI3K–Akt pathway [63] (Figure 3). Despite mediating different but similar signaling pathways, leptin and insulin are both known to be important modulators of adiposity and energy homeostasis. Studies have indicated that obesity, insulin resistance, hyperphagia, and hyperleptinemia observed in murine models are correlated with the disruption of insulin receptors (IRs) within the central nervous system [64]. Anorexigenic effects of these hormones are mediated by CNS-expressed IRs and leptin [65–67]. Leptin and insulin are known to enhance the activity of the anorexigenic POMC/CART (cocaine- and amphetamine-related transcript) neurons, while simultaneously exerting an inhibitory effect on the orexigenic NPY/AgRP neurons [67,68]. Recent research has also clarified how leptin and insulin interact with one another. For instance, insulin resistance might alter leptin signaling within a hypothalamic cell line, and leptin resistance could lead to the suppression of insulin signaling [63]. Also, insulin serves a pivotal function in enhancing the activation of STAT3 mediated by leptin, which is a transcription factor of considerable importance within a crucial signaling pathway designed to inhibit the development of obesity [69].

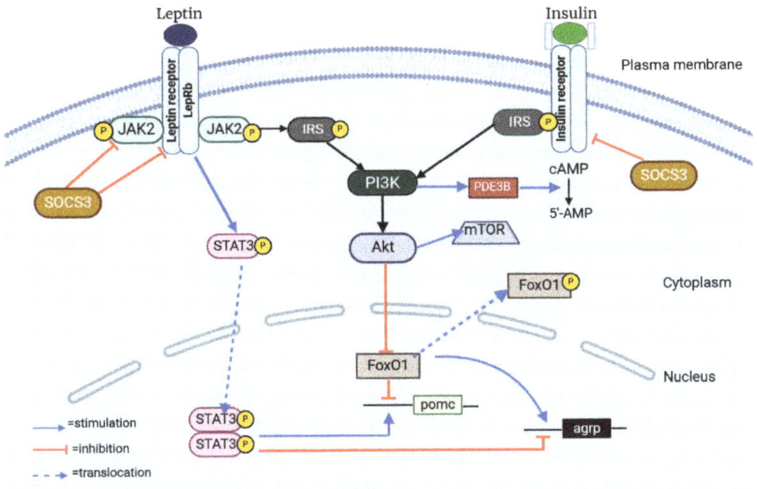

Figure 3. Insulin–leptin interplay in the hHypothalamus. SOCS3: Suppressor of Cytokine Signaling 3; JAK2: Janus Kinase 2; LepRb: Long isoform of Leptin Receptor B; STAT3: Signal Transducer and Activator of Transcription 3; IRS: Insulin Receptor Substrate 1; PI3K: Phosphatidylinositol 3 Kinase; FoxO1: Forkhead Box O1; mTOR: Mammalian Target of Rapamycin; PDE3B: Phosphodiesterase 3B; cAMP: cyclic Adenosine Monophosphate. Created with BioRender.com (accessed on 3 February 2025).

One feature of the signaling pathways common to ObRb (Leptin Receptor B, Obese Receptor B) and IR is the engagement of PI3K, suggesting that the interaction between IRS and PI3K might serve as a mechanism linking the regulatory effects of insulin and leptin on decreasing food consumption [70,71]. Mechanistically, when insulin triggers the PI3K/Akt signaling pathway, FoxO1, its downstream mediator, is phosphorylated and it becomes inactive and moves from the nucleus to the cytoplasm, allowing STAT3 to bind to the POMC or AgRP promoter [72–74]. The IRS/PI3K/Akt pathway plays a critical role in the central nervous system, being fundamental to the mechanisms of insulin and leptin [65,66]. Furthermore, weight loss and an increase in leptin sensitivity are the outcomes of FoxO1 deletion in POMC neurons [75], a fact that suggests that FoxO1 may serve as a mediator in the interaction between insulin and leptin in the regulation of food intake.

Protein Tyrosine Phosphatase 1B (PTP1B) is another mediator linked to the suppression of insulin and leptin signaling. Insulin and leptin signaling are both negatively regulated by PTP1B [76,77]. By dephosphorylating the activated insulin receptor, PTP1B inhibits the activity of insulin and leptin, respectively, through JAK2 [78]. Beyond PTP1B, the suppressor of cytokine signaling 3 (SOCS3) emerges as a significant negative regulator within the intricate networks of insulin and pathways [79]. When SOCS3 is overexpressed in POMC neurons, it triggers a cascade of physiological responses that culminate in hyperphagia and the development of obesity [80,81]. Conversely, the deletion of SOCS3 in hypothalamic neurons has demonstrated improvements in leptin sensitivity, a reduction in appetite, and protection against diet-induced obesity [82]. Also, according to some theories, SOCS3 inhibits IR signaling [79].

5. Pathophysiological Links Between COPD, Insulin, and Leptin

5.1. Leptin Dysregulation in COPD

5.1.1. Systemic and Local Inflammation

The mechanisms underlying lung inflammation and damage in COPD may be influenced by elevated circulating levels of leptin, given the highly vascularized nature of the lungs.

A distinctive pattern of inflammation has been delineated within each compartment of the lungs. The involvement of various types of inflammatory cells, including neutrophils, dendritic cells, CD^{8+} T-lymphocytes, and macrophages, has been associated with the progression of chronic inflammation [83]. In fact, Broekhuizen et al. [84] have elucidated that leptin is identifiable in the induced sputum specimens of individuals diagnosed with mild to moderate COPD, and their findings underscore a robust correlation between the concentration of leptin in sputum and the inflammatory biomarkers TNFα and C-reactive protein (CRP).

Cigarette smoke, a major stimulus of the innate immune response, causes inflammation and propels the pathophysiology of COPD, with subsequent host defense mechanisms being modified rather than suppressed. A recent investigation has been conducted to analyze the expression of leptin within peripheral lung tissue, and it has revealed that pulmonary leptin is primarily synthesized by bronchial epithelial cells, type II pneumocytes, and alveolar macrophages [85]. Furthermore, tobacco smoke appears to serve as a potential catalyst for the expression of pulmonary leptin, as demonstrated by the significantly elevated levels of leptin-expressing bronchial epithelial cells and alveolar macrophages observed in smokers, irrespective of their COPD status, in comparison to never-smokers [85]. These results suggest the existence of a potential autocrine and/or paracrine mechanism by which leptin may modulatively influence the activation of epithelial cells in the context of COPD. In fact, numerous intracellular signal transduction pathways, such as the JAK/STAT and MAPK pathways, have been demonstrated to be activated by leptin in bronchial epithelial cells [86]. Woo et al. demonstrated that leptin causes human airway epithelial cells to produce more mucin [86], which makes it more likely that leptin contributes to mucus buildup in inflammatory lung diseases.

Compared to healthy women, women with COPD have higher serum leptin concentrations [87]. Furthermore, women with COPD have higher levels of circulating leptin than men do, and these levels rise more in proportion to an increase in body fat than in men with COPD. Breyer et al. [88] demonstrated that there is a complex relationship between low-grade systemic inflammation in COPD and adipokine metabolism, with circulating leptin, CRP, and fibrinogen having a significant relationship. The BODE index, Body mass index, degree of airflow obstruction, dyspnea, and exercise capacity (E) along with the fat-free mass index (FFMI) are clearly linked to circulating levels of leptin in COPD patients, demonstrating a positive correlation with the BODE index and a negative correlation with FFMI [89]. Additionally, in these patients, leptin appears to be the primary predictor of low FFMI [90].

5.1.2. Leptin Resistance and COPD

Over one-third of individuals suffering from chronic obstructive pulmonary disease are obese [91], and obesity is linked to insulin resistance, dyslipidemia, and changes in immune function. Although the exact cause of these detrimental systemic changes in COPD is unknown, data from the COPD gene study indicate that obesity is linked to worse dyspnea, a shorter 6 min walk distance, a lower quality of life, and a higher risk of hospitalization for exacerbations [91]. Obese individuals specifically showed lower levels of Treg, which are key regulators of peripheral immune tolerance and have an inverse relationship with BMI and leptin levels [92].

Moreover, in patients with COPD who are overweight or obese, elevated insulin resistance is linked to obesity and metabolic syndrome [93]. The Bolton et al. [93] study implies that elevated levels of circulatory inflammatory mediators like IL-6 and high BMI in these patients both exacerbate insulin resistance. In individuals with COPD who present with excess body weight, there is a significant reduction in plasma adiponectin levels accompanied by markedly elevated levels of TNF-α, IL-6 and leptin [94]. Obesity in patients classified as GOLD Stages 1 and 2 is associated with a heightened risk of cardiovascular complications and overall mortality, much like the risks seen with metabolic syndrome and type 2 diabetes [95]. Conversely, overweight patients with significantly impaired lung function in GOLD Stages 3 and 4 exhibit a reduced relative mortality risk [96,97], an intriguing phenomenon commonly referred to as the "obesity paradox".

Leptin resistance is characterized by the inability to produce its anorexigenic effects. Molecular/cellular circulatory regulation, leptin autoregulation, genetic mutations, and limited tissue access are some of the mechanisms causing this [98]. The phenomenon of central leptin resistance is a key factor in the progression of obesity, and it extends its influence to peripheral tissues, including the liver, pancreas, platelets, vasculature, and myocardium [99]. Either resistance to leptin action in specific tissues or excessive leptin activity, associated with obesity-related hyperleptinemia, may cause metabolic and inflammatory damage.

Selective leptin resistance is a subtype of leptin resistance characterized by the absence of leptin's effects on appetite and body mass regulation, while the sympathetic nervous system remains responsive to leptin [100]. By enhancing the expression of uncoupling protein 1 (UCP1), leptin in this scenario continues to affect the sympathetic nervous system, resulting in thermogenesis in brown adipose tissue and the mobilization of lipids in white adipose tissue [101]. There are two plausible explanations: a malfunction may occur within the molecular signaling pathways responsible for mediating the effects of leptin locally rather than on a general scale, or the specific actions of leptin may be influenced by abnormalities within designated brain regions [100].

There are similarities between the mechanisms of obesity and COPD, including inflammation, and a connection between the modulation of lung function and the activation or deactivation of adipose tissue pathways. It is widely recognized that chronic obstructive pulmonary disease is linked to heightened levels of oxidative stress and reactive oxygen species, and these factors can alter signaling pathways and disrupt the function of antioxidant molecules, playing a significant role in the development of this pathology [102]. However, the association between obesity and related disorders, particularly insulin resistance and type 2 diabetes, is significantly influenced by heightened levels of reactive oxygen species [103].

5.2. Insulin Resistance and COPD

Insulin resistance is defined as a diminished responsiveness of insulin-targeting tissues to elevated levels of this hormone. This condition is regarded as a significant pathological contributor to a variety of health disorders, including metabolic syndrome, nonalcoholic fatty liver disease (NAFLD), atherosclerosis, and type 2 diabetes [104]. Non-physiologically elevated plasma glucose levels, the main clinical symptom of type 2 diabetes, is preceded by insulin resistance. In the prediabetic state, insulin levels increase to fulfill physiological demands, leading to chronic hyperinsulinemia and subsequent β cell dysfunction, which ultimately culminates in the development of type 2 diabetes [105].

The interaction of genetic and environmental factors contributes significantly to the pathogenesis of insulin resistance. The mechanism primarily consists of abnormalities in the immune environment, hypoxia, inflammation, lipotoxicity, and dysfunctional metabolic processes [106]. Genetic mutations affecting the insulin signaling pathway, abnormal insulin structures, substance metabolism-related genetic defects, and other related genetic defects are the categories of genetic factors linked to insulin resistance [106]. The hallmark of obesity-induced insulin resistance (IR) is compromised insulin function, which suppresses hepatic glucose production and increases muscle and adipose tissue glucose uptake [107]. It has been found that there is a causal relationship between obesity and insulin resistance and that changes in weight can either enhance or diminish insulin sensitivity [108].

IR and COPD have a pathophysiological connection, in part because they are associated with risk factors like smoking and inactivity. Furthermore, systemic effects, including inflammation and the exacerbation of physical inactivity and sedentary behavior, along with corticosteroid therapy, may also contribute to the challenges faced by patients with chronic obstructive pulmonary disease [109]. The principal mechanisms of inflammation associated with the development of insulin resistance (IR) encompass a range of inflammatory factors that markedly disrupt the signaling pathways of the insulin receptor [106]. Insulin sensitivity is directly impacted by pro-inflammatory mediators derived from macrophages, such as TNF-α and IL-1β [110]. TNF-α exerts a significant influence on insulin resistance within adipose tissue by eliciting aberrant signals on phosphorylated serine residues of insulin receptor substrate 1 (IRS1), interfering with its normal functioning, thereby compromising the integrity of insulin signaling pathways and contributing to metabolic dysfunction [111]. Furthermore, serine phosphorylation and kinase pathway defects may be two ways that TNF-α influences insulin signaling [112]. C-reactive protein is widely acknowledged as a significant indicator of inflammation that is correlated with insulin resistance (IR) and an array of metabolic disorders [106]. CRP exerts a profound influence on the regulation of energy homeostasis, insulin sensitivity, and glucose equilibrium through its interaction with leptin, thereby inhibiting the latter's signaling pathways and altering its central actions within the hypothalamic framework [113].

According to studies (Table 1), patients with COPD had higher insulin resistance than healthy, age-matched controls [114]. A significant number of individuals diagnosed with COPD are also affected by additional chronic conditions. Inflammatory mediators present in the bloodstream can contribute to or intensify comorbidities, such as type 2 diabetes mellitus (T2DM) and metabolic syndrome [115]. This syndrome encompasses a range of cardiovascular disease risk factors, including insulin resistance [116]. Moreover, IR is not influenced by the degree of airway obstruction; therefore, even in patients with COPD who are clinically stable, it increases the risk of metabolic and cardiovascular disorders [93].

Table 1. Key studies on leptin and insulin dysregulation in COPD patients.

Author (Year)	Main Outcomes
Bolton et al. (2007) [93]	COPD patients had greater insulin resistance than the healthy subjects
Breyer et al. (2011) [87]	Leptin is increased in COPD women when compared to healthy women and compared to COPD men and to a greater extent in overweight women with COPD
Breyer et al. (2012) [88]	Female COPD subjects had higher leptin and higher ratios of leptin/FM and leptin/adiponectin compared with male COPD subjects
Eker et al. (2010) [114]	Leptin levels were lower in COPD patients compared to controls. COPD patients had higher HOMA-IR scores
Minas et al. (2011) [117]	Patients with COPD and MetS show higher leptin levels and greater insulin resistance compared to those without MetS.
Takabatake et al. (1999) [118]	Serum leptin was lower in COPD patients compared to healthy controls, yet it remains physiologically regulated even amidst cachexia.
Schols et al. (1999) [25]	Emphysematous patients had lower leptin concentrations compared with bronchitic patients.
Broekhuizen et al. (2005) [119]	Leptin is detectable in COPD sputum, inversely correlates with plasma leptin, and is significantly linked to CRP and TNF-α.
Vernooy et al. (2009) [85]	Ex-smokers, with or without severe COPD, show higher leptin expression in bronchial epithelial cells and alveolar macrophages than never-smokers.
Gaki et al. (2011) [90]	In patients with COPD, both BODE index and FFMI presented significant positive and negative associations, respectively, with leptin levels.
Wells et al. (2016) [120]	Insulin resistance inversely correlates with quadricep strength, and patients with quadricep weakness exhibit significantly higher insulin resistance

BODE: body mass index, airflow obstruction, dyspnea, and exercise capacity; HOMA-IR: homeostasis model assessment insulin resistance; MetS: metabolic syndrome.

6. Crosstalk Between Insulin and Leptin in COPD Pathophysiology

6.1. Inflammation

Lung inflammation associated with COPD leads to an elevation in various biomarkers indicative of neutrophilic inflammation (neutrophils, elastase, MMP9, calprotectin, and neutrophils found in bronchoalveolar lavage) along with increased pro-inflammatory cytokines (C-reactive protein, TNF-α, IL-6, IL-1β, and IFNα within peripheral blood) [121]. The persistent increase in these inflammatory molecules leads to mild but ongoing systemic inflammation, which is significant in this scenario. In particular, cytokines such as IL-6, IL-1β, TNF-α, and CRP contribute to the development of insulin resistance [121].

Adipose tissue comprises adipocytes, macrophages, and endothelial cells, all of which have the capacity to produce and secrete various proteins: proinflammatory cytokines such as TNF-α, IL-6, and IFNγ; metabolic hormones like adiponectin, resistin, adipsin, and leptin; growth factors, including vascular endothelial growth factor (VEGF); blood pressure regulators such as PAI-1; and components of the renin–angiotensin system [121]. The pathological expansion of adipose tissue in individuals with obesity and COPD induces both adipocyte hypertrophy and hyperplasia. As adipocytes enlarge, they outstrip the available local oxygen supply and the rate of angiogenesis, and this discrepancy results in insufficient oxygenation and cellular hypoxia, subsequently triggering local inflammatory responses [122,123]. The concomitant presence of COPD and obesity has also been correlated with increased levels of IL-6, CRP, and TNF-α [121]. This correlation indicates that adipose tissue may serve as a substantial source of systemic inflammation in these individuals. Such findings illuminate the complex interactions between obesity and respiratory disorders, thereby underscoring the critical necessity for a multidimensional approach to the management of both conditions.

Cytokines released by adipocytes have a significant negative impact on metabolism and can exacerbate systemic inflammation. For instance, TNF-α manifests its effects by increasing insulin resistance through the stimulation of fatty acid release from adipose tissue into the bloodstream, directly affecting tissues such as muscle and liver [124]. Moreover, adipocytes respond to TNF-α by producing and releasing IL-6 and IL-8, which further stimulates lipolysis and the release of fatty acids from adipose tissue [125]. Also, it has been shown that TNF-α stimulates adipose tissue to produce leptin [126]. In rodent models, the expression of leptin mRNA in adipose tissue exhibits a dose-dependent increase, and the administration of endotoxins or pro-inflammatory cytokines, such as TNF-α, results in elevated concentrations of circulating leptin [127,128]. Therefore, a disrupted leptin feedback system may provide an explanation, at least partially, for elevated leptin levels, particularly during exacerbations when the systemic inflammatory response might be more pronounced than in stable patients [129]. Human airway smooth muscle cells, lung submucosa, and epithelial cells have been shown to express various leptin receptor isoforms [130]. Recent findings indicate that lung epithelial cells possess a functional leptin signaling pathway and elevated levels of leptin expression have been observed in the bronchial mucosa of patients with COPD [85].

Experimental studies suggest that airway inflammation diminishes the metabolic effects of insulin, leading to reduced glucose production in the liver and impaired glucose uptake in peripheral tissues, such as adipose tissue and muscle, ultimately affecting glucose metabolism. There were no obvious abnormalities in insulin receptor signaling that resulted in the reduced insulin action in these tissues. Accordingly, it has been shown that inflammation in the airway epithelium negatively impacts glucose metabolism by restricting blood flow to muscles and hindering microvascular recruitment without disrupting insulin signaling [131]. Moreover, elevated blood glucose levels have been correlated with the administration of corticosteroid therapy in individuals with COPD [132], and this relationship seems to be dose-dependent [133]. Since multiple studies have found no evidence of correlation between corticosteroid therapy and diabetes, there is debate regarding this topic.

6.2. Phenotype-Specific Pathways

COPD is a complex and heterogeneous condition characterized by multiple phenotypes, including emphysema and chronic bronchitis, each governed by distinct metabolic and inflammatory pathways influencing disease progression and comorbid burden. Recent omics-based research highlights glycerophospholipid and sphingolipid metabolism as pathways associated with worse airflow obstruction and more frequent exacerbations, whereas oxidative phosphorylation is strongly linked to the emphysematous phenotype [134]. Immune and inflammatory mechanisms also vary among phenotypes; T cell receptor signaling correlates with lung function outcomes, and antigen processing is associated with exacerbation frequency [134]. Hemostasis and immune signaling pathways, particularly in emphysema, suggest a shared immune response mechanism [135]. Additionally, gender-specific differences have been noted, with dysregulation of the phagocytosis–lysosomal axis more pronounced in female COPD patients, correlating with key clinical measures such as FEV1/FVC and disease severity [136].

Further genetic and molecular insights underscore the complexity of COPD. Microtubule transport and muscle adaptation, identified via genetic analyses, appear to be risk factors for COPD, although microtubule transport has not been previously linked to the disease [9]. Wnt signaling, a key biological pathway involved in regulating cell growth, tissue repair, and inflammation together with macrophage polarization are implicated in the development of emphysema and chronic bronchitis, reflecting their importance in inflammatory and tissue-remodeling processes [137]. Proteomic analyses point to markers such as KRT17 and DHRS9, which are highly expressed in the emphysematous phenotype and may be involved in wound healing and retinol metabolism, respectively [138]. Identifying biomarkers for specific endotypes, such as alpha-1 antitrypsin deficiency and eosinophilic COPD, could enhance targeted therapy development [138].

From a pathophysiological standpoint, the emphysema-predominant phenotype typically exhibits elevated oxidative stress, protease–antiprotease imbalance, and alveolar destruction, frequently driven by neutrophilic inflammation and high levels of reactive oxygen species. By contrast, chronic bronchitis is characterized by pronounced airway wall thickening, mucus hypersecretion, and increased levels of IL-8 and TNF-α [125]. Cachectic COPD phenotypes are marked by systemic inflammation (elevated IL-6 and TNF-α) and progressive muscle wasting, closely correlating with metabolic dysfunction and insulin resistance [121]. Meanwhile, the obese COPD phenotype shows a distinct metabolic–inflammatory pattern of elevated leptin levels, low-grade systemic inflammation, and reduced physical activity factors that collectively contribute to metabolic syndrome and elevated cardiovascular risk. These heterogeneous profiles underscore the importance of phenotype-specific therapeutic approaches targeting both the inflammatory and metabolic axes in COPD.

6.3. Hypoxia

In the context of COPD, there is a progressive increase in the risk of alveolar hypoxia, which subsequently leads to systemic hypoxia, as pulmonary function continues to decline over time [139]. Many of the extrapulmonary comorbidities and maladaptive processes that define COPD have been attributed to tissue hypoxia [140]. In fact, cellular metabolism and insulin sensitivity are significantly altered by prolonged hypoxia [141].

Hypoxia-inducible factor (HIF) is a transcription factor characterized by a basic helix–loop–helix structure, composed of α and β subunits, that mediates cellular responses to hypoxic conditions and has been found to promote insulin resistance in adipose tissue as a consequence of reduced oxygen availability [121]. The proline hydroxylation of HIF-α occurs in normoxic conditions, which causes the proteasome to degrade it, but hypoxia inactivates proline hydroxylases, leading to the accumulation of HIF-α and the formation of a heterodimeric transcription factor [142]. This activation subsequently reduces glucose transport in response to insulin by lowering insulin receptor phosphorylation and impairing downstream signaling mediated by Akt [143].

Hypoxia in adipose tissue results in a shift that promotes inflammation, characterized by an upregulation of adiponectin, concurrently downregulating various proinflammatory mediators, including TNF-α, IL-6, leptin, VEGF, macrophage migration inhibitory factor, tissue inhibitor of metalloproteinases-1, and monocyte chemotactic proteins [121]. Systemic hypoxia resulting from diminished pulmonary function is believed to be a key trigger for the expression of proinflammatory cytokines, alongside local adipose tissue hypoxia [144]. Chronic intermittent hypoxia is known to interfere with lipid biosynthesis [145], hinder insulin sensitivity [146], and disrupt the normal diurnal rhythm, leading to hyperglycemia and increasing the susceptibility of pancreatic β cells to damage induced by hypoxia [147].

It seems that hypoxia plays a more complex role in the liver. Despite an increase in hepatic lipid accumulation brought on by the activation of lipogenic genes [148,149], it has been demonstrated that HIF activation improves hepatic insulin sensitivity by inducing insulin receptor substrate 2 (IRS2) [150].

Insulin sensitivity is affected differently by hypoxia in skeletal muscle. Although it has been discovered that intermittent hypoxia causes insulin resistance [151], chronic hypoxia typically improves insulin action [152]. Remarkably, it has been demonstrated that skeletal muscle 5′ AMP-activated protein kinase (AMPK) pathway activation lessens the negative effects of intermittent hypoxia on whole-body glucose tolerance [152], suggesting that the adaptive response may be significantly influenced by AMPK. These results at least partially explain the positive correlation between lung function and insulin sensitivity [105].

6.4. Oxidative Stress

Undoubtedly, oxidative stress is a major factor in the development of COPD and may be the cause of several pathophysiological changes that occur [153]. Oxidative stress in the lungs following extended exposure to biomass fuels or cigarette smoke is most likely the primary etiologic factor driving this [154]. This stress occurs when the body's endogenous antioxidant defenses are either genetically weakened or overwhelmed by ROS [154].

The primary source of intracellular ROS in the airway epithelial cells of patients with COPD is malfunctioning, "leaky" mitochondria [155]. Nevertheless, the xanthine/xanthine oxidase system, membrane-bound reduced nicotinamide adenine dinucleotide phosphate (NADPH) oxidases (NOX), and neutrophil-derived myeloperoxidase (MPO) are additional contributors [153]. NOX is the primary source of superoxide anions, which are comparatively weak oxidizing agents but quickly transform into more harmful ROS species like the hydroxyl radical, H_2O_2, or the extremely reactive peroxynitrite radicals that are produced when NO is present [156]. MPO, which is released by activated neutrophils, creates the highly toxic hypochlorous acid that combines with protein tyrosine residues to form 3-chlorotyrosine, which is found in higher concentrations in the sputum of COPD patients [157]. Intracellular antioxidant defenses protect lung cells by preventing the production of ROS and preserving redox balance. Nevertheless, a number of endogenous antioxidants are diminished in COPD, which increases oxidative stress in the lungs [158]. Through the glycoxidation of sugars and lipid peroxidation, ROS produces reactive carbonyls, which in turn form aldehydes that carbonylated proteins [159]. Smokers' and COPD patients' lungs have higher levels of protein carbonylation, which is correlated with the severity of the illness [160].

The abnormal redox signaling also impacts insulin metabolic signaling, endothelial dysfunction, the development of cardiovascular and renal inflammation and fibrosis, and the promotion of pro-inflammatory and pro-fibrotic pathways, all of which result in harm to the target organs [161,162]. The accumulation of oxidants, particularly in skeletal muscle and adipose tissue, is linked to the complex development of insulin resistance, with a brief surge of H_2O_2 generated upon insulin release, exposing cells to reactive oxygen species at low concentrations for a short duration [163]. This may augment the insulin signaling cascade through the inhibition of tyrosine phosphatase activity, thereby elevating the basal level of tyrosine phosphorylation within the insulin receptor and its subsequent targets [164]. Research has demonstrated that oxidative stress causes insulin resistance by disrupting insulin signaling [164,165]. Among the theories that have been proposed to explain insulin resistance are the accumulation of specific lipid mediators, abnormal mitochondrial activity, an increase in the stress-activated protein c-Jun-N-terminal-kinase (JNK), and inflammatory pathways [166].

Leptin, adiponectin, visfatin, resistin, apelin, and plasminogen activator inhibitor type 1 are examples of bioactive substances that regulate oxidative stress in both physiological and pathological processes [167]. In addition to increasing oxidative stress, hyperleptinemia promotes monocyte and macrophage activation and proliferation, which results in the generation of TNF-α and IL-6 [168]. TNF-α controls the immune system, inflammatory response, oxidative stress, lipid metabolism, hepatic lipogenesis, adipose cell apoptosis, and insulin signaling [169–171]. IL-6 is involved in the regulation of inflammation and the maintenance of energy homeostasis, and its dysregulation is associated with the progression from acute to chronic inflammatory states, particularly in the contexts of obesity and insulin resistance [172]. Additionally, leptin stimulates the synthesis of reactive intermediates like H_2O_2 and OH free radicals and activates NOX [173].

Oxidative stress influences many signaling pathways that initiate or promote the release of chemokines and cytokines because they contain redox-sensitive molecular targets like the transcription factor nuclear factor-kappa B (NF-kB) and different signaling molecules like protein tyrosine phosphatases, Ras/Rac, Jun N-terminal kinase, and p38 mitogen-activated protein kinase [153]. By increasing systemic pro-inflammatory cytokines and activating activated protein kinase C (PKC), the NF-κB transcription factor contributes to immune and inflammatory responses [174,175]. COPD is associated with elevated NF-kB expression and activation, which is linked to airflow limitation [176].

As COPD advances, a variety of cell types, including macrophages, neutrophils, and T cells, become hyperactivated and release proinflammatory mediators [121]. Among these mediators are TNF-α, monocyte chemotactic protein-1 (MCP-1), reactive oxygen species, as well as chemotactic factors such as leukotriene B4 (LTB4) and IL-8. This response is primarily triggered by irritants, particularly cigarette smoke [121]. The recruitment of peripheral blood monocytes, neutrophils, and CD8+ cytotoxic T cells into the airway environments is facilitated by these mediators, thereby playing a crucial role in sustaining the inflammatory response. Emphysema and tissue destruction are caused by the release of proteases by these recruited cells, especially activated neutrophils and macrophages [177,178]. The oxidative insult that results from the ROS produced by the macrophages simultaneously damages tissue and causes inflammation in the lungs. During recurrent episodes of acute exacerbation, patients diagnosed with COPD become increasingly vulnerable to bacterial and viral infections. These infections can exacerbate lung inflammation and increase the production of ROS, ultimately leading to a rapid and significant decline in lung function [179].

6.5. Temporal Causality, Aging, and Epigenetic Impacts

COPD is intricately linked to aging and epigenetic changes, both of which shape the question of temporal causality whether metabolic dysregulation is a precursor to COPD pathogenesis or instead a consequence of persistent inflammation and oxidative stress. Aging-related cellular senescence, driven by oxidative stress and chronic inflammation, leads to telomere attrition and cell cycle arrest, reflecting key pathways such as telomere shortening, mitochondrial dysfunction, and stem cell exhaustion [180,181]. Additionally, epigenetic age acceleration, characterized by altered deoxyribonucleic acid (DNA) methylation patterns, has been identified as a risk factor for COPD, correlating with lung function decline and disease severity [182]. Differential DNA methylation in COPD can affect gene expression and contribute to pathogenesis, while microRNAs such as miR-125a-5p influence lung epithelial cell senescence [183,184]. Epigenetic biomarkers including DNA methylation signatures and histone modifications continue to show promise for improving diagnosis and treatment strategies [180,181]. Furthermore, gene–environment interactions play a vital role in disease trajectory, with the GETomics approach underscoring how lifetime exposures such as smoking can induce epigenetic changes, thereby exacerbating or triggering COPD [184]. These interactions between genetic predispositions and epigenetic modifications such as smoking-related DNA methylation, can intensify disease progression [185]. Recognizing these multifactorial influences is essential for disentangling the interplay among aging, epigenetics, and the temporal sequence of metabolic dysregulation in COPD, ultimately paving the way for more targeted, personalized therapeutic interventions [183–185].

6.6. Metabolomics and Lung Inflammation in Metabolic Dysregulation

Metabolomics, the study of small molecules in biological samples, offers insights into the metabolic dysregulation associated with COPD, particularly in relation to lung inflammation and metabolic pathways. COPD is associated with significant alterations in multiple metabolic pathways, including amino acid metabolism, energy production, and lipid metabolism. These disruptions contribute to systemic inflammation and oxidative stress, both central features of COPD pathogenesis [186,187]. Specifically, the dysregulation of amino acids such as histidine, creatine, and threonine has been documented, with these metabolites showing an inverse correlation with inflammatory markers like IL-6. Moreover, COPD patients exhibit an imbalance between aerobic and anaerobic energy metabolism, often favoring anaerobic pathways, a shift that accelerates lung injury and inflammation and is linked to disease progression [188]. This altered energy metabolism highlights potential therapeutic targets to manage COPD more effectively. Lipid metabolism is likewise notably affected, as changes in lipid mediators and synthesis pathways not only contribute to inflammation but also fulfill the heightened energy requirements of lung tissue, driving anabolic processes that further exacerbate disease. Additionally, sphingolipid dysregulation and alterations in other lipid molecules have been tied to specific COPD phenotypes, such as reduced lung function and emphysema [189].

Oxidative stress plays a crucial role in COPD, with metabolomic studies highlighting sex-associated differences in oxidative stress markers. Females with COPD show enhanced metabolic dysregulation related to oxidative stress compared to males, suggesting potential sex-specific therapeutic approaches. The autotaxin–lysoPA axis is also implicated in oxidative stress and inflammation in COPD [190].

Metabolomic analyses have identified significant alterations in the arginine and transsulfuration pathways, which are involved in nitric oxide production and oxidative stress. These changes are associated with increased levels of inflammatory markers and may serve as potential biomarkers for COPD management [191]. Metabolomic profiling offers potential for developing diagnostic tools to differentiate COPD from other respiratory conditions, such as asthma. The unique metabolic signatures identified in COPD patients could lead to more accurate diagnoses and personalized treatment strategies [192].

7. Clinical Implications of the Metabolic–Inflammatory Axis

7.1. COPD and Metabolic Syndrome

Metabolic syndrome (MetS) is a multifaceted condition that is clinically characterized by various risk factors, including abdominal obesity (BMI > 30 kg/m^2), elevated blood pressure, a dyslipidemic profile conducive to atherogenesis, and impaired fasting blood glucose, with or without insulin resistance [193]. The International Diabetes Federation (IDF) has established a general consensus indicating that neither cigarette smoke nor COPD are recognized as canonical risk factors for metabolic syndrome, nor is there definitive mechanistic evidence supporting a causal relationship between these conditions [121]. However, recent clinical findings suggest a strong association [194].

More than 30% of individuals diagnosed with COPD present with one or more components of MetS, a fact that might significantly impair patient prognosis [195]. COPD patients with MetS are more likely to be female, have a higher body mass index, and demonstrate higher FEV1 scores compared to those without MetS [123]. The heightened prevalence of MetS among patients with less severe airflow obstruction is likely attributable to the weight loss commonly observed in advanced stages of COPD, in conjunction with increased cardiovascular-related mortality associated with MetS in this population [196]. As a result, these patients may experience earlier death due to cardiovascular disease, preventing them from reaching end-stage COPD [195,197]. Moreover, insulin resistance is more prevalent in COPD patients with metabolic syndrome, which facilitates the progression to T2DM [117].

The etiology of MetS associated with COPD is complex, with several key factors contributing to its development, including inflammatory mediators, oxidative stress, and sedentary lifestyle [122]. There is compelling evidence indicating that the pathophysiology of COPD and its associated comorbidities, such as MetS, is profoundly influenced by elevated oxidative stress and the systemic dissemination of lung inflammation [121]. This dissemination, often referred to as "spill-over", occurs primarily due to increased membrane permeability; however, direct injury within the pulmonary environment can also arise from oxidants present in cigarette smoke, alongside heightened levels of reactive oxygen species and reactive nitrogen species generated by both pulmonary and systemic inflammatory responses [144]. In contrast, oxidative stress related to MetS predominantly results from the activation of specific biochemical pathways, including mitochondrial oxidative metabolism, elevated cellular synthesis due to inflammation, depletion of antioxidant systems, and lipid peroxidation, which is frequently observed in individuals with obesity [198]. Owing to its pro-inflammatory properties, oxidative stress has been proposed as the most likely cause of the elevated risk of cardiovascular comorbidity in both MetS and COPD [199].

As previously noted, proinflammatory cytokines, such as IL-1β, IL-6, TNF-α, and CRP, are persistently elevated in both serum and airway levels due to lung inflammation associated with COPD, and they also play a role in the development of T2DM [121]. Additionally, oxidative stress resulting from cigarette smoke or the body's inflammatory response further exacerbates insulin resistance [200]. It has been suggested that a vicious cycle exists between MetS and COPD: as lung function declines in COPD patients, increased physical inactivity heightens the risk of weight gain, which, in turn, accelerates lung function deterioration and further limits physical activity [95]. In contrast to patients with COPD who are not obese, these patients exhibit less tolerance to exercise and more severe dyspnea [201].

The inflammation of adipose tissue plays a pivotal role in the relationship between COPD and MetS. In macrophages, leptin functions as an acute-phase reactant, enhancing the secretion of proinflammatory cytokines such as TNF-α, IL-6, and IL-12 [202]. The inflammatory state is thereby encouraged by a feedback loop that raises leptin expression in adipose tissue and circulating leptin [98,203]. This association elucidates the intricate relationship between obesity and impaired cytokine production, increased levels of acute-phase reactants, and persistent proinflammatory signaling pathways, and it underscores the increased susceptibility to inflammatory diseases and immunity-related conditions [204]. Moreover, studies found that smokers had lower levels of leptin than non-smokers [205], while another study hypothesized that nicotine might directly affect insulin resistance by raising the levels of leptin in the blood [206]. All of these results suggest that the main factors influencing the onset and clinical progression of COPD and MetS are low-grade systemic inflammation and hormones linked to adipose tissue.

7.2. COPD and Type 2 Diabetes Mellitus

The prevalence of T2DM among individuals with COPD varies by study; however, it is generally higher, with approximately 18.7% of COPD patients affected compared to 5–10% in the general population [207,208]. Notably, there is a reciprocal relationship between these two conditions (Figure 4), as diabetes commonly coexists with COPD and patients with COPD face an increased risk of developing diabetes [209]. According to Oh et al. [210], smoking significantly increases the risk of diabetes, likely due to the worsening of insulin resistance caused by systemic inflammation and/or oxidative stress associated with smoking. Additionally, overweight and obese individuals face a greater likelihood of developing diabetes [211].

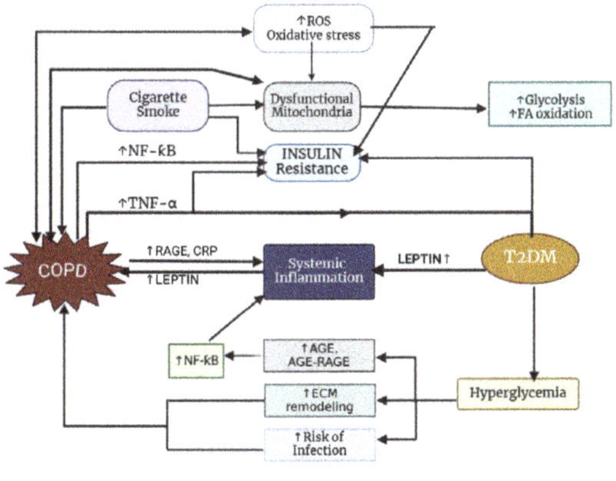

Figure 4. Pathways connecting COPD to type 2 diabetes mellitus.

Impaired lung function is one of the most common comorbidities among individuals diagnosed with T2DM [209]. According to Kinney et al. [212], there is a direct link between the severity of diabetes and the drop in FEV1 and FVC. There are several connections between diabetes and deterioration of lung function, including insulin resistance, glucotoxicity, and systemic inflammation. Inflammatory mediators like TNF-α, IL-6, and CRP are persistently elevated in T2DM [193], which may increase lung vascular permeability [213]. It has also been demonstrated that elevated glucose levels in airway secretions can lead to lung function impairment [214]. Hyperglycemia can also lead to the production of pro-inflammatory glycosylation endproducts (AGEs), which can hasten lung complications [215].

By promoting collagen release, proliferation, and contractions of airway smooth muscle cells through β catenin signaling, insulin remodels the pulmonary compartment and contributes to airway hyperresponsiveness [216]. Alveolar hypoxia and the ensuing hypoxemia (systemic hypoxia) are more likely to occur in the setting of COPD when pulmonary function deteriorates over time [139]. Diabetic patients diagnosed with COPD frequently experience hyperglycemia, occurring approximately 80% of the time during their hospital stay, a fact that is correlated with extended hospital stays and an increased risk of mortality when compared to non-diabetic patients [217,218].

In vivo research has shown that chronic hyperglycemia can cause endothelial dysfunction in diabetic patients' blood vessels through the excessive production of ROS, in addition to systemic inflammation [219]. Elevated levels of reactive oxygen species induced by hyperglycemia can trigger cellular stress, including pathways mediated by NFκB and MAPK, which may adversely affect pulmonary function [220]. Furthermore, hyperglycemia can lead to the presence of glucose in airway secretions, potentially increasing the risk of pulmonary infections by making the respiratory tracts more susceptible to infectious exacerbations [214,221]. Lastly, hyperglycemia-induced oxidative stress and inflammation can cause sarcomeric damage by activating proteolytic machinery, which results in contractile protein wasting and, ultimately, a reduction in the diaphragm fibers' ability to generate force in patients with COPD [222].

T2DM and insulin resistance are also connected to elevated leptin levels. The percentage of obesity, hypertension, and endothelial dysfunction is higher in this particular population, and hyperleptinemia is linked to an increased risk of cardiovascular diseases (CVD) [223]. As previously stated, leptin's impact on glucose homeostasis in obese or insulin-resistant individuals is linked to POMC-expressing neurons in the hypothalamic arcuate nucleus (ARC). Studies on animals with type 2 diabetes indicated that leptin replacement therapy improved insulin resistance and suppressed hepatic gluconeogenesis and fasting hyperglycemia [224]. T2DM, macroangiopathy, and insulin resistance have all been generally associated with hyperleptinemia. It is noteworthy that certain antidiabetic medications (metformin, pioglitazone, sitagliptin, liraglutide, and empagliflozin) have demonstrated the capacity to lower leptin levels [225,226], yet the comprehensive clinical implications of these medications remain to be fully elucidated. Moreover, existing research highlights that the distribution of adipose tissue plays a significant role in the development of insulin resistance, independent of the overall level of obesity [227].

7.3. COPD and Cardiovascular Disease

Numerous studies have shown that COPD patients have a higher incidence and prevalence of CVD than general population, making them especially susceptible to cardiovascular morbidity and mortality [228]. Research indicates that among patients with COPD, mortality from CVD is more prevalent than that from respiratory failure [229]. Moreover, patients with both COPD and CVD experience increased dyspnea and decreased exercise tolerance, along with a higher likelihood of hospitalization for either condition [229].

Common risk factors for both diseases include aging, cigarette smoking, and physical inactivity [230]. Hypoxemia, oxidative stress, lung hyperinflation, pulmonary hypertension, hypoxemia, and systemic inflammation represent key pathophysiological connections between cardiovascular disease and COPD [231]. An experimental study involving healthy participants found a significant reduction in left ventricular stroke volume, along with an increase in the end-diastolic radius curvature of the interventricular septum, linked to elevated dynamic hyperinflation induced by expiratory pressure [232]. The primary contributors to hypoxemia, pulmonary hypertension, and the subsequent development of right and left heart failure are ventilation/perfusion mismatches caused by progressive airflow obstruction and emphysema [231].

Low-grade inflammation appears to contribute significantly to the pathogenesis of cardiovascular comorbidities via the enhancement of atherosclerotic plaque formation and rupture, the proliferation of smooth muscle cells that results in increased arterial stiffness, increased platelet aggregation, the exacerbation of endothelial dysfunction, and a reduction in progenitor endothelial cells (CD^{34+}) [233]. In patients with stable COPD, exogenous stimuli have been shown to trigger both innate and adaptive activation [234], but cardiovascular events are especially risky during acute exacerbations. A five-day temporary elevated risk for acute myocardial infarction was linked to an acute exacerbation of COPD [235]. Procoagulant activity is also elevated in COPD patients due to inflammation. Coagulation, in turn, intensifies inflammation, and both are closely linked to the pathophysiology of atherothrombosis [236].

Cigarette smoke exposure is a major risk factor for the onset and progression of atherosclerosis due to its proinflammatory effects and ability to induce oxidative stress [237]. Studies have shown that smoking enhances systemic inflammation, leading to the destabilization of vulnerable plaques and promoting a prothrombotic environment in the vasculature [238,239]. Crucially, smoking causes both dyslipidemia and systemic inflammation. This interaction exacerbates dyslipidemia, resulting in detrimental cycles, while dyslipidemia enhances the availability of oxidized low-density lipoprotein (LDL), thereby contributing to the formation of atherosclerotic plaques, persistent systemic inflammation, and pulmonary dysfunction [237,239].

Additionally, leptin controls vascular and cardiac function through a NO-dependent mechanism [240]. Additionally, the onset of insulin resistance and hypertension has been associated with leptin resistance [241]. Hyperleptinemia is a strong predictor of acute myocardial infarction (AMI) and is considered an independent risk factor for coronary artery disease (CAD) [242]. In patients with CAD, elevated circulating leptin levels have been linked to a range of complications, including impaired diastolic function, short-term cardiac remodeling, acute coronary syndrome, stroke, heart failure, and cardiac death [243–247].

Emerging evidence suggests that long-acting muscarinic antagonists (LAMAs) and long-acting beta-agonists (LABAs) may potentially increase the risk of developing cardiovascular disease in susceptible populations or worsen preexisting cardiovascular disease, even though they have long been the standard pharmacological treatment for COPD [247,248]. While LABAs have a tendency to be beta 2-selective, the primary concern is with beta-adrenergic therapy, which can increase sympathetic nervous system activation [249] and cause cardiac rhythm abnormalities. LABAs and inhaled corticosteroids (ICSs) are frequently used in patients who are more likely to experience exacerbations. ICSs may exacerbate heart failure, ventricular arrhythmias, and atrial fibrillation, even though they are believed to lower cardiovascular mortality in COPD patients [248]. Clinical trial data indicate that inhaled COPD treatments do not significantly increase the risk of CVD, at least for those without cardiovascular comorbidities [248]. According to Gershon et al. [250], new users of LABA and LAMA had higher cardiovascular risk, as indicated by hospitalizations or ER visits for CVD. As a result, individuals with COPD and a history of heart disease may be more susceptible to atrial fibrillation and other cardiac conditions.

7.4. COPD, Muscle Wasting, and Dysfunction

Skeletal muscle wasting and dysfunction is another prevalent "scenario" associated with COPD, significantly impacting patients' survival and life quality [251]. The loss of muscle mass impacts approximately 40% of COPD patients, with both severity and prevalence of muscle wasting being more pronounced in those who are in advanced stages of the disease [97,119,252]. Research has established that, independent of the decline in pulmonary function, a low FFMI and diminished quadricep strength serve as critical predictors of mortality in COPD patients [253,254], emphasizing the role that muscle mass and functionality play within the broader pathophysiological context. Moreover, patients with COPD experience phenotypic alterations in their muscle fibers, characterized by a reduction in the proportion of slow, oxidative type I fibers and an increase in fast glycolytic type II fibers [255–258].

Insulin plays a vital role in the regulation of muscle protein metabolism, and when insulin resistance occurs, it can disrupt the delicate balance between protein synthesis and breakdown [120]. As previously highlighted, individuals diagnosed with COPD exhibit increased levels of insulin resistance in comparison to non-smoking matched controls [114]. Additionally, research indicates a significant negative correlation between insulin resistance and quadricep strength in both young [259] and old [260] adults who do not have COPD or diabetes mellitus. Although the mechanisms governing this association are complex, increased baseline insulin resistance is associated with a faster decline in skeletal muscle strength over the ensuing three years [261]. Moreover, insulin is essential for sustaining mitochondrial functional activity because it promotes the synthesis of proteins in the mitochondria [262].

Insulin resistance results in impaired vasodilation and endothelial dysfunction, which can impede the increase in blood flow to skeletal muscles during moderate exercise, ultimately contributing to exercise limitations [120]. Insulin resistance is linked to hyperglycemia, which affects skeletal muscle on its own. Hyperglycemia, when examined in vitro, activates pathways related to skeletal muscle atrophy through mechanisms such as caspase 3 activation, degradation of myofibrillar proteins, and the ubiquitin–proteasomal degradation pathway [263,264]. It is plausible that shared etiological factors account for the observed correlation between peripheral muscle weakness and insulin resistance [120]. Cigarette smoking decreases glucose absorption and hinders the action of insulin [265]. Additionally, physical inactivity, even in individuals with mild airflow obstruction, has been associated with quadricep wasting in COPD patients and is recognized as a significant risk factor for IR [197]. Intermuscular adipose infiltration is linked to decreased muscle strength and compromised physical function and is frequently seen in individuals with insulin resistance [266] or COPD [267].

It is important to note that both COPD and T2DM exhibit similar metabolic and mitochondrial alterations in skeletal muscle. These changes include shifts in fiber type, a reduction in oxidative capacity, decreased mitochondrial density, and alterations in peroxisome proliferator-activated receptor gamma co-activator 1 [120]. Moreover, both conditions show excessive production of ROS and increased oxidative damage to mitochondrial DNA [120].

The hypothesis suggesting that cachexia and muscle wasting in COPD caused by altered energy balance may arise from dysfunctions in the leptin feedback mechanism has been explored extensively in the literature [268]. Nonetheless, no statistically significant correlation has been identified between circulating leptin levels and the activated TNF-α system [269]. Researchers have not been able to demonstrate a consistent elevation of leptin levels in cachexic stable COPD patients [118]. However, when accounting for factors such as fat mass and the use of oral corticosteroids, certain studies have reported a significant partial correlation coefficient between leptin and soluble tumor necrosis factor receptor 55 (sTNF-R55) [269]. Moreover, leptin levels were determined to be linked to fat mass in patients with emphysematous COPD, which appears to support the feedback mechanism known to regulate body weight, while this correlation was not observed in patients with chronic bronchitis [25]. While it appears to be physiologically regulated, low levels of the hormone may be responsible for an increased risk of pulmonary infections in COPD patients [118].

Takabatake et al. [270] examined the circadian rhythm of circulating leptin in individuals with COPD to gain a deeper understanding of its dynamics. The study revealed that this circadian pattern is preserved in COPD patients with normal BMI, whereas it is absent in those exhibiting cachexia [269]. These findings indicate that the disruption of the physiological leptin release pattern in cachectic COPD patients may hold clinical significance concerning pathophysiological features, including abnormalities in the hypothalamic–pituitary axis and the autonomic nervous system, and this loss of rhythm may serve as a compensatory mechanism to help maintain body fat content [270].

7.5. COPD and Obesity

The "obesity paradox" in COPD refers to the intriguing observation that overweight and moderately obese COPD patients exhibit better survival outcomes compared to normal-weight individuals, particularly those with severe bronchial obstruction. This paradoxical relationship appears to diminish at extremely high BMI levels (>40 kg/m^2), suggesting a U-shaped association between BMI and mortality [271,272]. Potential mechanisms behind this paradox include beneficial mechanical changes in chest-wall dynamics that reduce lung hyperinflation. However, confounding factors such as reverse causation and variability in emphysema severity complicate interpretations [271].

Although leptin, a key regulator of body weight and energy balance, is generally lower in COPD patients compared to healthy controls, it correlates primarily with BMI and body composition rather than inflammation or cachexia-related markers. Notably, leptin levels do not consistently correlate with COPD-associated cachexia, questioning its role as a direct therapeutic target for managing weight loss in these patients. Due to these complexities, further research is essential to delineate specific obesity phenotypes, clarify leptin's mechanistic role, and evaluate the potential of leptin sensitizers or other targeted interventions to address obesity-related complications in COPD management [273].

Leptin plays a crucial role in the pathophysiology of COPD, notably influencing systemic inflammation, body composition, and disease progression. Elevated leptin levels observed in COPD patients, particularly during exacerbations, correlate closely with inflammatory markers such as CRP and TNF-α, indicating its involvement in systemic inflammatory responses [274]. In stable conditions, leptin concentrations correlate with body mass index and percent body fat, demonstrating preserved leptin regulation despite weight changes; however, this correlation weakens during disease exacerbations, suggesting a disruption in its normal regulatory function [275]. Gender differences are also evident, with higher leptin levels typically observed in women with COPD, particularly among those who are overweight, potentially impacting inflammation and disease progression uniquely [87]. Furthermore, age-related leptin resistance can amplify systemic inflammation, metabolic dysregulation, and muscle wasting in older COPD patients, exacerbating cachexia and reducing quality of life. Given these complex interactions, leptin not only holds promise as a biomarker for inflammation and disease monitoring but also represents a potential therapeutic target. Future research focusing on age- and gender-specific leptin dynamics could further clarify its mechanistic role and optimize personalized treatment strategies in COPD management [276].

8. COPD in Low- and Middle-Income Countries

Chronic obstructive pulmonary disease constitutes a considerable public health challenge in low- and middle-income countries (LMICs), where more than 90% of deaths attributable to COPD occur. Unlike in high-income nations, where tobacco smoking is the predominant risk factor, COPD in LMICs is strongly associated with indoor air pollution, occupational exposures, and inadequate healthcare infrastructure [277]. Many households in these regions rely on biomass fuels (charcoal, wood, and agricultural waste) for cooking and heating purposes, leading to chronic exposure to fine particulate matter and toxic pollutants. Prolonged inhalation of these pollutants triggers persistent airway inflammation, oxidative stress, and accelerated lung function decline, exacerbating COPD progression [278]. Biomass smoke exposure disproportionately impacts women and children due to their domestic roles, causing unique inflammatory patterns distinct from cigarette-induced COPD. Specifically, biomass smoke induces inflammation primarily through the IL-17F/IL-17RC pathway, resulting in bronchial hyperresponsiveness, bronchial anthracofibrosis, thicker pulmonary arterial intima, significant fibrosis, and typically less emphysema compared to tobacco-induced COPD [279]. Biomass-induced COPD is also characterized by lymphocyte-dominant airway inflammation and increased pigment deposition, reflecting different immune responses compared to the neutrophil-driven inflammation seen in cigarette-smoke COPD [279]. Additionally, pro-inflammatory diets, indicated by high Dietary Inflammatory Index (DII) scores, exacerbate COPD risk and correlate with decreased lung function. Addressing COPD in these regions necessitates interventions focused on improved ventilation to mitigate indoor biomass smoke exposure and dietary modifications emphasizing anti-inflammatory and antioxidant-rich foods, strategies that could significantly reduce disease severity and improve public health outcomes [280].

Additionally, rapid urbanization has led to increased exposure to industrial pollutants and vehicle emissions, further contributing to chronic respiratory inflammation [281].

Inflammatory markers such as CRP, IL-6, and TNF-α are consistently elevated in COPD patients from LMICs, indicating a higher systemic inflammatory burden. Frequent respiratory infections, including tuberculosis and bacterial pneumonias, are more common in these regions and further exacerbate airway inflammation [282]. Malnutrition, another prevalent issue in LMICs, weakens immune function and contributes to a heightened inflammatory state, worsening COPD symptoms and increasing the risk of severe exacerbations. Additionally, diets characterized by lower energy and protein intake, as well as deficiencies in micronutrients such as calcium, potassium, iron, folate, zinc, vitamin B6, retinol, and niacin, exacerbate the risk of malnutrition and negatively impact disease outcomes [283,284]. Poor dietary quality in COPD patients is frequently linked to disease-related symptoms such as breathlessness, anorexia, depression, and social factors including poverty and isolation. Western-style diets, high in processed meats and low in fiber-rich foods, further contribute to COPD risk and accelerated pulmonary decline; conversely, diets rich in fruits, vegetables, antioxidants, and dietary fiber have protective effects, particularly noted in middle-aged and elderly populations [283]. In LMICs, adherence to healthy dietary guidelines remains low due to economic, social, and cultural barriers that enhance the availability of unhealthy foods [285]. Suboptimal dietary practices significantly contribute to the global burden of non-communicable diseases (NCDs), with elevated sodium intake, low whole grain consumption, and inadequate fruit intake identified as leading risk factors [283]. Given these challenges, there is an urgent need for targeted nutritional interventions and policy frameworks in LMICs that prioritize healthy food access, improve dietary adherence, and address socio-economic determinants to effectively mitigate COPD and associated NCDs [278].

Additionally, metabolic comorbidities such as diabetes and cardiovascular disease, which are often underdiagnosed or poorly managed in LMICs, further contribute to disease progression.

A major challenge in managing COPD in LMICs is underdiagnosis and limited access to effective treatment. Spirometry, the gold standard for COPD diagnosis, is often unavailable in primary healthcare settings, leading to misclassification of COPD as asthma or chronic bronchitis [286]. Additionally, bronchodilators, inhaled corticosteroids, and pulmonary rehabilitation programs remain unaffordable for many patients due to financial constraints and limited healthcare funding. As a result, COPD patients in LMICs experience higher rates of severe exacerbations and hospitalizations, increasing the overall mortality burden [287].

To reduce the impact of COPD in LMICs, urgent public health interventions are needed [277]. Reducing household and outdoor air pollution through clean cooking technologies, stricter industrial emissions policies, and improved air quality monitoring could significantly lower the inflammatory burden in COPD patients. Expanding access to early diagnosis through training healthcare providers and increasing the availability of cost-effective medications are also crucial steps [1,6]. Additionally, public health initiatives promoting tobacco control, nutritional support, and vaccination programs (influenza and pneumococcus) could help mitigate COPD-related complications. Addressing these challenges holistically will be key to reducing COPD morbidity and mortality in low-income countries [1,8].

9. Therapeutic Management and Future Directions

COPD management currently revolves around symptom relief, exacerbation reduction, and improvement of overall quality of life. Conventional therapeutic strategies primarily include pharmacological treatments such as LAMAs, LABAs, inhaled corticosteroids, and systemic therapies for advanced disease stages. Pulmonary rehabilitation programs and lifestyle modifications, particularly smoking cessation and exercise, remain foundational. Despite the prevalence of COPD, current treatments like glucocorticoids and bronchodilators have limitations, including side effects and limited efficacy in halting disease progression. Consequently, there is significant interest in developing novel therapeutic agents that target the underlying mechanisms of COPD more effectively.

Recent research has focused on molecular targeted therapies that address specific pathways involved in COPD. Thioredoxin (Trx) is a promising agent that regulates redox status and protease/anti-protease balance, blocks NF-κB and MAPK signaling pathways, and improves steroid insensitivity by inhibiting macrophage migration inhibitory factor (MIF) production [288–290]. These mechanisms differ from traditional glucocorticoid-based treatments, offering a novel approach to managing COPD. Given the limited response of COPD to corticosteroids, novel anti-inflammatory drugs are being explored. These include agents that inhibit the recruitment and activation of inflammatory cells such as macrophages, neutrophils, and T-lymphocytes. Some promising candidates include chemokine receptor antagonists, matrix metalloproteinase inhibitors, and p38 MAPK inhibitors [288–290]. The monoclonal antibody dupilumab, which targets inflammatory pathways, has shown success in clinical trials, highlighting the potential of biologic agents in COPD treatment [291].

Antioxidants and anti-fibrotic compounds are also under investigation for their potential to mitigate oxidative stress and tissue remodeling in COPD. Compounds like N-acetyl-L-cysteine and other antioxidant enzyme mimetics are being studied for their ability to reduce oxidative damage. Additionally, anti-fibrotic agents aim to prevent airway remodeling, a key feature of COPD progression [292].

Glucagon-like peptide-1 receptor agonists (GLP-1RAs) and leptin sensitizers have shown potential, particularly for COPD patients with comorbid T2DM [293]. GLP-1RAs reduce inflammatory responses, oxidative stress, airway remodeling, and protease/anti-protease imbalance, improving airway mucus homeostasis. Studies indicate that GLP-1RAs significantly lower the risk of moderate and severe COPD exacerbations compared to other diabetes medications like dipeptidyl-peptidase 4 inhibitors (DPP-4i) and sulfonylureas, resulting in improved clinical outcomes and reduced healthcare utilization [294,295]. Furthermore, GLP-1 analogs are associated with improved pulmonary outcomes, including a lower risk of pneumonia, reduced oxygen dependence, and decreased all-cause mortality in COPD patients receiving single-inhaler triple therapy (SITT) [296]. GLP-1RAs also reduce leptin levels, potentially contributing to anti-inflammatory effects and mitigating inflammation-related lung damage, suggesting benefits beyond their glucose-lowering capabilities. While direct evidence on leptin sensitizers specifically in COPD is limited, the modulation of leptin levels by GLP-1RAs suggests a potential pathway for reducing inflammation and improving immune function in COPD patients [297]. This could be particularly relevant in managing COPD exacerbations and improving overall lung function.

Further studies could help refine treatment guidelines and improve patient outcomes by leveraging the dual benefits of these agents on metabolic and respiratory health [293].

Recent advancements have demonstrated the potential of interventional therapeutic approaches in managing COPD, particularly in advanced stages where pharmacological treatments alone may not suffice. Interventional therapies, including bronchoscopic lung volume reduction (BLVR), endobronchial valves, and lung volume reduction surgery (LVRS), have increasingly gained attention for their ability to substantially improve patient outcomes.

BLVR using endobronchial valves has shown significant improvements in lung function, exercise tolerance, and quality of life in patients with severe emphysema. Studies report increased forced expiratory volume in 1 s (FEV1), improved six-minute walking distance, and reduced dyspnea scores post-procedure [298]. The procedure is generally safe, with no significant increase in pneumonia rates or mortality compared to control groups, although there is a risk of complications such as pneumothorax [299].

LVRS has been shown to improve survival, lung function, and quality of life in selected patients with upper lobe-predominant emphysema and low exercise capacity. However, it is associated with significant complications, prolonged hospital stays, and high costs [300,301]. A randomized controlled trial comparing LVRS and BLVR found no substantial difference in outcomes at one year, suggesting that BLVR may be a viable alternative for patients who are suitable for both procedures [300].

Improving the quality of life (QoL) for patients with COPD involves a diverse array of therapeutic interventions. Self-management interventions (SMIs), particularly those targeting symptom control, physical activity, and mental health, have consistently demonstrated efficacy in enhancing health-related quality of life (HRQoL) and reducing emergency department visits across various patient subgroups, including those with severe symptoms and high body mass indices [302,303]. Telehealth approaches, while promising, have yielded mixed results, with only limited studies reporting significant improvements compared to standard care [304]. Although palliative care has not shown substantial direct benefits in QoL, it effectively reduces acute healthcare utilization, such as hospitalizations and intensive care admissions. Psychological interventions, especially cognitive behavioral therapy, have exhibited effectiveness primarily in reducing anxiety symptoms, though their overall impact on QoL remains limited. Integrated disease management programs, characterized by their multidisciplinary and multi-component nature, have emerged as effective strategies for improving disease-specific QoL, enhancing exercise capacity, and decreasing hospital admissions [305]. Additionally, web-based supportive interventions have proven valuable as supplementary options, significantly improving QoL when combined with usual care, despite not surpassing the effectiveness of face-to-face treatments [302].

Looking forward, therapeutic management strategies are likely to become increasingly personalized, with a greater emphasis on identifying phenotypes that respond best to specific interventional treatments. Technological advancements, alongside more refined patient-selection criteria, will continue to enhance the precision and effectiveness of COPD management, ultimately leading to improved patient-centric outcomes and reduced disease burden.

10. Conclusions

COPD extends well beyond the pulmonary compartment and is profoundly influenced by the interplay of metabolic, inflammatory, and epigenetic pathways, all of which can be further modulated by aging. Leptin and insulin, both key regulators of energy homeostasis, become dysregulated in COPD, contributing to muscle wasting, insulin resistance, and an increased risk of cardiometabolic comorbidities. Epigenetic modifications such as DNA methylation can amplify or alter these processes, shaping disease trajectory and therapeutic responses, especially when combined with environmental exposures like smoking or poor nutritional status.

The existing evidence underscores a pressing need for further research into how these metabolic and epigenetic factors converge to influence different COPD phenotypes, potentially uncovering novel biomarkers and patient-specific treatment strategies. By incorporating multi-omics approaches and focusing on the metabolic–inflammatory–epigenetic axis, personalized interventions and earlier therapeutic targets may emerge. Ultimately, refining our understanding of these multifaceted processes offers the prospect of reducing disease exacerbations and improving both respiratory and metabolic health outcomes for individuals suffering from this debilitating condition.

Author Contributions: Conceptualization, C.T.S. and O.M.C.; methodology, R.C.; software, O.M.C.; validation, C.T.S., R.C. and C.L.T.; formal analysis, A.F.N.; investigation, D.M.M.; resources, C.C.; data curation, R.C.; writing—original draft preparation, O.M.C.; writing—review and editing, O.M.C.; visualization, R.C.; supervision, C.T.S.; project administration, R.C. All authors have read and agreed to the published version of the manuscript.

Funding: The Article Processing Charges were funded by the University of Medicine and Pharmacy of Craiova, Romania.

Data Availability Statement: The data presented in this study are available from the corresponding author upon request.

Conflicts of Interest: The authors declare no conflicts of interest.

References

2025 GOLD Report—Global Initiative for Chronic Obstructive Lung Disease—GOLD. Available online: https://goldcopd.org/2025-gold-report/ (accessed on 4 February 2025).

Roth, G.A.; Abate, D.; Abate, K.H.; Abay, S.M.; Abbafati, C.; Abbasi, N.; Abbastabar, H.; Abd-Allah, F.; Abdela, J.; Abdelalim, A.; et al. Global, Regional, and National Age-Sex-Specific Mortality for 282 Causes of Death in 195 Countries and Territories, 1980–2017: A Systematic Analysis for the Global Burden of Disease Study 2017. *Lancet* **2018**, *392*, 1736. [CrossRef] [PubMed]

Lamprecht, B.; McBurnie, M.A.; Vollmer, W.M.; Gudmundsson, G.; Welte, T.; Nizankowska-Mogilnicka, E.; Studnicka, M.; Bateman, E.; Anto, J.M.; Burney, P.; et al. COPD in Never Smokers: Results from the Population-Based Burden of Obstructive Lung Disease Study. *Chest* **2011**, *139*, 752. [CrossRef]

FastStats—Chronic Lower Respiratory Disease. Available online: https://www.cdc.gov/nchs/fastats/copd.htm (accessed on 28 January 2025).

Lange, P.; Ahmed, E.; Lahmar, Z.M.; Martinez, F.J.; Bourdin, A. Natural History and Mechanisms of COPD. *Respirology* **2021**, *26*, 298–321. [CrossRef] [PubMed]

Adeloye, D.; Chua, S.; Lee, C.; Basquill, C.; Papana, A.; Theodoratou, E.; Nair, H.; Gasevic, D.; Sridhar, D.; Campbell, H.; et al. Global and Regional Estimates of COPD Prevalence: Systematic Review and Meta-Analysis. *J. Glob. Health* **2015**, *5*, 020415. [CrossRef]

7. Boers, E.; Barrett, M.; Su, J.G.; Benjafield, A.V.; Sinha, S.; Kaye, L.; Zar, H.J.; Vuong, V.; Tellez, D.; Gondalia, R.; et al. Global Burden of Chronic Obstructive Pulmonary Disease Through 2050. *JAMA Netw. Open* **2023**, *6*, e2346598. [CrossRef]
8. Fallahzadeh, A.; Sharifnejad Tehrani, Y.; Sheikhy, A.; Ghamari, S.H.; Mohammadi, E.; Saeedi Moghaddam, S.; Esfahani, Z. Nasserinejad, M.; Shobeiri, P.; Rashidi, M.M.; et al. The Burden of Chronic Respiratory Disease and Attributable Risk Factors in North Africa and Middle East: Findings from Global Burden of Disease Study (GBD) 2019. *Respir. Res.* **2022**, *23*, 268. [CrossRef] [PubMed]
9. Duan, R.R.; Hao, K.; Yang, T. Air Pollution and Chronic Obstructive Pulmonary Disease. *Chronic Dis. Transl. Med.* **2020**, *6*, 260–269. [CrossRef]
10. Nugmanova, D.; Feshchenko, Y.; Iashyna, L.; Gyrina, O.; Malynovska, K.; Mammadbayov, E.; Akhundova, I.; Nurkina, N.; Tariq L.; Makarova, J.; et al. The Prevalence, Burden and Risk Factors Associated with Chronic Obstructive Pulmonary Disease in Commonwealth of Independent States (Ukraine, Kazakhstan and Azerbaijan): Results of the CORE Study. *BMC Pulm. Med.* **2018**, *18*, 26. [CrossRef]
11. Chapmann, K.R.; Mannino, D.M.; Soriano, J.B.; Vermeire, P.A.; Buist, A.S.; Thun, M.J.; Connell, C.; Lee, T.A.; Miravitlles, M Aldington, S.; et al. Epidemiology and Costs of Chronic Obstructive Pulmonary Disease. *Eur. Respir. J.* **2006**, *27*, 188–207 [CrossRef]
12. Ho, T.; Cusack, R.P.; Chaudhary, N.; Satia, I.; Kurmi, O.P. Under- and over-Diagnosis of COPD: A Global Perspective. *Breathe* **2019**, *15*, 24. [CrossRef]
13. Decramer, M.; Janssens, W.; Miravitlles, M. Chronic Obstructive Pulmonary Disease. *Lancet* **2012**, *379*, 1341. [CrossRef] [PubMed]
14. Barnes, P.J.; Celli, B.R. Systemic Manifestations and Comorbidities of COPD. *Eur. Respir. J.* **2009**, *33*, 1165–1185. [CrossRef] [PubMed]
15. Zatloukal, J.; Brat, K.; Neumannova, K.; Volakova, E.; Hejduk, K.; Kocova, E.; Kudela, O.; Kopecky, M.; Plutinsky, M.; Koblizek V. Chronic Obstructive Pulmonary Disease—Diagnosis and Management of Stable Disease; a Personalized Approach to Care Using the Treatable Traits Concept Based on Clinical Phenotypes. Position Paper of the Czech Pneumological and Phthisiological Society. *Biomed. Pap. Med. Fac. Palacky Univ. Olomouc* **2020**, *164*, 325–356. [CrossRef]
16. Mannino, D.M.; Watt, G.; Hole, D.; Gillis, C.; Hart, C.; McConnachie, A.; Smith, G.D.; Upton, M.; Hawthorne, V.; Sin, D.D.; et al. The Natural History of Chronic Obstructive Pulmonary Disease. *Eur. Respir. J.* **2006**, *27*, 627–643. [CrossRef]
17. Miravitlles, M.; Ribera, A. Understanding the Impact of Symptoms on the Burden of COPD. *Respir. Res.* **2017**, *18*, 67. [CrossRef]
18. Vestbo, J.; Hurd, S.S.; Agustí, A.G.; Jones, P.W.; Vogelmeier, C.; Anzueto, A.; Barnes, P.J.; Fabbri, L.M.; Martinez, F.J.; Nishimura M.; et al. Global Strategy for the Diagnosis, Management, and Prevention of Chronic Obstructive Pulmonary Disease: GOLD Executive Summary. *Am. J. Respir. Crit. Care Med.* **2013**, *187*, 347–365. [CrossRef] [PubMed]
19. Rabe, K.F.; Wedzicha, J.A. Controversies in Treatment of Chronic Obstructive Pulmonary Disease. *Lancet* **2011**, *378*, 1038–1047 [CrossRef]
20. Sin, D.D.; Man, S.F.P. Impaired Lung Function and Serum Leptin in Men and Women with Normal Body Weight: A Population Based Study. *Thorax* **2003**, *58*, 695–698. [CrossRef]
21. Agusti, A. Thomas a. Neff Lecture. Chronic Obstructive Pulmonary Disease: A Systemic Disease. *Proc. Am. Thorac. Soc* **2006**, *3*, 478–481. [CrossRef]
22. Yanbaeva, D.G.; Dentener, M.A.; Creutzberg, E.C.; Wesseling, G.; Wouters, E.F.M. Systemic Effects of Smoking. *Chest* **2007**, *131*, 1557–1566. [CrossRef]
23. Kahnert, K.; Lucke, T.; Biertz, F.; Lechner, A.; Watz, H.; Alter, P.; Bals, R.; Behr, J.; Holle, R.; Huber, R.M.; et al. Transfer Factor for Carbon Monoxide in Patients with COPD and Diabetes: Results from the German COSYCONET Cohort. *Respir. Res.* **2017**, *18*, 14 [CrossRef] [PubMed]
24. Saltiel, A.R. Insulin Signaling in Health and Disease. *J. Clin. Investig.* **2021**, *131*, e142241. [CrossRef] [PubMed]
25. Schols, A.M.W.J.; Creutzberg, E.C.; Buurman, W.A.; Campfield, L.A.; Saris, W.H.M.; Wouters, E.F.M. Plasma Leptin Is Related to Proinflammatory Status and Dietary Intake in Patients with Chronic Obstructive Pulmonary Disease. *Am. J. Respir. Crit. Care Med.* **1999**, *160*, 1220–1226. [CrossRef]
26. Yamauchi, T.; Kamon, J.; Waki, H.; Terauchi, Y.; Kubota, N.; Hara, K.; Mori, Y.; Ide, T.; Murakami, K.; Tsuboyama-Kasaoka, N. et al. The Fat-Derived Hormone Adiponectin Reverses Insulin Resistance Associated with Both Lipoatrophy and Obesity. *Nat. Med.* **2001**, *7*, 941–946. [CrossRef]
27. Zhang, Y.; Proenca, R.; Maffei, M.; Barone, M.; Leopold, L.; Friedman, J.M. Positional Cloning of the Mouse Obese Gene and Its Human Homologue. *Nature* **1994**, *372*, 425–432. [CrossRef]
28. Sierra-Honigmann, M.R.; Nath, A.K.; Murakami, C.; García-Cardeña, G.; Papapetropoulos, A.; Sessa, W.C.; Madge L.A.; Schechner, J.S.; Schwabb, M.B.; Polverini, P.J.; et al. Biological Action of Leptin as an Angiogenic Factor. *Science* **1998**, *281*, 1683–1686. [CrossRef]
29. Emilsson, V.; Liu, Y.L.; Cawthorne, M.A.; Morton, N.M.; Davenport, M. Expression of the Functional Leptin Receptor MRNA in Pancreatic Islets and Direct Inhibitory Action of Leptin on Insulin Secretion. *Diabetes* **1997**, *46*, 313–316. [CrossRef] [PubMed]

Saladin, R.; De Vos, P.; Guerre-Millot, M.; Leturque, A.; Girard, J.; Staels, B.; Auwerx, J. Transient Increase in Obese Gene Expression after Food Intake or Insulin Administration. *Nature* **1995**, *377*, 527–528. [CrossRef]

Widjaja, A.; Schürmeyer, T.H.; Von Zur Mühlen, A.; Brabant, G. Determinants of Serum Leptin Levels in Cushing's Syndrome. *J. Clin. Endocrinol. Metab.* **1998**, *83*, 600–603. [CrossRef]

Pérez-Pérez, A.; Toro, A.; Vilariño-García, T.; Maymó, J.; Guadix, P.; Dueñas, J.L.; Fernández-Sánchez, M.; Varone, C.; Sánchez-Margalet, V. Leptin Action in Normal and Pathological Pregnancies. *J. Cell Mol. Med.* **2018**, *22*, 716–727. [CrossRef]

White, D.W.; Tartaglia, L.A. Leptin and OB-R: Body Weight Regulation by a Cytokine Receptor. *Cytokine Growth Factor Rev.* **1996**, *7*, 303–309. [CrossRef] [PubMed]

Harris, R.B.S. Leptin–Much More than a Satiety Signal. *Annu. Rev. Nutr.* **2000**, *20*, 45–75. [CrossRef] [PubMed]

Stephens, T.W.; Basinski, M.; Bristow, P.K.; Bue-Valleskey, J.M.; Burgett, S.G.; Craft, L.; Hale, J.; Hoffmann, J.; Hsiung, H.M.; Kriauciunas, A.; et al. The Role of Neuropeptide Y in the Antiobesity Action of the Obese Gene Product. *Nature* **1995**, *377*, 530–532. [CrossRef] [PubMed]

Fei, H.; Okano, H.J.; Li, C.; Lee, G.H.; Zhao, C.; Darnell, R.; Friedman, J.M. Anatomic Localization of Alternatively Spliced Leptin Receptors (Ob-R) in Mouse Brain and Other Tissues. *Proc. Natl. Acad. Sci. USA* **1997**, *94*, 7001. [CrossRef]

Li, M.D. Leptin and Beyond: An Odyssey to the Central Control of Body Weight. *Yale J. Biol. Med.* **2011**, *84*, 1.

Cowley, M.A.; Smart, J.L.; Rubinstein, M.; Cerdán, M.G.; Diano, S.; Horvath, T.L.; Cone, R.D.; Low, M.J. Leptin Activates Anorexigenic POMC Neurons through a Neural Network in the Arcuate Nucleus. *Nature* **2001**, *411*, 480–484. [CrossRef]

Coppari, R.; Ichinose, M.; Lee, C.E.; Pullen, A.E.; Kenny, C.D.; McGovern, R.A.; Tang, V.; Liu, S.M.; Ludwig, T.; Chua, S.C.; et al. The Hypothalamic Arcuate Nucleus: A Key Site for Mediating Leptin's Effects on Glucose Homeostasis and Locomotor Activity. *Cell Metab.* **2005**, *1*, 63–72. [CrossRef]

Rossi, J.; Balthasar, N.; Olson, D.; Scott, M.; Berglund, E.; Lee, C.E.; Choi, M.J.; Lauzon, D.; Lowell, B.B.; Elmquist, J.K. Melanocortin-4-Receptors Expressed by Cholinergic Neurons Regulate Energy Balance and Glucose Homeostasis. *Cell Metab.* **2011**, *13*, 195. [CrossRef]

Zhang, R.; Dhillon, H.; Yin, H.; Yoshimura, A.; Lowell, B.B.; Maratos-Flier, E.; Flier, J.S. Selective Inactivation of Socs3 in SF1 Neurons Improves Glucose Homeostasis Without Affecting Body Weight. *Endocrinology* **2008**, *149*, 5654. [CrossRef]

La Cava, A.; Matarese, G. The Weight of Leptin in Immunity. *Nat. Rev. Immunol.* **2004**, *4*, 371–379. [CrossRef]

Lord, G.M.; Matarese, G.; Howard, J.K.; Baker, R.J.; Bloom, S.R.; Lechler, R.I. Leptin Modulates the T-Cell Immune Response and Reverses Starvation-Induced Immunosuppression. *Nature* **1998**, *394*, 897–901. [CrossRef]

Faggioni, R.; Feingold, K.R.; Grunfeld, C. Leptin Regulation of the Immune Response and the Immunodeficiency of Malnutrition. *FASEB J.* **2001**, *15*, 2565–2571. [CrossRef] [PubMed]

Popa, C.; Netea, M.G.; Radstake, T.R.D.S.; Van Riel, P.L.; Barrera, P.; Van Der Meer, J.W.M. Markers of Inflammation Are Negatively Correlated with Serum Leptin in Rheumatoid Arthritis. *Ann. Rheum. Dis.* **2005**, *64*, 1195. [CrossRef] [PubMed]

Baumann, H.; Morella, K.K.; White, D.W.; Dembski, M.; Bailon, P.S.; Kim, H.; Lai, C.F.; Tartaglia, L.A. The Full-Length Leptin Receptor Has Signaling Capabilities of Interleukin 6-Type Cytokine Receptors. *Proc. Natl. Acad. Sci. USA* **1996**, *93*, 8374. [CrossRef] [PubMed]

Bjørbæk, C.; Elmquist, J.K.; Frantz, J.D.; Shoelson, S.E.; Flier, J.S. Identification of SOCS-3 as a Potential Mediator of Central Leptin Resistance. *Mol. Cell* **1998**, *1*, 619–625. [CrossRef]

Heinrich, P.C.; Behrmann, I.; Haan, S.; Hermanns, H.M.; Müller-Newen, G.; Schaper, F. Principles of Interleukin (IL)-6-Type Cytokine Signalling and Its Regulation. *Biochem. J.* **2003**, *374*, 1–20. [CrossRef]

Csajbók, É.A.; Tamás, G. Cerebral Cortex: A Target and Source of Insulin? *Diabetologia* **2016**, *59*, 1609–1615. [CrossRef]

Vasiljević, J.; Torkko, J.M.; Knoch, K.P.; Solimena, M. The Making of Insulin in Health and Disease. *Diabetologia* **2020**, *63*, 1981–1989. [CrossRef]

Suckale, J.; Solimena, M. The Insulin Secretory Granule as a Signaling Hub. *Trends Endocrinol. Metab.* **2010**, *21*, 599–609. [CrossRef]

Yang, B.Y.; Zhai, G.; Gong, Y.L.; Su, J.Z.; Peng, X.Y.; Shang, G.H.; Han, D.; Jin, J.Y.; Liu, H.K.; Du, Z.Y.; et al. Different Physiological Roles of Insulin Receptors in Mediating Nutrient Metabolism in Zebrafish. *Am. J. Physiol. Endocrinol. Metab.* **2018**, *315*, E38–E51. [CrossRef]

Taniguchi, C.M.; Emanuelli, B.; Kahn, C.R. Critical Nodes in Signalling Pathways: Insights into Insulin Action. *Nat. Rev. Mol. Cell Biol.* **2006**, *7*, 85–96. [CrossRef] [PubMed]

Baron, A.D.; Brechtel, G.; Wallace, P.; Edelman, S.V. Rates and Tissue Sites of Non-Insulin- and Insulin-Mediated Glucose Uptake in Humans. *Am. J. Physiol.* **1988**, *255*, E769–E774. [CrossRef]

Rahman, M.S.; Hossain, K.S.; Das, S.; Kundu, S.; Adegoke, E.O.; Rahman, M.A.; Hannan, M.A.; Uddin, M.J.; Pang, M.G. Role of Insulin in Health and Disease: An Update. *Int. J. Mol. Sci.* **2021**, *22*, 6403. [CrossRef] [PubMed]

Romijn, J.A.; Coyle, E.F.; Sidossis, L.S.; Gastaldelli, A.; Horowitz, J.F.; Endert, E.; Wolfe, R.R. Regulation of Endogenous Fat and Carbohydrate Metabolism in Relation to Exercise Intensity and Duration. *Am. J. Physiol.* **1993**, *265*, E380–E391. [CrossRef] [PubMed]

57. Defronzo, R.A. Banting Lecture. From the Triumvirate to the Ominous Octet: A New Paradigm for the Treatment of Type Diabetes Mellitus. *Diabetes* **2009**, *58*, 773–795. [CrossRef]
58. Smith, U. Impaired ('diabetic') Insulin Signaling and Action Occur in Fat Cells Long before Glucose Intolerance—Is Insuli Resistance Initiated in the Adipose Tissue? *Int. J. Obes.* **2002**, *26*, 897–904. [CrossRef]
59. Cignarelli, A.; Genchi, V.A.; Perrini, S.; Natalicchio, A.; Laviola, L.; Giorgino, F. Insulin and Insulin Receptors in Adipose Tissu Development. *Int. J. Mol. Sci.* **2019**, *20*, 759. [CrossRef]
60. Barac, A.; Campia, U.; Panza, J.A. Methods for Evaluating Endothelial Function in Humans. *Hypertension* **2007**, *49*, 748–76 [CrossRef]
61. Vicent, D.; Ilany, J.; Kondo, T.; Naruse, K.; Fisher, S.J.; Kisanuki, Y.Y.; Bursell, S.; Yanagisawa, M.; King, G.L.; Kahn, C.R. The Rol of Endothelial Insulin Signaling in the Regulation of Vascular Tone and Insulin Resistance. *J. Clin. Investig.* **2003**, *111*, 1373–138 [CrossRef]
62. Kim, K.J.; Kim, K.H.; Cheong, J.H. Hepatitis B Virus X Protein Impairs Hepatic Insulin Signaling Through Degradation of IRS and Induction of SOCS3. *PLoS ONE* **2010**, *5*, e8649. [CrossRef]
63. Kim, J.B.; Siddiqui, S.; Kim, K.W.; Hosoi, T.; Thon, M.; Ozawa, K. Possible Integrative Actions of Leptin and Insulin Signaling i the Hypothalamus Targeting Energy Homeostasis. *Front. Endocrinol.* **2016**, *7*, 138. [CrossRef]
64. Bruning, J.C.; Gautam, D.; Burks, D.J.; Gillette, J.; Schubert, M.; Orban, P.C.; Klein, R.; Krone, W.; Muller-Wieland, D.; Kahn, C. Role of Brain Insulin Receptor in Control of Body Weight and Reproduction. *Science* **2000**, *289*, 2122–2125. [CrossRef]
65. Baskin, D.G.; Breininger, J.F.; Schwartz, M.W. Leptin Receptor MRNA Identifies a Subpopulation of Neuropeptide Y Neuror Activated by Fasting in Rat Hypothalamus. *Diabetes* **1999**, *48*, 828–833. [CrossRef]
66. Cheung, C.C.; Clifton, D.K.; Steiner, R.A. Proopiomelanocortin Neurons Are Direct Targets for Leptin in the Hypothalamu *Endocrinology* **1997**, *138*, 4489–4492. [CrossRef] [PubMed]
67. Baskin, D.G.; Wilcox, B.J.; Figlewicz, D.P.; Dorsa, D.M. Insulin and Insulin-like Growth Factors in the CNS. *Trends Neurosc* **1988**, *11*, 107–111. [CrossRef]
68. Morton, G.J.; Cummings, D.E.; Baskin, D.G.; Barsh, G.S.; Schwartz, M.W. Central Nervous System Control of Food Intake an Body Weight. *Nature* **2006**, *443*, 289–295. [CrossRef] [PubMed]
69. Thon, M.; Hosoi, T.; Ozawa, K. Insulin Enhanced Leptin-Induced STAT3 Signaling by Inducing GRP78. *Sci. Rep.* **2016**, *6*, 3431 [CrossRef]
70. Niswender, K.D.; Schwartz, M.W. Insulin and Leptin Revisited: Adiposity Signals with Overlapping Physiological and Intracell lar Signaling Capabilities. *Front. Neuroendocrinol.* **2003**, *24*, 1–10. [CrossRef]
71. Benomar, Y.; Roy, A.F.; Aubourg, A.; Djiane, J.; Taouis, M. Cross Down-Regulation of Leptin and Insulin Receptor Expression an Signalling in a Human Neuronal Cell Line. *Biochem. J.* **2005**, *388*, 929. [CrossRef]
72. Kim, M.S.; Pak, Y.K.; Jang, P.G.; Namkoong, C.; Choi, Y.S.; Won, J.C.; Kim, K.S.; Kim, S.W.; Kim, H.S.; Park, J.Y.; et al. Role c Hypothalamic Foxo1 in the Regulation of Food Intake and Energy Homeostasis. *Nat. Neurosci.* **2006**, *9*, 901–906. [CrossRef]
73. Xu, A.W.; Kaelin, C.B.; Takeda, K.; Akira, S.; Schwartz, M.W.; Barsh, G.S. PI3K Integrates the Action of Insulin and Leptin o Hypothalamic Neurons. *J. Clin. Investig.* **2005**, *115*, 951. [CrossRef] [PubMed]
74. Niswender, K.D.; Morrison, C.D.; Clegg, D.J.; Olson, R.; Baskin, D.G.; Myers, M.G.; Seeley, R.J.; Schwartz, M.W. Insulin Activatio of Phosphatidylinositol 3-Kinase in the Hypothalamic Arcuate Nucleus: A Key Mediator of Insulin-Induced Anorexia. *Diabete* **2003**, *52*, 227–231. [CrossRef]
75. Plum, L.; Lin, H.V.; Dutia, R.; Tanaka, J.; Aizawa, K.S.; Matsumoto, M.; Kim, A.J.; Cawley, N.X.; Paik, J.H.; Loh, Y.P.; et al. Th Obesity Susceptibility Gene Carboxypeptidase E Links FoxO1 Signaling in Hypothalamic Pro–Opiomelanocortin Neurons wit Regulation of Food Intake. *Nat. Med.* **2009**, *15*, 1195. [CrossRef] [PubMed]
76. Cheng, A.; Uetani, N.; Simoncic, P.D.; Chaubey, V.P.; Lee-Loy, A.; McGlade, C.J.; Kennedy, B.P.; Tremblay, M.L. Attenuation c Leptin Action and Regulation of Obesity by Protein Tyrosine Phosphatase 1B. *Dev. Cell* **2002**, *2*, 497–503. [CrossRef]
77. Kenner, K.A.; Anyanwu, E.; Olefsky, J.M.; Kusari, J. Protein-Tyrosine Phosphatase 1B Is a Negative Regulator of Insulin- an Insulin-like Growth Factor-I-Stimulated Signaling. *J. Biol. Chem.* **1996**, *271*, 19810–19816. [CrossRef] [PubMed]
78. Elchebly, M.; Payette, P.; Michaliszyn, E.; Cromlish, W.; Collins, S.; Loy, A.L.; Normandin, D.; Cheng, A.; Himms-Hagen, J.; Cha C.C.; et al. Increased Insulin Sensitivity and Obesity Resistance in Mice Lacking the Protein Tyrosine Phosphatase-1B Gen *Science* **1999**, *283*, 1544–1548. [CrossRef]
79. Emanuelli, B.; Peraldi, P.; Filloux, C.; Sawka-Verhelle, D.; Hilton, D.; Van Obberghen, E. SOCS-3 Is an Insulin-Induced Negativ Regulator of Insulin Signaling. *J. Biol. Chem.* **2000**, *275*, 15985–15991. [CrossRef]
80. Reed, A.S.; Unger, E.K.; Olofsson, L.E.; Piper, M.L.; Myers, M.G.; Xu, A.W. Functional Role of Suppressor of Cytokine Signaling Upregulation in Hypothalamic Leptin Resistance and Long-Term Energy Homeostasis. *Diabetes* **2010**, *59*, 894–906. [CrossRef]
81. Ernst, M.B.; Wunderlich, C.M.; Hess, S.; Paehler, M.; Mesaros, A.; Koralov, S.B.; Kleinridders, A.; Husch, A.; Münzber H.; Hampel, B.; et al. Enhanced Stat3 Activation in POMC Neurons Provokes Negative Feedback Inhibition of Leptin an InsulinSignaling in Obesity. *J. Neurosci.* **2009**, *29*, 11582–11593. [CrossRef]

Kievit, P.; Howard, J.K.; Badman, M.K.; Balthasar, N.; Coppari, R.; Mori, H.; Lee, C.E.; Elmquist, J.K.; Yoshimura, A.; Flier, J.S. Enhanced Leptin Sensitivity and Improved Glucose Homeostasis in Mice Lacking Suppressor of Cytokine Signaling-3 in POMC-Expressing Cells. *Cell Metab.* **2006**, *4*, 123–132. [CrossRef]

Hogg, J.C. Pathophysiology of Airflow Limitation in Chronic Obstructive Pulmonary Disease. *Lancet* **2004**, *364*, 709–721. [CrossRef]

Broekhuizen, R.; Vernooy, J.H.J.; Schols, A.M.W.J.; Dentener, M.A.; Wouters, E.F.M. Leptin as Local Inflammatory Marker in COPD. *Respir. Med.* **2005**, *99*, 70–74. [CrossRef] [PubMed]

Vernooy, J.H.J.; Drummen, N.E.A.; Van Suylen, R.J.; Cloots, R.H.E.; Möller, G.M.; Bracke, K.R.; Zuyderduyn, S.; Dentener, M.A.; Brusselle, G.G.; Hiemstra, P.S.; et al. Enhanced Pulmonary Leptin Expression in Patients with Severe COPD and Asymptomatic Smokers. *Thorax* **2009**, *64*, 26–32. [CrossRef] [PubMed]

Woo, H.J.; Yoo, W.J.; Bae, C.H.; Song, S.Y.; Kim, Y.W.; Park, S.Y.; Kim, Y.D. Leptin Up-Regulates MUC5B Expression in Human Airway Epithelial Cells via Mitogen-Activated Protein Kinase Pathway. *Exp. Lung Res.* **2010**, *36*, 262–269. [CrossRef]

Breyer, M.K.; Rutten, E.P.A.; Vernooy, J.H.J.; Spruit, M.A.; Dentener, M.A.; Van Der Kallen, C.; Vangreevenbroek, M.M.J.; Wouters, E.F.M. Gender Differences in the Adipose Secretome System in Chronic Obstructive Pulmonary Disease (COPD): A Pivotal Role of Leptin. *Respir. Med.* **2011**, *105*, 1046–1053. [CrossRef]

Breyer, M.K.; Rutten, E.P.A.; Locantore, N.W.; Watkins, M.L.; Miller, B.E.; Wouters, E.F.M. Dysregulated Adipokine Metabolism in Chronic Obstructive Pulmonary Disease. *Eur. J. Clin. Investig.* **2012**, *42*, 983–991. [CrossRef] [PubMed]

Vernooy, J.H.J.; Ubags, N.D.J.; Brusselle, G.G.; Tavernier, J.; Suratt, B.T.; Joos, G.F.; Wouters, E.F.M.; Bracke, K.R. Leptin as Regulator of Pulmonary Immune Responses: Involvement in Respiratory Diseases. *Pulm. Pharmacol. Ther.* **2013**, *26*, 464. [CrossRef]

Gaki, E.; Kontogianni, K.; Papaioannou, A.I.; Bakakos, P.; Gourgoulianis, K.I.; Kostikas, K.; Alchanatis, M.; Papiris, S.; Loukides, S. Associations between BODE Index and Systemic Inflammatory Biomarkers in COPD. *COPD J. Chronic Obstr. Pulm. Dis.* **2011**, *8*, 408–413. [CrossRef]

Lambert, A.A.; Putcha, N.; Drummond, M.B.; Boriek, A.M.; Hanania, N.A.; Kim, V.; Kinney, G.L.; McDonald, M.L.N.; Brigham, E.P.; Wise, R.A.; et al. Obesity Is Associated With Increased Morbidity in Moderate to Severe COPD. *Chest* **2016**, *151*, 68. [CrossRef]

Matarese, G.; Procaccini, C.; De Rosa, V.; Horvath, T.L.; La Cava, A. Regulatory T Cells in Obesity: The Leptin Connection. *Trends Mol. Med.* **2010**, *16*, 247–256. [CrossRef]

Bolton, C.E.; Evans, M.; Ionescu, A.A.; Edwards, S.M.; Morris, R.H.K.; Dunseath, G.; Luzio, S.D.; Owens, D.R.; Shale, D.J. Insulin Resistance and Inflammation—A Further Systemic Complication of COPD. *COPD J. Chronic Obstr. Pulm. Dis.* **2007**, *4*, 121–126. [CrossRef] [PubMed]

Poulain, M.; Doucet, M.; Major, G.C.; Drapeau, V.; Sériès, F.; Boulet, L.P.; Tremblay, A.; Maltais, F. The Effect of Obesity on Chronic Respiratory Diseases: Pathophysiology and Therapeutic Strategies. *CMAJ Can. Med. Assoc. J.* **2006**, *174*, 1293. [CrossRef]

Franssen, F.M.E.; O'Donnell, D.E.; Goossens, G.H.; Blaak, E.E.; Schols, A.M.W.J. Obesity and the Lung: 5. Obesity and COPD. *Thorax* **2008**, *63*, 1110–1117. [CrossRef]

Landbo, C.; Prescott, E.; Lange, P.; Vestbo, J.; Almdal, T.P. Prognostic Value of Nutritional Status in Chronic Obstructive Pulmonary Disease. *Am. J. Respir. Crit. Care Med.* **1999**, *160*, 1856–1861. [CrossRef]

Vestbo, J.; Prescott, E.; Almdal, T.; Dahl, M.; Nordestgaard, B.G.; Andersen, T.; Sørensen, T.I.A.; Lange, P. Body Mass, Fat-Free Body Mass, and Prognosis in Patients with Chronic Obstructive Pulmonary Disease from a Random Population Sample: Findings from the Copenhagen City Heart Study. *Am. J. Respir. Crit. Care Med.* **2006**, *173*, 79–83. [CrossRef] [PubMed]

Pérez-Pérez, A.; Sánchez-Jiménez, F.; Vilariño-García, T.; Sánchez-Margalet, V. Role of Leptin in Inflammation and Vice Versa. *Int. J. Mol. Sci.* **2020**, *21*, 5887. [CrossRef] [PubMed]

Martin, S.S.; Qasim, A.; Reilly, M.P. Leptin Resistance: A Possible Interface of Inflammation and Metabolism in Obesity-Related Cardiovascular Disease. *J. Am. Coll. Cardiol.* **2008**, *52*, 1201. [CrossRef]

)0. Vilariño-García, T.; Polonio-González, M.L.; Pérez-Pérez, A.; Ribalta, J.; Arrieta, F.; Aguilar, M.; Obaya, J.C.; Gimeno-Orna, J.A.; Iglesias, P.; Navarro, J.; et al. Role of Leptin in Obesity, Cardiovascular Disease, and Type 2 Diabetes. *Int. J. Mol. Sci.* **2024**, *25*, 2338. [CrossRef]

)1. Frederich, R.C.; Hamann, A.; Anderson, S.; Löllmann, B.; Lowell, B.B.; Flier, J.S. Leptin Levels Reflect Body Lipid Content in Mice: Evidence for Diet-Induced Resistance to Leptin Action. *Nat. Med.* **1995**, *1*, 1311–1314. [CrossRef]

)2. McGuinness, A.J.A.; Sapey, L. Oxidative Stress in COPD: Sources, Markers, and Potential Mechanisms. *J. Clin. Med.* **2017**, *6*, 21. [CrossRef]

)3. McMurray, F.; Patten, D.A.; Harper, M.E. Reactive Oxygen Species and Oxidative Stress in Obesity-Recent Findings and Empirical Approaches. *Obesity* **2016**, *24*, 2301–2310. [CrossRef]

)4. Zimmet, P.; Alberti, K.G.M.M.; Shaw, J. Global and Societal Implications of the Diabetes Epidemic. *Nature* **2001**, *414*, 782–787. [CrossRef]

)5. Abstracts 2007. *Diabetologia* **2007**, *50*, 1–538. [CrossRef] [PubMed]

106. Zhao, X.; An, X.; Yang, C.; Sun, W.; Ji, H.; Lian, F. The Crucial Role and Mechanism of Insulin Resistance in Metabolic Disease *Front. Endocrinol.* **2023**, *14*, 1149239. [CrossRef] [PubMed]
107. Saltiel, A.R.; Kahn, C.R. Insulin Signalling and the Regulation of Glucose and Lipid Metabolism. *Nature* **2001**, *414*, 799–806 [CrossRef] [PubMed]
108. Freidenberg, G.R.; Reichart, D.; Olefsky, J.M.; Henry, R.R. Reversibility of Defective Adipocyte Insulin Receptor Kinase Activity in Non-Insulin-Dependent Diabetes Mellitus. Effect of Weight Loss. *J. Clin. Investig.* **1988**, *82*, 1398. [CrossRef]
109. Machado, F.V.C.; Pitta, F.; Hernandes, N.A.; Bertolini, G.L. Physiopathological Relationship between Chronic Obstructive Pulmonary Disease and Insulin Resistance. *Endocrine* **2018**, *61*, 17–22. [CrossRef]
110. Donath, M.Y.; Dalmas, É.; Sauter, N.S.; Böni-Schnetzler, M. Inflammation in Obesity and Diabetes: Islet Dysfunction and Therapeutic Opportunity. *Cell Metab.* **2013**, *17*, 860–872. [CrossRef]
111. Nieto-Vazquez, I.; Fernández-Veledo, S.; Krämer, D.K.; Vila-Bedmar, R.; Garcia-Guerra, L.; Lorenzo, M. Insulin Resistance Associated to Obesity: The Link TNF-Alpha. *Arch. Physiol. Biochem.* **2008**, *114*, 183–194. [CrossRef]
112. Samuel, V.T.; Shulman, G.I. Integrating Mechanisms for Insulin Resistance: Common Threads and Missing Links. *Cell* **2012**, *148*, 852. [CrossRef]
113. Chen, K.; Li, F.; Li, J.; Cai, H.; Strom, S.; Bisello, A.; Kelley, D.E.; Friedman-Einat, M.; Skibinski, G.A.; McCrory, M.A.; et al. Induction of Leptin Resistance through Direct Interaction of C-Reactive Protein with Leptin. *Nat. Med.* **2006**, *12*, 425–432 [CrossRef] [PubMed]
114. Eker, S.; Ayaz, L.; Tamer, L.; Ulubas, B. Leptin, Visfatin, Insulin Resistance, and Body Composition Change in Chronic Obstructive Pulmonary Disease. *Scand. J. Clin. Lab. Investig.* **2010**, *70*, 40–44. [CrossRef] [PubMed]
115. Streba, L.; Popovici, V.; Mihai, A.; Mititelu, M.; Lupu, C.E.; Matei, M.; Vladu, I.M.; Iovănescu, M.L.; Cioboată, R.; Călărașu, C.; et al. Integrative Approach to Risk Factors in Simple Chronic Obstructive Airway Diseases of the Lung or Associated with Metabolic Syndrome-Analysis and Prediction. *Nutrients* **2024**, *16*, 1851. [CrossRef] [PubMed]
116. Hayden, M.R. Overview and New Insights into the Metabolic Syndrome: Risk Factors and Emerging Variables in the Development of Type 2 Diabetes and Cerebrocardiovascular Disease. *Medicina* **2023**, *59*, 561. [CrossRef]
117. Minas, M.; Kostikas, K.; Papaioannou, A.I.; Mystridou, P.; Karetsi, E.; Georgoulias, P.; Liakos, N.; Pournaras, S.; Gourgoulianis, K.I. The Association of Metabolic Syndrome with Adipose Tissue Hormones and Insulin Resistance in Patients with COPD without Co-Morbidities. *COPD J. Chronic Obstr. Pulm. Dis.* **2011**, *8*, 414–420. [CrossRef]
118. Takabatake, N.; Nakamura, H.; Abe, S.; Hino, T.; Saito, H.; Yuki, H.; Kato, S.; Tomoike, H. Circulating Leptin in Patients with Chronic Obstructive Pulmonary Disease. *Am. J. Respir. Crit. Care Med.* **1999**, *159*, 1215–1219. [CrossRef]
119. Schols, A.M.; Broekhuizen, R.; Weling-Scheepers, C.A.; Wouters, E.F. Body Composition and Mortality in Chronic Obstructive Pulmonary Disease. *Am. J. Clin. Nutr.* **2005**, *82*, 53–59. [CrossRef]
120. Wells, C.E.; Polkey, M.I.; Baker, E.H. Insulin Resistance Is Associated with Skeletal Muscle Weakness in COPD. *Respirology* **2016**, *21*, 689–696. [CrossRef] [PubMed]
121. Chan, S.M.H.; Selemidis, S.; Bozinovski, S.; Vlahos, R. Pathobiological Mechanisms Underlying Metabolic Syndrome (MetS) in Chronic Obstructive Pulmonary Disease (COPD): Clinical Significance and Therapeutic Strategies. *Pharmacol. Ther.* **2019**, *198*, 160–188. [CrossRef]
122. Clini, E.; Crisafulli, E.; Radaeli, A.; Malerba, M. COPD and the Metabolic Syndrome: An Intriguing Association. *Intern. Emerg. Med.* **2013**, *8*, 283–289. [CrossRef]
123. Díez-Manglano, J.; Barquero-Romero, J.; Almagro, P.; Cabrera, F.J.; López García, F.; Montero, L.; Soriano, J.B. COPD Patients with and Without Metabolic Syndrome: Clinical and Functional Differences. *Intern. Emerg. Med.* **2014**, *9*, 419–425. [CrossRef] [PubMed]
124. Gregor, M.F.; Hotamisligil, G.S. Inflammatory Mechanisms in Obesity. *Annu. Rev. Immunol.* **2011**, *29*, 415–445. [CrossRef]
125. Bruun, J.M.; Pedersen, S.B.; Kristensen, K.; Richelsen, B. Opposite Regulation of Interleukin-8 and Tumor Necrosis Factor-Alpha by Weight Loss. *Obes. Res.* **2002**, *10*, 499–506. [CrossRef]
126. Zumbach, M.S.; Boehme, M.W.J.; Wahl, P.; Stremmel, W.; Ziegler, R.; Nawroth, P.P. Tumor Necrosis Factor Increases Serum Leptin Levels in Humans. *J. Clin. Endocrinol. Metab.* **1997**, *82*, 4080–4082. [CrossRef]
127. Grunfeld, C.; Zhao, C.; Fuller, J.; Pollock, A.; Moser, A.; Friedman, J.; Feingold, K.R. Endotoxin and Cytokines Induce Expression of Leptin, the Ob Gene Product, in Hamsters. *J. Clin. Investig.* **1996**, *97*, 2152–2157. [CrossRef] [PubMed]
128. Sarraf, P.; Frederich, R.C.; Turner, E.M.; Ma, G.; Jaskowiak, N.T.; Rivet, D.J.; Flier, J.S.; Lowell, B.B.; Fraker, D.L.; Alexander, H.R. Multiple Cytokines and Acute Inflammation Raise Mouse Leptin Levels: Potential Role in Inflammatory Anorexia. *J. Exp. Med.* **1997**, *185*, 171–175. [CrossRef]
129. Saetta, M.; Di Stefano, A.; Maestrelli, P.; Turato, G.; Ruggieri, M.P.; Roggeri, A.; Calcagni, P.; Mapp, C.E.; Ciaccia, A.; Fabbri, L.M. Airway Eosinophilia in Chronic Bronchitis During Exacerbations. *Am. J. Respir. Crit. Care Med.* **1994**, *150*, 1646–1652. [CrossRef] [PubMed]

0. Nair, P.; Radford, K.; Fanat, A.; Janssen, L.J.; Peters-Golden, M.; Cox, P.G. The Effects of Leptin on Airway Smooth Muscle Responses. *Am. J. Respir. Cell Mol. Biol.* **2008**, *39*, 475–481. [CrossRef]
1. Clerk, L.H.; Vincent, M.A.; Jahn, L.A.; Liu, Z.; Lindner, J.R.; Barrett, E.J. Obesity Blunts Insulin-Mediated Microvascular Recruitment in Human Forearm Muscle. *Diabetes* **2006**, *55*, 1436–1442. [CrossRef]
2. Barnes, P.J. Chronic Obstructive Pulmonary Disease: Effects Beyond the Lungs. *PLoS Med.* **2010**, *7*, e1000220. [CrossRef]
3. Price, D.B.; Russell, R.; Mares, R.; Burden, A.; Skinner, D.; Mikkelsen, H.; Ding, C.; Brice, R.; Chavannes, N.H.; Kocks, J.W.H.; et al. Metabolic Effects Associated with ICS in Patients with COPD and Comorbid Type 2 Diabetes: A Historical Matched Cohort Study. *PLoS ONE* **2016**, *11*, e0162903. [CrossRef]
4. Cruickshank-Quinn, C.I.; Jacobson, S.; Hughes, G.; Powell, R.L.; Petrache, I.; Kechris, K.; Bowler, R.; Reisdorph, N. Metabolomics and Transcriptomics Pathway Approach Reveals Outcome-Specific Perturbations in COPD. *Sci. Rep.* **2018**, *8*, 17132. [CrossRef] [PubMed]
5. Morrow, J.D.; Chase, R.P.; Parker, M.M.; Glass, K.; Seo, M.; Divo, M.; Owen, C.A.; Castaldi, P.; Demeo, D.L.; Silverman, E.K.; et al. RNA-Sequencing across Three Matched Tissues Reveals Shared and Tissue-Specific Gene Expression and Pathway Signatures of COPD. *Respir. Res.* **2019**, *20*, 65. [CrossRef] [PubMed]
6. Yang, M.; Kohler, M.; Heyder, T.; Forsslund, H.; Garberg, H.K.; Karimi, R.; Grunewald, J.; Berven, F.S.; Nyrén, S.; Magnus Sköld, C.; et al. Proteomic Profiling of Lung Immune Cells Reveals Dysregulation of Phagocytotic Pathways in Female-Dominated Molecular COPD Phenotype. *Respir. Res.* **2018**, *19*, 39. [CrossRef] [PubMed]
7. Bai, S.; Ye, R.; Wang, C.; Sun, P.; Wang, D.; Yue, Y.; Wang, H.; Wu, S.; Yu, M.; Xi, S.; et al. Identification of Proteomic Signatures in Chronic Obstructive Pulmonary Disease Emphysematous Phenotype. *Front. Mol. Biosci.* **2021**, *8*, 650604. [CrossRef]
8. Garudadri, S.; Woodruff, P.G. Targeting Chronic Obstructive Pulmonary Disease Phenotypes, Endotypes, and Biomarkers. *Ann. Am. Thorac. Soc.* **2018**, *15*, S234–S238. [CrossRef]
9. Vogelmeier, C.F.; Criner, G.J.; Martinez, F.J.; Anzueto, A.; Barnes, P.J.; Bourbeau, J.; Celli, B.R.; Chen, R.; Decramer, M.; Fabbri, L.M.; et al. Global Strategy for the Diagnosis, Management, and Prevention of Chronic Obstructive Lung Disease 2017 Report. GOLD Executive Summary. *Am. J. Respir. Crit. Care Med.* **2017**, *195*, 557–582. [CrossRef]
0. Kent, B.D.; Mitchell, P.D.; Mcnicholas, W.T. Hypoxemia in Patients with COPD: Cause, Effects, and Disease Progression. *Int. J. Chronic Obstr. Pulm. Dis.* **2011**, *6*, 199–208. [CrossRef]
1. Gileles-Hillel, A.; Kheirandish-Gozal, L.; Gozal, D. Biological Plausibility Linking Sleep Apnoea and Metabolic Dysfunction. *Nat. Rev. Endocrinol.* **2016**, *12*, 290–298. [CrossRef]
2. Kim, J.W.; Tchernyshyov, I.; Semenza, G.L.; Dang, C.V. HIF-1-Mediated Expression of Pyruvate Dehydrogenase Kinase: A Metabolic Switch Required for Cellular Adaptation to Hypoxia. *Cell Metab.* **2006**, *3*, 177–185. [CrossRef]
3. Regazzetti, C.; Peraldi, P.; Grémeaux, T.; Najem-Lendom, R.; Ben-Sahra, I.; Cormont, M.; Bost, F.; Marchand-Brustel, Y.L.; Tanti, J.F.; Giorgetti-Peraldi, S. Hypoxia Decreases Insulin Signaling Pathways in Adipocytes. *Diabetes* **2009**, *58*, 95–103. [CrossRef] [PubMed]
4. Bernardo, I.; Bozinovski, S.; Vlahos, R. Targeting Oxidant-Dependent Mechanisms for the Treatment of COPD and Its Comorbidities. *Pharmacol. Ther.* **2015**, *155*, 60–79. [CrossRef] [PubMed]
5. Li, J.; Grigoryev, D.N.; Ye, S.Q.; Thorne, L.; Schwartz, A.R.; Smith, P.L.; O'Donnell, C.P.; Polotsky, V.Y. Chronic Intermittent Hypoxia Upregulates Genes of Lipid Biosynthesis in Obese Mice. *J. Appl. Physiol.* **2005**, *99*, 1643–1648. [CrossRef]
6. Murphy, A.M.; Thomas, A.; Crinion, S.J.; Kent, B.D.; Tambuwala, M.M.; Fabre, A.; Pepin, J.L.; Roche, H.M.; Arnaud, C.; Ryan, S. Intermittent Hypoxia in Obstructive Sleep Apnoea Mediates Insulin Resistance through Adipose Tissue Inflammation. *Eur. Respir. J.* **2017**, *49*, 1601731. [CrossRef]
7. Yokoe, T.; Alonso, L.C.; Romano, L.C.; Rosa, T.C.; O'Doherty, R.M.; Garcia-Ocana, A.; Minoguchi, K.; O'Donnell, C.P. Intermittent Hypoxia Reverses the Diurnal Glucose Rhythm and Causes Pancreatic Beta-Cell Replication in Mice. *J. Physiol.* **2008**, *586*, 899–911. [CrossRef] [PubMed]
8. Qu, A.; Taylor, M.; Xue, X.; Matsubara, T.; Metzger, D.; Chambon, P.; Gonzalez, F.J.; Shah, Y.M. Hypoxia-Inducible Transcription Factor 2α Promotes Steatohepatitis through Augmenting Lipid Accumulation, Inflammation, and Fibrosis. *Hepatology* **2011**, *54*, 472–483. [CrossRef]
9. Taniguchi, C.M.; Finger, E.C.; Krieg, A.J.; Wu, C.; Diep, A.N.; Lagory, E.L.; Wei, K.; McGinnis, L.M.; Yuan, J.; Kuo, C.J.; et al. Cross-Talk between Hypoxia and Insulin Signaling through Phd3 Regulates Hepatic Glucose and Lipid Metabolism and Ameliorates Diabetes. *Nat. Med.* **2013**, *19*, 1325–1330. [CrossRef]
0. Wei, K.; Piecewicz, S.M.; McGinnis, L.M.; Taniguchi, C.M.; Wiegand, S.J.; Anderson, K.; Chan, C.W.M.; Mulligan, K.X.; Kuo, D.; Yuan, J.; et al. A Liver Hif-2α-Irs2 Pathway Sensitizes Hepatic Insulin Signaling and Is Modulated by Vegf Inhibition. *Nat. Med.* **2013**, *19*, 1331–1337. [CrossRef]
1. Thomas, A.; Belaidi, E.; Moulin, S.; Horman, S.; Van Der Zon, G.C.; Viollet, B.; Levy, P.; Bertrand, L.; Pepin, J.L.; Godin-Ribuot, D.; et al. Chronic Intermittent Hypoxia Impairs Insulin Sensitivity but Improves Whole-Body Glucose Tolerance by Activating Skeletal Muscle AMPK. *Diabetes* **2017**, *66*, 2942–2951. [CrossRef]

152. Gamboa, J.L.; Garcia-Cazarin, M.L.; Andrade, F.H. Chronic Hypoxia Increases Insulin-Stimulated Glucose Uptake in Mous Soleus Muscle. *Am. J. Physiol.-Regul. Integr. Comp. Physiol.* **2011**, *300*, R85–R91. [CrossRef]
153. Kirkham, P.A.; Barnes, P.J. Oxidative Stress in COPD. *Chest* **2013**, *144*, 266–273. [CrossRef]
154. Taniguchi, A.; Tsuge, M.; Miyahara, N.; Tsukahara, H. Reactive Oxygen Species and Antioxidative Defense in Chronic Obstructiv Pulmonary Disease. *Antioxidants* **2021**, *10*, 1537. [CrossRef]
155. Van Der Toorn, M.; Rezayat, D.; Kauffman, H.F.; Bakker, S.J.L.; Gans, R.O.B.; Koëter, G.H.; Choi, A.M.K.; Van Oosterhout, A.J.M Slebos, D.J. Lipid-Soluble Components in Cigarette Smoke Induce Mitochondrial Production of Reactive Oxygen Species in Lur Epithelial Cells. *Am. J. Physiol. Lung Cell Mol. Physiol.* **2009**, *297*, L109–L114. [CrossRef]
156. Osoata, G.O.; Hanazawa, T.; Brindicci, C.; Ito, M.; Barnes, P.J.; Kharitonov, S.; Ito, K. Peroxynitrite Elevation in Exhaled Breat Condensate of COPD and Its Inhibition by Fudosteine. *Chest* **2009**, *135*, 1513–1520. [CrossRef] [PubMed]
157. O'Donnell, C.; Newbold, P.; White, P.; Thong, B.; Stone, H.; Stockley, R.A. 3-Chlorotyrosine in Sputum of COPD Patient Relationship with Airway Inflammation. *COPD J. Chronic Obstr. Pulm. Dis.* **2010**, *7*, 411–417. [CrossRef] [PubMed]
158. Miklós, Z.; Horváth, I. The Role of Oxidative Stress and Antioxidants in Cardiovascular Comorbidities in COPD. *Antioxidan* **2023**, *12*, 1196. [CrossRef] [PubMed]
159. Negre-Salvayre, A.; Coatrieux, C.; Ingueneau, C.; Salvayre, R. Advanced Lipid Peroxidation End Products in Oxidative Damag to Proteins. Potential Role in Diseases and Therapeutic Prospects for the Inhibitors. *Br. J. Pharmacol.* **2008**, *153*, 6–20. [CrossRef
160. Kirkham, P.A.; Caramori, G.; Casolari, P.; Papi, A.A.; Edwards, M.; Shamji, B.; Triantaphyllopoulos, K.; Hussain, F.; Pinart, M Khan, Y.; et al. Oxidative Stress–Induced Antibodies to Carbonyl-Modified Protein Correlate with Severity of Chronic Obstructiv Pulmonary Disease. *Am. J. Respir. Crit. Care Med.* **2011**, *184*, 796. [CrossRef]
161. Touyz, R.M.; Rios, F.J.; Alves-Lopes, R.; Neves, K.B.; Camargo, L.L.; Montezano, A.C. Oxidative Stress: A Unifying Paradigm i Hypertension. *Can. J. Cardiol.* **2020**, *36*, 659–670. [CrossRef]
162. Devallance, E.; Li, Y.; Jurczak, M.J.; Cifuentes-Pagano, E.; Pagano, P.J. The Role of NADPH Oxidases in the Etiology of Obesity an Metabolic Syndrome: Contribution of Individual Isoforms and Cell Biology. *Antioxid. Redox Signal.* **2019**, *31*, 687–709. [CrossRe
163. Masenga, S.K.; Kabwe, L.S.; Chakulya, M.; Kirabo, A. Mechanisms of Oxidative Stress in Metabolic Syndrome. *Int. J. Mol. Sc* **2023**, *24*, 7898. [CrossRef] [PubMed]
164. Petersen, M.C.; Shulman, G.I. Mechanisms of Insulin Action and Insulin Resistance. *Physiol. Rev.* **2018**, *98*, 2133–2223. [CrossRe [PubMed]
165. Kolka, C.M.; Bergman, R.N. The Endothelium in Diabetes: Its Role in Insulin Access and Diabetic Complications. *Rev. Endoc Metab. Disord.* **2013**, *14*, 13–19. [CrossRef]
166. Tarantino, G.; Caputi, A. JNKs, Insulin Resistance and Inflammation: A Possible Link between NAFLD and Coronary Arter Disease. *World J. Gastroenterol. WJG* **2011**, *17*, 3785. [CrossRef]
167. Marseglia, L.; Manti, S.; D'Angelo, G.; Nicotera, A.; Parisi, E.; Di Rosa, G.; Gitto, E.; Arrigo, T. Oxidative Stress in Obesit A Critical Component in Human Diseases. *Int. J. Mol. Sci.* **2014**, *16*, 378–400. [CrossRef]
168. Savini, I.; Catani, M.V.; Evangelista, D.; Gasperi, V.; Avigliano, L. Obesity-Associated Oxidative Stress: Strategies Finalized t Improve Redox State. *Int. J. Mol. Sci.* **2013**, *14*, 10497–10538. [CrossRef]
169. Colak, E.; Pap, D. The Role of Oxidative Stress in the Development of Obesity and Obesity-Related Metabolic Disorders. *J. Me Biochem.* **2021**, *40*, 1–9. [CrossRef]
170. Glass, C.K.; Olefsky, J.M. Inflammation and Lipid Signaling in the Etiology of Insulin Resistance. *Cell Metab.* **2012**, *15*, 635–64 [CrossRef] [PubMed]
171. Aras, M.; Tchang, B.G.; Pape, J. Obesity and Diabetes. *Nurs. Clin. N. Am.* **2021**, *56*, 527–541. [CrossRef]
172. Recinella, L.; Orlando, G.; Ferrante, C.; Chiavaroli, A.; Brunetti, L.; Leone, S. Adipokines: New Potential Therapeutic Target fc Obesity and Metabolic, Rheumatic, and Cardiovascular Diseases. *Front. Physiol.* **2020**, *11*, 578966. [CrossRef]
173. Manna, P.; Jain, S.K. Obesity, Oxidative Stress, Adipose Tissue Dysfunction, and the Associated Health Risks: Causes an Therapeutic Strategies. *Metab. Syndr. Relat. Disord.* **2015**, *13*, 423–444. [CrossRef] [PubMed]
174. Lingappan, K. NF-KB in Oxidative Stress. *Curr. Opin. Toxicol.* **2018**, *7*, 81–86. [CrossRef]
175. Tangvarasittichai, S. Oxidative Stress, Insulin Resistance, Dyslipidemia and Type 2 Diabetes Mellitus. *World J. Diabete* **2015**, *6*, 456. [CrossRef] [PubMed]
176. Di Stefano, A.; Caramori, G.; Oates, T.; Capelli, A.; Lusuardi, M.; Gnemmi, I.; Ioli, F.; Chung, K.F.; Donner, C.F.; Barnes, P.J.; et a Increased Expression of Nuclear Factor-KappaB in Bronchial Biopsies from Smokers and Patients with COPD. *Eur. Respir.* **2002**, *20*, 556–563. [CrossRef]
177. Barnes, P.J. Cellular and Molecular Mechanisms of Asthma and COPD. *Clin. Sci.* **2017**, *131*, 1541–1558. [CrossRef]
178. Fabbri, L.M.; Rabe, K.F. From COPD to Chronic Systemic Inflammatory Syndrome? *Lancet* **2007**, *370*, 797–799. [CrossRef]
179. Decramer, M.; Rennard, S.; Troosters, T.; Mapel, D.W.; Giardino, N.; Mannino, D.; Wouters, E.; Sethi, S.; Cooper, C.B. COPD as Lung Disease with Systemic Consequences—Clinical Impact, Mechanisms, and Potential for Early Intervention. *COPD J. Chron Obstr. Pulm. Dis.* **2008**, *5*, 235–256. [CrossRef]

0. Easter, M.; Bollenbecker, S.; Barnes, J.W.; Krick, S. Targeting Aging Pathways in Chronic Obstructive Pulmonary Disease. *Int. J. Mol. Sci.* **2020**, *21*, 6294. [CrossRef] [PubMed]
1. Hernandez Cordero, A.I.; Yang, C.X.; Milne, S.; Li, X.; Hollander, Z.; Chen, V.; Ng, R.; Tebbutt, S.J.; Leung, J.M.; Sin, D.D. Epigenetic Blood Biomarkers of Ageing and Mortality in COPD. *Eur. Respir. J.* **2021**, *58*, 2101890. [CrossRef]
2. Breen, M.; Nwanaji-Enwerem, J.C.; Karrasch, S.; Flexeder, C.; Schulz, H.; Waldenberger, M.; Kunze, S.; Ollert, M.; Weidinger, S.; Colicino, E.; et al. Accelerated Epigenetic Aging as a Risk Factor for Chronic Obstructive Pulmonary Disease and Decreased Lung Function in Two Prospective Cohort Studies. *Aging* **2020**, *12*, 16539–16554. [CrossRef]
3. Górski, P.; Białas, A.J.; Piotrowski, W.J. Aging Lung: Molecular Drivers and Impact on Respiratory Diseases—A Narrative Clinical Review. *Antioxidants* **2024**, *13*, 1480. [CrossRef] [PubMed]
4. Pellegrino, D.; Casas-Recasens, S.; Faner, R.; Palange, P.; Agusti, A. When GETomics Meets Aging and Exercise in COPD. *Respir. Med.* **2023**, *216*, 107294. [CrossRef]
5. Martino, D.J.; Bui, D.S.; Li, S.; Idrose, S.; Perret, J.; Lowe, A.J.; Lodge, C.J.; Bowatte, G.; Moodley, Y.; Thomas, P.S.; et al. Genetic and Epigenetic Associations with Pre-COPD Lung Function Trajectories. *Am. J. Respir. Crit. Care Med.* **2023**, *208*, 1135–1137. [CrossRef]
6. Feng, Y.; Xie, M.; Liu, Q.; Weng, J.; Wei, L.; Chung, K.F.; Adcock, I.M.; Chang, Q.; Li, M.; Huang, Y.; et al. Changes in Targeted Metabolomics in Lung Tissue of Chronic Obstructive Pulmonary Disease. *J. Thorac. Dis.* **2023**, *15*, 2544–2558. [CrossRef]
7. Diao, W.; Labaki, W.W.; Han, M.K.; Yeomans, L.; Sun, Y.; Smiley, Z.; Kim, J.H.; McHugh, C.; Xiang, P.; Shen, N.; et al. Disruption of Histidine and Energy Homeostasis in Chronic Obstructive Pulmonary Disease. *Int. J. Chronic Obstr. Pulm. Dis.* **2019**, *14*, 2015–2025. [CrossRef] [PubMed]
8. Xue, M.; Zeng, Y.; Lin, R.; Qu, H.Q.; Zhang, T.; Zhang, X.D.; Liang, Y.; Zhen, Y.; Chen, H.; Huang, Z.; et al. Metabolomic Profiling of Anaerobic and Aerobic Energy Metabolic Pathways in Chronic Obstructive Pulmonary Disease. *Exp. Biol. Med.* **2021**, *246*, 1586–1596. [CrossRef]
9. Kim, J.; Suresh, B.; Lim, M.N.; Hong, S.H.; Kim, K.S.; Song, H.E.; Lee, H.Y.; Yoo, H.J.; Kim, W.J. Metabolomics Reveals Dysregulated Sphingolipid and Amino Acid Metabolism Associated with Chronic Obstructive Pulmonary Disease. *Int. J. Chronic Obstr. Pulm. Dis.* **2022**, *17*, 2343–2353. [CrossRef] [PubMed]
0. Naz, S.; Kolmert, J.; Yang, M.; Reinke, S.N.; Kamleh, M.A.; Snowden, S.; Heyder, T.; Levänen, B.; Erle, D.J.; Sköld, C.M.; et al. Metabolomics Analysis Identifies Sex-Associated Metabotypes of Oxidative Stress and the Autotaxin–LysoPA Axis in COPD. *Eur. Respir. J.* **2017**, *49*, 1602322. [CrossRef]
1. Zinellu, A.; Mangoni, A.A. Arginine, Transsulfuration, and Folic Acid Pathway Metabolomics in Chronic Obstructive Pulmonary Disease: A Systematic Review and Meta-Analysis. *Cells* **2023**, *12*, 2180. [CrossRef]
2. Adamko, D.J.; Nair, P.; Mayers, I.; Tsuyuki, R.T.; Regush, S.; Rowe, B.H. Metabolomic Profiling of Asthma and Chronic Obstructive Pulmonary Disease: A Pilot Study Differentiating Diseases. *J. Allergy Clin. Immunol.* **2015**, *136*, 571–580.e3. [CrossRef]
3. Saltiel, A.R.; Olefsky, J.M. Inflammatory Mechanisms Linking Obesity and Metabolic Disease. *J. Clin. Investig.* **2017**, *127*, 1–4. [CrossRef] [PubMed]
4. Mihai, A.; Mititelu, M.; Matei, M.; Lupu, E.C.; Streba, L.; Vladu, I.M.; Iovănescu, M.L.; Cioboată, R.; Călărașu, C.; Busnatu, Ș.S.; et al. Assessment of Behavioral Risk Factors in Chronic Obstructive Airway Diseases of the Lung Associated with Metabolic Syndrome. *J. Clin. Med.* **2024**, *13*, 1037. [CrossRef] [PubMed]
5. Cebron Lipovec, N.; Beijers, R.J.H.C.G.; van den Borst, B.; Doehner, W.; Lainscak, M.; Schols, A.M.W.J. The Prevalence of Metabolic Syndrome in Chronic Obstructive Pulmonary Disease: A Systematic Review. *COPD J. Chronic Obstr. Pulm. Dis.* **2016**, *13*, 399–406. [CrossRef] [PubMed]
6. Vujic, T.; Nagorni Obradovic, L.; Maric, G.; Popovic, L.; Jankovic, J. Metabolic Syndrome in Patients with Chronic Obstructive Pulmonary Disease: Frequency and Relationship with Systemic Inflammation. *Hippokratia* **2016**, *20*, 110.
7. Watz, H.; Waschki, B.; Kirsten, A.; Müller, K.C.; Kretschmar, G.; Meyer, T.; Holz, O.; Magnussen, H. The Metabolic Syndrome in Patients with Chronic Bronchitis and COPD: Frequency and Associated Consequences for Systemic Inflammation and Physical Inactivity. *Chest* **2009**, *136*, 1039–1046. [CrossRef]
8. Furukawa, S.; Fujita, T.; Shimabukuro, M.; Iwaki, M.; Yamada, Y.; Nakajima, Y.; Nakayama, O.; Makishima, M.; Matsuda, M.; Shimomura, I. Increased Oxidative Stress in Obesity and Its Impact on Metabolic Syndrome. *J. Clin. Investig.* **2004**, *114*, 1752–1761. [CrossRef]
9. Hutcheson, R.; Rocic, P. The Metabolic Syndrome, Oxidative Stress, Environment, and Cardiovascular Disease: The Great Exploration. *Exp. Diabetes Res.* **2012**, *2012*, 271028. [CrossRef] [PubMed]
0. Cyphert, T.J.; Morris, R.T.; House, L.M.; Barnes, T.M.; Otero, Y.F.; Barham, W.J.; Hunt, R.P.; Zaynagetdinov, R.; Yull, F.E.; Blackwell, T.S.; et al. NF-KB-Dependent Airway Inflammation Triggers Systemic Insulin Resistance. *Am. J. Physiol.-Regul. Integr. Comp. Physiol.* **2015**, *309*, R1144–R1152. [CrossRef]
1. Monteiro, F.; Camillo, C.A.; Vitorasso, R.; Sant'Anna, T.; Hernandes, N.A.; Probst, V.S.; Pitta, F. Obesity and Physical Activity in the Daily Life of Patients with COPD. *Lung* **2012**, *190*, 403–410. [CrossRef]

202. Kawai, T.; Autieri, M.V.; Scalia, R. Adipose Tissue Inflammation and Metabolic Dysfunction in Obesity. *Am. J. Physiol. Cell Physic* **2020**, *320*, C375–C391. [CrossRef]
203. Sánchez-Margalet, V.; Fernández-Riejos, P.; Najib, S.; Santos-Alvarez, J.; Martín-Romero, C.; Pérez-Pérez, A.; González-Yanes, C Role of Leptin in the Activation of Immune Cells. *Mediat. Inflamm.* **2010**, *2010*, 568343. [CrossRef]
204. Pérez-Pérez, A.; Vilariño-García, T.; Fernández-Riejos, P.; Martín-González, J.; Segura-Egea, J.J.; Sánchez-Margalet, V. Role o Leptin as a Link Between Metabolism and the Immune System. *Cytokine Growth Factor Rev.* **2017**, *35*, 71–84. [CrossRef] [PubMed
205. Hodge, A.M.; Westerman, R.A.; De Courten, M.P.; Collier, G.R.; Zimmet, P.Z.; Alberti, K.G.M.M. Is Leptin Sensitivity the Lin between Smoking Cessation and Weight Gain? *Int. J. Obes.* **1997**, *21*, 50–53. [CrossRef]
206. Eliasson, B.; Smith, U. Leptin Levels in Smokers and Long-Term Users of Nicotine Gum. *Eur. J. Clin. Investig.* **1999**, *29*, 145–15 [CrossRef] [PubMed]
207. Cazzola, M.; Bettoncelli, G.; Sessa, E.; Cricelli, C.; Biscione, G. Prevalence of Comorbidities in Patients with Chronic Obstructiv Pulmonary Disease. *Respiration* **2010**, *80*, 112–119. [CrossRef]
208. Yin, H.L.; Yin, S.Q.; Lin, Q.Y.; Xu, Y.; Xu, H.W.; Liu, T. Prevalence of Comorbidities in Chronic Obstructive Pulmonary Diseas Patients: A Meta-Analysis. *Medicine* **2017**, *96*, e6863. [CrossRef]
209. Cazzola, M.; Rogliani, P.; Calzetta, L.; Lauro, D.; Page, C.; Matera, M.G. Targeting Mechanisms Linking COPD to Type 2 Diabete Mellitus. *Trends Pharmacol. Sci.* **2017**, *38*, 940–951. [CrossRef]
210. Oh, J.Y.; Sin, D.D. Lung Inflammation in COPD: Why Does It Matter? *F1000 Med. Rep.* **2012**, *4*, 23. [CrossRef]
211. Cravo, J.; Esquinas, A.M. Obesity and COPD Exacerbations—It's Not That Simple. *Respir. Med.* **2017**, *125*, 103. [CrossRef]
212. Kinney, G.L.; Black-Shinn, J.L.; Wan, E.S.; Make, B.; Regan, E.; Lutz, S.; Soler, X.; Silverman, E.K.; Crapo, J.; Hokansor J.E. Pulmonary Function Reduction in Diabetes with and Without Chronic Obstructive Pulmonary Disease. *Diabetes Car* **2014**, *37*, 389–395. [CrossRef]
213. Sedgwick, J.B.; Menon, I.; Gern, J.E.; Busse, W.W. Effects of Inflammatory Cytokines on the Permeability of Huma Lung Microvascular Endothelial Cell Monolayers and Differential Eosinophil Transmigration. *J. Allergy Clin. Immuno* **2002**, *110*, 752–756. [CrossRef] [PubMed]
214. McKeever, T.M.; Weston, P.J.; Hubbard, R.; Fogarty, A. Lung Function and Glucose Metabolism: An Analysis of Data from th Third National Health and Nutrition Examination Survey. *Am. J. Epidemiol.* **2005**, *161*, 546–556. [CrossRef]
215. Sparvero, L.J.; Asafu-Adjei, D.; Kang, R.; Tang, D.; Amin, N.; Im, J.; Rutledge, R.; Lin, B.; Amoscato, A.A.; Zeh, H.J.; et al. RAG (Receptor for Advanced Glycation Endproducts), RAGE Ligands, and Their Role in Cancer and Inflammation. *J. Transl. Mec* **2009**, *7*, 17. [CrossRef]
216. Singh, S.; Bodas, M.; Bhatraju, N.K.; Pattnaik, B.; Gheware, A.; Parameswaran, P.K.; Thompson, M.; Freeman, M.; Mabalirajar U.; Gosens, R.; et al. Hyperinsulinemia Adversely Affects Lung Structure and Function. *Am. J. Physiol. Lung Cell Mol. Physio* **2016**, *310*, L837–L845. [CrossRef]
217. Baker, E.H.; Janaway, C.H.; Philips, B.J.; Brennan, A.L.; Baines, D.L.; Wood, D.M.; Jones, P.W. Hyperglycaemia Is Associated wit Poor Outcomes in Patients Admitted to Hospital with Acute Exacerbations of Chronic Obstructive Pulmonary Disease. *Thora* **2006**, *61*, 284–289. [CrossRef] [PubMed]
218. Parappil, A.; Depczynski, B.; Collett, P.; Marks, G.B. Effect of Comorbid Diabetes on Length of Stay and Risk of Death in Patient Admitted with Acute Exacerbations of COPD. *Respirology* **2010**, *15*, 918–922. [CrossRef]
219. Ceriello, A. Oxidative Stress and Diabetes-Associated Complications. *Endocr. Pract.* **2006**, *12* (Suppl. S1), 60–62. [CrossRef]
220. Tiengo, A.; Fadini, G.P.; Avogaro, A. The Metabolic Syndrome, Diabetes and Lung Dysfunction. *Diabetes Metab.* **2008**, *34*, 447–45 [CrossRef] [PubMed]
221. Cazzola, M.; Calzetta, L.; Rogliani, P.; Lauro, D.; Novelli, L.; Page, C.P.; Kanabar, V.; Matera, M.G. High Glucose Enhance Responsiveness of Human Airways Smooth Muscle via the Rho/ROCK Pathway. *Am. J. Respir. Cell Mol. Biol.* **2012**, *47*, 509–51 [CrossRef]
222. Ottenheijm, C.A.C.; Heunks, L.M.A.; Dekhuijzen, R.P.N. Diaphragm Adaptations in Patients with COPD. *Respir. Res.* **2008**, *9*, 1 [CrossRef]
223. Friedman, J. 20 Years of Leptin: Leptin at 20: An Overview. *J. Endocrinol.* **2014**, *223*, T1–T8. [CrossRef]
224. Schwartz, M.W.; Seeley, R.J.; Campfield, L.A.; Burn, P.; Baskin, D.G. Identification of Targets of Leptin Action in Rat Hypothalamus *J. Clin. Investig.* **1996**, *98*, 1101–1106. [CrossRef] [PubMed]
225. German, J.P.; Thaler, J.P.; Wisse, B.E.; Oh-I, S.; Sarruf, D.A.; Matsen, M.E.; Fischer, J.D.; Taborsky, G.J.; Schwartz, M.W.; Morton G.J. Leptin Activates a Novel CNS Mechanism for Insulin-Independent Normalization of Severe Diabetic Hyperglycemia *Endocrinology* **2011**, *152*, 394–404. [CrossRef]
226. Tang, X.; Li, J.; Xiang, W.; Cui, Y.; Xie, B.; Wang, X.; Xu, Z.; Gan, L. Metformin Increases Hepatic Leptin Receptor and Decrease Steatosis in Mice. *J. Endocrinol.* **2016**, *230*, 227–237. [CrossRef]
227. Hocking, S.; Samocha-Bonet, D.; Milner, K.L.; Greenfield, J.R.; Chisholm, D.J. Adiposity and Insulin Resistance in Humans: The Role of the Different Tissue and Cellular Lipid Depots. *Endocr. Rev.* **2013**, *34*, 463–500. [CrossRef] [PubMed]

8. Sin, D.D.; Man, S.F.P. Chronic Obstructive Pulmonary Disease as a Risk Factor for Cardiovascular Morbidity and Mortality. *Proc. Am. Thorac. Soc.* **2005**, *2*, 8–11. [CrossRef] [PubMed]
9. André, S.; Conde, B.; Fragoso, E.; Boléo-Tomé, J.P.; Areias, V.; Cardoso, J. COPD and Cardiovascular Disease. *Pulmonology* **2019**, *25*, 168–176. [CrossRef]
0. Howe, M.; Leidal, A.; Montgomery, D.; Jackson, E. Role of Cigarette Smoking and Gender in Acute Coronary Syndrome Events. *Am. J. Cardiol.* **2011**, *108*, 1382–1386. [CrossRef]
1. Mariniello, D.F.; D'Agnano, V.; Cennamo, D.; Conte, S.; Quarcio, G.; Notizia, L.; Pagliaro, R.; Schiattarella, A.; Salvi, R.; Bianco, A.; et al. Comorbidities in COPD: Current and Future Treatment Challenges. *J. Clin. Med.* **2024**, *13*, 743. [CrossRef]
2. Cheyne, W.S.; Gelinas, J.C.; Eves, N.D. Hemodynamic Effects of Incremental Lung Hyperinflation. *Am. J. Physiol.-Heart Circ. Physiol.* **2018**, *315*, H474–H481. [CrossRef]
3. Rabe, K.F.; Hurst, J.R.; Suissa, S. Cardiovascular Disease and COPD: Dangerous Liaisons? *Eur. Respir. Rev.* **2018**, *27*, 180057. [CrossRef] [PubMed]
4. Cosio, M.G.; Saetta, M.; Agusti, A. Immunologic Aspects of Chronic Obstructive Pulmonary Disease. *N. Engl. J. Med.* **2009**, *360*, 2445–2454. [CrossRef] [PubMed]
5. Donaldson, G.C.; Hurst, J.R.; Smith, C.J.; Hubbard, R.B.; Wedzicha, J.A. Increased Risk of Myocardial Infarction and Stroke Following Exacerbation of COPD. *Chest* **2010**, *137*, 1091–1097. [CrossRef]
6. Hansson, G.K. Inflammation, Atherosclerosis, and Coronary Artery Disease. *N. Engl. J. Med.* **2005**, *352*, 1685–1695. [CrossRef] [PubMed]
7. Athyros, V.G.; Katsiki, N.; Doumas, M.; Karagiannis, A.; Mikhailidis, D.P. Effect of Tobacco Smoking and Smoking Cessation on Plasma Lipoproteins and Associated Major Cardiovascular Risk Factors: A Narrative Review. *Curr. Med. Res. Opin.* **2013**, *29*, 1263–1274. [CrossRef]
8. Man, S.F.P.; Van Eeden, S.; Sin, D.D. Vascular Risk in Chronic Obstructive Pulmonary Disease: Role of Inflammation and Other Mediators. *Can. J. Cardiol.* **2012**, *28*, 653–661. [CrossRef]
9. Mirrakhimov, A.E.; Mirrakhimov, E.M. Chronic Obstructive Pulmonary Disease and Vascular Risk: Should We Account for Diabetes Mellitus and Renal Disease? *Can. J. Cardiol.* **2013**, *29*, 639.e9. [CrossRef]
0. Dong, M.; Ren, J. What Fans the Fire: Insights into Mechanisms of Leptin in Metabolic Syndrome-Associated Heart Diseases. *Curr. Pharm. Des.* **2014**, *20*, 652–658. [CrossRef]
1. Katsiki, N.; Mikhailidis, D.P.; Banach, M. Leptin, Cardiovascular Diseases and Type 2 Diabetes Mellitus. *Acta Pharmacol. Sin.* **2018**, *39*, 1176. [CrossRef]
2. Ren, J. Leptin and Hyperleptinemia—From Friend to Foe for Cardiovascular Function. *J. Endocrinol.* **2004**, *181*, 1–10. [CrossRef]
3. Puurunen, V.P.; Kiviniemi, A.; Lepojärvi, S.; Piira, O.P.; Hedberg, P.; Junttila, J.; Ukkola, O.; Huikuri, H. Leptin Predicts Short-Term Major Adverse Cardiac Events in Patients with Coronary Artery Disease. *Ann. Med.* **2017**, *49*, 448–454. [CrossRef]
4. Puurunen, V.P.; Lepojärvi, E.S.; Piira, O.P.; Hedberg, P.; Junttila, M.J.; Ukkola, O.; Huikuri, H.V. High Plasma Leptin Levels Are Associated with Impaired Diastolic Function in Patients with Coronary Artery Disease. *Peptides* **2016**, *84*, 17–21. [CrossRef] [PubMed]
5. Farcaş, A.D.; Rusu, A.; Stoia, M.A.; Vida-Simiti, L.A. Plasma Leptin, but Not Resistin, TNF-α and Adiponectin, Is Associated with Echocardiographic Parameters of Cardiac Remodeling in Patients with Coronary Artery Disease. *Cytokine* **2018**, *103*, 46–49. [CrossRef]
6. Chen, M.C.; Wang, J.H.; Lee, C.J.; Hsu, B.G. Association between Hyperleptinemia and Cardiovascular Outcomes in Patients with Coronary Artery Disease. *Ther. Clin. Risk Manag.* **2018**, *14*, 1855. [CrossRef] [PubMed]
7. Decramer, M.; Janssens, W. Chronic Obstructive Pulmonary Disease and Comorbidities. *Lancet Respir. Med.* **2013**, *1*, 73–83. [CrossRef] [PubMed]
8. Lahousse, L.; Verhamme, K.M.; Stricker, B.H.; Brusselle, G.G. Cardiac Effects of Current Treatments of Chronic Obstructive Pulmonary Disease. *Lancet Respir. Med.* **2016**, *4*, 149–164. [CrossRef]
9. Heindl, S.; Lehnert, M.; Criée, C.P.; Hasenfuss, G.; Andreas, S. Marked Sympathetic Activation in Patients with Chronic Respiratory Failure. *Am. J. Respir. Crit. Care Med.* **2001**, *164*, 597–601. [CrossRef]
0. Gershon, A.; Croxford, R.; Calzavara, A.; To, T.; Stanbrook, M.B.; Upshur, R.; Stukel, T.A. Cardiovascular Safety of Inhaled Long-Acting Bronchodilators in Individuals with Chronic Obstructive Pulmonary Disease. *JAMA Intern. Med.* **2013**, *173*, 1175–1184. [CrossRef]
1. Passey, S.L.; Hansen, M.J.; Bozinovski, S.; McDonald, C.F.; Holland, A.E.; Vlahos, R. Emerging Therapies for the Treatment of Skeletal Muscle Wasting in Chronic Obstructive Pulmonary Disease. *Pharmacol. Ther.* **2016**, *166*, 56–70. [CrossRef]
2. Sergi, G.; Coin, A.; Marin, S.; Vianello, A.; Manzan, A.; Peruzza, S.; Inelmen, E.M.; Busetto, L.; Mulone, S.; Enzi, G. Body Composition and Resting Energy Expenditure in Elderly Male Patients with Chronic Obstructive Pulmonary Disease. *Respir. Med.* **2006**, *100*, 1918–1924. [CrossRef]

253. Schols, A.M.W.J. Body Composition in COPD.; Stepping Back or Moving Forward? *Respir. Med.* **2010**, *104*, 157–158. [CrossRe [PubMed]
254. Swallow, E.B.; Reyes, D.; Hopkinson, N.S.; Man, W.D.C.; Porcher, R.; Cetti, E.J.; Moore, A.J.; Moxham, J.; Polkey, M.I. Quadricep Strength Predicts Mortality in Patients with Moderate to Severe Chronic Obstructive Pulmonary Disease. *Thorax* **2007**, *62*, 115–12 [CrossRef] [PubMed]
255. Debigaré, R.; Côté, C.H.; Hould, F.S.; LeBlanc, P.; Maltais, F. In Vitro and In Vivo Contractile Properties of the Vastus Laterali Muscle in Males with COPD. *Eur. Respir. J.* **2003**, *21*, 273–278. [CrossRef]
256. Jobin, J.; Maltais, F.; Doyon, J.F.; LeBlanc, P.; Simard, P.M.; Simard, A.A.; Simard, C. Chronic Obstructive Pulmonary Diseas Capillarity and Fiber-Type Characteristics of Skeletal Muscle. *J. Cardiopulm. Rehabil. Prev.* **1998**, *18*, 432–437. [CrossRef]
257. Vogiatzis, I.; Terzis, G.; Stratakos, G.; Cherouveim, E.; Athanasopoulos, D.; Spetsioti, S.; Nasis, I.; Manta, P.; Roussos, C Zakynthinos, S. Effect of Pulmonary Rehabilitation on Peripheral Muscle Fiber Remodeling in Patients with COPD in GOL Stages II to IV. *Chest* **2011**, *140*, 744–752. [CrossRef]
258. Whittom, F.; Jobin, J.; Simard, P.M.; Leblanc, P.; Simard, C.; Bernard, S.; Belleau, R.; Maltais, F. Histochemical and Morphologica Characteristics of the Vastus Lateralis Muscle in Patients with Chronic Obstructive Pulmonary Disease. *Med. Sci. Sports Exer* **1998**, *30*, 1467–1474. [CrossRef] [PubMed]
259. Gysel, T.; Cambier, D.; Roman De Mettelinge, T. Association Between Insulin Resistance, Lean Mass and Muscle Torque/Force i Proximal Versus Distal Body Parts in Healthy Young Men. *J. Musculoskelet. Neuronal Interact.* **2014**, *14*, 41–49.
260. Barzilay, J.I.; Cotsonis, G.A.; Walston, J.; Schwartz, A.V.; Satterfield, S.; Miljkovic, I.; Harris, T.B. Insulin Resistance Is Associate With Decreased Quadriceps Muscle Strength in Nondiabetic Adults Aged $\geq$ 70 Years. *Diabetes Care* **2009**, *32*, 736. [CrossRef]
261. Seok, W.P.; Goodpaster, B.H.; Strotmeyer, E.S.; Kuller, L.H.; Broudeau, R.; Kammerer, C.; De Rekeneire, N.; Harris, T.B.; Schwart A.V.; Tylavsky, F.A.; et al. Accelerated Loss of Skeletal Muscle Strength in Older Adults with Type 2 Diabetes: The Health, Agin and Body Composition Study. *Diabetes Care* **2007**, *30*, 1507–1512. [CrossRef]
262. Guillet, C.; Boirie, Y. Insulin Resistance: A Contributing Factor to Age-Related Muscle Mass Loss? *Diabetes Meta* **2005**, *31*, 5S20–5S26. [CrossRef]
263. Du, J.; Wang, X.; Miereles, C.; Bailey, J.L.; Debigare, R.; Zheng, B.; Price, S.R.; Mitch, W.E. Activation of Caspase-3 Is an Initial Ste Triggering Accelerated Muscle Proteolysis in Catabolic Conditions. *J. Clin. Investig.* **2004**, *113*, 115–123. [CrossRef] [PubMed]
264. Russell, S.T.; Rajani, S.; Dhadda, R.S.; Tisdale, M.J. Mechanism of Induction of Muscle Protein Loss by Hyperglycaemia. *Exp. Ce Res.* **2009**, *315*, 16–25. [CrossRef] [PubMed]
265. Attvall, S.; Fowelin, J.; Lager, I.; Von Schenck, H.; Smith, U. Smoking Induces Insulin Resistance—A Potential Link with th Insulin Resistance Syndrome. *J. Intern. Med.* **1993**, *233*, 327–332. [CrossRef]
266. Boettcher, M.; Machann, J.; Stefan, N.; Thamer, C.; Häring, H.U.; Claussen, C.D.; Fritsche, A.; Schick, F. Intermuscular Ad pose Tissue (IMAT): Association with Other Adipose Tissue Compartments and Insulin Sensitivity. *J. Magn. Reson. Imagin* **2009**, *29*, 1340–1345. [CrossRef]
267. Shields, G.S.; Coissi, G.S.; Jimenez-Royo, P.; Gambarota, G.; Dimber, R.; Hopkinson, N.S.; Matthews, P.M.; Brown, A.P.; Polke M.I. Bioenergetics and Intermuscular Fat in Chronic Obstructive Pulmonary Disease-Associated Quadriceps Weakness. *Musc Nerve* **2015**, *51*, 214–221. [CrossRef]
268. Andreas, S.; Anker, S.D.; Scanlon, P.D.; Somers, V.K. Neurohumoral Activation as a Link to Systemic Manifestations of Chron Lung Disease. *Chest* **2005**, *128*, 3618–3624. [CrossRef] [PubMed]
269. Malli, F.; Papaioannou, A.I.; Gourgoulianis, K.I.; Daniil, Z. The Role of Leptin in the Respiratory System: An Overview. *Resp Res.* **2010**, *11*, 152. [CrossRef]
270. Takabatake, N.; Nakamura, H.; Minamihaba, O.; Inage, M.; Inoue, S.; Kagaya, S.; Yamaki, M.; Tomoike, H. A Novel Pathophysi logic Phenomenon in Cachexic Patients with Chronic Obstructive Pulmonary Disease: The Relationship Between the Circadia Rhythm of Circulating Leptin and the Very Low-Frequency Component of Heart Rate Variability. *Am. J. Respir. Crit. Care Me* **2001**, *163*, 1314–1319. [CrossRef]
271. Yao, S.; Zeng, L.; Wang, F.; Chen, K. Obesity Paradox in Lung Diseases: What Explains It? *Obes. Facts* **2023**, *16*, 411–426. [CrossRe
272. Tenda, E.D.; Henrina, J.; Setiadharma, A.; Felix, I.; Yulianti, M.; Pitoyo, C.W.; Kho, S.S.; Tay, M.C.K.; Purnamasari, D.S.; Soejon C.H.; et al. The Impact of Body Mass Index on Mortality in COPD: An Updated Dose–Response Meta-Analysis. *Eur. Respir. Re* **2024**, *33*, 230261. [CrossRef]
273. Obradovic, M.; Sudar-Milovanovic, E.; Soskic, S.; Essack, M.; Arya, S.; Stewart, A.J.; Gojobori, T.; Isenovic, E.R. Leptin an Obesity: Role and Clinical Implication. *Front. Endocrinol.* **2021**, *12*, 585887. [CrossRef] [PubMed]
274. Savchenko, L.; Mykytiuk, M.; Cinato, M.; Tronchere, H.; Kunduzova, O.; Kaidashev, I.P. IL-26 in the Induced Sputum Is Associate with the Level of Systemic Inflammation, Lung Functions and Body Weight in COPD Patients. *Int. J. Chronic Obstr. Pulm. Di* **2018**, *13*, 2569–2575. [CrossRef] [PubMed]

75. Çalikoglu, M.; Şahin, G.; Unlu, A.; Ozturk, C.; Tamer, L.; Ercan, B.; Kanik, A.; Atik, U. Leptin and TNF-Alpha Levels in Patients with Chronic Obstructive Pulmonary Disease and Their Relationship to Nutritional Parameters. *Respiration* **2004**, *71*, 45–50. [CrossRef] [PubMed]
76. Zhou, L.; Yuan, C.; Zhang, J.; Yu, R.; Huang, M.; Adcock, I.M.; Yao, X. Circulating Leptin Concentrations in Patients with Chronic Obstructive Pulmonary Disease: A Systematic Review and Meta-Analysis. *Respiration* **2013**, *86*, 512–522. [CrossRef]
77. Halpin, D.M.G.; Celli, B.R.; Criner, G.J.; Frith, P.; López Varela, M.V.; Salvi, S.; Vogelmeier, C.F.; Chen, R.; Mortimer, K.; Montes de Oca, M.; et al. The GOLD Summit on Chronic Obstructive Pulmonary Disease in Low- and Middle-Income Countries. *Int. J. Tuberc. Lung Dis.* **2019**, *23*, 1131–1141. [CrossRef]
78. Meghji, J.; Mortimer, K.; Agusti, A.; Allwood, B.W.; Asher, I.; Bateman, E.D.; Bissell, K.; Bolton, C.E.; Bush, A.; Celli, B.; et al. Improving Lung Health in Low-Income and Middle-Income Countries: From Challenges to Solutions. *Lancet* **2021**, *397*, 928–940. [CrossRef]
79. Perret, J.L.; Abramson, M.J. Biomass Smoke COPD: A Phenotype or a Different Disease? *Respirology* **2018**, *23*, 124–125. [CrossRef]
80. Ramírez-Venegas, A.; Montiel-Lopez, F.; Lara-Albisua, J.L.P.; Aranda-Chávez, A.; Perea-Gutiérrez, H.; Falfán-Valencia, R.; Pérez-Rubio, G.; Pérez-Padilla, R.; Ramírez-Díaz, M.; Martínez-Gómez, M.L.; et al. Association between Chronic Obstructive Pulmonary Disease and Biomass Smoke in Rural Areas. *Int. J. Tuberc. Lung Dis.* **2022**, *26*, 1191–1193. [CrossRef]
81. Ozoh, O.B.; Ayo-Olagunju, T.; Mortimer, K. Meeting Unmet Needs in Chronic Obstructive Pulmonary Disease Diagnosis and Treatment in Low- and Middle-Income Countries. *Am. J. Respir. Crit. Care Med.* **2023**, *208*, 352–354. [CrossRef]
82. Florman, K.E.H.; Siddharthan, T.; Pollard, S.L.; Alupo, P.; Barber, J.A.; Chandyo, R.K.; Flores-Flores, O.; Kirenga, B.; Mendes, R.G.; Miranda, J.J.; et al. Unmet Diagnostic and Therapeutic Opportunities for Chronic Obstructive Pulmonary Disease in Low- and Middle-Income Countries. *Am. J. Respir. Crit. Care Med.* **2023**, *208*, 442–450. [CrossRef]
83. Lim, H.; Kim, D.-Y.; Park, J.H.; Lim, H. The Global Non-Communicable Diseases Epidemic and Association Between Dietary Factors and Non-Communicable Diseases by Income Levels. *Proc. Nutr. Soc.* **2020**, *79*, E606. [CrossRef]
84. Van Iersel, L.E.J.; Beijers, R.J.H.C.G.; Gosker, H.R.; Schols, A.M.W.J. Nutrition as a Modifiable Factor in the Onset and Progression of Pulmonary Function Impairment in COPD: A Systematic Review. *Nutr. Rev.* **2022**, *80*, 1434–1444. [CrossRef]
85. Leme, A.C.B.; Hou, S.; Fisberg, R.M.; Fisberg, M.; Haines, J. Adherence to Food-Based Dietary Guidelines: A Systemic Review of High-Income and Low- and Middle-Income Countries. *Nutrients* **2021**, *13*, 1038. [CrossRef]
86. Alupo, P.; Baluku, J.; Bongomin, F.; Siddharthan, T.; Katagira, W.; Ddungu, A.; Hurst, J.R.; van Boven, J.F.M.; Worodria, W.; Kirenga, B.J. Overcoming Challenges of Managing Chronic Obstructive Pulmonary Disease in Low- and Middle-Income Countries. *Expert Rev. Respir. Med.* **2024**, *18*, 873–882. [CrossRef]
87. Beran, D.; Zar, H.J.; Perrin, C.; Menezes, A.M.; Burney, P. Burden of Asthma and Chronic Obstructive Pulmonary Disease and Access to Essential Medicines in Low-Income and Middle-Income Countries. *Lancet Respir. Med.* **2015**, *3*, 159–170. [CrossRef] [PubMed]
88. Gross, N.J. Novel Antiinflammatory Therapies for COPD. *Chest* **2012**, *142*, 1300–1307. [CrossRef] [PubMed]
89. Cazzola, M.; Hanania, N.A.; Page, C.P.; Matera, M.G. Novel Anti-Inflammatory Approaches to COPD. *Int. J. Chronic Obstr. Pulm. Dis.* **2023**, *18*, 1333–1352. [CrossRef] [PubMed]
90. Matera, M.G.; Cazzola, M.; Page, C. Prospects for COPD Treatment. *Curr. Opin. Pharmacol.* **2020**, *56*, 74–84. [CrossRef]
91. Bolger, G.B. Therapeutic Targets and Precision Medicine in COPD: Inflammation, Ion Channels, Both, or Neither? *Int. J. Mol. Sci.* **2023**, *24*, 17363. [CrossRef]
92. Lo Bello, F.; Hansbro, P.M.; Donovan, C.; Coppolino, I.; Mumby, S.; Adcock, I.M.; Caramori, G. New Drugs Under Development for COPD. *Expert Opin. Emerg. Drugs* **2020**, *25*, 419–431. [CrossRef]
93. Ray, A.; Paik, J.M.; Wexler, D.J.; Sreedhara, S.K.; Bykov, K.; Feldman, W.B.; Patorno, E. Glucose-Lowering Medications and Risk of Chronic Obstructive Pulmonary Disease Exacerbations in Patients with Type 2 Diabetes. *JAMA Intern. Med.* **2025**, *185*, 399–410. [CrossRef] [PubMed]
94. Huang, J.; Yi, H.; Zhao, C.; Zhang, Y.; Zhu, L.; Liu, B.; He, P.; Zhou, M. Glucagon-like Peptide-1 Receptor (GLP-1R) Signaling Ameliorates Dysfunctional Immunity in COPD Patients. *Int. J. Chronic Obstr. Pulm. Dis.* **2018**, *13*, 3191–3202. [CrossRef]
95. Wang, W.; Mei, A.; Qian, H.; Li, D.; Xu, H.; Chen, J.; Yang, H.; Min, X.; Li, C.; Cheng, L.; et al. The Role of Glucagon-Like Peptide-1 Receptor Agonists in Chronic Obstructive Pulmonary Disease. *Int. J. Chronic Obstr. Pulm. Dis.* **2023**, *18*, 129–137. [CrossRef] [PubMed]
96. See, X.Y.; Xanthavanij, N.; Lee, Y.-C.; Ong, T.E.; Wang, T.-H.; Ahmed, O.; Chang, Y.-C.; Peng, C.-Y.; Chi, K.-Y.; Chang, Y.-C.; et al. Pulmonary Outcomes of Incretin-Based Therapies in COPD Patients Receiving Single-Inhaler Triple Therapy. *ERJ Open Res.* **2024**, 00803–02024. [CrossRef]
97. Simental-Mendía, L.E.; Sánchez-García, A.; Linden-Torres, E.; Simental-Mendía, M. Effect of Glucagon-like Peptide-1 Receptor Agonists on Circulating Levels of Leptin and Resistin: A Meta-Analysis of Randomized Controlled Trials. *Diabetes Res. Clin. Pract.* **2021**, *177*, 108899. [CrossRef]

298. Borg, M.; Ibsen, R.; Hilberg, O.; Løkke, A. Real-Life Nationwide Outcomes of Bronchoscopic Lung Volume Reduction wit Endobronchial Valves in Severe COPD. *Respiration* **2024**, *103*, 322–331. [CrossRef]
299. Zhong, C.; You, Z.; Li, S. Application and Innovation of Bronchoscopic Lung Volume Reduction with Endobronchial Valv *Zhonghua Jie He He Hu Xi Za Zhi* **2024**, *47*, 1015–1018. [CrossRef]
300. Buttery, S.C.; Banya, W.; Bilancia, R.; Boyd, E.; Buckley, J.; Greening, N.J.; Housley, K.; Jordan, S.; Kemp, S.V.; Kirk, A.J.B.; et a Lung Volume Reduction Surgery versus Endobronchial Valves: A Randomised Controlled Trial. *Eur. Respir. J.* **2023**, *61*, 220206 [CrossRef]
301. Simoff, M.J.; Diaz-Mendoza, J.I.; Khan, A.Y.; Bechara, R.I. Bronchoscopic Lung Volume Reduction. *Clin. Chest Me* **2013**, *34*, 445–457. [CrossRef]
302. Calvache-Mateo, A.; López-López, L.; Heredia-Ciuró, A.; Martín-Núñez, J.; Rodríguez-Torres, J.; Ortiz-Rubio, A.; Valenza, M.C Efficacy of Web-Based Supportive Interventions in Quality of Life in COPD Patients, a Systematic Review and Meta-Analysis. *In J. Environ. Res. Public Health* **2021**, *18*, 12692. [CrossRef]
303. Jonkman, N.H.; Westland, H.; Trappenburg, J.C.A.; Groenwold, R.H.H.; Bischoff, E.W.M.A.; Bourbeau, J.; Bucknall, C.E.; Coulta D.; Effing, T.W.; Epton, M.J.; et al. Do Self-Management Interventions in COPD Patients Work and Which Patients Benefit Most An Individual Patient Data Meta-Analysis. *Int. J. Chronic Obstr. Pulm. Dis.* **2016**, *11*, 2063–2074. [CrossRef] [PubMed]
304. Gregersen, T.L.; Green, A.; Frausing, E.; Ringbæk, T.; Brøndum, E.; Ulrik, C.S. Do Telemedical Interventions Improve Quality o Life in Patients with COPD? A Systematic Review. *Int. J. Chronic Obstr. Pulm. Dis.* **2016**, *11*, 809–822. [CrossRef]
305. Newham, J.J.; Presseau, J.; Heslop-Marshall, K.; Russell, S.; Ogunbayo, O.J.; Netts, P.; Hanratty, B.; Kaner, E. Features of Sel Management Interventions for People with COPD Associated with Improved Health-Related Quality of Life and Reduce Emergency Department Visits: A Systematic Review and Meta-Analysis. *Int. J. Chronic Obstr. Pulm. Dis.* **2017**, *12*, 1705–172 [CrossRef] [PubMed]

Journal of
Clinical Medicine

MDPI

view

;entral Sleep Apnea in Adults: An Interdisciplinary Approach to)iagnosis and Management—A Narrative Review

pár Csipor Fodor [1], Dragoş Huţanu [2], Corina Eugenia Budin [3], Maria Beatrice Ianoşi [4,*], Delia Liana Rachiş [4], édi-Katalin Sárközi [2], Mara Andreea Vultur [2] and Gabriela Jimborean [2]

1 Pulmonology Department, County Emergency Hospital Miercurea-Ciuc, 530173 Miercurea-Ciuc, Romania; sfnkcaj@gmail.com
2 Pulmonology Department, "George Emil Palade" University of Medicine, Pharmacy, Science and Technology of Târgu Mureş, 540139 Târgu Mureş, Romania; hutanudragos1@gmail.com (D.H.); hedi.balog@umfst.ro (H.-K.S.); mara.vultur@umfst.ro (M.A.V.); gabriela.jimborean@umfst.ro (G.J.)
3 Pathophysiology Department, "George Emil Palade" University of Medicine, Pharmacy, Science and Technology of Târgu Mureş, 540139 Târgu Mureş, Romania; corina.budin@umfst.ro
4 Pulmonology Clinic, Mureş County Clinical Hospital, 540011 Târgu Mureş, Romania; rachis.delia-liana.23@stud.umfst.ro
* Correspondence: ianosi.maria-beatrice@stud18.umfst.ro

Abstract: Central sleep apnea (CSA) is a heterogeneous group of sleep-related breathing disorders characterized by intermittent absence of respiratory effort during sleep. CSA results from impaired neurological signaling from the respiratory centers to the respiratory muscles, leading to airflow cessation for at least 10 s. Major causes include heart failure, opioid use, central neurological disorders, and altitude exposure. This review outlines the pathophysiology of CSA, emphasizing ventilatory instability and brainstem dysfunction as key mechanisms. It details the classification of CSA subtypes, including Cheyne–Stokes respiration, high-altitude CSA, and drug-induced CSA. Clinical manifestations range from excessive daytime sleepiness to cardiovascular complications. Diagnostic approaches encompass polygraphy, polysomnography, and various laboratory tests to evaluate comorbidities. Treatment requires a multidisciplinary approach, addressing underlying conditions while utilizing positive airway pressure (PAP) therapy, adaptive servo-ventilation (ASV), supplemental oxygen, and pharmacological interventions. Newer modalities, such as phrenic nerve stimulation, offer promising outcomes for CSA management. This review underscores the necessity of an individualized, interdisciplinary strategy to improve patient outcomes in CSA.

Keywords: sleep apnea; central sleep apnea; Cheyne-stokes Apnea

1. Introduction

Central sleep apnea (CSA) comprises a heterogeneous group of sleep-related breathing disorders in which respiratory effort is absent intermittently during sleep. CSA is defined as the absence of airflow/very severe decrease in airflow at the nose and mouth level for at least 10 s during sleep in an adult (repeated >5 events/hour), caused by the absence of neurological impulses from the respiratory centers to the respiratory muscles; therefore, no thoracal/abdominal effort can be observed during the events [1].

The most common possible causes of CSA are systolic heart failure, opioid abuse, central neurological disorders, exposure to altitude variations, or CSA associated with severe obstructive sleep apnea (OSA). The International Classification of Sleep Disorders, Third

Edition (ICSD-3rd) describes five different CSA entities that affect adults with different clinical and polysomnographic (PSG) features [2]:

- Primary CSA;
- Central Cheyne–Stokes Apnea (CC-SA);
- High-altitude CSA;
- CSA due to medical conditions other than Cheyne–Stokes;
- CSA due to drugs or other noxious substances.

2. Mechanisms of CSA Production and Main Causes

The mechanism of CSA production, unlike OSA (which presents respiratory effort), consists in the lack of transmission of nervous impulses from the respiratory centers to the respiratory muscles to trigger periodic breathing [2–4]. CSA is found in approximately 5% of all cases of sleep apnea [4]. Normal ventilation is tightly regulated to maintain arterial oxygen (PaO_2) and carbon dioxide ($PaCO_2$) levels within narrow normal ranges. This is achieved through feedback phenomena through the intervention of several components: peripheral and central chemoreceptors, intrapulmonary vagal receptors, respiratory control-centers in the brainstem, and respiratory muscles [3].

During wakefulness, signals from the cortex influence breathing through behavioral control. During sleep, behavioral control is lost, and chemical control is the major mechanism for regulating ventilation, with $PaCO_2$ being the major stimulus for ventilation. CSA is most often observed during non-rapid eye movement (NREM) sleep, when behavioral influence is minimal. Sleep associates increased $PaCO_2$ and a higher $PaCO_2$ apnea threshold. Reductions in $PaCO_2$ of only a few mmHg can lead to apnea [3,4]. Two major pathophysiological events cause CSA: (1) Ventilatory instability; (2) Depression of brainstem respiratory-centers or chemoreceptors [5,6].

Ventilatory instability is the mechanism behind CSA, CC-SA, high altitude periodic breathing, and primary CSA [3–5]. Ventilation is particularly at risk for instability when resting $PaCO_2$ approaches the apneic threshold of $PaCO_2$. Patients with hypocapnia and heart failure and those ascending to high altitudes often develop these conditions, with predisposition to a periodic breathing pattern. Hypoxia increases the ventilatory response to changes in $PaCO_2$ and predisposes to ventilatory instability. During wakefulness, breathing is regulated by both behavioral and chemical control mechanisms, but upon sleep onset, behavioral control is lost, making ventilation entirely dependent on chemical feedback. This transition increases the apneic threshold, meaning that smaller drops in $PaCO_2$ can suppress respiratory drive, promoting sleep-onset central apneas. In conditions like heart failure and high altitude, CO_2 regulation is further altered. Heart failure leads to chronic hyperventilation and hypocapnia due to increased chemoreceptor sensitivity, predisposing patients to Cheyne–Stokes respiration and central sleep apnea. Similarly, at high altitude, hypoxia-driven hyperventilation lowers $PaCO_2$, shifting it closer to the apneic threshold, increasing the risk of periodic breathing. These conditions also elevate loop gain, a measure of ventilatory control instability, where heightened sensitivity to CO_2 fluctuations results in exaggerated ventilatory responses, making individuals more prone to central apnea events [6–8].

CSA-hypoventilation syndromes, such as those associated with narcotic use or brainstem lesions, are due to disturbances in the respiratory centers and/or peripheral chemoreceptors that may become more apparent during sleep due to the suppression of wakefulness.

Narcotics (heroin, morphine, and methadone) cause respiratory depression by stimulating opioid receptors on neurons located in the respiratory centers of the medulla. Although tolerance to many of the central nervous system effects of opioids develops, studies [9,10] have demonstrated abnormal hypercapnic and hypoxic ventilatory responses in chronic narcotic users. CSA is common especially in individuals who use opioids long-term [11,12].

Sometimes the mechanisms responsible for CSA and OSA overlap, and patients with CSA often present obstructive events. Studies have shown that the hypopharynx can be significantly narrowed during a CSA event. During normal inspiration, neuronal stimulation occurs in the diaphragm and upper airway muscles (UAMs) that stiffen and dilate the pharynx to keep it open. If there is a decrease in activity in both the diaphragm and the UAM dilators, the result could be CSA or OSA. If the UAMs remain open, the event will be CSA. If the UAMs are closed during CSA and diaphragmatic activity resumes before pharyngeal dilator muscle tone is restored, a mixed apnea results [12]. Thus, susceptibility to UAM collapse may determine whether OSA occurs due to ventilatory instability.

CSA is more common in the elderly than in the middle-aged, and it is quite rare compared to OSA (about 2–3% of all sleep apnea) [5,9]. CSA is prevalent in men and less common in postmenopausal women. The explanation for this discrepancy is the presence of a lower apneic threshold of $PaCO_2$ in women compared to men. Thus, women require a greater reduction in $PaCO_2$ to initiate apnea than men [8].

Medical causes (associated with CC-SA or CSA) [13–15] (Box 1).

- Heart failure, severe arrhythmias;
- Renal failure;
- Stroke, brain tumors, encephalitis, Parkinson's disease, lesions of the medullary centers by neoplasms, infarctions, infections;
- "Shy Drager" syndrome with orthostatic hypotension and extrapyramidal syndrome;
- Post-poliomyelitis syndrome (progressive muscle weakness);
- Muscular dystrophy, myasthenia gravis.
- Diabetes mellitus;
- Hypothyroidism; acromegaly;
- "Arnold Chiari" syndrome types I–III (congenital condition of the cerebellum that herniates into a neighboring anatomical compartment);
- "Prader Willi" syndrome (genetic disease with muscle hypotonia, slowed development and growth, obsessive–compulsive behavior, hyperphagia, and obesity).

Box 1. ICSD 3 Criteria for Cheyne–Stokes respiration [1,2].

A. Presence of one or more symptoms—drowsiness, difficulty maintaining or inducing sleep, frequent awakenings and restless sleep, awakening due to shortness of breath;
B. Association with atrial fibrillation/flutter, heart failure, neurological disorder (stroke/tumors);
C. PSG polysomnography (during diagnosis or CPAP titration) shows the following:
1. $\geq$5 central apneas and hypopneas/hour of sleep.
2. The total number of CSA and/or CSH is >50% of the total number of apneas and hypopneas.
3. The ventilatory "pattern" meets the criteria for CC-SA (at least a series of 3 consecutive CSA/CSH separated by periods of crescendo–decrescendo breathing with a cycle length from the onset of the apnea to the onset of the next of $\geq$40 s).
D. The illness cannot be better explained by another sleep disorder, medical or neurological disorder, or the use of a medication or substance.

High-altitude CSA can occur above $\geq$5000 m altitude. The breathing patterns are Cheyne–Stokes type with a shorter cycle of apnea and hyperventilation (15–35 s) [1,3,4].

Use of opioids and other central nervous system depressants [10,11] is easily diagnosed by history. Of the participants in a stable methadone maintenance program, 30% had a CSA index >5 and 20% >10. Methadone blood concentration was significantly associated with CSA severity.

Primary (idiopathic) CSA has an unknown etiology characterized by CSA without CC-SA pattern [10,16,17]. It can be described when $\geq$5 CSA occur, each >10 s/h of sleep. $PaCO_2$ is normal or low. CSA ends abruptly with a large breath and without associated hypoxemia. It is rare (one study highlights 3.8% of 650 CSA diagnosed by PSG) [18]. In the history of the sleep laboratory of the Pulmonology Clinic of Targu Mures, the cases were severe and were associated with cognitive decline/dementia and arrhythmias without being able to establish a link between them as triggering factors or as consequences of CSA.

CSA associated with titration or CPAP therapy (emergent CSA, previously referred to as "complex sleep apnea") may occur during the first CPAP titration for primary OSA (6.5%), and it is mainly due to ventilatory instability caused by CPAP's effect on carbon dioxide regulation. Only 1.5% of patients develop persistent CSA associated with long-term persistent CPAP therapy. Key pathways leading to central apnea in complex sleep apnea are characterized by relief of upper airway obstruction, when CPAP therapy eliminates airway obstruction, leading to increased ventilation causing excess CO_2 elimination, lowering arterial $PaCO_2$. If $PaCO_2$ drops below the apneic threshold, the brainstem's respiratory drive is inhibited, resulting in central apnea. Another causing mechanism can be the over-titration of CPAP pressure, when excessively high CPAP pressure can overstimulate lung stretch receptors, which triggers a central apneustic response, possibly leading to central apneas. Furthermore, factors such as sleep fragmentation, arousals, and underlying ventilatory instability can further contribute to CO_2 fluctuations. An unstable sleep state with frequent arousals may increase the likelihood of $PaCO_2$ dropping below the apneic threshold, leading to central apnea (Figure 1) [1,15].

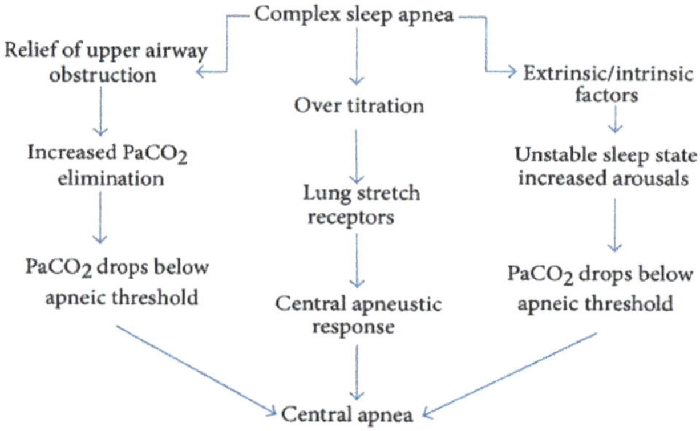

Figure 1. Complex sleep apnea syndrome/emergent CSA detection algorithm [1,15].

Most apneas resolve after a few weeks of proper treatment of OSA [15]. CSA also occurs in healthy individuals during the wake–sleep transition, when chemoreceptors reset and instability of ventilatory control occurs, with the events being brief and not associating with significant O_2 desaturation. Once the wake–sleep transition is completed, normal individuals should not present more than 5 events/h of sleep during the night [15,19,20].

Common risk factors for CSA are frequently encountered as complex forms of heart failure due to systolic deficit, significant rhythm disturbances, cerebrovascular and central nervous diseases in general, and in case of opioid use [19].

3. Symptoms of Central Sleep Apnea

CSA presents daytime and nocturnal symptoms, but also evident etiological factors and complications, such as the following [4]:

- Excessive daytime sleepiness (less than OSA); lack of energy and daytime fatigue;
- Insomnia or awakenings—restless sleep;
- Apnea reported by sleep partners;
- Paroxysmal nocturnal dyspnea;

- Signs of underlying causes with frequent association with the following:
  - Cardiovascular disorders (atrial fibrillation, flutter, ventricular ectopy, other nocturnal arrhythmias, heart failure) [14–16,21];
  - Neurological diseases (stroke, tumors, Parkinson's disease, encephalitis);
  - Neuromuscular disorders, muscular dystrophy, myasthenia gravis;
  - Chronic kidney disease;
  - Living at high altitude or recent variations in altitude;
  - Drug abuse (methadone, opioids);
  - Presence of obesity (BMI > 30 kg/m^2) more strongly correlates with OSA rather than CSA.

4. Specific Laboratory Investigations in Sleep Apnea

Sleep apnea should be investigated in patients with the help of the following:

- Questionnaires for suspicion of daytime sleepiness (Epworth) and sleep apnea risk (Stop Bang Questionnaire, Berlin) should be applied to all patients with sleep apnea suspicion, before correctly differentiating OSA from CSA through more complex sleep study investigations;
- Pulse oximetry; blood gas analysis;
- Polygraphy/home sleep testing/level 3 testing (PG) and polysomnography/level 1 testing (PSG) with the following findings:
  (a) Central sleep apnea CSA (Figure 2) [1–4]:
    - Lack of airflow at nose and mouth level for >10 s during sleep in an adult;
    - Lack of respiratory effort of the thoracic and abdominal muscles;
    - Nocturnal micro-awakenings;
    - Hypoxemia +/− hypercapnia.

  (b) Central sleep hypopnea CSH [1–4]:
    - Decrease in airflow at the nose or mouth over 30% of the pre-event value, ≥10 s, together with absence of inspiratory effort and desaturation of +3% with or without arousal associated to the event; this is important to report, while frequently difficult to identify, due to multiple factors overlapping, such as the presence of insufficient respiratory effort or even lack in sensitivity of monitoring devices.

  (c) Cheyne–Stokes respiration/Central Cheyne–Stokes Apnea (CC-SA) (periodic ventilation) is characterized by respiratory events during sleep (succession of at least 3 events), with a progressive periodic amplification of ventilation "crescendo/decrescendo pattern" and then, with its progressive decrease, alternating with CSA/CSH [1,2]. The duration of the respiratory cycle from the onset of ventilation to the onset of another ventilation is ≥40 s [1].

  (d) Mixed apnea (MSA) is characterized by apnea during sleep that begins as a CSA (without thoraco-abdominal effort) and is followed by an OSA (ventilatory movements of the chest and abdomen).
- Associated tests for causes and comorbidities: serological tests—glycemia, glycosylated Hb, LDL, HDL, uric acid, anti-acetylcholine receptor antibodies, blood gas analysis, renal function tests, ENT examination, EKG, cardiological examination, cardiac ultrasound, coronary angiography, spirometry, COPD Assessment test (CAT), 6-min-walk-test, imaging tests (MRI, brain CT), neurological and endocrinological examination, capnography.
- Blood gas analysis may reveal respiratory alkalosis ($PaCO_2$ < 40 mm Hg while awake) in patients with primary CSA, high-altitude periodic breathing, and CC-SA.

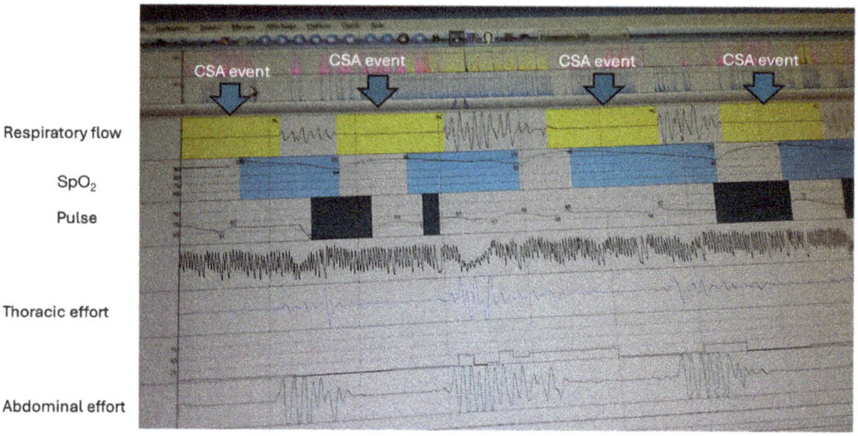

Figure 2. Central sleep apnea (polygraphy—Pulmonology Clinic Mureș). Absence of airflow, absence of respiratory movements of the chest and abdomen. CSA—central sleep apnea; SpO_2—blood oxygen saturation.

4.1. Cardio-Respiratory Ventilatory Polygraphy (PG)

PG evaluates several parameters (through 4–6 channels) during sleep [1,22–24]: nasal/oral airflow; respiratory effort (respiratory movements of the chest and abdomen); SaO_2; patient position during sleep; and pulse and pulse variability.

Advantages of PG: PG is accepted in the diagnosis of uncomplicated sleep apnea in which the clinical examination is suggestive [2]; it is portable and has a high accessibility; it is relatively inexpensive. PG can benefit from additional channels (EKG, video camera, body position and snoring sensors, EEG channels). The reading and validation of sleep curves is performed in a short time compared to PSG (30 min). Disadvantages of PG could be that it does not measure sleep stages, it cannot assess the sleep architecture, and it cannot detect micro-awakenings or limb movements. The exact moment when patients fall asleep and exact duration of sleep cannot be accurately determined and neither can patient behavior during sleep be investigated through PG [1,2,22–24].

4.2. Polysomnography (PSG)

Polysomnography is considered to be the reference/gold standard sleep study tool, by allowing the diagnosis of complex sleep disorders and breathing disorders during sleep, providing comprehensive data on sleep architecture, arousals, and respiratory events. It is performed in dedicated centers (sleep laboratories) where medical teams with high expertise collaborate. PSG associates complex equipment for recording different parameters during sleep [1,2,23,25]. Parameters monitored with PSG are the following:

1. Sleep structure: electrical brain activity (electroencephalography—EEG) that identifies sleep stages, microarousals; electrooculogram (EOG); chin electromyogram (EMG); anterior tibial electromyogram that can prove limb movement or atonia during sleep.
2. Respiratory events—detection of nose/mouth air flow and another sensor for snoring detection.
3. Thoracal and abdominal movements detected by 2 strips attached to the patient.
4. Repercussions of respiratory events: (a) Consequences on sleep structure (sleep fragmentation); (b) Gasometry (nocturnal SaO_2 and $PaCO_2$) and cardiovascular repercussions through EKG; pulse measurement should be considered when identifying the potential mechanism of CSA.

5. Patient behavior recorded by PSG-associated camera and by a position sensor ("positional sleep apnea", actigraphy).

PSG allows the diagnosis of various sleep disorders: central apneas, narcolepsy, parasomnias, complex apneas, behavioral disorders during REM sleep, aspects related to legal medicine, periodic limb movements, restless legs syndrome, insomnia, circadian rhythm disorders, and hypoxia of various causes [23,25].

CSA is more common in stages 1 and 2 of sleep, and awakenings are frequent, which fragments sleep and prevents patients from entering into deep delta-sleep. Events are less often encountered in REM. The duration of an apnea/ventilation cycle is <45 s [10]. In the CC-SA cycle in heart failure, CSA is determined by awakening and increased tidal volume associated with decreased $PaCO_2$. As the patient falls asleep, the apnea threshold also rises, and the PaO_2 and ventilation oscillates around this threshold. The duration of a ventilatory cycle (apnea–hyperpnea) is $\geq$45 s and depends on cardiac output [2]. Altitude CSA occurs in NREM sleep and improves within a few days with altitude adaptation. Substance-induced CSA occurs in NREM sleep [11].

5. Assessment of Comorbidities

1. Investigation of the cardiovascular system:
    a. EKG, cardiorespiratory exercise test, blood pressure, pulse measurement;
    b. Cardiac ultrasound (often the ejection fraction is <40%);
    c. Imaging investigations—ultrasound, magnetic resonance imaging, positron emission tomography of myocardial perfusion;
    d. Coronary angiography;
2. Investigation of metabolic syndrome (BMI, waist circumference), blood count, blood sugar, glycosylated Hb, expanded lipidogram;
3. Neuropsychiatric consultation.

6. Treatment of Central Apnea

The treatment of CSA should be managed by a multidisciplinary team—pulmonologist, cardiologist, physiotherapist, and specialist of the internal medicine (to treat underlying cause of CSA) when secondary causes of CSA might be present and treatment and recommendations from a sleep specialist could overlook the presence of significant comorbidities. The main objectives are to stabilize sleep and treat the causes that led to CSA. The treatment of CSA is more difficult than the treatment of OSA and will be personalized for each patient.

Positive airway pressure (PAP) devices are the standard treatment and are initiated alongside treatment of the underlying cause of CSA. Treatment of underlying conditions—heart failure, renal failure, OSA, descent to lower altitudes (in those living at higher altitudes), tapering of opioid medications—is important (the dose may be reduced). Exercise has no direct effect on CSA linked to heart failure [26]. Other useful treatments include oxygen therapy and some pharmacological agents.

6.1. Treatment with Positive Airway Pressure (PAP)

Devices can be initiated as CPAP—continuous PAP, bilevel PAP therapy, and adaptive servoventilation (ASV). Studies have shown that CPAP and BPAP are more effective for the management of CSA in heart failure and opioid use [27,28].

(a) Continuous positive airway pressure (CPAP) devices

CPAP is widely used to treat OSA: the device used during sleep delivers continuous air under pressure into the airway via a mask to keep the upper airways (UAW) open. CPAP can prevent the closure of UAW, which can trigger CSA. Several types of masks are available to ameliorate patient comfort. The air pressure can be adjusted considering the needs of each patient.

CPAP devices should be initiated, firstly in patients where CSA and OSA coexist, with positive pressure treating the obstructive component of sleep apnea and therefore stabilizing ventilation, which can reduce the central events. Furthermore, when dealing with patients with CSA due to heart failure, CPAP reduces nocturnal hypoxia, reduces left ventricular afterload, and stabilizes ventilation, therefore stabilizing PCO_2 fluctuations that can trigger central events. However, studies show that overall survival was not improved significantly in these patients, as proved in the CANPAP trial [29].

A reference study showed that CPAP improves symptoms of CSA, cardiac performance, heart transplant-related mortality, and quality of life [27]. Other studies show that CPAP in patients with congestive heart failure was associated with improvement in CSA, improvement in nocturnal oxygenation and ejection fraction, and improvement in 6-min-walk-test distance [28–34].

The increase in dead space can be done by attaching a 400–800 mL piece to the mask that increases the $PaCO_2$ in the inspired air and the expiratory rebreathing space, and raises the $PaCO_2$ threshold for a stable ventilation (a threshold that is too low could cause CSA) [34].

(b) Bilevel positive airway pressure (BPAP)

Devices may be an alternative for those who cannot tolerate CPAP (and who might need very high CPAP pressures that interfere with expiration) or who do not respond to CPAP. Bilevel PAP devices create a positive pressure difference (between IPAP and EPAP) and are recommended especially for patients with hypercapnic CSA with hypoventilation and for those who require high PAP values. Also, some patients with CC-SA, heart failure or primary CSA may benefit from BPAP [32], as well as those with CSA related to opioid use [33].

BPAP devices are set with inspiratory positive airway pressure levels (IPAP) and expiratory positive airway pressure levels (EPAP).

IPAP provides ventilatory support during inspiration (increases alveolar volume), in the following ways:

- Decreases respiratory effort (takes over the effort of the inspiratory muscles);
- Increases tidal volume and ventilation/minute;
- Improves gas exchange;
- Decreases the apnea–hypopnea index.

EPAP is the pressure provided by the ventilator while the patient exhales.

- Keeps the upper airways (UAW) open during sleep in those with unstable CC-SA;
- Reduces the mechanical work and respiratory effort due to end-expiratory pressure;
- Recruits alveoli and improves oxygenation;
- Eliminates obstructive apneas.

Back-up respiratory frequency (BRF) is useful in long apneas, ensuring a desired respiratory frequency if the patient has no trigger for a period of time, or when he is in apnea as well as when the patient's inspiration effort is not effective [35]. The bed will be inclined at 45–60° (in those who require high pressures), and all devices should benefit from a humidifier and personalized masks (preferred oronasal) that lead to an increase in comfort, and thus in patient compliance [36,37].

(c) Adaptive servo ventilation (ASV)

The ASV device provides individualized ventilatory support (IPAP and EPAP) based on the detection of apneas (IPAP is increased compared to EPAP ensuring ventilatory support). The ASV principle is based on continuous monitoring of patients' breathing patterns, together with dynamic pressure titration [37]. It is recommended for patients with respiratory failure (especially with CC-SA or opioid use) but with preserved cardiac ejection fraction (EFLV). Several studies have shown that in patients with low EFLV (NYHA 2–4, EFLV $\leq$ 45), ASV may increase mortality [38,39]; however, more recent research has shown that ASV does not impact all-cause mortality in these patients [40]. However, observing this controversy, the recommendation of ASV in patients with symptomatic heart failure should be considered by balancing the pros and cons, inside a multidisciplinary team, in order to avoid all risks. ASV has been effective and superior to CPAP in patients with preserved EF. ASV detects CSA, and provides an IPAP that compensates the lack of nerve impulses to the muscles and a back-up respiratory rate, improving AHI, EFLV, symptoms, and sleep architecture and decreasing daytime sleepiness [41,42]. ASV decreases heart rate and heart rate variability as well as CC-SA. ASV has been proven to decrease brain-natriuretic peptides in people with heart failure [43]. Monitoring of the effects of ASV by clinical exam, PSG, and cardiac ultrasound is necessary.

6.2. Other Treatment Recommendations

Nocturnal supplemental oxygen is beneficial in patients with heart failure by increasing EFLV, reducing hypoxemia and hyperventilation secondary to changes in $PaCO_2$, minimizing the respiratory effort, and overall improving quality of life [37,44]. Oxygen is also beneficial in CSA caused by altitude factors, by allowing patients to maintain normal levels of PO_2 and PCO_2 when in high altitude locations.

Drugs that can improve CSA include acetazolamide, theophylline, and some hypnotic agents. Unfortunately, they do not have approval for common use in CSA and remain investigational drugs [45].

Acetazolamide is a carbonic anhydrase inhibitor that causes metabolic acidosis and increases basal ventilation. It would be useful (although is not indicated prophylactically) in primary CSA and in CC-SA caused by heart failure and altitude. It allows acclimatization to reduce the risk of cerebral edema and altitude sickness [45]. Some hypnotics (temazepam, zolpidem) can reduce wakefulness, unstable sleep, and arousals, especially in the period of sleep–wake transition [46]. Zolpidem was useful both in initiating sleep and in maintaining it. It reduced CSA and AHI without producing or worsening OSA [45]. Mirtazepam and Buspirone seem to have encouraging results [47,48] in reducing hypocapnia in people with spinal cord injuries. Theophylline is useful in CSA due to heart failure and altitude-induced CSA [49].

Some invasive procedures have been shown to reduce CSA and obstructive CSA (overdrive atrial pacing in patients with pacemakers for bradycardia) [50]. A newer therapy for CSA is electrical stimulation of the phrenic nerve. An FDA-approved device from the USA delivers an electrical impulse to the phrenic nerve for diaphragm contractions. The device is implanted under the skin, unilaterally; it is battery-powered and has been shown to reduce AHI by over 50%, decrease nocturnal awakenings, improve symptoms at 1 year (in 45%), decrease daytime sleepiness (in 44%), fatigue, and snoring (in 60% of cases), and improve overall sleep and quality of life [51,52].

6.3. Treatment Algorithms

When engaging in treatment strategies, the underlying cause for CSA syndrome should be taken in consideration, as follows [28–30,32–35,41–45]:

- For Primary CSA, the recommended approach is to trial CPAP first; if CSA worsens, adaptive servo-ventilation (ASV) should be considered, and if ASV fails, oxygen therapy or acetazolamide may be used.

- In Heart Failure-Related CSA, the priority is optimizing heart failure therapy; if CSA persists, ASV is recommended for patients with a left ventricular ejection fraction (LVEF) above 45%, while oxygen therapy or phrenic nerve stimulation may be considered if ASV fails.
- Emergent CSA from CPAP therapy should be monitored for 8–12 weeks; if it persists, reducing CPAP pressure or switching to BiPAP is advised, followed by ASV if necessary, and, in refractory cases, oxygen therapy or acetazolamide may be introduced.
- Opioid-Induced CSA should be managed primarily by reducing opioid dosage; if CSA persists, CPAP or BiPAP can be used, escalating to ASV if needed, with acetazolamide as an alternative if ASV fails.
- High-Altitude CSA is best addressed with acetazolamide as first-line treatment, followed by oxygen therapy if CSA persists, and CPAP or BiPAP for patients with ongoing symptoms.

7. Conclusions

Central sleep apnea (CSA) is a complex sleep-related breathing disorder with multiple underlying causes, including heart failure, opioid use, neurological conditions, and altitude exposure. The pathophysiology primarily involves ventilatory instability and brainstem dysfunction, leading to intermittent cessation of respiratory effort during sleep. Diagnosis relies on polysomnography and polygraphy, with treatment requiring a multidisciplinary approach. While positive airway pressure (PAP) therapy remains the standard treatment, newer modalities such as adaptive servo-ventilation (ASV), oxygen therapy, pharmacological agents, and phrenic nerve stimulation offer additional therapeutic options. Given the heterogeneity of CSA, individualized management strategies are crucial to optimizing patient outcomes and improving quality of life. Further research is needed to refine treatment protocols and explore novel interventions for CSA.

Author Contributions: Conceptualization, A.C.F., M.B.I. and G.J.; Methodology, A.C.F., D.H., C.E.B., M.B.I. and G.J.; Software, D.H., C.E.B., D.L.R., H.-K.S. and M.A.V.; Validation, A.C.F. and G.J.; Formal Analysis, A.C.F., M.B.I. and G.J.; Investigation, A.C.F., D.H., C.E.B., M.B.I., D.L.R., H.-K.S., M.A.V. and G.J.; Resources, A.C.F. and G.J.; Data Curation, D.H., C.E.B., D.L.R., H.-K.S. and M.A.V.; Writing—Original Draft Preparation, A.C.F., D.H., C.E.B., M.B.I., D.L.R., H.-K.S., M.A.V. and G.J.; Writing—Review and Editing, A.C.F., D.H., C.E.B., M.B.I. and G.J.; Visualization, A.C.F., D.H., C.E.B., M.B.I., D.L.R., H.-K.S., M.A.V. and G.J.; Supervision, A.C.F. and G.J. Project Administration, A.C.F., M.B.I. and G.J.; All authors have read and agreed to the published version of the manuscript.

Funding: This research received no external funding.

Conflicts of Interest: The authors declare no conflicts of interest.

References

1. Simmonds, A.; de Backer, W. *ERS Handbook of Respiratory Sleep Medicine*; European Respiratory Society: Sheffield, UK, 201[illegible] Available online: http://www.ers-education.org/publications/handbook-series/ers-handbook-of-respiratory-sleep-medicin[illegible] aspx (accessed on 17 January 2025).
2. American Academy of Sleep Medicine. *International Classification of Sleep Disorders*, 3rd ed.; Text Revision; American Academy o[illegible] Sleep Medicine: Darian, IL, USA, 2023.
3. White, D.P. Pathogenesis of Obstructive and Central Sleep Apnea. *Am. J. Respir. Crit. Care Med.* **2005**, *172*, 1363–1370. [CrossRef] [PubMed]
4. Eckert, D.J.; Jordan, A.S.; Merchia, P.; Malhotra, A. Central Sleep Apnea: Pathophysiology and Treatment. *Chest* **2007**, *13*[illegible] 595–607.
5. Johansson, P.; Alehagen, U.; Svanborg, E.; Dahlström, U.; Broström, A. Sleep disordered breathing in an elderly community-livin[illegible] population: Relationship to cardiac function, insomnia symptoms and daytime sleepiness. *Sleep Med.* **2009**, *10*, 1005–101[illegible] [CrossRef] [PubMed]

Donovan, L.M.; Kapur, V.K. Prevalence and Characteristics of Central Compared to Obstructive Sleep Apnea: Analyses from the Sleep Heart Health Study Cohort. *Sleep* **2016**, *39*, 1353–1359. [CrossRef] [PubMed]

Arzt, M.; Harth, M.; Luchner, A.; Muders, F.; Holmer, S.R.; Blumberg, F.C.; Riegger, G.A.; Pfeifer, M. Enhanced Ventilatory Response to Exercise in Patients with Chronic Heart Failure and Central Sleep Apnea. *Circulation* **2003**, *107*, 1998–2003. [CrossRef] [PubMed]

Zhou, X.S.; Shahabuddin, S.; Zahn, B.R.; Babcock, M.A.; Badr, M.S. Effect of gender on the development of hypocapnic apnea/hypopnea during NREM sleep. *J. Appl. Physiol.* **2000**, *89*, 192–199. [CrossRef]

Bixler, E.O.; Vgontzas, A.N.; Have, T.T.; Tyson, K.; Kales, A. Effects of Age on Sleep Apnea in Men: I. Prevalence and Severity. *Am. J. Respir. Crit. Care Med.* **1998**, *157*, 144–148. [CrossRef]

Beker, K. Central Sleep Apnea Syndromes. Available online: https://emedicine.medscape.com/article/304967-overview#a7 (accessed on 24 January 2025).

Walker, J.M.; Farney, R.J.; Rhondeau, S.M.; Boyle, K.M.; Valentine, K.; Cloward, T.V.; Shilling, K.C. Chronic Opioid Use is a Risk Factor for the Development of Central Sleep Apnea and Ataxic Breathing. *J. Clin. Sleep Med.* **2007**, *3*, 455–461. [CrossRef]

Verbraecken, J.A.; De Backer, W.A. Upper airway mechanics. *Respiration* **2009**, *78*, 121–133.

Grunstein, R.R.; Ho, K.Y.; Sullivan, C.E. Sleep apnea in acromegaly. *Ann. Intern. Med.* **1991**, *115*, 527–532. [CrossRef]

Leung, R.S.T.; Huber, M.A.; Rogge, T.; Maimon, N.; Chiu, K.-L.; Bradley, T.D. Association Between Atrial Fibrillation and Central Sleep Apnea. *Sleep* **2005**, *28*, 1543–1546. [CrossRef] [PubMed]

Khan, M.T.; Franco, R.A. Complex Sleep Apnea Syndrome. *Sleep Disord.* **2014**, *2014*, 798487. [CrossRef] [PubMed] [PubMed Central]

Javaheri, S. Central Sleep Apnea in Congestive Heart Failure: Prevalence, Mechanisms, Impact, and Therapeutic Options. *Semin. Respir. Crit. Care Med.* **2005**, *26*, 44–55. [CrossRef] [PubMed]

Javaheri, S.; Brown, L.K. Positive airway pressure therapy for hyperventilatory CSA: Idiopathic, heart failure, cerebrovascular disease, and high altitude. *Sleep Med. Clin.* **2017**, *12*, 565–572. [CrossRef]

Kouri, I.; Kolla, B.P.; Morgenthaler, T.I.; Mansukhani, M.P. Frequency and outcomes of primary central sleep apnea in a population-based study. *Sleep Med.* **2019**, *68*, 177–183. [CrossRef]

Wang, J.; Wang, Y.; Feng, J.; Chen, B.-Y.; Cao, J. Complex sleep apnea syndrome. *Patient Prefer. Adherence* **2013**, *7*, 633–641. [CrossRef]

Bitter, T.; Westerheide, N.; Hossain, M.S.; Lehmann, R.; Prinz, C.; Kleemeyer, A.; Horstkotte, D.; Oldenburg, O. Complex sleep apnoea in congestive heart failure. *Thorax* **2011**, *66*, 402–407. [CrossRef]

Luo, Q.; Zhang, H.-L.; Tao, X.-C.; Zhao, Z.-H.; Yang, Y.-J.; Liu, Z.-H. Impact of untreated sleep apnea on prognosis of patients with congestive heart failure. *Int. J. Cardiol.* **2010**, *144*, 420–422. [CrossRef]

van de Water, A.T.M.; Holmes, A.; Hurley, D.A. Objective measurements of sleep for non-laboratory settings as alternatives to polysomnography—A systematic review. *J. Sleep Res.* **2011**, *20*, 183–200. [CrossRef]

Jimborean, G.; Arghir, O.; Postolache, P. Capitol în Tulburările Respiratorii în Timpul Somnului—Tratat de Diagnostic și Tratament. In *Poligrafia în Timpul Somnului*; Constanța, M., Ed.; 2017; ISBN 978-973-692-406-4. Available online: https://books.google.com.au/books/about/Tulbur%C4%83rile_respiratorii_%C3%AEn_timpul_som.html?id=6e8J0AEACAAJ&redir_esc=y (accessed on 12 January 2025).

Kapur, V.K.; Auckley, D.H.; Chowdhuri, S.; Kuhlmann, D.C.; Mehra, R.; Ramar, K.; Harrod, C.G. Clinical Practice Guideline for Diagnostic Testing for Adult Obstructive Sleep Apnea: An American Academy of Sleep Medicine Clinical Practice Guideline. *J. Clin. Sleep Med.* **2017**, *13*, 479–504. [CrossRef]

Deutsch, P.A.; Simmons, M.S.; Wallace, J.M. Cost-Effectiveness of Split-Night Polysomnography and Home Studies in the Evaluation of Obstructive Sleep Apnea Syndrome. *J. Clin. Sleep Med.* **2006**, *2*, 145–153. [CrossRef] [PubMed]

Ueno, L.M.; Drager, L.F.; Rodrigues, A.C.T.; Rondon, M.U.P.B.; Braga, A.M.F.W.; Mathias, W.; Krieger, E.M.; Barretto, A.C.P.; Middlekauff, H.R.; Lorenzi-Filho, G.; et al. Effects of Exercise Training in Patients with Chronic Heart Failure and Sleep Apnea. *Sleep* **2009**, *32*, 637–647. [CrossRef] [PubMed]

Sadeghi, Y.; Sedaghat, M.; Majedi, M.A.; Pakzad, B.; Ghaderi, A.; Raeisi, A. Comparative Evaluation of Therapeutic Approaches to Central Sleep Apnea. *Adv. Biomed. Res.* **2019**, *8*, 13. [CrossRef]

Jamil, S.M.; Owens, R.L.; Lipford, M.C.; Marron, R.M.; Vega Sanchez, M.E.; Lam, M.T.; Sunwoo, B.Y.; Schmickl, C.; Orr, J.E.; Sharma, S.; et al. ATS Core Curriculum 2020. Adult Sleep Medicine. *ATS Sch.* **2020**, *1*, 476–494. [PubMed]

Bradley, T.D.; Logan, A.G.; Kimoff, R.J.; Sériès, F.; Morrison, D.; Ferguson, K.; Belenkie, I.; Pfeifer, M.; Fleetham, J.; Hanly, P.; et al. Continuous Positive Airway Pressure for Central Sleep Apnea and Heart Failure. *N. Engl. J. Med.* **2005**, *353*, 2025–2033. [CrossRef]

30. Sin, D.D.; Logan, A.G.; Fitzgerald, F.S.; Liu, P.P.; Bradley, T.D. Effects of Continuous Positive Airway Pressure on Cardiovascula Outcomes in Heart Failure Patients with and Without Cheyne-Stokes Respiration. *Circulation* **2000**, *102*, 61–66. [CrossRef]
31. Ruttanaumpawan, P.; Logan, A.G.; Floras, J.S.; Bradley, T.D.; for the CANPAP Investigators. Effect of Continuous Positive Airwa Pressure on Sleep Structure in Heart Failure Patients with Central Sleep Apnea. *Sleep* **2009**, *32*, 91–98. [CrossRef]
32. Dohi, T.; Kasai, T.; Narui, K.; Ishiwata, S.; Ohno, M.; Yamaguchi, T.; Momomura, S.-I. Bi-Level Positive Airway Pressure Ventilatio for Treating Heart Failure with Central Sleep Apnea That is Unresponsive to Continuous Positive Airway Pressure. *Circ. J.* **200** *72*, 1100–1105. [CrossRef]
33. Schoebel, C.; Ghaderi, A.; Amra, B.; Soltaninejad, F.; Penzel, T.; Fietze, I. Comparison of Therapeutic Approaches to Addicte Patients with Central Sleep Apnea. *Tanaffos* **2018**, *17*, 155–162.
34. Gilmartin, G.; McGeehan, B.; Vigneault, K.; Daly, R.W.; Manento, M.; Weiss, J.W.; Thomas, R.J. Treatment of Positive Airwa Pressure Treatment-Associated Respiratory Instability with Enhanced Expiratory Rebreathing Space (EERS). *J. Clin. Sleep Me* **2010**, *6*, 529–538. [CrossRef]
35. Arnal, J.-M.; Thevenin, C.-P.; Couzinou, B.; Texereau, J.; Garnero, A. Setting up home noninvasive ventilation. *Chronic Respir. Di* **2019**, *16*, 1479973119844090. [CrossRef]
36. Javaheri, S.; Malik, A.; Smith, J.; Chung, E. Adaptive pressure support servoventilation: A novel treatment for sleep apne associated with use of opioids. *J. Clin. Sleep Med.* **2008**, *4*, 305–310. [CrossRef]
37. D'Elia, E.; Vanoli, E.; La Rovere, M.T.; Fanfulla, F.; Maggioni, A.; Casali, V.; Damiano, S.; Specchia, G.; Mortara, A. Adaptive serv ventilation reduces central sleep apnea in chronic heart failure patients: Beneficial effects on autonomic modulation of heart rat *J. Cardiovasc. Med.* **2013**, *14*, 296–300. [CrossRef] [PubMed]
38. Cowie, M.R.; Woehrle, H.; Wegscheider, K.; Angermann, C.; D'ortho, M.-P.; Erdmann, E.; Levy, P.; Simonds, A.K.; Somers, V.K Zannad, F.; et al. Adaptive Servo-Ventilation for Central Sleep Apnea in Systolic Heart Failure. *N. Engl. J. Med.* **2015**, *37* 1095–1105. [CrossRef]
39. American Academy of Sleep Medicine. Special Safety Notice: ASV Therapy for Central Sleep Apnea Patients with Hear Failure. Available online: https://aasm.org/special-safety-notice-asv-therapy-for-central-sleep-apnea-patients-with-hear failure/ (accessed on 12 January 2025).
40. Fukumoto, Y.; Tada, T.; Suzuki, H.; Nishimoto, Y.; Moriuchi, K.; Arikawa, T.; Adachi, H.; Momomura, S.-I.; Seino, Y.; Yasumur Y.; et al. Chronic Effects of Adaptive Servo-Ventilation Therapy on Mortality and the Urgent Rehospitalization Rate in Patient Experiencing Recurrent Admissions for Heart Failure—A Multicenter Prospective Observational Study (SAVIOR-L). *Circ. J.* **202** *88*, 692–702. [CrossRef] [PubMed]
41. Philippe, C.; Stoïca-Herman, M.; Drouot, X.; Raffestin, B.; Escourrou, P.; Hittinger, L.; Michel, P.-L.; Rouault, S.; D'ortho, M.- Compliance with and effectiveness of adaptive servoventilation versus continuous positive airway pressure in the treatment o Cheyne-Stokes respiration in heart failure over a six month period. *Heart* **2005**, *92*, 337–342. [CrossRef] [PubMed]
42. Allam, J.S.; Olson, E.J.; Gay, P.C.; Morgenthaler, T.I. Efficacy of Adaptive Servoventilation in Treatment of Complex and Centra Sleep Apnea Syndromes. *Chest* **2007**, *132*, 1839–1846. [CrossRef]
43. Randerath, W.J.; Nothofer, G.; Priegnitz, C.; Anduleit, N.; Treml, M.; Kehl, V.; Galetke, W. Long-term auto servo-ventilatio or constant positive pressure in heart failure and co-existing central with obstructive sleep apnea. *Chest* **2012**, *142*, 440–44 [CrossRef]
44. Sasayama, S.; Izumi, T.; Matsuzaki, M.; Matsumori, A.; Asanoi, H.; Momomura, S.-I.; Seino, Y.; Ueshima, K.; The CHF-HOT Stud Group. Improvement of Quality of Life with Nocturnal Oxygen Therapy in Heart Failure Patients With Central Sleep Apne *Circ. J.* **2009**, *73*, 1255–1262. [CrossRef]
45. Rocha, A.; Pinto, A.C.P.N.; Pachito, D.V.; Drager, L.F.; Lorenzi-Filho, G.; Atallah, Á.N. Pharmacological treatment for central slee apnoea in adults. *Cochrane Database Syst. Rev.* **2023**, *2023*, CD012922. [CrossRef]
46. Quadri, S.; Drake, C.; Hudgel, D.W. Improvement of idiopathic central sleep apnea with zolpidem. *J. Clin. Sleep Med.* **2009**, 122–129. [PubMed]
47. Prowting, J.; Maresh, S.; Vaughan, S.; Kruppe, E.; Alsabri, B.; Badr, M.S.; Sankari, A. Mirtazapine reduces susceptibility t hypocapnic central sleep apnea in males with sleep-disordered breathing: A pilot study. *J. Appl. Physiol.* **2021**, *131*, 414–42 [CrossRef] [PubMed]
48. Maresh, S.; Prowting, J.L.; Vaughan, S.; Kruppe, E.; Alsabri, B.; Yarandi, H.; Badr, M.S.; Sankari, A. Buspirone decrease susceptibility to hypocapnic central sleep apnea in chronic SCI patients. *J. Appl. Physiol.* **2020**, *129*, 675–682. [CrossRef] [PubMed
49. Javaheri, S.; Parker, T.; Wexler, L.; Liming, J.; Lindower, P.; Roselle, G. Effect of Theophylline on Sleep-Disordered Breathing i Heart Failure. *N. Engl. J. Med.* **1996**, *335*, 562–567. [CrossRef]
50. Garrigue, S.; Bordier, P.; Jaïs, P.; Shah, D.C.; Hocini, M.; Raherison, C.; De Lara, M.T.; Haïssaguerre, M.; Clementy, J. Benefit o Atrial Pacing in Sleep Apnea Syndrome. *N. Engl. J. Med.* **2002**, *346*, 404–412. [CrossRef]

Lowes, R. Implant to Treat Central Sleep Apnea Approved by FDA. *Medscape Medical News*. 6 October 2017. Available online: https://www.medscape.com/viewarticle/886744?nlid=118337_3901&src=wnl_newsalrt_171006_MSCPEDIT&uac=106950CX&impID=1451417&faf=1 (accessed on 10 October 2024).
Hill, L.; Meyer, T.; McKane, S.; Lainscak, M.A.; Ahmed, Q. Transvenous phrenic nerve stimulation to treat central sleep apnoea in patients with heart failure may improve sleep, quality of life, and symptoms. *Eur. J. Cardiovasc. Nurs.* **2022**, *22*, 489–497. [CrossRef]

Journal of
Clinical Medicine

MDPI

Systematic Review

Indoor Air Pollution and Lung Cancer Risk—A Systematic Review and Meta-Analysis

Stefan-Roberto Rusoiu [1,2], Norbert Wellmann [1,2,3,*], Ana Adriana Trusculescu [2,3,*], Andreea Roxana Durdan [1,2], Dorotea Carmen Cioanca [1,2], Alexandra Bosoanca [1,2], Cristian Oancea [2,3] and Monica Steluta Marc [2,3]

[1] Doctoral School, "Victor Babes" University of Medicine and Pharmacy, 2 Eftimie Murgu Square, RO-300041 Timisoara, Romania; stefan.rusoiu@rezident.umft.ro (S.-R.R.)
[2] Pulmonology University Clinic, Clinical Hospital of Infectious Diseases and Pneumophthisiology "Dr. Victor Babes", 13 Gheorghe Adam Street, RO-300310 Timisoara, Romania
[3] Center of Research and Innovation in Personalized Medicine of Respiratory Diseases (CRIPMRD), "Victor Babes" University of Medicine and Pharmacy, 2 Eftimie Murgu Square, RO-300041 Timisoara, Romania
* Correspondence: norbert.wellmann@umft.ro (N.W.); ana.trusculescu@umft.ro (A.A.T.)

Abstract

Background/Objectives: Indoor air pollution is an increasingly recognized cause of lung cancer, yet evidence remains fragmented across exposure categories. This systematic review aimed to consolidate epidemiological findings on the relationship between household pollutants and lung cancer risk across diverse settings. **Methods:** A systematic search of PubMed, Web of Science, Scopus, and Cochrane was conducted to identify observational studies published between 2015 and 2025. Eligible articles evaluated indoor exposure in relation to primary lung cancer. Maximally adjusted effect estimates were extracted. Random effects models were used to calculate pooled odds ratios (ORs) and hazard ratios (HRs) when appropriate. Study quality was assessed using the Newcastle–Ottawa Scale. **Results:** Thirty-eight studies comprising 475,565 participants were included. Environmental tobacco smoke (ETS) was associated with lung cancer risk (pooled OR 1.97, 95% CI 1.63–2.37; pooled HR 1.44, 95% CI 1.19–1.74). Cooking oil fumes showed a pooled OR of 1.83 (95% CI 1.53–2.21). Solid fuel and biomass combustion were also associated with increased lung cancer risk, with pooled estimates indicating elevated odds and hazard ratios (pooled OR 2.26, 95% CI 1.36–3.77; pooled HR 1.66, 95% CI 1.37–2.02). Incense burning was evaluated in a single study (OR 3.05, 95% CI 1.06–8.84), with wide confidence intervals. Two studies explored gene–environment interactions, suggesting possible variability in susceptibility, although statistical robustness was limited. **Conclusions:** Across multiple exposure categories, indoor air pollution was consistently associated with lung cancer risk, although the effect magnitude and precision varied between studies. Given the observational nature of the evidence and methodological heterogeneity, further prospective research with standardized exposure assessment is needed to clarify the strength and consistency of these associations.

Keywords: indoor air pollution; lung cancer risk; environmental tobacco smoke; cooking oil fumes; biomass; solid fuel; household exposure

1. Introduction

The first evidence connecting second-hand smoke with lung cancer came from Japan, from the Six-Prefecture Cohort Study by Takeshi Hirayama [1]. At the time, the idea that non-smokers could develop lung cancer simply by living with a smoker was unexpected. Hirayama's work proved this association, revealing the carcinogenic nature of environmental tobacco smoke (ETS). It changed how passive exposure to second-hand smoke was viewed worldwide [2]. In the years that followed, several international studies confirmed these results across diverse populations, eventually shaping smoke-free policies in public and occupational settings [3–5].

Over half a century later, this message has evolved into a broader, more urgent concern: the air inside our homes, workplaces, and schools can itself be carcinogenic [6,7]. Today, scientists increasingly recognize that it is not only tobacco smoke that poses a risk. A variety of indoor pollutants—from the smoke produced by solid fuels to the vapors released during high-temperature cooking and everyday volatile organic compounds (VOCs)—are now linked to lung cancer [8–10]. This issue is particularly pressing in regions where biomass combustion and high-temperature cooking remain common, exposing women and other non-smoking groups to invisible yet persistent risks.

Globally, lung cancer is the leading cause of cancer-related mortality, claiming 1.8 million lives annually. Although smoking continues to account for most cases, 15–25% occurs in people who have never smoked [11]. For these individuals, chronic exposure to indoor air pollution represents one of the most plausible and often overlooked pathways. Indoors, carcinogenic compounds such as polycyclic aromatic hydrocarbons, aldehydes, nitrosamines, and fine particulate matter can accumulate to levels capable of inducing biological harm. More and more studies show that repeated inhalation of these pollutants triggers oxidative DNA injury, chromosomal instability, and dysregulation of genes involved in epithelial repair [12–14]. Taken together, these mechanisms explain how household or workplace exposures can, over time, contribute to lung carcinogenesis in people who have never smoked.

Although awareness of indoor air pollution has grown in recent years, its role in lung cancer has still received far less attention than smoking or outdoor air quality. For many years, research examined these exposures separately, even though real-world exposure is rarely isolated. Earlier reviews also faced significant limitations, such as different exposure measurement methods and rarely documented ventilation or housing conditions, which made comparisons difficult. Only a small number explored whether genetic susceptibility might intensify, alter, or decrease these risks. Together, these gaps have left the overall picture fragmented, contributing to persistent uncertainty about how indoor pollutants shape lung cancer risk across different settings.

This systematic review brings together the most recent evidence on how indoor air pollution contributes to lung cancer risk. Using clearly defined inclusion criteria and a consistent approach to quality and data extraction, we examined findings across major exposure domains: ETS, cooking oil fumes (COFs), use of solid fuels and biomass, and a small group of other domestic pollutants. Where studies allowed, we also considered how genetic susceptibility may modify these associations. Our goal was to assemble a coherent view of a field often fragmented by differing methods and contexts, and to highlight the gaps that still limit prevention efforts and the development of effective public health policy.

2. Materials and Methods

2.1. Study Design and Search Strategy

This systematic review was conducted in accordance with PRISMA 2020 recommendations, and the PRISMA checklist is included in the Supplementary Material Table S1.

https://doi.org/10.3390/jcm15051854

The review protocol was not prospectively registered. In October 2025, we performed a literature search across four databases: PubMed, Web of Science, Scopus, and the Cochrane Library. No date limits were applied at the search stage; however, as part of the predefined eligibility criteria, we restricted inclusion to studies published from 2015 onward to enhance the comparability of exposure definitions and multivariable adjustment practices in the contemporary indoor air pollution literature (e.g., clearer specification of household exposure metrics, ventilation-related variables, and more consistent reporting of adjusted effect estimates).

For PubMed, we used a predefined query combining MeSH terms and free-text keywords related to indoor air pollution and lung cancer as follows: ("Air Pollution, Indoor"[Mesh] OR "Household air pollution"[tiab] OR "indoor air pollution"[tiab] OR "cooking fumes"[tiab] OR biomass[tiab] OR "solid fuel"[tiab] OR coal[tiab] OR "wood smoke"[tiab] OR Incense[tiab] OR kerosene[tiab] OR "cooking oil fumes"[tiab] OR "particulate matter"[tiab] OR PM2.5[tiab] OR PM10[tiab] OR VOC[tiab] OR "volatile organic compounds"[tiab] OR "Tobacco Smoke Pollution"[Mesh] OR "environmental tobacco smoke"[tiab] OR "second-hand smoke"[tiab] OR "passive smoking"[tiab] OR "involuntary smoking"[tiab]) AND ("Lung Neoplasms"[Mesh] OR "lung cancer"[tiab] OR "pulmonary carcinoma"[tiab]) AND ("case-control"[tiab] OR "case control"[tiab] OR cohort[tiab] OR "nested case-control"[tiab] OR "case-cohort"[tiab]) NOT (radon[tiab] OR "in vitro"[tiab] OR animal[tiab] OR mice[tiab] OR rats[tiab] OR outdoor[tiab] OR traffic[tiab] OR "ambient air"[tiab]). The search yielded 565 records in PubMed.

The Web of Science Core Collection was queried in the Topic field (title, abstract, author keywords, keywords plus) using terms the terms "indoor air pollution", "household air pollution", "cooking fumes", "solid fuel", "wood smoke", "biomass", "coal", "incense", and "kerosene", combined with "lung cancer", "lung neoplasms", "pulmonary carcinoma", and "pulmonary neoplasms". This yielded 268 records. The Scopus database was searched in the TITLE-ABS-KEY fields with the same exposure terms. The search was filtered to case–control or cohort designs, and excluded radon, in vitro, animal, and outdoor pollution studies. This search retrieved 344 records. The Cochrane Library was queried using equivalent exposure and outcome terms, and 10 records were returned; all were excluded during screening for not meeting the eligibility criteria. The full texts of potentially relevant studies were then assessed.

The search strategy was initially developed for PubMed and subsequently adapted to the field structure and indexing systems of the other databases, while preserving the same exposure and outcome concepts and Boolean logic to ensure methodological consistency across platforms.

2.2. Eligibility Criteria

The pre-established exclusion criteria were as follows:

1. Articles not published in English;
2. Publications dated before 2015;
3. Studies conducted exclusively on non-human models or unrelated laboratory settings;
4. Research addressing only radon, outdoor air pollution, or occupational exposure;
5. Studies reporting non-neoplastic respiratory outcomes;
6. Research on malignancies other than lung cancer;
7. Reviews, editorials, commentaries, letters, conference abstracts only, or duplicate records.

2.3. Study Selection and Data Extraction

All records identified through database searches were imported into a reference management system, and duplicate entries were removed prior to screening. Titles and abstracts

https://doi.org/10.3390/jcm15051854

were screened using Rayyan (Rayyan Systems Inc., Cambridge, MA, USA), a web-based systematic review management platform. Two reviewers independently screened titles and abstracts to assess eligibility. Full-text articles were evaluated against predefined exclusion criteria. Any discrepancies were resolved through discussion and, when necessary, consultation with a third reviewer to reach consensus. Full-text articles were excluded primarily due to exclusive focus on outdoor or occupational air pollution, non-neoplastic outcomes, or non-human study designs. Studies not meeting any of the exclusion criteria were considered eligible for inclusion if they evaluated indoor air pollution exposures in relation to lung cancer risk in human populations and reported effect estimates suitable for quantitative synthesis. The methodological quality and risk of bias of all included studies were assessed using the Newcastle–Ottawa Scale (NOS) for observational studies, with detailed scoring for each study provided in Supplementary Tables S2 and S3.

The overall search process is summarized in the PRISMA flow diagram (Figure 1), which provides a step-by-step visual overview of how records were identified, screened, excluded, and, finally, included in the review. The main characteristics of the eligible studies are summarized in Table 1.

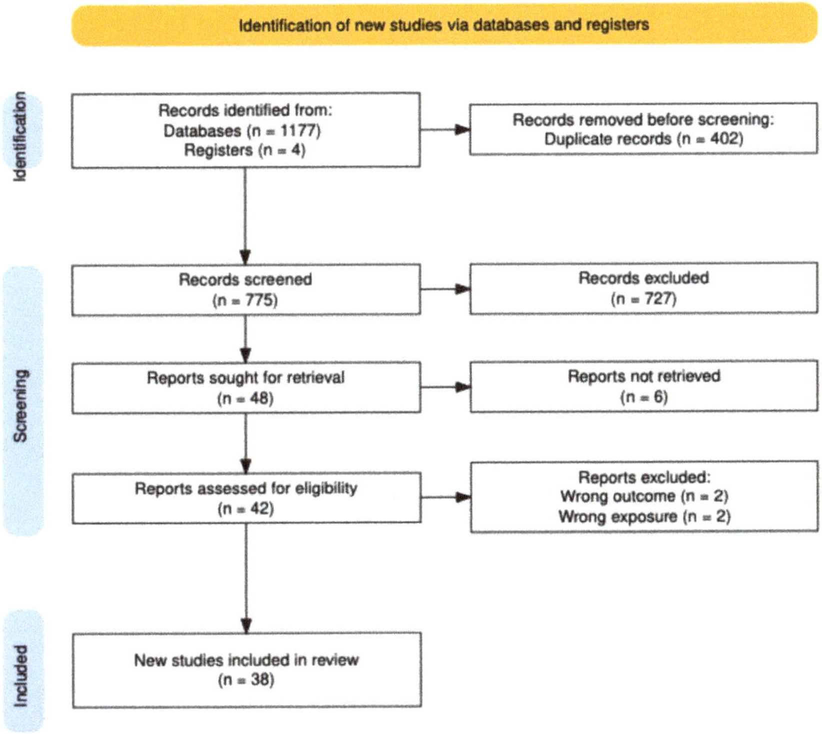

Figure 1. Prisma flowchart. Literature review.

Data extraction was independently performed by two reviewers using a standardized data collection table. For each eligible study, we recorded study design, population characteristics, exposure definition and assessment method, outcome definition (primary lung cancer), covariates included in multivariable models, and maximally adjusted effect estimates with corresponding confidence intervals. When studies reported stratified analyses, particularly by smoking status, we extracted effect estimates among never-smokers to minimize confounding by active tobacco use and to better isolate the impact of indoor

https://doi.org/10.3390/jcm15051854

environmental exposures. When specific estimates for never-smokers were unavailable, the fully adjusted overall estimates were retained. Any discrepancies in extracted data were resolved through discussion and, when necessary, consultation with a third reviewer.

Table 1. Main characteristics of the eligible studies.

Author, Year	Country	Study Design	Exposure	Effect Estimate (95% CI)	N	Summary
Blechter et al., 2023 [15]	Taiwan	Case–control	ETS	OR 1.49 (1.24–1.80)	2048 (1024 cases; 1024 controls)	Female lifetime never-smokers; matched on age, sex, ethnicity; adjusted for age and 10 principal components; lung adenocarcinoma
Das et al., 2017 [16]	India	Hospital-based case series (prospective)	ETS	No comparative effect estimate reported	495	Descriptive; no OR/HR; limited generalizability
Erhumunneese L et al., 2022 [17]	USA	Prospective cohort	ETS	HR 1.96 (1.23–3.13)	37,650 (77 LC cases)	Never-smoking Black women; no matching; age, BMI, health insurance, education, income, ETS at home, PM2.5; incident lung cancer overall
Fang F et al., 2025 [18]	China	Population-based case–control	ETS	OR 1.84 (1.58–2.15)	10,890 (2871 cases; 8019 controls)	Adjusted for age, sex, income (10 y prior), education, county, family history of LC, smoking status, alcohol; mutual IAP adjustment; lung cancer overall
Hansen MS et al., 2021 [19]	Norway	Prospective cohort	ETS	HR 1.34 (0.89–2.01)	142,508 (1507 LC cases)	Never-smoking women, adjusted for age, education, and alcohol consumption; no significant association found; lung cancer overall
He F et al., 2017 [20]	China (Fujian)	Hospital case–control	ETS	OR 2.96 (2.47–3.55)	2206 (1096 cases; 1110 controls)	Adjusted for age, sex, education, occupation, marital status, BMI; primary lung cancer overall
Kim CH et al., 2015 [21]	USA (ILCCO pooled)	Pooled case–control	ETS	OR 1.45 (1.00–2.12)	3205 (170 cases; 3035 controls)	Female never-smokers; adjusted for age, sex, race/ethnicity; lung adenocarcinoma in situ; minimally invasive adenocarcinoma (AIS/MIA); heterogeneity reported
Li et al., 2020 [22]	China (Shanghai)	Prospective cohort	ETS	HR 1.29 (0.98–1.71)	23,415 (255 LC cases)	No significant association after full adjustment; adjusted for age, gender, education, income, smoking status, pack-years, BMI, alcohol, fat intake, fruit/vegetables; family history, lung cancer overall
Liang D et al., 2019 [23]	China (Hebei)	Matched case–control	ETS	OR 1.93 (1.62–2.31)	3248 (1086 cases; 2172 controls)	Never-smokers; conditional logistic regression; adjusted for sociodemographics, lifestyle factors, ETS, cooking, occupation, diet; lung cancer overall
Lotfi F et al., 2024 [24]	Iran	Multicenter case–control	ETS	OR 1.69 (1.13–2.52)	4104 (627 cases; 3477 controls)	Never-smokers; adjusted for age, sex, province, and SES; lung cancer overall
Masood et al., 2016 [25]	Pakistan	Case–control	ETS	Not reported separately	522 (252 cases; 270 controls)	No fully adjusted OR for ETS provided; lung cancer overall
Mbeje NP et al., 2022 [26]	South Africa	Case–control	ETS	aOR 3.28 (1.48–7.30)	234 (75 cases; 159 controls)	General population; adjusted for age, gender, race, marital status, education, alcohol, siblings, and history of lung cancer; lung cancer overall

https://doi.org/10.3390/jcm1505185

Table 1. *Cont.*

Author, Year	Country	Study Design	Exposure	Effect Estimate (95% CI)	N	Summary
Soeroso et al., 2021 [27]	Indonesia	Hospital case–control	ETS + CYP2A13 CT	OR 2.70 (1.07–7.16)	106 (53 cases; 53 controls)	Female never-smokers; no confounders specified (crude OR); lung cancer overall
Torres-Durán et al., 2015 [28]	Spain	Case–control	ETS + AAT SS genotype	OR 12.10 (1.18–123.77)	530 (5 SS cases out of 212; 318 controls)	Never-smokers; adjusted for age, gender, residential radon exposure; lung cancer overall
Wang A et al., 2015 [29]	USA (NIH centers)	Prospective cohort	ETS $\geq$ 30 years	HR 1.61 (1.00–2.58)	39,771	Never-smokers; adjusted for age, ethnicity, BMI, prior lung cancer, family cancer history, education, vitamin D, occupation, hormone therapy, lifestyle; lung cancer overall
Zhuang et al., 2022 [30]	China (Fujian)	Case–control	ETS	OR 2.23 (1.78–2.79)	1608 (623 cases; 985 controls)	Never-smokers; adjusted for age, nationality, education, marital status, BMI, alcohol, tea, lung disease history, occupation, family history of cancer; lung cancer overall
Pan JL et al., 2018 [31]	China (Shandong)	Case–control	COFs	OR 1.50 (1.02–2.20)	526 (261 cases; 265 controls)	Non-smoking women; adjusted for age, nationality, education, BMI, income, family history, passive smoking, occupation, soot; lung cancer overall
He F et al., 2017 [32]	China (Fujian)	Hospital case–control	COFs	OR 2.63 (1.91–3.61)	956 (477 cases; 479 controls)	Non-smoking women; Crude OR; lung cancer overall
Fang X et al., 2016 [33]	China (Shenyang)	Hospital case–control	COFs	OR 2.13 (1.42–3.21)	468 (224 cases; 244 controls)	Non-smoking women; age-adjusted; lung cancer overall
Chen et al., 2020 [34]	Taiwan	Case–control	Cooking time years (11–60 vs. $\leq$10)	OR 1.63 (1.20–2.23)	2604 (1302 cases; 1302 controls)	Non-smoking women; adjusted for age, education, family lung cancer, ETS exposure, HRT, oral contraceptive use, homemaker status, history of being a chef; mostly adenocarcinoma (84.6%)-1101
Jang J et al., 2025 [35]	Korea	Nationwide retrospective cohort	School kitchen COFs	HR 1.72 (1.14–2.60)	23,778	Female school cooks; adjusted for age, BMI, smoking, income, and CCI; PSM on age, BMI and CCI; lung cancer overall
Yin Z et al., 2015 [36]	China	Case–control	COFs	OR 1.52 (1.06–2.17)	568 (258 cases; 310 controls)	Non-smoking women; adjustment not specified for main COF model; adenocarcinoma (194), squamous cell carcinoma (34), other types (30)
Yin Z et al., 2016 [37]	China	Case–control	COFs	OR 1.80 (1.24–2.62)	534 (268 cases; 266 controls)	Non-smokers; adjustment not specified; 197 adenocarcinoma, 44 squamous cell, 27 other lung cancer types
Blechter et al., 2021 [38]	China (Shanghai, Shenyang)	GWAS-based case–control	Household coal use (ever vs. never)	OR 1.29 (1.01–1.64)	2297 (1183 cases; 1114 controls)	Never-smoking women; adjusted for age and study; adenocarcinoma
Maurya et al., 2023 [39]	India (W. Maharashtra)	Case–control	Smoke-generating fuel	OR 4.00 (1.5–10.0)	136 (68 cases; 68 controls)	Crude OR; hospital-based sample; small sample size
Kim C et al., 2015 [40]	China (Shanghai)	Prospective cohort	Coal use + poor ventilation	HR 1.69 (1.22–2.35)	71,320	Never-smoking women; adjusted for age, education, income, ETS, history of lung disease, occupation; incident lung cancer overall

https://doi.org/10.3390/jcm15051854

Table 1. *Cont.*

Author, Year	Country	Study Design	Exposure	Effect Estimate (95% CI)	N	Summary
Leng S et al., 2022 [41]	USA (New Mexico)	Prospective cohort	Wood smoke exposure (≥1 year)	HR 1.53 (0.92–2.55)	2372	Ever-smokers; adjusted for age, smoking status and PY, sex, ethnicity; non-significant association; incident lung cancer overall
Mehta SS et al., 2023 [42]	USA (Sister Study)	Prospective cohort	Indoor wood-burning ≥30 days/year	HR 1.68 (1.27–2.20)	50,226 women	Adjusted for race, ethnicity, education, residential status, smoking, PY, ETS, marital status, income; incident primary lung cancer;
Vermeulen R et al., 2019 [43]	China (Xuanwei & Fuyuan)	Case–control	Smoky coal exposure (PAH25 per 1 SD)	OR 2.21 (1.67–2.87)	1500 (1015 cases; 485 controls)	Never-smoking women; adjusted for age, ETS, SES (food sufficiency); overall lung cancer
Wong JYY et al., 2019 [44]	China (Xuanwei & Fuyuan)	Case–control	Smoky coal exposure (by geologic deposit)	OR 33.40 (13.07–85.34)	1524 (1031 cases; 493 controls)	Female never-smokers; adjusted for age and food sufficiency before marriage or age; extreme effect estimate
Liu L et al., 2020 [45]	China (Yunnan)	Case–control	Smoky coal exposure (high vs. low exposure)	OR 6.63 (4.72–9.32)	3000 (684 cases; 2316 controls)	Adjusted for age, sex, heating method, occupation, diet, alcohol, lung disease history, family history, education; overall lung cancer
Mhimbira et al., 2015 [46]	Asia (FLC Cons.)	Pooled case–control	Coal use (ever vs. never)	OR 1.30 (1.00–1.60)	3080 (1731 cases; 1349 controls)	Never-smoking women; adjusted for age and study; lung cancer overall
Raspanti GA et al., 2016 [47]	Nepal	Hospital-based case–control	Biomass burning	OR 1.77 (1.00–3.14)	1212 (606 cases; 606 controls)	Adjusted for age, sex, ethnicity, tobacco use, ETS, SES, tobacco status + PY; lung cancer overall
Yang L et al., 2015 [48]	China	Case–control	Solid fuel use; Southern China	OR 1.42 (1.06–1.90)	2112 (1056 cases; 1056 controls)	Adjusted for age, sex, BMI, education; lung cancer overall
Yang R et al., 2025 [49]	China (Beijing)	Matched case–control	HAP + indoor time spent (>23 h/day for ≥10 years)	OR 3.84 (1.63–9.05)	286 (143 cases; 143 controls)	Female never-smokers; adjusted for age, sex, BMI, diet; lung adenocarcinoma
Chen et al., 2022 [50]	Taiwan	Case–control	Incense burning	OR 3.05 (1.06–8.84)	79 (39 cases; 40 controls)	Age-adjusted; wide CI; small sample size; lung adenocarcinoma
Ren Y et al., 2015 [51]	China (Liaoning)	Case–control	Gene–COF interaction	OR 0.34 (0.12–0.98)	585 (272 cases; 313 controls)	Age-adjusted logistic regression only; interaction not significant after Bonferroni correction; lung adenocarcinoma
Wang G et al., 2019 [52]	China (Dongfeng–Tongji)	Prospective cohort	Gene–cooking time interaction	HR 2.48 (1.03–5.97)	33868 (5178 genotyped)	Adjusted for age, gender, marital status, education, smoking, alcohol, exercise, BMI, family history of cancer, benign lung disease, housing characteristics, and occupational factors; incident lung cancer overall

Abbreviations: AAT, alpha-1 antitrypsin; AIS, adenocarcinoma in situ; MIA, minimally invasive adenocarcinoma; CCI, Charlson Comorbidity Index; CI, confidence interval; COF, cooking oil fume; ETS, environmental tobacco smoke; GWAS, genome-wide association study; HR, hazard ratio; ILCCO, International Lung Cancer Consortium; OR, odds ratio; PAH, polycyclic aromatic hydrocarbons; PM2.5, particulate matter ≤ 2.5 µm; PSM, propensity score matching; PY, pack-years; SD, standard deviation; SES, socioeconomic status.

Exposure assessment methods varied across studies. Most investigations relied on structured or interviewer-administered questionnaires capturing exposure history, duration, and intensity. Several studies incorporated additional components such as genetic profiling, biomarker analyses, registry linkage, or exposure modeling approaches, while direct environmental monitoring was infrequently reported. This heterogeneity was documented during data extraction.

2.4. Statistical Analysis

Effect measures were transformed to the natural logarithm scale, and standard errors were derived from the reported 95% intervals. Pooled estimates were calculated separately for ORs and HRs using random-effects models (DerSimonian–Laird method). Between-study heterogeneity was evaluated using Cochran's Q statistic and quantified with the I^2 metric. The robustness of pooled results was explored through leave-one-out sensitivity analyses, in which each study was sequentially omitted to assess the stability of the summary estimate. Detailed results of the sensitivity are presented in the Supplementary Tables (Tables S4–S8). Given the limited number of studies within certain exposure categories and substantial heterogeneity in exposure assessment and adjustment strategies, additional modeling approaches were not undertaken. All statistical analyses were performed using MedCalc Statistical Software version 23.4.9 (MedCalc Software Ltd., Ostend, Belgium).

3. Results

We used Rayyan as a tool that facilitated paper screening. A total of 38 studies met the eligibility criteria and were included in the final synthesis, comprising 475,565 participants across Asia, Europe, North America, and Africa. The evidence base included both case–control and cohort study designs, between 2015 and 2025. Across studies, exposure assessment captured five distinct categories of indoor pollutants: ETS, COFs, solid fuels/biomass, incense exposure, and gene–environment interactions. The distribution of studies according to exposure category, study design, and reported lung cancer histology is summarized in Table 2. The following sections present the findings structured by exposure type.

Table 2. Distribution of included studies by indoor pollutant category, study design, and reported cancer histology.

Exposure Category	No. of Studies (*n*)	Study Design	Reported Histology
ETS	16	Case–control (*n* = 12); Cohort (*n* = 4)	Primary lung cancer (overall); adenocarcinoma
COF	7	Case–control (*n* = 6); Cohort (*n* = 1)	Primary lung cancer (overall); adenocarcinoma, squamous cell carcinoma, other
Solid fuels/biomass	12	Case–control (*n* = 9); Cohort (*n* = 3)	Primary lung cancer (overall); adenocarcinoma
Incense	1	Case–control (*n* = 1)	Adenocarcinoma
Gene–environment interactions	2	Case–control (*n* = 1); Cohort (*n* = 1)	Primary lung cancer (overall); adenocarcinoma

All outcomes refer to primary lung cancer. Where histology was reported, subtypes are specified.

3.1. Environmental Tobacco Smoke (ETS)

3.1.1. Principal Findings and Interpretation

Across sixteen epidemiological studies, environmental tobacco smoke (ETS) was consistently associated with an increased risk of lung cancer. Excluding one descriptive hospital-based series from India, ten case–control studies contributed adjusted odds ratios for ETS exposure. The random-effects model yielded a pooled OR of 1.97 (95% CI 1.63–2.37), indicating that individuals exposed to ETS had approximately double the odds of developing lung cancer compared with unexposed participants. The heterogeneity was

https://doi.org/10.3390/jcm15051854

substantial (I^2 = 77.9%), consistent with notable methodological variability across studies, including differences in exposure definitions, assessment periods, and population characteristics. Four cohort studies reported hazard ratios for ETS exposure. The random-effects model produced a pooled HR of 1.44 (95% CI 1.19–1.74), and unlike the OR-based evidence, heterogeneity across cohort studies was negligible (I^2 = 0%), suggesting high internal consistency of ETS effects on lung cancer incidence across longitudinal designs. Leave-one-out sensitivity analyses confirmed the stability of the pooled estimates, with no single study altering the direction or statistical significance of the associations (Supplementary Tables S4 and S5).

We constructed separate forest plots for pooled odds ratios and hazard ratios to facilitate comparison across studies; these are presented in Figures 2 and 3, respectively. Zhuang et al. [30] reported an overall ETS OR of 2.23 (95% CI 1.78–2.79), with sex-specific estimates of 2.22 in household-exposed women and 2.45 in workplace-exposed men. Similar magnitudes were observed by Liang D et al. [23], where both household and workplace ETS yielded ORs of 1.93 (95% CI 1.62–2.31) for home exposure and 1.93 (95% CI 1.53–2.42) for workplace exposure. He et al. [20] reported an adjusted OR of 2.96 (95% CI 2.47–3.55) for ETS in China, while Mbeje et al. [26] observed an aOR of 3.28 (95% CI 1.48–7.30) in a South African population. In the Iranian multicenter IROPICAN study, Lotfi F et al. reported an adjusted OR of 1.69 (95% CI 1.13–2.52) for exposure to second-hand tobacco smoke among never-smokers, further supporting a positive association between ETS and lung cancer risk.

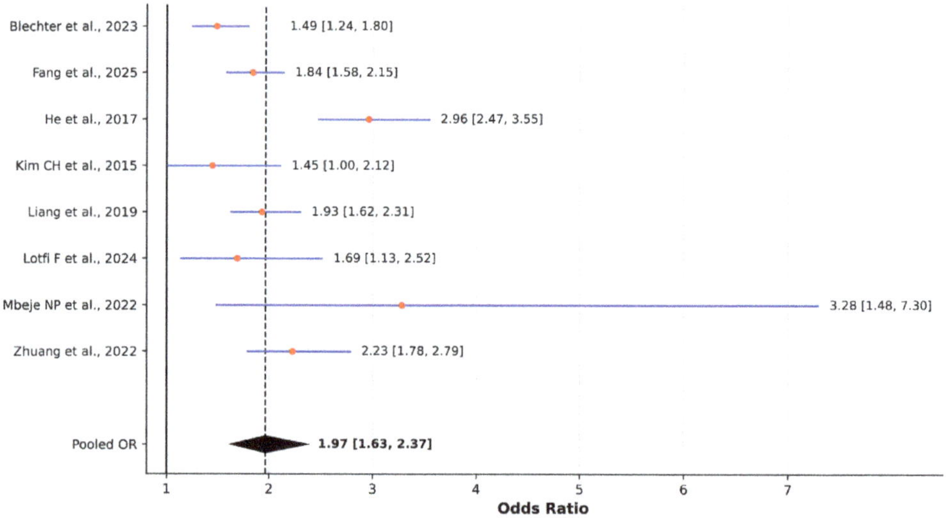

Figure 2. Forest plot of odds ratios (ORs) for environmental tobacco smoke (ETS) exposure and lung cancer risk in case–control studies [15,18,20,21,23,24,26,30]. Pooled estimates were calculated using a random-effects model (DerSimonian–Laird method). Red dots represent individual study effect estimates and blue lines indicate 95% confidence intervals. The diamond represents the pooled estimate with its 95% confidence interval. Between-study heterogeneity was assessed using Cochran's Q test and I^2 statistic.

Moderate risk associations were observed in prospective cohorts, such as those reported by Wang A et al. [29] with an HR 1.61 (95% CI 1.00–2.58) for 30 years or more of exposure, and Li J et al. (2020) [22], where ETS in never-smokers produced an HR 1.27 (0.98–1.71) after full adjustment, indicating a non-significant trend toward increased risk.

https://doi.org/10.3390/jcm1505185

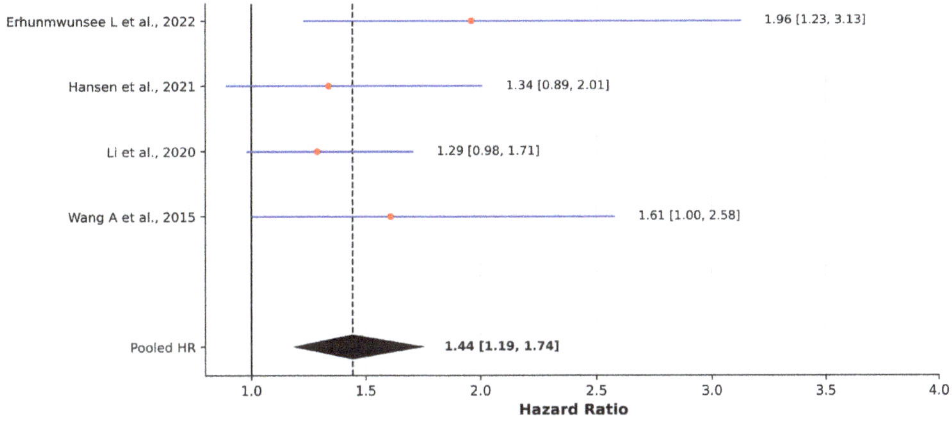

Figure 3. Forest plot of hazard ratios (HRs) for environmental tobacco smoke (ETS) exposure and lung cancer incidence in cohort studies [17,19,22,29]. Pooled estimates were calculated using a random-effects model (DerSimonian–Laird method). Red dots represent individual study effect estimates and blue lines indicate 95% confidence intervals. The diamond represents the pooled estimate with its 95% confidence interval. Between-study heterogeneity was assessed using Cochran's Q test and I^2 statistic.

Overall, the direction and magnitude of associations were consistent with an increased lung cancer risk associated with environmental tobacco smoke exposure across diverse populations.

3.1.2. Subgroup Trends and Effect Modifiers

When analyzed by sex, the risk was higher in women, particularly in household environments where exposure intensity and duration tend to be greater. Dose–response gradients were present in several studies, for example, Lotfii F et al. [24] reported an increasing OR with more prolonged daily exposure, reaching 2.29 (95% CI 1.20–4.37) for more than 3 h per day.

Genetic profile studies further contributed to heterogeneity. Soeroso et al. [27] shows an OR of 2.70 (95% CI 1.07–7.16) among the population with the CYP2A13 CT genotype, while Torres-Duran et al. [28] identified a striking synergy between the AAT SS genotype and 20 or more years of ETS exposure, resulting in an OR of 12.10 (95% CI 1.18–123.77); however, the wide confidence interval indicates limited precision and likely reflects sparse data due to the rarity of the genotype.

Despite these modifiers, the association remained directionally consistent across studies, including those adjusting for co-exposures such as cooking fumes or biomass fuels.

3.2. Cooking Oil Fumes (COFs)

3.2.1. Principal Findings and Interpretation

Evidence from the seven eligible studies shows a consistent association between cooking oil fume (COF) exposure and increased lung cancer risk. Six case–control studies contributed effect estimates to the quantitative synthesis. Using a random-effects model, the pooled OR was 1.83 (95% CI 1.53–2.21), indicating a positive association across study settings. Between-study heterogeneity was low to moderate (I^2 = 37.31%), likely reflecting differences in exposure assessment methods, cooking intensity metrics, and population characteristics. Leave-one-out sensitivity analyses did not materially alter the pooled estimate, and heterogeneity remained negligible upon sequential exclusion of individual

https://doi.org/10.3390/jcm15051854

studies (Supplementary Table S6), supporting the stability of the findings. The forest plot is displayed in Figure 4. One nationwide cohort study further examined occupational exposure to cooking fumes and reported an adjusted HR of 1.72 (95% CI 1.14–2.60), consistent in direction and magnitude with the pooled ORs from the case–control designs.

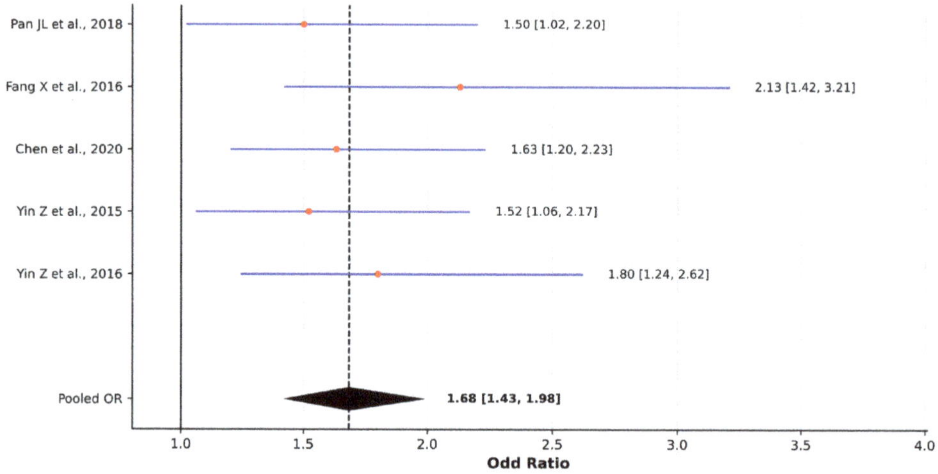

Figure 4. Forest plot of odds ratios (ORs) for cooking oil fume (COF) exposure and lung cancer risk in case–control studies [31,33,34,36,37]. Pooled estimates were calculated using a random-effects model (DerSimonian–Laird method). Red dots represent individual study effect estimates and blue lines indicate 95% confidence intervals. The diamond represents the pooled OR estimate with its 95% confidence interval. Between-study heterogeneity was assessed using Cochran's Q test and I^2 statistic.

Hospital-based case–control studies in China reported some of the highest risks, with He F et al. [32] finding an OR of 2.63 (95% CI 1.91–3.61) for COF exposure in non-smoking women, reporting a positive association between COF exposure and lung cancer; however, as COFs were not the primary exposure and the degree of multivariable adjustment was insufficiently detailed, this estimate was excluded from the pooled analysis. Fang X et al. [33] reported an OR of 2.13 (95% CI 1.42–3.21) for cumulative COF exposure. In Taiwan, Chen et al. [34] showed a dose–response pattern with medium cumulative exposure to COFs being associated with an OR of 1.63 (95% CI 1.20–2.23), with higher risk at the upper end of exposure and partial risk reduction among long-term users of fume removers.

Occupational evidence pointed in the same direction, with a nationwide cohort of female school cooks (Jang J et al.) [35] observing a hazard ratio of 1.72 (95% CI 1.14–2.60) compared with clerks, suggesting that chronic occupational exposure to cooking fumes in institutional kitchens carries a risk of a similar magnitude to heavy domestic exposure.

Additional studies from the Liaoning region by Yin et al., 2015 [36] and Yin et al. 2016 [37] reported ORs of 1.52 and 1.80, respectively, again consistent with the broader evidence in this direction. Overall, the pattern across all eligible studies is coherent across different populations, designs, and strategies, converging on a harmful effect of COFs on lung cancer risk.

3.2.2. Subgroup Trends and Effect Modifiers

Higher risks were generally seen in situations where people cooked for long periods, used high-heat methods, or worked in kitchens with limited ventilation. Studies that measured total cooking hours or captured specific habits such as frequent stir-frying or

https://doi.org/10.3390/jcm15051854

pan-frying showed clearer exposure–response trends than those using only broad frequency categories. In Chen et al., 2020 [34], both frequent pan-frying and greater lifetime cooking duration were associated with a higher risk, whereas regular use of a kitchen hood appeared to reduce the risk, with an adjusted OR close to 0.5.

Genetic susceptibility added further nuance, with several polymorphisms in miRNA-related genes and other loci showing higher combined risks when present together with COF exposure, but formal tests for interaction on additive or multiplicative scales were not always statistically significant.

Taken together, the main-effect signal for COFs remains stable across subgroups, with modifiers such as ventilation, cumulative exposure, and genetic background influencing the magnitude, rather than the presence, of excess risk.

3.3. Solid Fuels and Biomass

3.3.1. Principal Findings and Interpretation

Based on the 12 eligible studies evaluating solid fuel and biomass exposure, the direction of association was generally consistent, with most investigations reporting elevated effect estimates: individuals who relied on coal, wood, or other smoke-generating fuels faced a higher risk of lung cancer than those using cleaner combustion sources. Most studies reported elevated adjusted odds ratios, while investigations conducted in high-exposure settings showed markedly stronger associations. Despite variability in exposure definitions and regional fuel characteristics, pooled analyses demonstrated a statistically significant association between solid fuel/biomass exposure and lung cancer risk. For case–control studies, the pooled OR was 2.26 (95% CI 1.36–3.77), with substantial between-study heterogeneity ($I^2 = 83\%$). In contrast, cohort-based estimates showed a pooled HR of 1.66 (95% CI 1.37–2.02) with no evidence of statistical heterogeneity ($I^2 = 0\%$). Leave-one-out sensitivity analyses confirmed the stability of both models (Supplementary Tables S7 and S8).

In the Shanghai cohort, Kim C et al. [40] found an HR of 1.69 (95% CI 1.22–2.35), indicating that lung cancer risk increased when coal was used under poor kitchen ventilation, underscoring the combined relevance of fuel type and airflow conditions. Mehta SS et al. [42], using prospective data from the Sister Study, reported an HR of 1.68 (1.27–2.20), meaning that women engaging in indoor wood-burning for 30 days or more per year experienced a significantly increased incidence of lung cancer, highlighting that even intermittent domestic combustion in otherwise low-pollution environments may contribute to risk. To aid interpretation, we constructed separate forest plots for odds ratio and hazard ratio estimates, shown in Figures 5 and 6, which outline the pattern of elevated risk across studies.

Two studies from China quantified exposure to smoky coal, historically highest risk fuel. Vermeulen R et al. [43] reported that the PAH25 exposure cluster was positively associated with lung cancer among never-smoking women (OR 2.21, 95% CI 1.67–2.87 per one standard deviation increase), after adjustment for age, second-hand smoke and socioeconomic status. Wong JYY et al. [44], with an OR of 33.40 (95% CI 13.07–85.34), identified extremely elevated odds ratios in households using high-emission deposits such as Laibin coal. However, the magnitude of this estimate likely reflects highly specific exposure conditions and regional fuel characteristics, and should be interpreted in the context of localized extreme emission profiles rather than generalized biomass exposure. Additional insights come from a recent matched case–control study by Yang R et al. [49], which reported an OR of 3.84 (95% CI 1.63–9.05), suggesting that prolonged indoor time may further modify the effective exposure dose beyond fuel type alone.

https://doi.org/10.3390/jcm15051854

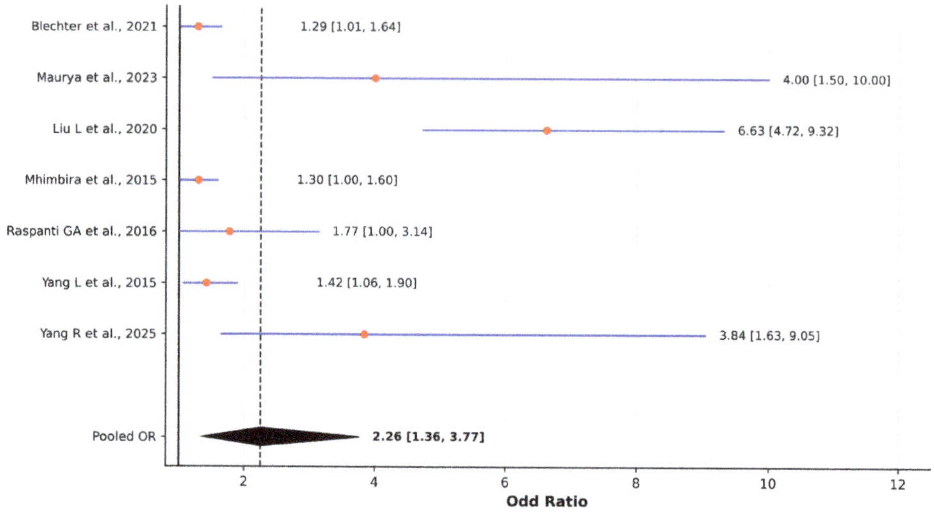

Figure 5. Forest plot of pooled odds ratios for the association between solid fuel/biomass exposure and lung cancer risk in case–control studies [38,39,45–49]. Pooled estimates were calculated using a random-effects model (DerSimonian–Laird method). Red dots represent individual study effect estimates and blue lines indicate 95% confidence intervals. The diamond represents the pooled effect estimate with 95% confidence interval. Between-study heterogeneity was assessed using Cochran's Q test and I^2 statistic.

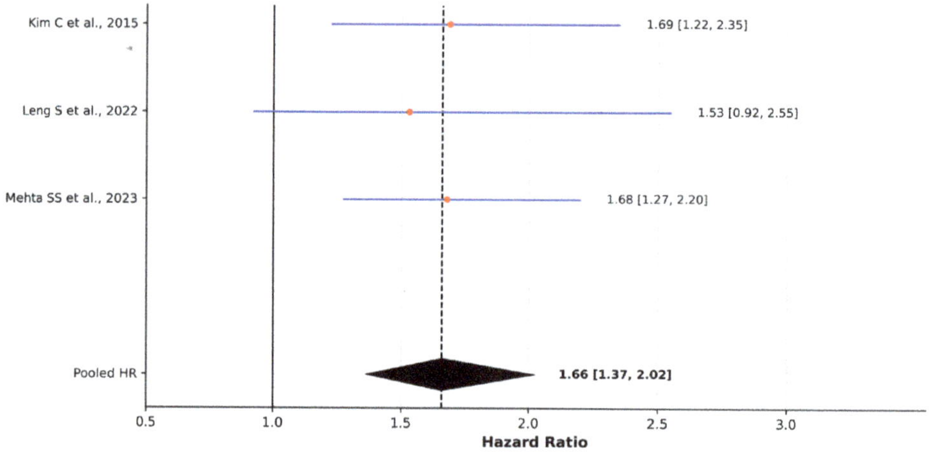

Figure 6. Forest plot of hazard ratios (HRs) for the association between solid fuel/biomass exposure and lung cancer risk in cohort studies [40–42]. Pooled estimates were calculated using a random-effects model (DerSimonian–Laird). Red dots represent individual study effect estimates and blue lines indicate 95% confidence intervals. The diamond represents the pooled effect estimate with 95% confidence interval. Between-study heterogeneity was assessed using Cochran's Q test and I^2 statistic.

3.3.2. Subgroup Trends and Effect Modifiers

Several factors influenced the strength of the observed associations for solid fuel and biomass exposure. Poor ventilation consistently amplified risk, as shown in Kim C et al. [40], where coal use in enclosed kitchens produced higher estimates than in well-ventilated

https://doi.org/10.3390/jcm1505185

settings. Fuel characteristics also played an important role, with studies from Xuanwei (Vermeulen et al. [43]; Wong JYY et al. [44]) demonstrating that smoky coal varieties carried a greater risk than smokeless coal, reflecting their higher emission profiles.

Behavioral context also further modified exposure. Yang R et al. found that individuals who spent more extended periods indoors accumulated higher effective doses, even when using similar fuels. Mehta SS et al. showed that repeated wood-burning in domestic environments may also contribute to risk over time [42].

Taken together, the evidence indicates a directionally consistent association between solid fuel combustion and lung cancer risk, with the magnitude of estimates influenced by the fuel's emission characteristics, local ventilation conditions, and the time individuals spend indoors.

3.4. *Incense Burning and Gene–Environment Interactions*

3.4.1. Incense Burning

Among the included studies, incense burning was identified as a distinct indoor exposure, particularly prevalent in certain cultural contexts. However, this exposure category was represented by a single case–control study (Chen et al. [50]). In that study, habitual incense use was associated with lung adenocarcinoma, with an adjusted OR of 3.05 (95% CI 1.06–8.84). A higher point estimate was observed among women (aOR 6.01), although the corresponding confidence interval was wide, indicating limited precision. Given that the evidence derives from a single study and exhibits imprecision, these findings should be interpreted cautiously and considered hypothesis-generating rather than confirmatory.

3.4.2. Gene–Environment Interactions

Two studies evaluated whether genetic susceptibility modifies the association between indoor air pollution and lung cancer.

Ren Y et al. [51] examined the interaction between cooking oil fume exposure and TGFβ-1 polymorphisms in lung adenocarcinoma. In stratified analyses, individuals exposed to cooking oil fumes carrying the TGFβ-1 C509T TT genotype showed a reduced risk compared with the CC genotype (age-adjusted OR 0.36, 95% CI 0.15–0.88). Logistic regression models evaluating gene–environment interactions also yielded a reduced odds ratio for TT carriers exposed to COFs (age-adjusted OR 0.34, 95% CI 0.12–0.98), with a reported interaction p value of 0.046. However, after Bonferroni correction for multiple comparisons, these associations were no longer statistically significant. The findings, therefore, suggest possible effect modification, although statistical robustness was limited.

Wang G et al. [52] reported that longer daily cooking duration was associated with increased lung cancer incidence in a large prospective Chinese cohort. Participants who cooked for more than 2 h per day had an adjusted hazard ratio of 2.05 (95% CI 1.20–3.53) compared with non-cooking individuals. Joint effect analyses further indicated that carriers of the rs2395185 GT + TT genotype who cooked >2 h/day were associated with an adjusted hazard ratio of 2.48 (95% CI 1.03–5.97) compared with non-cooking individuals with the GG genotype, and similar elevated joint estimates were reported for rs3817963 variants. However, multiplicative interaction tests were not statistically significant. These findings suggest potential combined effects of prolonged cooking exposure and genetic background, although confirmation in larger cohorts is warranted.

Overall, although based on a limited number of studies, the findings suggest potential variability in risk estimates across genetic backgrounds.

https://doi.org/10.3390/jcm15051854

4. Discussions

Indoor air pollution has long been overshadowed by the overwhelming impact of cigarette smoking on lung cancer epidemiology, but evidence accumulated over the past decade suggests that a proportion of lung cancer cases, especially among never-smokers, may be associated with household and environmental exposures [53]. The findings of this review support this perspective by demonstrating generally consistent associations across several exposure categories, although the magnitude and precision of estimates varied between studies.

The first and well-established determinant is environmental tobacco smoke (ETS). Most studies in our review reported an elevated risk, particularly in settings where exposure occurred over long periods in the home or indoor environment with inadequate ventilation. These results align with earlier pooled analyses [54] and continue to suggest that involuntary smoke exposure remains a relevant risk factor in populations where active smoking prevalence has declined. Sensitivity analyses using leave-one-out procedures did not materially alter the direction or statistical significance of pooled estimates, supporting the robustness of the association.

Cooking oil fumes were also associated with increased lung cancer risk in multiple studies, an important risk factor in regions where high-temperature frying, poor ventilation, and extended daily cooking durations are common. These findings are supported by studies demonstrating that hot oil aerosols contain aldehydes, PAHs, particulate matter, and other reactive species capable of inducing oxidative DNA damage and epithelial stress [55,56]. The fact that association patterns remain stable across domestic and occupational settings, as in large cohorts of school cooks, further underscores their robustness. Leave-one-out analyses confirmed the stability of pooled estimates, with minimal impact of any single study on overall effect size.

Solid fuel and biomass combustion were similarly associated with elevated lung cancer risk across most studies, particularly in poorly ventilated settings. When quantitatively synthesized, pooled estimates indicated a significantly increased risk. Substantial heterogeneity was observed in the case–control synthesis, likely reflecting differences in fuel types, combustion characteristics, exposure intensity, and regional contexts, whereas cohort-based estimates showed minimal statistical heterogeneity. Although heterogeneity was substantial in case–control studies, sensitivity analyses indicated that the association remained statistically significant even after excluding individual studies. In several high-emission settings, particularly coal-dependent regions, effect estimates were markedly elevated, suggesting that risk magnitude may depend strongly on exposure profile and environmental conditions.

Although supported by only a single eligible study, incense burning was identified as a distinct domestic exposure. The available evidence remains limited and does not allow firm conclusions. The observed association is biologically plausible, as incense combustion generates aromatic hydrocarbons and fine particulate matter that have been implicated in oxidative and inflammatory airway responses [57–59]. However, given the absence of replication and the wide confidence intervals reported, these findings should be interpreted cautiously and warrant further investigations.

Two studies addressed gene–environment interactions in the context of indoor air pollution and lung cancer. In one case–control study, associations between the TGFβ-1 polymorphisms and lung adenocarcinoma appeared to vary by cooking oil fume exposure. However, statistical significance did not persist after correction for multiple testing. In the prospective cohort study, prolonged daily cooking duration was independently associated with increased lung cancer incidence, and joint exposure–genotype analyses suggested higher risk estimates in selected polymorphism strata, although formal interaction tests

https://doi.org/10.3390/jcm15051854

were not statistically significant. Taken together, these findings indicate possible heterogeneity in susceptibility, but the evidence remains limited and statistically fragile. Larger, adequately powered studies with prespecified interaction evidence analyses are required before firm conclusions regarding gene–environment modification can be drawn.

4.1. Limitations

Despite the overall consistency of associations across exposure types, several methodological constraints limit the precision of the available estimates. Additionally, covariate adjustment strategies differed across studies. Age was consistently included in multivariable models, and most investigations adjusted for sex and active smoking status or cumulative pack-years. However, adjustment for socioeconomic indicators, body mass index, family history of lung cancer, occupational exposures, and comorbid lung disease was inconsistent. Only a subset of studies incorporated environmental co-exposures such as outdoor PM2.5, ventilation conditions, or concurrent indoor pollutants. This heterogeneity in confounder control limits the direct comparability of effect estimates and may partly explain the variability in magnitude across exposure categories. Residual confounding, therefore, cannot be excluded and should be considered when interpreting both pooled and narrative findings.

Most studies relied on self-reported exposure histories, introducing nondifferential misclassification that likely attenuates true risks. Objective exposure measures, such as airborne particulate monitoring or biomarker validation, were rarely used, and critical determinants, such as ventilation, stove efficiency, and housing structure, were inconsistently reported. Selection bias remains a concern in hospital-based case–control designs, while unmeasured or imperfectly captured co-exposures may also have influenced effect estimates.

An additional limitation relates to the geographical distribution of the included studies. A substantial proportion of investigations, particularly those evaluating cooking oil fumes and solid fuel/biomass exposure, were conducted in Asian populations. While this distribution reflects the higher prevalence of these exposure sources in specific regions, it may constrain the external validity of the findings in settings where household fuel types, cooking practices, ventilation standards, and background environmental exposures differ. Broader representation from underrepresented regions would strengthen the global applicability of future evidence.

Even so, the overall direction of associations was largely consistent across exposure categories, although the magnitude and precision of estimates varied substantially. In several studies, wide confidence intervals reflected limited sample size or rare exposure patterns, further contributing to statistical uncertainty. Associations observed for ETS, COFs, and solid fuel/biomass combustion are directionally consistent across multiple populations, although the magnitude varied. Evidence also suggests that combined or overlapping exposures may yield higher cumulative risk than single-pollutant models imply. Future studies should prioritize standardized exposure assessment, incorporate objective measurement strategies, and integrate behavioral, structural, and genetic modifiers to improve causal inference and support refined risk stratification for lung cancer prevention.

4.2. Clinical Relevance and Implications for Practice

The findings of this systematic review may have clinical relevance, particularly in the evaluation of lung cancer risk among individuals who fall outside traditional smoking-based risk frameworks. Lung cancer in never-smokers is increasingly recognized as a distinct clinical entity, characterized by specific epidemiological patterns and molecular features [60]. In this context, chronic indoor air pollution represents a potential exposure domain that may contribute to individualized risk assessment.

https://doi.org/10.3390/jcm15051854

Although the associations observed across environmental tobacco smoke, cooking oil fumes, and solid fuel or biomass combustion were generally consistent, they derive predominantly from observational designs and varied in magnitude and precision. Therefore, indoor exposure histories should not be considered independent diagnostic criteria, but rather contextual factors that may complement established risk models.

Systematic inquiry into indoor exposure patterns, including household smoking, cooking practices, fuel type, ventilation conditions, and cumulative indoor time, may contribute to a more comprehensive contextual assessment of lung cancer risk, particularly among women and older adults, in whom non-tobacco-related lung cancer represents a meaningful proportion of cases [53,61]. Such exposure-aware evaluation may be informative when evaluating persistent respiratory symptoms, unexplained radiological abnormalities, or indeterminate pulmonary nodules in never-smokers, where pre-test probability of malignancy may otherwise be underestimated, and diagnostic delays can occur [62].

Overall, these findings support careful consideration of indoor exposure histories in clinical reasoning, while acknowledging that further prospective research is needed before formal integration into structured risk stratification frameworks.

5. Conclusions

Indoor air pollution was consistently associated with lung cancer risk across the studies included in this review. Adjusted effect estimates for the major exposure categories generally fell within a comparable range, although the magnitudes and precision varied substantially across studies.

From a public health perspective, these findings support continued investigation of indoor exposures as potentially modifiable risk factors. However, the current evidence remains predominantly observational, and further prospective research with standardized exposure assessment is required before integration into formal screening or risk stratification frameworks is considered.

In summary, the available evidence indicates that indoor air pollution represents a relevant exposure domain in lung cancer epidemiology. Greater awareness of household exposure patterns may contribute to improved contextual risk assessment, particularly among never-smokers and individuals outside traditional smoking-based risk categories.

Supplementary Materials: The following supporting information can be downloaded at: https://www.mdpi.com/article/10.3390/jcm15051854/s1, File S1: Research protocol; Table S1: PRISMA Checklist [63]; Table S2: Newcastle–Ottawa Assessment Scale for case–control studies [15,18,20,21,23,24,26–28,30–34,36–39,43–51]; Table S3: Newcastle–Ottawa Assessment Scale for cohort studies [17,19,22,29,35,40–42,52]; Table S4: Leave-one-out for pooled ORs of ETS case-control studies [15,18,20,21,23,24,26,30]; Table S5: Leave-one-out for pooled HRs of ETS cohort studies [17,19,22,29]; Table S6: Leave-one-out for pooled ORs of COF case-control studies [31,33,34,36,37]; Table S7: Leave-one-out for pooled ORs of solid fuels/biomass case-control studies [38,39,45–49]; Table S8: Leave-one-out for pooled HRs of solid fuels/biomass cohort studies [40–42].

Author Contributions: Conceptualization, S.-R.R. and M.S.M.; methodology, S.-R.R.; software, S.-R.R.; validation, S.-R.R., N.W. and M.S.M.; formal analysis, S.-R.R.; investigation, S.-R.R., A.A.T. and A.B.; resources, C.O. and M.S.M.; data curation, S.-R.R., A.R.D. and D.C.C.; writing—original draft preparation, S.-R.R.; writing—review and editing, N.W., A.A.T., A.R.D., D.C.C., A.B., C.O. and M.S.M.; visualization, S.-R.R.; supervision, C.O. and M.S.M.; project administration, M.S.M. All authors have read and agreed to the published version of the manuscript.

Funding: This research received no external funding. The article processing charges (APCs) were covered by institutional funding from the Victor Babeș University of Medicine and Pharmacy, Timișoara, Romania, according to Decision No 5/4270/04.03.2025 regarding the publication of scientific articles approved by the Administrative Council.

Informed Consent Statement: Not applicable.

Acknowledgments: During the preparation of this manuscript, the authors used ChatGPT version 5.0 (OpenAI, San Francisco, CA, USA) to improve language and readability, text structuring and clarification of scientific content. Rayyan (Rayyan Systems Inc., Cambridge, MA, USA), was used to support screening and management of records during the systematic review process. All decisions regarding study selection, data extraction, interpretation, and manuscript content were made by the authors. The authors have reviewed and edited the output and take full responsibility for the content of this publication. We thank the Victor Babeș University of Medicine and Pharmacy for institutional support.

Conflicts of Interest: The authors declare no conflicts of interest.

References

1. Akiba, S.; Kinjo, Y. Japanese Legacy Cohorts: Six-Prefecture Cohort Study (Hirayama Cohort Study). *J. Epidemiol.* **2020**, *30*, 111–115. [CrossRef]
2. Ong, E.; Glantz, S.A. Hirayama's Work Has Stood the Test of Time. *Bull. World Health Organ.* **2000**, *78*, 938–939.
3. Jinot, J.; Bayard, S. Respiratory Health Effects of Passive Smoking: EPA's Weight-of-Evidence Analysis. *J. Clin. Epidemiol.* **1994**, *47*, 339–349; discussion 351–353. [CrossRef]
4. OEHHA. Health Effects of Exposure to Environmental Tobacco Smoke: Final Report. Available online: https://oehha.ca.gov/air/report/health-effects-exposure-environmental-tobacco-smoke-final-report (accessed on 12 November 2025).
5. Chapman, S.; Borland, R.; Scollo, M.; Brownson, R.C.; Dominello, A.; Woodward, S. The Impact of Smoke-Free Workplaces on Declining Cigarette Consumption in Australia and the United States. *Am. J. Public Health* **1999**, *89*, 1018–1023. [CrossRef]
6. Household Air Pollution. Available online: https://www.who.int/news-room/fact-sheets/detail/household-air-pollution-and-health (accessed on 12 November 2025).
7. Straif, K.; Cohen, A.; Samet, J. *Air Pollution and Cancer*; International Agency for Research on Cancer: Lyon, France, 2013.
8. Pope, C.A.; Burnett, R.T.; Turner, M.C.; Cohen, A.; Krewski, D.; Jerrett, M.; Gapstur, S.M.; Thun, M.J. Lung Cancer and Cardiovascular Disease Mortality Associated with Ambient Air Pollution and Cigarette Smoke: Shape of the Exposure–Response Relationships. *Environ. Health Perspect.* **2011**, *119*, 1616–1621. [CrossRef] [PubMed]
9. Hosgood, H.D.; Boffetta, P.; Greenland, S.; Lee, Y.-C.A.; McLaughlin, J.; Seow, A.; Duell, E.J.; Andrew, A.S.; Zaridze, D.; Szeszenia-Dabrowska, N.; et al. In-Home Coal and Wood Use and Lung Cancer Risk: A Pooled Analysis of the International Lung Cancer Consortium. *Environ. Health Perspect.* **2010**, *118*, 1743–1747. [CrossRef]
10. Lissowska, J.; Bardin-Mikolajczak, A.; Fletcher, T.; Zaridze, D.; Szeszenia-Dabrowska, N.; Rudnai, P.; Fabianova, E.; Cassidy, A.; Mates, D.; Holcatova, I.; et al. Lung Cancer and Indoor Pollution from Heating and Cooking with Solid Fuels: The IARC International Multicentre Case-Control Study in Eastern/Central Europe and the United Kingdom. *Am. J. Epidemiol.* **2005**, *162*, 326–333. [CrossRef] [PubMed]
11. Cheng, E.S.; Weber, M.; Steinberg, J.; Yu, X.Q. Lung Cancer Risk in Never-Smokers: An Overview of Environmental and Genetic Factors. *Chin. J. Cancer Res.* **2021**, *33*, 548–562. [CrossRef] [PubMed]
12. Weng, M.; Lee, H.-W.; Park, S.-H.; Hu, Y.; Wang, H.-T.; Chen, L.-C.; Rom, W.N.; Huang, W.C.; Lepor, H.; Wu, X.-R.; et al. Aldehydes Are the Predominant Forces Inducing DNA Damage and Inhibiting DNA Repair in Tobacco Smoke Carcinogenesis. *Proc. Natl. Acad. Sci. USA* **2018**, *115*, E6152–E6161. [CrossRef]
13. Luo, K.; Stepanov, I.; Hecht, S.S. Chemical Biomarkers of Exposure and Early Damage from Potentially Carcinogenic Airborne Pollutants. *Ann. Cancer Epidemiol.* **2019**, *3*, 5. [CrossRef]
14. Albano, G.D.; Montalbano, A.M.; Gagliardo, R.; Anzalone, G.; Profita, M. Impact of Air Pollution in Airway Diseases: Role of the Epithelial Cells (Cell Models and Biomarkers). *Int. J. Mol. Sci.* **2022**, *23*, 2799. [CrossRef]
15. Blechter, B.; Chien, L.-H.; Chen, T.-Y.; Chang, I.-S.; Choudhury, P.P.; Hsiao, C.-F.; Shu, X.-O.; Wong, J.Y.Y.; Chen, K.-Y.; Chang, G.-C.; et al. Polygenic Risk Score, Environmental Tobacco Smoke, and Risk of Lung Adenocarcinoma in Never-Smoking Women in Taiwan. *JAMA Netw. Open* **2023**, *6*, e2339254. [CrossRef] [PubMed]
16. Krishnamurthy, A.; Das, A.; Ramshankar, V.; Sagar, T.; Swaminathan, R. Swaminathan R The Increasing Challenge of Never Smokers with Adenocarcinoma Lung: Need to Look beyond Tobacco Exposure. *Indian J. Cancer* **2017**, *54*, 172–177. [CrossRef]
17. Erhunmwunsee, L.; Wing, S.E.; Zou, X.; Coogan, P.; Palmer, J.R.; Wong, F.L. Neighborhood Disadvantage and Lung Cancer Risk in a National Cohort of Never Smoking Black Women. *Lung Cancer* **2022**, *173*, 21–27. [CrossRef] [PubMed]
18. Fang, F.; Zhou, J.-Y.; Kim, C.H.; Jin, Z.-Y.; Liu, X.; Li, L.; Mu, L.; Wu, M.; Zhao, J.-K.; Zhang, Z.-F. The Association Between Indoor Air Pollution and Lung Cancer Risk in a Chinese Population. *Indoor Air* **2025**, *2025*, 9937960. [CrossRef]

https://doi.org/10.3390/jcm15051854

19. Hansen, M.S.; Licaj, I.; Braaten, T.; Lund, E.; Gram, I.T. The Fraction of Lung Cancer Attributable to Smoking in the Norwegian Women and Cancer (NOWAC) Study. *Br. J. Cancer* **2021**, *124*, 658–662. [CrossRef]
20. Fei, H.E.; Qi, Q.I.; Xu, L.I.; Rendong, X.I.A.O.; Qiuping, X.U.; Zhiqiang, L.I.U.; Lin, C.A.I. Association of Indoor Air Pollution Single Nucleotide Polymorphism of HIF-1α Gene with Susceptibility to Lung Cancer in Han Population in Fujian Province *Zhongguo Fei Ai Za Zhi Chin. J. Lung Cancer* **2017**, *20*, 149–156. [CrossRef]
21. Kim, C.H.; Lee, Y.-C.A.; Hung, R.J.; Boffetta, P.; Xie, D.; Wampfler, J.A.; Cote, M.L.; Chang, S.-C.; Ugolini, D.; Neri, M.; et al. Secondhand Tobacco Smoke Exposure and Lung Adenocarcinoma In Situ/Minimally Invasive Adenocarcinoma (AIS/MIA) *Cancer Epidemiol. Biomark. Prev.* **2015**, *24*, 1902–1906. [CrossRef]
22. Li, J.; Xu, H.-L.; Yao, B.-D.; Li, W.-X.; Fang, H.; Xu, D.-L.; Zhang, Z.-F. Environmental Tobacco Smoke and Cancer Risk, a Prospective Cohort Study in a Chinese Population. *Environ. Res.* **2020**, *191*, 110015. [CrossRef]
23. Liang, D.; Wang, J.; Li, D.; Shi, J.; Jing, J.; Shan, B.; He, Y. Lung Cancer in Never-Smokers: A Multicenter Case-Control Study in North China. *Front. Oncol.* **2019**, *9*, 1354. [CrossRef]
24. Lotfi, F.; Rashidian, H.; Hadji, M.; Mohebbi, E.; Marzban, M.; Naghibzadeh-Tahami, A.; Pukkala, E.; Boffetta, P.; Etemadi, A. Zendehdel, K. Zendehdel K Exposure to Second-Hand Smoke and Risk of Lung Cancer among Iranian Population: A Multicenter Case-Control Study. *PLoS ONE* **2024**, *19*, e0306517. [CrossRef]
25. Masood, N.; Taseer, B.; Yasmin, A. Association of GSTM1 and GSTT1 Deletion with Lung Cancer Development in Pakistani Population. *J. Cancer Res. Ther.* **2016**, *12*, 731–734. [CrossRef] [PubMed]
26. Mbeje, N.P.; Ginindza, T.; Jafta, N. Epidemiological Study of Risk Factors for Lung Cancer in KwaZulu-Natal, South Africa. *Int. J. Environ. Res. Public Health* **2022**, *19*, 6752. [CrossRef] [PubMed]
27. Soeroso, N.; Zain-Hamid, R.; Bihar, S.; Tarigan, S.P.; Ananda, F.R. Genetic Polymorphism of Cyp2a6 and Cyp2a13 Genes and Environmental Tobacco Smoke Induced Lung Cancer Risk in Indonesian Female Never Smokers. *Open Access Maced. J. Med. Sci.* **2021**, *9*, 1219–1225. [CrossRef]
28. Torres-Durán, M.; Ruano-Ravina, A.; Parente-Lamelas, I.; Abal-Arca, J.; Leiro-Fernández, V.; Montero-Martínez, C.; Pena, C. Castro-Añón, O.; Golpe-Gómez, A.; González-Barcala, F.J.; et al. Alpha-1 Antitrypsin Deficiency and Lung Cancer Risk: A Case-Control Study in Never-Smokers. *J. Thorac. Oncol.* **2015**, *10*, 1279–1284. [CrossRef]
29. Wang, A.; Kubo, J.; Luo, J.; Desai, M.; Hedlin, H.; Henderson, M.; Chlebowski, R.; Tindle, H.; Chen, C.; Gomez, S.; et al. Active and Passive Smoking in Relation to Lung Cancer Incidence in the Women's Health Initiative Observational Study Prospective Cohort. *Ann. Oncol. Off. J. Eur. Soc. Med. Oncol.* **2015**, *26*, 221–230. [CrossRef]
30. Zhuang, J.; Liu, Z.; Xiao, R.; Xu, Q.; Xiong, W.; Li, X.; Cai, L.; He, F. Association between Smoking and Environmental Tobacco Smoke with Lung Cancer Risk: A Case-Control Study in the Fujian Chinese Population. *J. Public Health-Heidelb.* **2022**, *30*, 2047–2057. [CrossRef]
31. Pan, J.-L.; Gao, J.; Hou, J.-H.; Hu, D.-Z.; Li, L. Interaction Between Environmental Risk Factors and Catechol-O-Methyltransferase (COMT) and X-Ray Repair Cross-Complementing Protein 1 (XRCC1) Gene Polymorphisms in Risk of Lung Cancer Among Non-Smoking Chinese Women: A Case-Control Study. *Med. Sci. Monit. Int. Med. J. Exp. Clin. Res.* **2018**, *24*, 5689–5697. [CrossRef]
32. He, F.; Xie, J.-X.; Liu, C.-L.; Xiong, W.-M.; Xu, Q.-P.; Liu, Z.-Q.; Lin, T.; Xiao, R.-D.; Li, X.; Cai, L. The Relationship of Lung Cancer with Menstrual and Reproductive Factors May Be Influenced by Passive Smoking, Cooking Oil Fumes, and Tea Intake: A Case-Control Study in Chinese Women. *Medicine* **2017**, *96*, e8816. [CrossRef]
33. Fang, X.; Yin, Z.; Li, X.; Xia, L.; Zhou, B. Polymorphisms in GEMIN4 and AGO1 Genes Are Associated with the Risk of Lung Cancer: A Case-Control Study in Chinese Female Non-Smokers. *Int. J. Environ. Res. Public Health* **2016**, *13*, 939. [CrossRef]
34. Chen, T.; Fang, Y.; Chen, H.; Chang, C.; Huang, H.; Chen, Y.; Liao, K.; Wu, H.; Chang, G.; Tsai, Y.; et al. Impact of Cooking Oil Fume Exposure and Fume Extractor Use on Lung Cancer Risk in Non-Smoking Han Chinese Women. *Sci. Rep.* **2020**, *10*, 6774. [CrossRef]
35. Jang, J.; Kim, E.M.; Kim, J.; Min, J.; Kim, I. Lung Cancer Risk in Female School Cooks: A Nationwide Retrospective Cohort Study in the Republic of Korea. *Saf. Health Work* **2025**, *16*, 105–112. [CrossRef]
36. Yin, Z.; Cui, Z.; Guan, P.; Li, X.; Wu, W.; Ren, Y.; He, Q.; Zhou, B. Interaction between Polymorphisms in Pre-MiRNA Genes and Cooking Oil Fume Exposure on the Risk of Lung Cancer in Chinese Non-Smoking Female Population. *PLoS ONE* **2015**, *10*, e0128572. [CrossRef]
37. Yin, Z.; Cui, Z.; Li, H.; Ren, Y.; Qian, B.; Rothman, N.; Lan, Q.; Zhou, B. Polymorphisms in miR-135a-2, miR-219-2 and miR-211 as Well as Their Interaction with Cooking Oil Fume Exposure on the Risk of Lung Cancer in Chinese Nonsmoking Females: A Case-Control Study. *BMC Cancer* **2016**, *16*, 751. [CrossRef] [PubMed]
38. Blechter, B.; Wong, J.Y.Y.; Agnes Hsiung, C.; Mhimbira, H.D.; Yin, Z.; Shu, X.-O.; Zhang, H.; Shi, J.; Song, L.; Song, M. Sub Multiplicative Interaction between Polygenic Risk Score and Household Coal Use in Relation to Lung Adenocarcinoma among Never-Smoking Women in Asia. *Environ. Int.* **2021**, *147*, 105975. [CrossRef]
39. Maurya, A.; Kumar, R.; Khera, A.; Singh, D.K.; Dudeja, P. A Case-Control Study of Lung Cancer at a Tertiary Care Hospital of Western Maharashtra, India. *Med. J. Dr. Patil Vidyapeeth* **2023**, *16*, 336–342. [CrossRef]

https://doi.org/10.3390/jcm15051854

Kim, C.; Gao, Y.; Xiang, Y.; Barone-Adesi, F.; Zhang, Y.; Hosgood, H.D.; Ma, S.; Shu, X.; Ji, B.; Chow, W.; et al. Home Kitchen Ventilation, Cooking Fuels, and Lung Cancer Risk in a Prospective Cohort of Never Smoking Women in Shanghai, China. *Int. J. Cancer* **2015**, *136*, 632–638. [CrossRef]
Leng, S.; Picchi, M.A.; Meek, P.M.; Jiang, M.; Bayliss, S.H.; Zhai, T.; Bayliyev, R.I.; Tesfaigzi, Y.; Campen, M.J.; Kang, H.; et al. Wood Smoke Exposure Affects Lung Aging, Quality of Life, and All-Cause Mortality in New Mexican Smokers. *Respir. Res.* **2022**, *23*, 236. [CrossRef] [PubMed]
Mehta, S.S.; Hodgson, M.E.; Lunn, R.M.; Ashley, C.E.; Arroyave, W.D.; Sandler, D.P.; White, A.J. Indoor Wood-Burning from Stoves and Fireplaces and Incident Lung Cancer among Sister Study Participants. *Environ. Int.* **2023**, *178*, 108128. [CrossRef] [PubMed]
Vermeulen, R.; Downward, G.S.; Zhang, J.; Hu, W.; Portengen, L.; Bassig, B.A.; Hammond, S.K.; Wong, J.Y.; Li, J.; Reiss, B.; et al. Constituents of Household Air Pollution and Risk of Lung Cancer among Never-Smoking Women in Xuanwei and Fuyuan, China. *Environ. Health Perspect.* **2019**, *127*, 97001. [CrossRef]
Wong, J.Y.; Downward, G.S.; Hu, W.; Portengen, L.; Seow, W.J.; Silverman, D.T.; Bassig, B.A.; Zhang, J.; Xu, J.; Ji, B.; et al. Lung Cancer Risk by Geologic Coal Deposits: A Case-Control Study of Female Never-Smokers from Xuanwei and Fuyuan, China. *Int. J. Cancer* **2019**, *144*, 2918–2927. [CrossRef]
Liu, L.; Liu, X.; Ma, X.; Ning, B.; Wan, X. Analysis of the Associations of Indoor Air Pollution and Tobacco Use with Morbidity of Lung Cancer in Xuanwei, China. *Sci. Total Environ.* **2020**, *717*, 135232. [CrossRef]
Mhimbira, H.D.; Song, M.; Hsiung, C.A.; Yin, Z.; Shu, X.-O.; Wang, Z.; Chaterjee, N.; Zheng, W.; Caporaso, N.; Burdett, L. Interactions between Household Air Pollution and GWAS-Identified Lung Cancer Susceptibility Markers in the Female Lung Cancer Consortium in Asia (FLCCA). *Hum. Genet.* **2015**, *134*, 333–341. [CrossRef]
Raspanti, G.A.; Hashibe, M.; Siwakoti, B.; Wei, M.; Thakur, B.K.; Pun, C.B.; Al-Temimi, M.; Lee, Y.-C.A.; Sapkota, A. Household Air Pollution and Lung Cancer Risk among Never-Smokers in Nepal. *Environ. Res.* **2016**, *147*, 141–145. [CrossRef]
Yang, L.; Lu, X.; Deng, J.; Zhou, Y.; Huang, D.; Qiu, F.; Yang, X.; Yang, R.; Fang, W.; Ran, P.; et al. Risk Factors Shared by COPD and Lung Cancer and Mediation Effect of COPD: Two-Center Case-Control Studies. *Cancer Causes Control CCC* **2015**, *26*, 11–24. [CrossRef]
Yang, R.; Mu, X.; Wang, G.; Tang, D.; Wang, B.; Li, Z.; Kan, H.; Lin, N.; Tao, S. Urban-Rural Inequality in Lung Cancer Risk from Indoor Air Pollution: Prolonged Indoor Time Amplifies the Risks of Solid Fuel Use. *J. Environ. Manag.* **2025**, *393*, 127084. [CrossRef]
Chen, K.; Tsai, S.; Shie, R.; Zeng, C.; Yang, H. Indoor Air Pollution Increases the Risk of Lung Cancer. *Int. J. Environ. Res. Public Health* **2022**, *19*, 1164. [CrossRef] [PubMed]
Ren, Y.; Yin, Z.; Li, K.; Wan, Y.; Li, X.; Wu, W.; Guan, P.; Zhou, B. TGFβ-1 and TGFBR2 Polymorphisms, Cooking Oil Fume Exposure and Risk of Lung Adenocarcinoma in Chinese Nonsmoking Females: A Case Control Study. *BMC Med. Genet.* **2015**, *16*, 22. [CrossRef] [PubMed]
Wang, G.; Bai, Y.; Fu, W.; Feng, Y.; Chen, W.; Li, G.; Wu, X.; Meng, H.; Liu, Y.; Wei, W.; et al. Daily Cooking Duration and Its Joint Effects with Genetic Polymorphisms on Lung Cancer Incidence: Results from a Chinese Prospective Cohort Study. *Environ. Res.* **2019**, *179*, 108747. [CrossRef]
Samet, J.M.; Avila-Tang, E.; Boffetta, P.; Hannan, L.M.; Olivo-Marston, S.; Thun, M.J.; Rudin, C.M. Lung Cancer in Never Smokers: Clinical Epidemiology and Environmental Risk Factors. *Clin. Cancer Res.* **2009**, *15*, 5626–5645. [CrossRef] [PubMed]
Ni, X.; Xu, N.; Wang, Q. Meta-Analysis and Systematic Review in Environmental Tobacco Smoke Risk of Female Lung Cancer by Research Type. *Int. J. Environ. Res. Public Health* **2018**, *15*, 1348. [CrossRef]
Yao, Z.; Li, J.; Wu, B.; Hao, X.; Yin, Y.; Jiang, X. Characteristics of PAHs from Deep-Frying and Frying Cooking Fumes. *Environ. Sci. Pollut. Res.* **2015**, *22*, 16110–16120. [CrossRef]
Chang, L.W.; Lo, W.-S.; Lin, P. Trans, Trans-2,4-Decadienal, a Product Found in Cooking Oil Fumes, Induces Cell Proliferation and Cytokine Production Due to Reactive Oxygen Species in Human Bronchial Epithelial Cells. *Toxicol. Sci.* **2005**, *87*, 337–343. [CrossRef]
Lee, C.-W.; Vo, T.T.T.; Wee, Y.; Chiang, Y.-C.; Chi, M.-C.; Chen, M.-L.; Hsu, L.-F.; Fang, M.-L.; Lee, K.-H.; Guo, S.-E.; et al. The Adverse Impact of Incense Smoke on Human Health: From Mechanisms to Implications. *J. Inflamm. Res.* **2021**, *14*, 5451–5472. [CrossRef]
Bălă, G.-P.; Râjnoveanu, R.-M.; Tudorache, E.; Motișan, R.; Oancea, C. Air Pollution Exposure—The (in)Visible Risk Factor for Respiratory Diseases. *Environ. Sci. Pollut. Res.* **2021**, *28*, 19615–19628. [CrossRef]
Niu, X.; Jones, T.; BéruBé, K.; Chuang, H.-C.; Sun, J.; Ho, K.F. The Oxidative Capacity of Indoor Source Combustion Derived Particulate Matter and Resulting Respiratory Toxicity. *Sci. Total Environ.* **2021**, *767*, 144391. [CrossRef]
Planchard, D.; Besse, B. Lung Cancer in Never-Smokers. *Eur. Respir. J.* **2015**, *45*, 1214–1217. [CrossRef] [PubMed]
Couraud, S.; Zalcman, G.; Milleron, B.; Morin, F.; Souquet, P.-J. Lung Cancer in Never Smokers—A Review. *Eur. J. Cancer* **2012**, *48*, 1299–1311. [CrossRef] [PubMed]

https://doi.org/10.3390/jcm15051854

62. Ellis, P.M.; Vandermeer, R. Delays in the Diagnosis of Lung Cancer. *J. Thorac. Dis.* **2011**, *3*, 183–188. [CrossRef] [PubMed]
63. Page, M.J.; McKenzie, J.E.; Bossuyt, P.M.; Boutron, I.; Hoffmann, T.C.; Mulrow, C.D.; Shamseer, L.; Tetzlaff, J.M.; Akl, E.A Brennan, S.E.; et al. The PRISMA 2020 statement: An updated guideline for reporting systematic reviews. *BMJ* **2021**, *372*, n7 [CrossRef]

https://doi.org/10.3390/jcm150518

Journal of
Clinical Medicine

MDPI

pinion

esson from COVID-19—Adapting Respiratory Rehabilitation hrough Early Multidisciplinary Care: An Opinion Paper from etrospective Data

derica Bellone [1], Adriana Tisano [1], Giulia Leonardi [2], Daniela Amato [2], Daniele Borzelli [3], Giuseppe Santoro [3], ngelo Alito [3], Francesca Cucinotta [4,*] and Simona Portaro [2]

1 Department of Clinical and Experimental Medicine, University of Messina, 98125 Messina, Italy; federica.bellone@unime.it (F.B.); atisano@unime.it (A.T.)
2 Physical Rehabilitation Medicine Department, University Hospital A.O.U. "G. Martino", 98124 Messina, Italy; giulia.leonardi@polime.it (G.L.); daniela.amato@polime.it (D.A.); simonaportaro@hotmail.it (S.P.)
3 Department of Biomedical, Dental Sciences and Morphological and Functional Images, University of Messina, 98125 Messina, Italy; daniele.borzelli@unime.it (D.B.); giuseppe.santoro@unime.it (G.S.); alitoa@unime.it (A.A.)
4 IRCCS Centro Neurolesi Bonino-Pulejo, 98124 Messina, Italy
* Correspondence: francesca.cucinotta@irccsme.it

Abstract: The COVID-19 pandemic significantly challenged healthcare systems worldwide, highlighting the critical role of early and multidisciplinary rehabilitation interventions. There remains uncertainty about whether these rehabilitation principles developed in response to COVID-19 can be effectively generalized to chronic respiratory diseases. This opinion paper evaluates retrospective data from early stages of the COVID-19 pandemic to propose a comprehensive early multidisciplinary rehabilitation model, potentially applicable across various chronic respiratory conditions. We retrospectively analyzed data from 62 COVID-19 patients hospitalized at the University Hospital of Messina, Italy, between March and June 2020. The patients underwent structured multidisciplinary rehabilitation sessions initiated upon achieving clinical stability. Functional improvements were assessed weekly using the Barthel Index (BI). Significant correlations were observed between initial BI scores and functional improvements at discharge ($p < 0.001$) and between functional gains and the number of rehabilitation sessions administered ($p = 0.025$). Early physiatric evaluation significantly enhanced functional recovery ($p = 0.036$). Early structured multidisciplinary rehabilitation during acute hospitalization demonstrated clear benefits in COVID-19 patients, indicating potential for broad applicability in chronic respiratory disease management. Systematic implementation could improve clinical outcomes, reduce healthcare resource utilization, and enhance patients' quality of life.

Keywords: Barthel Index; COVID-19; chronic respiratory diseases; early rehabilitation; functional assessment; multidisciplinary care

1. Introduction

The emergence of Severe Acute Respiratory Syndrome Coronavirus 2 (SARS-CoV-2) in December 2019 strongly challenged healthcare systems worldwide [1–3]. Coronavirus disease 2019 (COVID-19) presented with various clinical manifestations, from mild influenza-like symptoms to severe forms characterized by acute respiratory distress syndrome (ARDS), multisystem organ failure, and extended periods of critical illness [4,5].

While COVID-19 primarily affects respiratory function, extensive evidence suggests it should be regarded as a systemic condition impacting multiple organ systems, including cardiovascular, neurological, hematopoietic, and immune systems [6–8].

Rehabilitation strategies developed in response to the COVID-19 crisis may offer valuable insights into the management of respiratory diseases.

Can these strategies serve as a translational model for managing chronic respiratory diseases?

Recent literature underscores that early and multidisciplinary rehabilitation initiated during acute illness, including intensive care unit (ICU) stays, significantly improves long-term patient outcomes, reducing disability and promoting faster functional recovery [6,9]. The exceptional contexts of the COVID-19 pandemic imposed rapid innovation and adaptation, providing a unique opportunity to reconsider established rehabilitation protocols and explore novel multidisciplinary approaches [10,11]. This perspective offers interesting possibilities for the transfer of these findings to chronic respiratory diseases, such as chronic obstructive pulmonary disease (COPD), idiopathic pulmonary fibrosis (IPF), and post-ARDS sequelae of various etiologies.

Furthermore, contemporary studies indicate a clear necessity to optimize healthcare resources by implementing early interventions that improve patient outcomes while concurrently reducing hospital stays, readmission rates, and overall healthcare costs [12,13]. Rehabilitation programs traditionally implemented during later stages of chronic respiratory disease progression have limited impact on reversing significant functional decline [14]. Conversely, early structured interventions may considerably correct patient paths, reduce subsequent healthcare utilization, and enhance quality of life, presenting significant economic benefits for strained healthcare systems [15].

These findings raise the possibility that what we have learned under the pressure of the pandemic could evolve into a new paradigm, offering a potential way forward to better support people living with chronic and disabling respiratory conditions.

Initiating pulmonary rehabilitation programs after hospital discharge or during the stable chronic phase limits their effectiveness in reversing deconditioning and impairs long-term prognosis [16]. Furthermore, many healthcare systems still lack multidisciplinary integration, which is often limited by logistical, economic, or structural issues.

The 2023 Global Initiative for Chronic Obstructive Lung Disease (GOLD) report emphasizes the importance of multidisciplinary and early interventions but provides few practical guidelines for implementing these strategies during acute hospitalizations [17].

Recent studies have shown that early physiotherapy and mobilization during hospitalization may improve outcomes for patients with chronic respiratory disease [18], but randomized evidence remains scarce, and structured protocols applicable to broader populations are lacking. The pandemic presented an unexpected opportunity to advance the implementation of early, intensive, and multidisciplinary rehabilitation approaches, even for critically ill patients. It has been shown that these interventions, which were driven by necessity, are safe, feasible, and potentially impactful [19,20].

Early rehabilitation intervention is crucial for optimizing outcomes for respiratory patients [21]. A recent study found that starting respiratory rehabilitation within four days of admission significantly reduced disease progression and mortality, even among critically ill patients. Multimodal approaches are safe and feasible in acute care, reinforcing the value of early rehabilitation for chronic respiratory diseases [19].

The effective delivery of such interventions depends on the coordinated involvement of a multidisciplinary team. This typically includes the medical team, physiatrists, physiotherapists, respiratory therapists, nurses, and intensive care specialists working closely with psychologists and occupational therapists. The integration of these professionals allows for a comprehensive and patient-centered approach that addresses not only respiratory and functional impairments but also the neurocognitive, psychological, and nutritional sequelae of COVID-19 [20,22]. Shared clinical protocols and continuous interdisciplinary communication are essential to adapt rehabilitation strategies to the evolving clinical course of the patient and to maximize safety and functional recovery while minimizing complications.

This opinion paper aims to retrospectively describe the functional outcomes associated with an early, structured, multidisciplinary rehabilitation program administered to hospitalized patients with acute SARS-CoV-2 infection. A secondary aim is to explore potential associations between rehabilitation variables (i.e., timing, number of sessions, early approach) and improvements in functional status. In addition, this paper aims not only to challenge existing paradigms but also to encourage proactive adoption of tailored rehabilitation strategies with demonstrable cost-effectiveness and enhanced patient-centered outcomes.

2. Materials, Methods, and Results

We retrospectively reviewed data from 62 patients admitted to the University Hospital of Messina (Italy) between March and June 2020 with a confirmed COVID-19 diagnosis (Ethical Committee approved the study on 9 November 2021 (protocol number 40-21 10 March 2021)). Eligible patients were identified in intensive care units (ICU, n = 25) and acute care units (internal medicine, pulmonology, infectious diseases departments, n = 37). Demographic and functional data are provided in Table 1. Once patients were clinically stabilized during hospitalization in the ICU or acute care units, the physiatrist assessed their physical and neurological condition, blood exams, ventilation type, oxygen saturation, and the absence of any contraindications to start rehabilitation. According to the literature [23], the exclusion criteria for starting rehabilitation were (1) signs of respiratory distress; (2) the need for respiratory support with a fraction of inspired oxygen (FiO_2) > 60%; (3) the need for continuous positive airway pressure (CPAP); (4) signs of cardiovascular instability or chest compression; and (5) psychomotor agitation or resistance to treatment. Rehabilitation interventions began upon achieving stable respiratory and hemodynamic parameters, irrespective of nasopharyngeal swab positivity, until hospital discharge.

The patients participated in daily rehabilitation sessions (~40 min), and functional assessments were performed weekly using the Barthel Index (BI).

In the ICU, rehabilitation started as soon as respiratory and hemodynamic stability was achieved. The physiotherapy plan was personalized and guided by the level of consciousness, ventilatory support, and clinical parameters. Core interventions included passive and active assisted mobilization, frequent postural changes (including sitting or semi-orthopedic positions), early verticalization when possible, trunk control exercises, and static standing balance. Respiratory rehabilitation focused on improving deep lung ventilation and secretion clearance. Exercises were performed with rest periods to compensate for fatigue, and continuous monitoring was required to interrupt treatment in the event of fever, oxygen desaturation (SpO_2 < 90%), dyspnea, or clinical deterioration. If possible and tolerated by the patient, muscle strengthening, stretching, and ambulation exercises helped with gradual recovery.

The patients on acute wards often had significant deconditioning due to immobilization, inflammation, and prolonged oxygen therapy. Physiotherapy focused on restoring functional autonomy and endurance through active mobilization, progressive resistance exercises, coordination tasks, and respiratory muscle training. Out-of-bed sitting, sit-to-stand training, early gait re-education, and ADL retraining were progressively introduced. Trunk control and dynamic balance exercises supported neuromotor recovery, while oxygen saturation and other clinical parameters guided intensity. Volume-based breathing strategies, including deep, slow inspirations with inspiration, supported lung recruitment.

In all settings, interventions were tailored to each patient's clinical status, with particular attention to respiratory, cardiovascular, musculoskeletal, and cognitive functions.

Respiratory techniques, such as diaphragmatic or pursed-lip breathing, were avoided in the acute phase. The treatment plan and exercises were tailored to each patient's clinical condition, comorbidities, and tolerance levels to ensure safety and maximize functional recovery. Figure 1 shows a schematic representation of the different rehabilitation pathways.

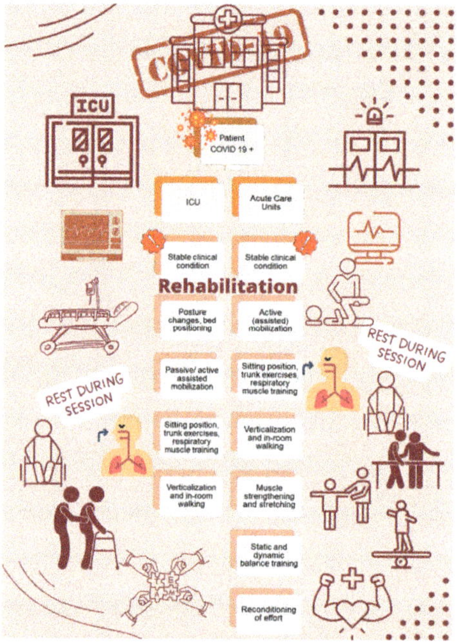

Figure 1. Rehabilitation pathways for patients with COVID-19, based on clinical setting and stability. This flowchart illustrates the different approaches to rehabilitation for hospitalized COVID-19 patients. Once clinical stability has been achieved, rehabilitation is introduced progressively with tailored interventions. The figure highlights the importance of rest during sessions and emphasizes the need for a multidisciplinary team approach to ensure safe, personalized progression.

A linear model (Matlab® v2023b function fitlm) tested the effects of the following factors on the BI at discharge: (i) BI at the first physiatric evaluation, (ii) days of hospitalization before physiatric examination, (iii) number of physiotherapy treatments administrated, (iv) age, and (v) sex. Our data showed that the days before physiatric examination affected the BI at discharge but not linearly. Therefore, the effect of the days before physiatric examination was modelled as a dummy variable, whose value was equal to 1 if the patient was examined in less than d days, where d ranged from 5 to 43, and 0 otherwise. A different linear model was built with each d, while the other tested effects were (a) BI at the first physiatric evaluation, (b) number of physiotherapy treatments administrated, (c) age, and (d) sex.

The linear model showed that, as expected, the discharge BI was significantly influenced by the BI measured on admission ($p < 0.001$, Figure 2, left panel, black line) and by the number of treatments given to the patient ($p = 0.025$, Figure 2, right panel, black line), with each additional treatment resulting in an average improvement of 1.55 in the discharge BI. In contrast, the discharge BI was not affected by age ($p = 0.481$), sex ($p = 0.319$), or days prior to the medical examination ($p = 0.324$).

Table 1. Demographic features and functional evaluation of patients.

	ICU	Acute Care Units	Total
Number of patients	25	37	62
Age (y)	65.84 ± 11.55	72.19 ± 12.53	70.50 ± 12.31
Sex	14 M/11 F	10 M/27 F	24 M/38 F
LOS	49.32 ± 29.67	34.13 ± 13.87	40.26 ± 22.90
Tracheostomy	12 (48%)	2 (5.41%)	12 (48%)
Number of treatments	10.92 ± 7.91	6.70 ± 5.22	8.40 ± 6.77
Dead	3 (12%)	2 (5.41%)	5 (8.06%)
Comorbidities (%)			
Arterial hypertension	15 (60%)	28 (75.68%)	43 (69.35%)
Diabetes mellitus	9 (36%)	14 (37.84%)	23 (37.10%)
Dyslipidemia	3 (12%)	8 (21.62%)	11 (17.74%)
Obesity	4 (16%)	8 (21.62%)	12 (19.35%)
Neuromuscular diseases	1 (4%)	5 (13.51%)	6 (9.68%)
Functional assessment			
Days before first physiatric evaluation	23 ± 14	19 ± 12	21 ± 13
BI on admission	8 ± 8	19 ± 15	15.28 ± 14.32
BI at discharge	16 ± 15	29 ± 21	24.17 ± 21.84

BI: Barthel Index; ICU: intensive care unit; LOS: length of stay.

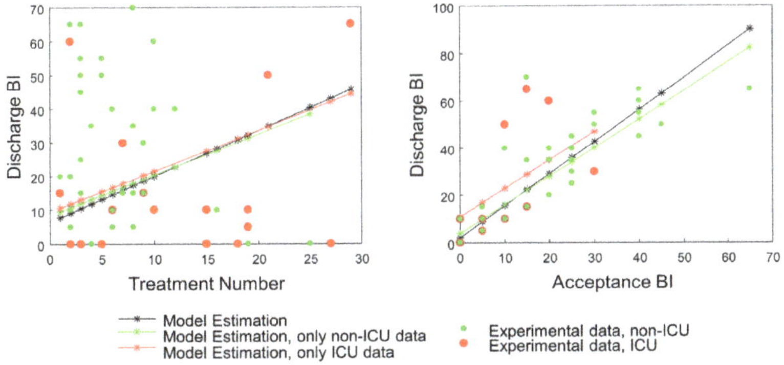

Figure 2. Experimental data and linear model of discharge BI. Experimental data collected from patients who underwent ICU treatment are shown as red dots; data from patients who did not are shown as green dots. The black line with asterisks represents the linear model fitted to data from all patients. The red and green lines with asterisks represent the linear models fitted to data from patients who underwent ICU treatment and those who did not, respectively. (**Left panel**): effect of treatment number on discharge BI. (**Right panel**): effect of admission BI on discharge BI.

A further stratification was performed by dividing the patients who underwent ICU treatment from those who did not. Accordingly, linear models were built on two separate datasets: one comprising the patients who underwent ICU treatment and the other comprising those who did not. The effects of the following factors on the BI at discharge were tested: (i) BI at the first physiatric evaluation, (ii) days of hospitalization before physiatric examination, (iii) number of physiotherapy treatments administrated, (iv) age, and (v) sex.

In line with the model built on the full dataset, discharge BI was significantly influenced by BI at admission in both groups: the patients who underwent ICU treatment

(p = 0.011; Figure 2, left panel, red line) and those who did not (p < 0.001; Figure 2, left panel, green line). Similarly, discharge BI was not affected by age (p = 0.405 and p = 0.993, respectively, for ICU and non-ICU groups), sex (p = 0.728 and p = 0.285), or days before the medical examination (p = 0.167 and p = 0.824). Interestingly, the number of physiotherapy treatments significantly affected discharge BI only in the patients who underwent ICU treatment (p = 0.037; Figure 2, right panel, red line) but not in those who did not (p = 0.485; Figure 2, right panel, green line).

However, linear models testing the effect of days to examination as a dummy variable identified a significant effect on discharge BI, with an average 8.8 higher value if the examination was performed within 30 days (p = 0.036). Examinations performed within fewer days had no effect on discharge BI (see Table 1). The effect of the other parameters did not change with the different threshold in days to examination, and while the number of treatments (p < 0.037 in all conditions) and the admission BI (p < 0.001 in all conditions) showed a significant effect on the discharge BI, age (p > 0.302 in all conditions) and sex (p > 0.218 in all conditions) did not.

3. Discussion

The retrospective data strongly support the effectiveness of an early, structured, multidisciplinary rehabilitation protocol, inviting broader consideration of how acute care pathways for chronic respiratory diseases could be restructured beyond the immediate context of the pandemic. The significant improvements in functional outcomes highlight the necessity and effectiveness of early initiation of rehabilitation, even in intensive care settings. Recent literature reinforces that initiating rehabilitation early in ICU settings significantly reduces morbidity, decreases the length of hospital stay, and improves overall functional recovery [24,25]. Continuous rehabilitation through subsequent inpatient settings further consolidates these functional gains, highlighting the importance of seamless rehabilitation care transitions [26].

BI is confirmed as a reliable prognostic tool for both mortality and functional outcomes, particularly in older patients with COVID-19. Our findings are consistent with data from the Italian RePoSI Registry, in which, in a cohort of 4714 elderly hospitalized patients, alongside glycemia level $\geq$ 250 mg/dL, Cumulative Illness rating Scale (CIRS-SI), and male sex, a BI $\leq$ 40 was a stronger predictor of in-hospital mortality for older patients admitted in general wards [27].

Early physiatric evaluation is critical for the timely and targeted initiation of rehabilitation in patients with acute respiratory failure. It allows for early identification of functional limitations and guides the integration of rehabilitation into the acute care pathway, helping to prevent complications such as deconditioning and prolonged immobility and ensuring continuity of care from admission to post-acute recovery [28].

BI assessment enables the identification of individuals at higher risk of disability and poor prognosis, while its longitudinal use provides valuable insight into rehabilitation response and functional progression. The utility of the BI extends beyond mortality prediction, offering a valuable means of evaluating functional outcomes such as post-intensive care syndrome (PICS). Its routine application in clinical practice could facilitate more precise rehabilitation planning and contribute to a more efficient allocation of healthcare resources [29,30].

The principles of early mobilization and structured respiratory physiotherapy reinforce our rehabilitation protocol. Early mobilization addresses the severe muscular and cardiovascular deconditioning prevalent in critically ill respiratory patients, suggesting similar benefits could extend effectively to chronic conditions like COPD and IPF [31,32].

The application of respiratory physiotherapy, including postural drainage and respiratory muscle training, is well supported by current literature as essential in managing chronic respiratory diseases, reducing complications, and improving pulmonary function [33]. Implementing early multidisciplinary rehabilitation for chronic respiratory diseases would require redefining the timing, roles, and resource allocation across clinical settings. This would entail structured training programs, early physiatric involvement, and protocols for individualized progression. Most importantly, it would demand a cultural shift in how we approach chronic disability in respiratory patients, moving from a reactive to an anticipatory care model.

The multidisciplinary approach involving physiotherapists, respiratory therapists, psychologists, and physicians significantly contributed to comprehensive, patient-tailored rehabilitation [34,35], improving patient adherence, optimizing healthcare resources, and improving outcomes across a range of respiratory diseases through the speculative but practical integration of such multidisciplinary care across the board.

The COVID-19 pandemic has served as a strong catalyst for the development of early pulmonary rehabilitation strategies for hospitalized patients with acute respiratory failure. Recent studies consistently highlight multidisciplinary interventions as essential to improving chronic respiratory disease management outcomes. A multidisciplinary approach significantly enhances the quality of life and health outcomes for individuals with COPD [36]. The 2023 Global Initiative for Chronic Obstructive Lung Disease (GOLD) report emphasizes integrated multidisciplinary care as necessary for effective COPD management [17].

Based on the extensive clinical data collected during the pandemic, a structured model of pulmonary rehabilitation has emerged that has demonstrated significant benefits in improving functional outcomes, reducing disease progression, and improving overall quality of care. Given the similarities in pathophysiology and rehabilitation needs, this model may be applicable to other respiratory diseases, such as acute exacerbation of COPD, ARDS, or severe pneumonia.

This protocol can be broadly divided into three related phases. The initial stabilization phase focuses on ventilatory efficiency, and the prevention of complications related to immobility. Semi-orthopneic or sitting positions are recommended to improve the ventilation/perfusion ratio and pulmonary mechanics. In selected patients with refractory hypoxemia, prone positioning for at least four hours daily may further improve oxygenation, although careful monitoring of hemodynamic and cardiac status is essential during this intervention.

The pulmonary optimization phase focuses on airway clearance and lung recruitment strategies. Airway clearance therapy (ACT), including vibratory positive expiratory pressure and high-frequency chest wall oscillation, is indicated in the presence of rough crackles or high sputum burden, especially in the presence of bacterial coinfection. Respiratory resistance training using incentive spirometry is particularly beneficial in cases with radiological evidence of atelectasis or consolidation. Studies have shown that the inclusion of at least two different pulmonary rehabilitation interventions is associated with greater improvements in respiratory parameters and clinical outcomes [37].

Once respiratory and hemodynamic parameters have stabilized, the patient enters the mobilization and functional recovery phase, where early physical rehabilitation becomes central. Gradual progression from bed-based exercises to sitting, standing, and assisted ambulation forms the basis of this phase. Progressive resistance training, trunk control, and gait retraining are implemented with continuous clinical monitoring. Patients are also encouraged to perform simple activities of daily living, such as sitting up for meals and walking short distances, to increase autonomy and prevent ICU-acquired weakness. Patient safety must guide all phases of rehabilitation. Continuous monitoring of vital signs, especially oxygen saturation, heart rate, and blood pressure, is essential. In patients with cardiovascular comorbidities, baseline cardiac assessment is recommended to minimize the risk of adverse events during exercise. Any clinical deterioration should prompt immediate reassessment or cessation of the intervention.

Functional outcomes should be monitored using validated tools, while improvements in respiratory status can be assessed by changes in the PaO_2/FiO_2 ratio.

This structured model, developed during the COVID-19 pandemic, can provide a safe, flexible, and evidence-based framework for pulmonary rehabilitation. When applied within a multidisciplinary team, it can be effectively adapted to other acute respiratory conditions to enhance recovery, reduce disability, and improve patient outcomes.

The authors acknowledge that the retrospective nature of this study, the limited sample size, and the absence of a concurrent control group limit the ability to draw causal relationships. It is important to note that this evidence includes results from retrospective cohort studies, which have inherent limitations, such as potential selection bias and possibly unmeasured confounders. The findings align with existing literature supporting early multidisciplinary rehabilitation, but unmeasured confounders may have influenced the outcomes. These factors highlight the need for caution when interpreting the results as evidence of efficacy. The pandemic experience highlights significant challenges, including logistical constraints and limited resources, emphasizing the need for flexible and adaptable rehabilitation strategies broadly applicable across healthcare systems. Future research should focus on prospective randomized controlled trials on a large scale to validate the proposed rehabilitation model and to improve generalizability across various populations, assessing both clinical effectiveness and cost–benefit sustainability.

4. Conclusions

While the findings of this retrospective analysis highlight the potential benefits of early, structured, multidisciplinary rehabilitation in acute respiratory settings, they should consider the limitations. Nevertheless, the observed functional improvements and the feasibility of early intervention suggest that this model should be explored further in broader clinical contexts.

Integrating early rehabilitation into standard respiratory care pathways holds significant translational potential. However, generalizing this approach requires caution due to the heterogeneity of conditions such as COPD, IPF, and post-ARDS syndromes as well as variability in individual patient profiles. Meanwhile, careful implementation in well-resourced settings, with the right training and monitoring, could be a practical way to improve respiratory care.

Author Contributions: Conceptualization, A.T., A.A. and S.P.; methodology, F.B., D.B. and F.C.; software, D.B.; validation, F.C., G.S. and A.A.; formal analysis, D.B.; investigation, D.A., A.T. and S.P.; data curation, G.L.; writing—original draft preparation, A.A., G.L., G.S., D.A. and S.P.; writing—review and editing, F.B., D.B. and A.T.; visualization, G.S.; supervision, A.A. and S.P. All authors have read and agreed to the published version of the manuscript.

Funding: This study was supported by Current Research Funds 2025, Ministry of Health, Italy.

Institutional Review Board Statement: This study was conducted in accordance with the Declaration of Helsinki and approved by the Ethics Committee of Messina (protocol number 40-21 10 March 2021).

Informed Consent Statement: Informed consent was obtained from all subjects involved in this study.

Data Availability Statement: The data presented in this study are available within this article.

Conflicts of Interest: The authors declare no conflicts of interest.

Abbreviations

The following abbreviations are used in this manuscript:

SARS-CoV-2	Severe Acute Respiratory Syndrome Coronavirus 2
COVID-19	Coronavirus disease 2019
ARDS	Acute respiratory distress syndrome
ICU	Intensive care unit
COPD	Chronic obstructive pulmonary disease
IPF	Idiopathic pulmonary fibrosis
PICS	Post-intensive care syndrome
GOLD	Global Initiative for Chronic Obstructive Lung Disease

References

El Zowalaty, M.E.; Järhult, J.D. From SARS to COVID-19: A previously unknown SARS- related coronavirus (SARS-CoV-2) of pandemic potential infecting humans—Call for a One Health approach. *One Health* **2020**, *9*, 100124. [CrossRef] [PubMed]

Lai, C.C.; Shih, T.P.; Ko, W.C.; Tang, H.J.; Hsueh, P.R. Severe acute respiratory syndrome coronavirus 2 (SARS-CoV-2) and coronavirus disease-2019 (COVID-19): The epidemic and the challenges. *Int. J. Antimicrob. Agents* **2020**, *55*, 105924. [CrossRef]

Carta, M.; Orrù, G.; Littera, R.; Firinu, D.; Chessa, L.; Cossu, G.; Del Giacco, S.; Tramontano, E.; Manocchio, N.; Buonomo, C.; et al. Comparing the responses of countries and National Health Systems to the COVID-19 pandemic- a critical analysis with a case-report series. *Eur. Rev. Med. Pharmacol. Sci.* **2023**, *27*, 7868–7880. [CrossRef]

Asselah, T.; Durantel, D.; Pasmant, E.; Lau, G.; Schinazi, R.F. COVID-19: Discovery, diagnostics and drug development. *J. Hepatol.* **2021**, *74*, 168–184. [CrossRef]

Yang, X.; Yu, Y.; Xu, J.; Shu, H.; Xia, J.; Liu, H.; Wu, Y.; Zhang, L.; Yu, Z.; Fang, M.; et al. Clinical course and outcomes of critically ill patients with SARS-CoV-2 pneumonia in Wuhan, China: A single-centered, retrospective, observational study. *Lancet Respir. Med.* **2020**, *8*, 475–481. [CrossRef]

Bangash, M.N.; Patel, J.; Parekh, D. COVID-19 and the liver: Little cause for concern. *Lancet Gastroenterol. Hepatol.* **2020**, *5*, 529–530. [CrossRef]

Driggin, E.; Madhavan, M.V.; Bikdeli, B.; Chuich, T.; Laracy, J.; Biondi-Zoccai, G.; Brown, T.S.; Der Nigoghossian, C.; Zidar, D.A.; Haythe, J.; et al. Cardiovascular Considerations for Patients, Health Care Workers, and Health Systems During the COVID-19 Pandemic. *J. Am. Coll. Cardiol.* **2020**, *75*, 2352–2371. [CrossRef]

Bellone, F.; Gaudio, A.; Bellone, I.G.; Stagno, A.; Catalano, A. An unusual bilateral groin pain after COVID-19 infection in an 82-year-old man. *Intern. Emerg. Med.* **2023**, *18*, 1217–1219. [CrossRef]

Brugliera, L.; Spina, A.; Castellazzi, P.; Cimino, P.; Tettamanti, A.; Houdayer, E.; Arcuri, P.; Alemanno, F.; Mortini, P.; Iannaccone, S. Rehabilitation of COVID-19 patients. *J. Rehabil. Med.* **2020**, *52*, jrm00046. [CrossRef]

10. Chang, R.; Elhusseiny, K.M.; Yeh, Y.C.; Sun, W.Z. COVID-19 ICU and mechanical ventilation patient characteristics and outcomes- A systematic review and meta-analysis. *PLoS ONE* **2021**, *16*, e0246318. [CrossRef]
11. Cavallaro, F.; Portaro, S.; Pintaudi, T.; Ceccio, M.; Alito, A. Remote Cognitive Therapeutic Exercise in Facial Nerve Palsy Rehabilitation: Pandemic Tips and Tricks. *Innov. Clin. Neurosci.* **2023**, *20*, 10–12. [PubMed]
12. Hodgson, C.L.; Stiller, K.; Needham, D.M.; Tipping, C.J.; Harrold, M.; Baldwin, C.E.; Bradley, S.; Berney, S.; Caruana, L.R.; Elliott, D.; et al. Expert consensus and recommendations on safety criteria for active mobilization of mechanically ventilated critically ill adults. *Crit. Care* **2014**, *18*, 658. [CrossRef]
13. Wang, E.; Liu, A.; Wang, Z.; Shang, X.; Zhang, L.; Jin, Y.; Ma, Y.; Zhang, L.; Bai, T.; Song, J.; et al. The prognostic value of the Barthel Index for mortality in patients with COVID-19: A cross-sectional study. *Front. Public Health* **2022**, *10*, 978237. [CrossRef]
14. Chen, D.; Curtis, J.L.; Chen, Y. Twenty years of changes in the definition of early chronic obstructive pulmonary disease. *Chin. Med. J. Pulm. Crit. Care Med.* **2023**, *1*, 84–93. [CrossRef]
15. Troosters, T.; Janssens, W.; Demeyer, H.; Rabinovich, R.A. Pulmonary rehabilitation and physical interventions. *Eur. Respir. Rev.* **2023**, *32*, 220222. [CrossRef]
16. Jenkins, A.; Burtin, C.; Camp, P.; Lindenauer, P.; Carlin, B.; Alison, J.; Rochester, C.; Holland, A. Do pulmonary rehabilitation programmes improve outcomes in patients with COPD posthospital discharge for exacerbation: A systematic review and meta-analysis. *Thorax* **2024**, *79*, 2023. [CrossRef]
17. Agustí, A.; Celli, B.R.; Criner, G.J.; Halpin, D.; Anzueto, A.; Barnes, P.; Bourbeau, J.; Han, M.K.; Martinez, F.J.; Montes de Oca, M.; et al. Global Initiative for Chronic Obstructive Lung Disease 2023 Report: GOLD Executive Summary. *Am. J. Respir. Crit. Care Med.* **2023**, *207*, 819–837. [CrossRef]
18. Nair, S.P.; Augustine, A.; Panchabhai, C.; Patil, S.; Parmar, K.; Panhale, V.P. Safety and feasibility of pulmonary rehabilitation in patients hospitalized with post-COVID-19 fibrosis: A feasibility study. *PM&R* **2024**, *16*, 848–855. [CrossRef]

19. Wang, X.; Ma, H.; He, X.; Gu, X.; Ren, Y.; Yang, H.; Tong, Z. Efficacy of early pulmonary rehabilitation in severe and critically il COVID-19 patients: A retrospective cohort study. *BMC Pulm. Med.* **2025**, *25*, 203. [CrossRef]
20. Carvalho, A.C.; Moreira, J.; Cubelo, P.; Cantista, P.; Aguiar Branco, C.; Guimarães, B. Multidisciplinary rehabilitation in intensiv care for COVID-19: Randomised controlled trial. *ERJ Open Res.* **2023**, *9*, 00350–2022. [CrossRef]
21. Khwaja, S.A., Sr.; Habib, M.A.; Gupta, R.; Singla, D.; Basista, R. Implementing Early Rehabilitation Strategies for Chroni Obstructive Pulmonary Disease (COPD) Patients Undergoing Mechanical Ventilation in the Intensive Care Unit. *Cureus* **2024** *16*, e72847. [CrossRef]
22. Weigl, M.; Beeck, S.; Kraft, E.; Stubbe, H.C.; Adorjan, K.; Ruzicka, M.; Lemhöfer, C. Multidisciplinary rehabilitation with a focu on physiotherapy in patients with Post Covid19 condition: An observational pilot study. *Eur. Arch. Psychiatry Clin. Neurosci.* **2024** *274*, 2003–2014. [CrossRef]
23. Curci, C.; Pisano, F.; Bonacci, E.; Camozzi, D.M.; Ceravolo, C.; Bergonzi, R.; De Franceschi, S.; Moro, P.; Guarnieri, R.; Ferrillo, M et al. Early rehabilitation in post-acute COVID-19 patients: Data from an Italian COVID-19 Rehabilitation Unit and proposal of a treatment protocol. *Eur. J. Phys. Rehabil. Med.* **2020**, *56*, 633–641. [CrossRef]
24. Green, M.; Marzano, V.; Leditschke, I.A.; Mitchell, I.; Bissett, B. Mobilization of intensive care patients: A multidisciplinary practical guide for clinicians. *J. Multidiscip. Healthc.* **2016**, *9*, 247–256. [CrossRef]
25. Thomas, P.; Baldwin, C.; Bissett, B.; Boden, I.; Gosselink, R.; Granger, C.L.; Hodgson, C.; Jones, A.Y.; Kho, M.E.; Moses, R.; et al. Physiotherapy management for COVID-19 in the acute hospital setting: Clinical practice recommendations. *J. Physiother.* **2020**, *66* 73–82. [CrossRef]
26. Zang, K.; Chen, B.; Wang, M.; Chen, D.; Hui, L.; Guo, S.; Ji, T.; Shang, F. The effect of early mobilization in critically ill patients: A meta-analysis. *Nurs. Crit. Care* **2020**, *25*, 360–367. [CrossRef]
27. Corrao, S.; Nobili, A.; Natoli, G.; Mannucci, P.M.; Perticone, F.; Pietrangelo, A.; Argano, C. Hyperglycemia at admission comorbidities, and in-hospital mortality in elderly patients hospitalized in internal medicine wards: Data from the RePoS Registry. *Acta Diabetol.* **2021**, *58*, 1225–1236. [CrossRef]
28. Yu, P.; Wei, Q.; He, C. Early Rehabilitation for Critically Ill Patients With COVID-19: More Benefits Than Risks. *Am. J. Phys. Med Rehabil.* **2020**, *99*, 468–469. [CrossRef]
29. Pfoh, E.R.; Wozniak, A.W.; Colantuoni, E.; Dinglas, V.D.; Mendez-Tellez, P.A.; Shanholtz, C.; Ciesla, N.D.; Pronovost, P.J. Needham, D.M. Physical declines occurring after hospital discharge in ARDS survivors: A 5-year longitudinal study. *Intensive Care Med.* **2016**, *42*, 1557–1566. [CrossRef]
30. Cox, N.S.; Bondarenko, J.; Chong, M.; Marceu, T.; Perryman, J.; Holland, A.E. Rapid real-world implementation of pulmonary telerehabilitation: Good fortune or COVID-19 luck? *ERJ Open Res.* **2024**, *10*, 00820–02023. [CrossRef]
31. Reis, N.; Costa Dias, M.J.; Sousa, L.; Canedo, F.; Rico, M.T.; Henriques, M.A.; Baixinho, C.L. Telerehabilitation Intervention in Transitional Care for People with COVID-19: Pre-Post Study with a Non-Equivalent Control Group. *Healthcare* **2023**, *11*, 2561 [CrossRef] [PubMed]
32. Yang, J.; Li, H.; Zhao, H.; Xie, Y.; Li, J.; Wang, M. Effectiveness of telerehabilitation in patients with post-COVID-19: A systemati review and meta-analysis of randomised controlled trials. *BMJ Open* **2024**, *14*, e074325. [CrossRef] [PubMed]
33. Spruit, M.A.; Singh, S.J.; Garvey, C.; ZuWallack, R.; Nici, L.; Rochester, C.; Hill, K.; Holland, A.E.; Lareau, S.C.; Man, W.D. et al. An official American Thoracic Society/European Respiratory Society statement: Key concepts and advances in pulmonary rehabilitation. *Am. J. Respir. Crit. Care Med.* **2013**, *188*, e13–e64. [CrossRef]
34. Chuang, H.J.; Hsiao, M.Y.; Wang, T.G.; Liang, H.W. A multi-disciplinary rehabilitation approach for people surviving severe COVID-19—A case series and literature review. *J. Formos. Med. Assoc.* **2022**, *121*, 2408–2415. [CrossRef]
35. Fontana, J.M.; Alito, A.; Piterà, P.; Verme, F.; Cattaldo, S.; Cornacchia, M.; Mai, S.; Brunani, A.; Capodaglio, P. Whole-Body Cryostimulation in Post-COVID Rehabilitation for Patients with Obesity: A Multidisciplinary Feasibility Study. *Biomedicines* **2023** *11*, 3092. [CrossRef]
36. Hekking, P.P.; van Meggelen, M.; Lie, W.J.; Hoek, R.A.S.; van Ranst, D.; van der Kleij, S.C.J.; Seghers, L.; Kappen, J.; Braunstahl G.J.; In 't Veen, J. Severe COPD: Multidisciplinary Consultation to Get the Right Care at the Right Place. *Int. J. Chron. Obstruct Pulm. Dis.* **2024**, *19*, 749–752. [CrossRef]
37. Zhang, H.; Hu, D.; Xu, Y.; Wu, L.; Lou, L. Effect of pulmonary rehabilitation in patients with chronic obstructive pulmonary disease: A systematic review and meta-analysis of randomized controlled trials. *Ann. Med.* **2022**, *54*, 262–273. [CrossRef]

MDPI AG
Grosspeteranlage 5
4052 Basel
Switzerland
Tel.: +41 61 683 77 34

Journal of Clinical Medicine Editorial Office
E-mail: jcm@mdpi.com
www.mdpi.com/journal/jcm

www.ingramcontent.com/pod-product-compliance
Lightning Source LLC
LaVergne TN
LVHW070538071126
851858LV00011BA/200
* 9 7 8 3 7 2 5 8 8 2 7 5 5 *

New Advances and Perspectives in Ophthalmology: Progress and Modern Challenges

New Advances and Perspectives in Ophthalmology: Progress and Modern Challenges

Guest Editor

Livio Vitiello

MDPI

Basel • Beijing • Wuhan • Barcelona • Belgrade • Novi Sad • Cluj • Manchester

Guest Editor
Livio Vitiello
Eye Unit, "Luigi Curto" Hospital
Azienda Sanitaria Locale Salerno
Polla
Italy

Editorial Office
MDPI AG
Grosspeteranlage 5
4052 Basel, Switzerland

This is a reprint of the Special Issue, published open access by the journal *Journal of Personalized Medicine* (ISSN 2075-4426), freely accessible at: https://www.mdpi.com/journal/jpm/special_issues/L47SKVR7OM.

For citation purposes, cite each article independently as indicated on the article page online and as indicated below:

Lastname, A.A.; Lastname, B.B. Article Title. *Journal Name* **Year**, *Volume Number*, Page Range.

ISBN 978-3-7258-8333-2 (Hbk)
ISBN 978-3-7258-8334-9 (PDF)
https://doi.org/10.3390/books978-3-7258-8334-9

Contents

About the Editor

Livio Vitiello

Livio Vitiello is a general ophthalmologist affiliated with the Eye Unit of "Luigi Curto" Hospital (Azienda Sanitaria Locale Salerno, Polla, Italy). His clinical and research interests relate to medical retina, with particular emphasis on macular diseases and ocular ultrasound. He is currently completing a Master's degree in posterior segment imaging of the eye at the "Cattolica del Sacro Cuore" University in Rome.

Journal of
Personalized Medicine

MDPI

torial

ew Advances and Perspectives in Ophthalmology: Progress ıd Modern Challenges Toward Personalized Eye Care

io Vitiello

Eye Unit, "Luigi Curto" Hospital, Azienda Sanitaria Locale Salerno, 84035 Polla, Italy; livio.vitiello@gmail.com

1. Recent Developments in Ophthalmology

Over the past two decades, ophthalmology has been reshaped by the convergence of high-resolution multimodal imaging, pharmacological innovation and the broader paradigm of personalized medicine. Swept-source optical coherence tomography (OCT), OCT angiography, ultra-widefield retinal imaging and high-frequency ocular ultrasound now enable in vivo, micrometer-scale phenotyping of virtually every ocular structure [1], while artificial intelligence (AI) and deep learning turn these imaging outputs into quantitative biomarkers suitable for automated risk stratification [2,3]. In parallel, the therapeutic armamentarium has expanded from intravitreal anti-VEGF biologics—now available in longer-acting formulations and individualized treat-and-extend regimens [4]—to gene and cell therapies for inherited retinal dystrophies [5,6], and to increasingly refined cataract, refractive and oculoplastic platforms. Underlying these advances is a conceptual shift: ophthalmic diseases are no longer treated as homogeneous entities, but rather as heterogeneous clusters of phenotypes, each with their own risk profiles and optimal management.

2. Knowledge Gaps Addressed by This Special Issue

Despite this progress, several important gaps remain: real-world long-term data on individualized anti-VEGF regimens are still limited; ROP screening is inequitably distributed and logistically demanding; AI-based screening tools often lack prospective validation and safe-failure mechanisms [7]; IOL calculation remains problematic in post-refractive eyes [8]; predictors of surgical success in strabismus are poorly standardized; postural and dynamic components of intraocular pressure (IOP) are rarely integrated into routine glaucoma risk assessment; ocular imaging biomarkers of systemic disease are still being defined [9]; subclinical dysfunction in "inactive" orbitopathy is underdiagnosed; and the nutritional management of age-related macular degeneration (AMD) has evolved beyond the original AREDS framework without a consensus on individualized protocols. The sixteen contributions collected in this Special Issue directly address these gaps and sketch a coherent roadmap toward more personalized ophthalmic care.

3. Key Findings and Contributions

3.1. Retinal Vascular Disease and Anti-VEGF Personalization

Diabetic retinopathy (DR) remains a paradigmatic setting for personalized medicine. Zhou et al. (contribution 1) report 1-year outcomes of the VOYAGE extension study: in patients who had completed the PANORAMA trial and received 2 mg intravitreal aflibercept every 16 weeks as needed, less frequent dosing between PANORAMA exit and VOYAGE enrollment was associated with a measurable deterioration of the Diabetic Retinopathy Severity Scale score, best-corrected visual acuity and central subfield thickness, which subsequently stabilized or improved once regular, individualized treatment resumed. These findings are real-world evidence that anti-VEGF schedules must be tailored to ongoing disease activity. Ivanescu et al. (contribution 2) profiled 105 patients with type 1 or type 2 diabetes (77 with diabetic macular edema) in Western Romania, describing a high-risk cohort with median age 65 years, 15-year mean disease duration, HbA1c 7.5% and universal comorbidities (hypertension 100%, dyslipidemia 62.3%)—reinforcing the need for screening pathways integrated with systemic risk stratification.

3.2. Retinopathy of Prematurity: From Universal Screening to Tailored Pathways

Two complementary studies address retinopathy of prematurity. Christodoulou et al. (contribution 3) evaluated incidence, treatment patterns and risk factors for type 1 ROP in a national tertiary NICU in Cyprus, translating local epidemiology into a personalized screening-to-therapy pathway. Al-Abaiji et al. (contribution 4) demonstrated the feasibility of telescreening in Denmark using the ICON GO® widefield camera operated by a non-physician healthcare professional: across 415 sessions in 165 neonates, on-site/off-site agreement was almost perfect for overall outcome ($\kappa = 0.82$) and substantial for stage and disease ($\kappa = 0.69$), with treatment needed in 3.6% of children. These findings provide evidence that delegated, tele-supported screening is safe, scalable, and a concrete step toward equitable neonatal care.

3.3. Artificial Intelligence and Glaucoma Screening

Hitzl et al. (contribution 5) leveraged a longitudinal dataset of 6889 subjects, with 585 completing an average 11.1-year follow-up period, to train two neural-network models equipped with a "reject option" that allows the algorithm to withhold a prediction in ambiguous cases. The clinical and economic rationale is to identify, already at baseline, the large proportion of screened individuals who remain free of open-angle glaucoma for up to 10 years and can therefore safely be excluded from intensive monitoring—a concrete translation of precision screening into everyday practice.

3.4. Precision in Refractive, Cataract and Strabismus Surgery

Tailored surgical planning is the focus of two studies. Lin et al. (contribution 6) compared the calibration accuracy of the Symfony extended depth-of-focus (EDOF) intraocular lens in eyes with and without previous LASIK, combining optical biometry with the SRK/T formula in non-LASIK eyes and Haigis-L in post-LASIK eyes—a clinically actionable framework for IOL power selection in complex refractive histories. Lino, de Aguiar and Cunha (contribution 7) retrospectively analyzed 258 children (mean age 11.2 years) with basic-type intermittent exotropia or divergence excess who underwent bilateral lateral rectus recession, identifying pre-operative predictors of post-operative alignment stability and refining the individualized surgical dosing needed to improve on the historical ~75% success rate.

3.5. Intraocular Pressure, Biometrics and Glaucoma Biomechanics

De Bernardo et al. (contribution 8) measured IOP across sitting, supine, prone and standing postures in 124 eyes of 62 healthy subjects: the prone–supine differential was the largest (+2.24 mmHg; $p < 0.001$), followed by supine–sitting (+1.30 mmHg), while standing produced a significant IOP decrease relative to supine (−1.43 mmHg). Such postural profiles, which a single in-office measurement cannot capture, argue for a more individualized interpretation of IOP in selected glaucoma suspects. Gioia et al. (contribution 9) correlated the corrected axial length—a refinement addressing the systematic biometric error of cataractous eyes—with choroidal thickness, refining the quantitative framework for myopic and degenerative risk stratification.

https://doi.org/10.3390/jpm160603

3.6. Imaging Biomarkers and the Ocular–Systemic Interface

Three contributions use imaging biomarkers as windows onto systemic disease. Isleyen et al. (contribution 10) applied swept-source OCT to 67 patients with vasovagal syncope versus 61 controls, demonstrating a significantly thicker choroid in affected subjects without changes in peripapillary retinal nerve fiber layer (RNFL), showing that the choroidal vasculature is sensitive to autonomic dysregulation. Lixi et al. (contribution 11) reviewed the spectrum of ocular manifestations of patent foramen ovale, from transient visual disturbances and migraine with aura to oculomotor deficits and rare endogenous endophthalmitis from paradoxical embolism, reinforcing the need for a multidisciplinary ophthalmology–cardiology–neurology pathway. In 67 patients with inactive Graves' orbitopathy, Lixi, Giannaccare and co-authors (contribution 12) combined orbital ultrasound with the Red Filter Test and detected latent diplopia in 49.25% of subjects despite no reported double vision—a strong case for sensitivity-based reassessment in a disease too often labeled "burnt out".

3.7. Genomics and Precision Medicine in Inherited Retinal Disease

Two contributions address the genomic frontier of personalized ophthalmology. Dhivagaran et al. (contribution 13) provide a comprehensive review of precision medicine in inherited retinal diseases (IRDs), tracing the evolution from clinical phenotyping to next-generation sequencing (NGS)-based diagnostics and mutation-specific therapies. The review details how NGS has transformed the diagnostic landscape by enabling precise identification of causative variants across the more than 300 genes implicated in IRDs, and examines the patient-selection protocols—integrating genetic confirmation, structural retinal evaluation and genetic counseling—that underpin targeted interventions such as voretigene neparvovec (Luxturna) for RPE65-related disease. The authors also map the remaining barriers to broader adoption: high costs, uneven access to specialist services, and the interpretive complexity of variants of uncertain significance. Bakhamees et al. (contribution 14) complement this perspective with a cross-sectional survey of 115 ophthalmologists across Saudi Arabia, assessing knowledge, attitudes and practices toward genomic medicine. While 99% correctly recognized autosomal recessive inheritance and 90% endorsed the clinical value of genetic testing, confidence in practical tasks such as test selection and pre-test counselling was low (mean 4.7/10), and only 9% answered DNA base-pairing questions correctly. Taken together, these two contributions delineate a critical gap between the rapid maturation of genomic tools and the readiness of the clinical workforce to deploy them—and underscore the urgency of integrating genetics into ophthalmology training programs.

3.8. Diagnostic Imaging and Tailored Medical Therapy

Two narrative reviews complete this Special Issue. Coppola et al. (contribution 15) synthesized the literature on ocular ultrasound for optic neuropathies, emphasizing its bedside availability and particular value in patients unable to undergo magnetic resonance imaging, while acknowledging the methodological heterogeneity that still characterizes the field [10–12]. D'Angelo et al. (contribution 16) reviewed the evolving evidence on oral supplementation in AMD—the third leading cause of global visual impairment—mapping the interplay between oxidative stress, neuroinflammation and ocular ischemia, and discussing AREDS-based formulations alongside emerging compounds such as astaxanthin and melatonin. Their synthesis supports the move from one-size-fits-all supplementation toward individualized antioxidant strategies.

https://doi.org/10.3390/jpm16060333

4. Future Research Directions

The contributions collected here open several avenues that will shape the next phase of personalized ophthalmology. First, imaging biomarkers—from choroidal thickness and RNFL to corrected axial length and extraocular muscle measurements—need cross-platform standardization, with consensus on acquisition protocols, reference ranges and reproducibility thresholds, before they can reliably guide individual decisions. Second, machine learning models should undergo prospective, multicenter validation in ethnically and demographically heterogeneous populations, ideally with confidence-aware outputs and human-in-the-loop oversight. Third, the integration of telemedicine, AI and portable imaging must be evaluated not only for diagnostic accuracy but also for cost-effectiveness and equity of access, particularly in vulnerable populations. Fourth, evidence on postural IOP, subclinical ocular motility dysfunction and ocular signs of systemic disease calls for the systematic integration of ophthalmology into cardio-, neuro- and endocrine-ophthalmology pathways. Fifth, pharmacological and nutritional management should move beyond population-average recommendations toward genotype-, phenotype- and biomarker-guided regimens for anti-VEGF therapy in DR/DME, IOL selection in complex refractive histories and antioxidant supplementation in AMD. Finally, patient-reported outcomes and adherence metrics must be prospectively incorporated into personalized protocols, so that success is defined not only by anatomical and functional endpoints but also by what matters most to patients.

5. Concluding Remarks

Collectively, the sixteen contributions in this Special Issue trace a coherent trajectory for contemporary ophthalmology: broader and earlier screening underpinned by telemedicine and AI; finer phenotyping supported by multimodal imaging and advanced biometrics; and more individualized therapeutic choices, from anti-VEGF regimens and IOL calculations to surgical dosing and antioxidant supplementation. The work presented here offers concrete building blocks for a genuinely personalized ophthalmic practice—and a clear agenda for the studies that will follow.

Funding: This research received no external funding.

Acknowledgments: As Guest Editor, I am grateful to all the authors who contributed their high-quality work, to the reviewers whose rigor sustains the scientific standards of the *Journal of Personalized Medicine*, and to the editorial staff for their constant support throughout the preparation of this Special Issue.

Conflicts of Interest: The author declares no conflicts of interest.

List of Contributions:

1. Zhou, A.W.; Teagle, G.M.; Baumann, L.M.; Cao, J.A.; Emanuelli, A.; Hu, A.Y.; Berger, A.S.; Major, J.C., Jr.; Lee, S.Y.; Huddleston, S.M.; et al. Intravitreal Aflibercept for the Treatment of Diabetic Retinopathy Among Patients Who Completed PANORAMA: 1-Year Outcomes from the VOYAGE Extension Study. *J. Pers. Med.* **2025**, *15*, 555. https://doi.org/10.3390/jpm15110555.
2. Ivanescu, A.; Popescu, S.; Roman, D.; Dragomir, M.; Timar, R. Diabetic Macular Edema in the Western Part of Romania: Screening to Improve Patient Outcomes. *J. Pers. Med.* **2025**, *15*, 106. https://doi.org/10.3390/jpm15030106.
3. Christodoulou, S.; Herodotou, F.; Quattrocchi, A.; Potamitis, T.; Choleva, V. From Screening to Therapy: A Personalized Approach to ROP in a National NICU Setting. *J. Pers. Med.* **2025**, *15*, 388. https://doi.org/10.3390/jpm15080388.

4. Al-Abaiji, H.A.; Bangsgaard, R.; Kofod, M.; Faber, C.; Larsen, A.-C.; Brost, A.G.; Slidsborg, C.; Klemp, K.; Breindahl, M.; la Cour, M.D.d.; et al. Evaluating the Feasibility of a Telescreening Program for Retinopathy of Prematurity (ROP) in Denmark. *J. Pers. Med.* **2024**, *14*, 1020. https://doi.org/10.3390/jpm14101020.
5. Hitzl, W.; Lenzhofer, M.; Hohensinn, M.; Reitsamer, H.A. Two Machine Learning Models to Economize Glaucoma Screening Programs: An Approach Based on Neural Nets. *J. Pers. Med.* **2025**, *15*, 361. https://doi.org/10.3390/jpm15080361.
6. Lin, I.-H.; Chao, C.-C.; Chang, C.-K. Effect of Prior Laser-Assisted In Situ Keratomileusis on the Calibration Accuracy of Extended Depth of Focus Intraocular Lenses: A Direct Comparative Study. *J. Pers. Med.* **2025**, *15*, 301. https://doi.org/10.3390/jpm15070301.
7. Lino, P.; de Aguiar, P.V.; Cunha, J.P. Success of Strabismus Surgery in Intermittent Exotropia. *J. Pers. Med.* **2025**, *15*, 333. https://doi.org/10.3390/jpm15080333.
8. De Bernardo, M.; Cione, F.; De Pascale, I.; Pagliarulo, S.; Rosa, N. Intraocular Pressure Measurements in Standing, Sitting, Prone, and Supine Positions. *J. Pers. Med.* **2024**, *14*, 826. https://doi.org/10.3390/jpm14080826.
9. Gioia, M.; De Bernardo, M.; Cione, F.; De Luca, M.; Rosa, N. Corrected Axial Length and Choroidal Thickness: A Correlation Analysis for Scientific Purposes. *J. Pers. Med.* **2025**, *15*, 15. https://doi.org/10.3390/jpm15010015.
10. Isleyen, H.B.; Kanar, B.G.; Akcay, G.; Demir, S.; Kanar, H.S.; Yazicioglu, M.V. Evaluation of the Choroidal Thickness and Retinal Nerve Fiber Layer Thickness in Patients with Vasovagal Syncope. *J. Pers. Med.* **2025**, *15*, 259. https://doi.org/10.3390/jpm15060259.
11. Lixi, F.; Cuccu, A.; Giannaccare, G.; Onnis, M.; Timofte Zorila, M.M.; Mariotti, S.; Vacca, R.; Meloni, P.E.; Pisu, M.; Mura, C.; et al. Subclinical Ocular Motility Dysfunction and Extraocular Muscle Changes in Inactive Graves' Orbitopathy. *J. Pers. Med.* **2024**, *14*, 848. https://doi.org/10.3390/jpm14080848.
12. Lixi, F.; Fazzini, L.; Cannas, C.; Montisci, R.; Giannaccare, G. Ocular Manifestations and Complications of Patent Foramen Ovale: A Narrative Review. *J. Pers. Med.* **2024**, *14*, 695. https://doi.org/10.3390/jpm14070695.
13. Dhivagaran, T.; Butt, F.R.; Grover, K.; Devgan, K.; Sachdeva, K.; Dhivagaran, V.; Abid, F.; Tao, B.K.; Balas, M.; Dimopoulos, I.; et al. Precision Medicine in Inherited Retinal Disease: Advances, Challenges, and Future Directions. *J. Pers. Med.* **2026**, *16*, 292. https://doi.org/10.3390/jpm16060292.
14. Bakhamees, W.; Alsafran, H.; ALBalawi, H.B.; Alali, N.M.; Alotaibi, Y.A.; Magliyah, M.S. Genomic Medicine Among Ophthalmologists: Knowledge, Current Practice, and Barriers. *J. Pers. Med.* **2026**, *16*, 267. https://doi.org/10.3390/jpm16050267.
15. Coppola, A.; Abbinante, G.; De Pascale, I.; Gagliardi, V.; Salerno, G.; Pellegrino, A.; Vitiello, L. Ocular Ultrasound in the Diagnosis of Optic Neuropathies: A Review of the Literature. *J. Pers. Med.* **2024**, *14*, 949. https://doi.org/10.3390/jpm14090949.
16. D'Angelo, A.; Vitiello, L.; Gagliardi, V.; Salerno, G.; De Pascale, I.; Coppola, A.; Abbinante, G.; Pellegrino, A.; Giannaccare, G. The Role of Oral Supplementation for the Management of Age-Related Macular Degeneration: A Narrative Review. *J. Pers. Med.* **2024**, *14*, 653. https://doi.org/10.3390/jpm14060653.

eferences

Wong, Q.Y.; Sim, R.; Ang, M. Anterior Segment Optical Coherence Tomography with Angiography for the Cornea and Ocular Surface. *J. Clin. Med.* **2026**, *15*, 2402. [CrossRef] [PubMed]

Parravano, M.; Cennamo, G.; Di Antonio, L.; Grassi, M.O.; Lupidi, M.; Rispoli, M.; Savastano, M.C.; Veritti, D.; Vujosevic, S. Multimodal imaging in diabetic retinopathy and macular edema: An update about biomarkers. *Surv. Ophthalmol.* **2024**, *69*, 893–904. [CrossRef] [PubMed]

Rispoli, M.; Cennamo, G.; Antonio, L.D.; Lupidi, M.; Parravano, M.; Pellegrini, M.; Veritti, D.; Vujosevic, S.; Savastano, M.C. Practical guidance for imaging biomarkers in exudative age-related macular degeneration. *Surv. Ophthalmol.* **2023**, *68*, 615–627. [CrossRef] [PubMed]

https://doi.org/10.3390/jpm16060333

4. Menna, F.; De Luca, L.; Meduri, A.; Baldascino, A.; Lupo, S.; Vingolo, E.M. New Clinical Trials and Therapeutic Advanc with Faricimab and Aflibercept 8 mg in Neovascular Age-Related Macular Degeneration: A Durability-Oriented Comparativ Perspective. *Biomedicines* **2026**, *14*, 773. [CrossRef] [PubMed]
5. Ekemiri, K.; Daniel, E.; Seemongal-Dass, R.; Ekemiri, C.; Victor, V.; Amobi, M.; Adebo, O.; Tekalign, T. Advanced therapeut approaches for inherited retinal diseases: An umbrella review. *BMJ Open* **2026**, *16*, e102647. [CrossRef] [PubMed]
6. Britten-Jones, A.C.; Jin, R.; Gocuk, S.A.; Cichello, E.; O'Hare, F.; Hickey, D.G.; Edwards, T.L.; Ayton, L.N. The safety and efficac of gene therapy treatment for monogenic retinal and optic nerve diseases: A systematic review. *Genet. Med.* **2022**, *24*, 521–53 [CrossRef] [PubMed]
7. Savastano, M.C.; Rizzo, C.; Fossataro, C.; Bacherini, D.; Giansanti, F.; Savastano, A.; Arcuri, G.; Rizzo, S.; Faraldi, F. Artifici intelligence in ophthalmology: Progress, challenges, and ethical implications. *Prog. Retin. Eye Res.* **2025**, *107*, 101374. [CrossRe [PubMed]
8. Cione, F.; De Bernardo, M.; Di Stasi, M.; De Luca, M.; Albano, R.; Rosa, N. Lens Factor Choice in IOL Power Calculation aft Laser Refractive Surgery: The Right Constant for Advanced Lens Measurement Approach (ALMA). *J. Clin. Med.* **2024**, *13*, 518 [CrossRef] [PubMed]
9. Crincoli, E.; Savastano, M.C.; Savastano, A.; Carlà, M.M.; Giannuzzi, F.; Catania, F.; Kilian, R.; Rizzo, C.; Rizzo, S. Artifici intelligence and neurodegeneration: State of the art and explainability. *Int. J. Retin. Vitr.* **2026**. [CrossRef] [PubMed]
10. De Bernardo, M.; Vitiello, L.; Rosa, N. A-scan ultrasonography and optic nerve sheath diameter assessment during acu elevations in intra-abdominal pressure. *Surgery* **2020**, *167*, 1023–1024. [CrossRef] [PubMed]
11. De Bernardo, M.; Vitiello, L.; Capone, M.; Rosa, N. A-scan ultrasonography and optic nerve sheath diameter evaluation i children with acute liver failure. *Liver Int.* **2020**, *40*, 1504. [CrossRef] [PubMed]
12. De Bernardo, M.; Vitiello, L.; Rosa, N. Optic nerve sheath diameter ultrasonography in differentiation of ischemic and hemorrhag strokes. *Am. J. Emerg. Med.* **2019**, *37*, 1384–1385. [CrossRef] [PubMed]

https://doi.org/10.3390/jpm160603

Journal of
Personalized Medicine

MDPI

view

recision Medicine in Inherited Retinal Disease: Advances, hallenges, and Future Directions

** anansayan Dhivagaran [1,†], Fahad R. Butt [1,†], Krystal Grover [2], Krish Devgan [2], Kyran Sachdeva [3], rounan Dhivagaran [4], Fatima Abid [5], Brendan K. Tao [6], Michael Balas [6], Ioannis Dimopoulos [7] and Adil Bhatti [7,*]**

1 Schulich School of Medicine & Dentistry, University of Western Ontario, London, ON N6A 5C1, Canada
2 Faculty of Health Sciences, McMaster University, Hamilton, ON L8S 4L8, Canada
3 Faculty of Medicine, University of Ottawa, Ottawa, ON K1H 8M5, Canada
4 Faculty of Sciences, McMaster University, Hamilton, ON L8S 4K1, Canada
5 Faculty of Science, Toronto Metropolitan University, Toronto, ON M5B 2K3, Canada
6 Department of Ophthalmology & Vision Sciences, University of Toronto, Toronto, ON M4N 3M5, Canada
7 Department of Ophthalmology, University of Ottawa, Ottawa, ON K1H 1C4, Canada
* Correspondence: abhatti@toh.ca
† These authors contributed equally to this work.

Abstract

Background/Objectives: Inherited retinal diseases (IRDs) represent a group of rare conditions characterized by significant clinical and genetic heterogeneity. Historically, the diagnosis of these conditions relied primarily on clinical presentation and imaging techniques. This literature review aims to discuss the current state of progress and ongoing challenges in applying precision medicine approaches to IRDs and to examine how advances in genetic testing have transformed diagnostics and opened new therapeutic avenues. **Methods**: This review examines the application of genetic testing methods to IRDs, with particular focus on next-generation sequencing (NGS) technologies. The review also evaluates current patient selection protocols that combine genetic confirmation, retinal structural evaluation, and detailed genetic counselling to achieve optimal therapeutic outcomes. **Results**: The implementation of NGS has significantly enhanced diagnostic capabilities for IRDs by enabling precise identification of specific genetic mutations. This advancement has paved the way for targeted therapeutic strategies, exemplified by Luxturna for RPE65-related IRDs. However, several barriers to broader adoption of precision medicine persist, including high costs, varied access to services, and complexities in interpreting genetic variants. **Conclusions**: While the continued development of innovative therapeutic modalities offers promise for expanding treatment options for IRDs, fully harnessing the potential of current and emerging therapeutic technologies requires addressing existing economic, technological, educational, and infrastructural challenges.

Keywords: precision medicine; inherited retinal diseases gene therapies; retina

1. Introduction

Inherited retinal diseases (IRDs) are a group of rare, progressive conditions that can result in visual deficits or blindness due to dysfunction, degeneration, or abnormal development of the photoreceptors or the retinal pigment epithelium. IRDs encompass a wide range of disorders that differ in severity, age of onset, and rate of progression. They may affect central or peripheral vision and can present from early childhood to late adulthood. Although individually rare, IRDs are collectively important because of their chronic nature and long-term impact on vision and quality of life [1].

IRDs show significant clinical and genetic heterogeneity. For example, two patients with the same clinical diagnosis may experience different ages of onset, rates of progression, and severity of symptoms, while others with similar clinical presentations may have entirely different genetic mutations underlying their disease. These differences can come from principles such as allelic heterogeneity, where different mutations in the same gene can cause similar conditions, or locus heterogeneity, where mutations in different genes result in the same disease. This variability demonstrates why IRDs require a precision medicine approach [1].

In recent years, genetic testing has improved, changing the way clinicians approach IRDs. Rather than only relying on clinical features and imaging, there is now an increasing emphasis on identifying the genetic basis of disease in order to inform the diagnostic plan for the patient. This shift is one of the goals of precision medicine. Because IRDs are caused by a wide range of mutations across many genes, gene therapy aims to overcome this heterogeneity by targeting specific, disease-causing variants, either by replacing the defective gene, correcting the mutation, or modulating gene expression. This precision-based strategy enables more targeted and potentially effective treatments for patients [2].

The application of precision medicine for the treatment of IRDs is especially promising. However, understanding the results of genetic testing when variants of uncertain significance are involved is more challenging for doctors and patients. Exploring the techniques and methods used for interpreting IRDs and understanding the difficulty of linking genetic information with clinical outcomes is essential for advancements in precision medicine [2].

2. Background

The following section briefly outlines examples of IRDs to show this variability in clinical presentation and genetic mechanisms.

2.1. Retinitis Pigmentosa (RP)

Early signs of RP often include trouble seeing in low light (nyctalopia) and peripheral vision loss, which can later affect central vision as well. However, the age of onset and severity vary widely, and patients may also experience photophobia, near-sightedness, or colour vision defects. With over 80 genes implicated, RP can be inherited in autosomal dominant (20–25%), autosomal recessive (15–20%), or X-linked (10–15%) patterns, and rare cases of digenic inheritance have been reported. Even within the same gene, different mutations may have differing clinical presentations. For example, *ABCA4* and *BEST1* mutations can cause RP alongside other retinal dystrophies, and the same pathogenic variant can also present in a variety of ways across families [3].

2.2. Leber Congenital Amaurosis (LCA)

This IRD is a severe early-onset retinal dystrophy, which typically presents with visual impairment or blindness in infancy, though the severity of the disease and its symptoms, such as nystagmus, photophobia, or refractive errors, differ between patients. Additionally, fundus appearance and progression can differ, and extra-ocular features may occasionally be present in some patients. The condition is genetically diverse, with at least 20 genes involved, including *CEP290*, *CRB1*, *GUCY2D*, and *RPE65*. These genes affect different retinal pathways, such as phototransduction or ciliary function. Most cases are inherited in an autosomal recessive manner, though some rare forms follow an autosomal dominant pattern. This variation makes diagnosis complex, but also allows for new approaches to gene-specific therapy [4].

https://doi.org/10.3390/jpm1606029

2.3. Stargardt Disease (STGD)

STGD is the most common inherited macular dystrophy, varying in the age of onset, severity, fundus appearance, and progression [5]. Some individuals present in childhood with rapid vision loss and impairments, while others are diagnosed in adulthood with slower decline [6]. Yellow-white pisciform flecks and macular atrophy may be absent early on, complicating diagnosis. Furthermore, full-field ERG and imaging findings differ across patients [6]. STGD is most commonly caused by mutations in *ABCA4*, but even among patients with similar mutations, phenotypes can vary [3].

Due to the high level of variability seen among different genotypes implicated in IRDs and how the condition clinically presents, precision medicine is a promising method of therapy for these unique conditions [3].

3. Genetics (WES/WGS, VUS)

Diagnosing inherited retinal diseases has become more reliant on genetic testing, as these diseases usually have mutations across a wide range of genes. With the growing availability of gene panels, whole-exome sequencing (WES), and whole-genome sequencing (WGS), clinicians now have more methods to uncover the molecular basis of retinal degeneration. Moreover, the cost of sequencing, particularly for WGS, has decreased dramatically in recent years, falling from over $4000 to approximately $200 per genome, thereby increasing its accessibility for clinical diagnostic use. However, these advances have challenges, especially when genetic findings do not clearly explain a patient's symptoms. Variants of uncertain significance (VUS) further add to this complexity, making it hard to distinguish between benign variation and disease-causing mutations. At the same time, improved genetic resolution plays an important role in identifying patients eligible for new gene therapies, many of which are designed to target specific mutations or pathways involved in IRDs [7].

Gene panel sequences curated a list of genes known to be associated with IRDs. They are cost-effective and good for detecting known pathogenic variants, especially in populations with well-characterized mutation spectra. However, Panels can miss novel or rare variants outside the selected genes, which limits their use in highly heterogeneous populations or for discovering new disease genes [8].

WES sequences all protein-coding regions, capturing both known and novel variants across hundreds of IRD-associated genes [9]. WES is particularly valuable in genetically diverse populations or when initial gene panel testing is inconclusive [9]. It enables the discovery of new disease-causing genes and expands the mutation spectrum, which is seen in many IRD cohorts. However, WES may not detect deep intronic or regulatory variants and structural rearrangements [9].

WGS covers the entire genome, including coding, non-coding, and regulatory regions, and can identify variants which goes undetected by other methods [9]. WGS is being used more frequently for unresolved cases after panel or WES testing, although cost and data analysis still pose challenges [9].

Identifying clear links between different genetic variants and clinical features, known as genotype-phenotype correlations, is an important step in understanding inherited retinal diseases [10]. These correlations can allow researchers to understand how a disease might progress and help shape genetic counselling for families [10]. For example, individuals who carry two copies of a disease-causing mutation (homozygous variants) often present with more extreme symptoms or earlier onset when compared to individuals with only one copy (heterozygous) [10]. This pattern has been seen across multiple IRDs, including retinitis pigmentosa (RP), Leber congenital amaurosis (LCA), and Stargardt disease [10]. However, the relationship between genotype and phenotype is not always straightforward [10].

https://doi.org/10.3390/jpm16060292

Certain genes, such as *PROM1, USH2A*, and *ABCA4*, have been associated with a wide range of clinical outcomes [9]. Sometimes, the same gene can lead to differing conditions, which are dependent on the specific mutation involved and whether it is inherited in a dominant or recessive manner [9]. Despite the growing availability of genetic testing, strong genotype-phenotype matches are still only found in a fraction of patients [9]. One large study conducted in an Indian population, for example, reported clear correlations in just 35% of cases, which shows the ongoing challenges in interpreting gene data and the influence of other factors, such as modifier genes or environmental exposures, on clinical presentation [9]. A major hurdle in the genetic diagnosis of IRDs is the high number of variants that are classified as variants of uncertain significance (VUS) [11]. These are genetic changes for which there is not enough evidence to determine whether they are actually involved in causing disease or are simply benign differences [11]. In one study, nearly 45% of all IRD-related variants were categorized this way, emphasizing how often clinicians are left with ambiguous results [11]. This uncertainty complicates not only how clinicians approach diagnosis but also how they support patients in making sense of their results, as it is challenging to offer confident answers about prognosis, recurrence risk, or eligibility for gene-specific therapies [11]. Sometimes, added steps like functional assays, segregation studies in relatives, or analysis of variant frequency in populations that are diverse can help clarify whether a VUS is likely to be harmful [11]. Still, these follow-up investigations are not always possible, especially in resource-limited environments or when family members are unavailable [11].

Beyond VUS, several other factors make genetic diagnosis of IRDs complex. Many IRDs share overlapping clinical features, making it hard to tell them apart just from symptoms alone. At the same time, extensive genetic heterogeneity means that mutations in dozens to hundreds of different genes can lead to similar retinal findings. The situation becomes harder to untangle when considering population genetics. For example, genetic differences might be more frequently observed in specific communities or in areas with high rates of consanguinity, which affects both how common the disease is and how it appears in individuals. Despite growing reliance on newer sequencing technologies, a portion of IRD cases remain without a clear genetic explanation. This points to missing genes still to be discovered, deep intronic or structural variants not captured by standard tests, or more complex modes of inheritance that are not fully understood as of right now, and need further research [8].

4. Therapies and Trials

Luxturna (voretigene neparvovec), developed by Spark Therapeutics, is the first gene therapy approved by the FDA for any inherited disease, specifically targeting vision loss caused by biallelic mutations in the *RPE65* gene [11]. This therapy is indicated for patients with Leber congenital amaurosis (LCA) and certain forms of retinitis pigmentosa (RP) due to *RPE65* mutations [11].

With regard to its mechanism of action, Luxturna uses an adeno-associated viral (AAV2) vector to insert the *RPE65* gene into retinal cells via subretinal injection, restoring the ability to produce the critical enzyme required for the visual cycle [11]. In clinical trials, Luxturna led to significant and durable improvements in functional vision, light sensitivity, and visual function, with benefits persisting for at least three years [11]. Many patients were able to get back some independence, such as navigating without canes and recognizing faces [11]. The FDA approved Luxturna in December 2017 following unanimous advisory committee support, representing a major turning point in the treatment of inherited retinal diseases [12]. The approval of Luxturna has accelerated progress for therapies for other

https://doi.org/10.3390/jpm1606029

IRDs. Several promising clinical trials are underway for genes implicated in RP, LCA, and related disorders:

RPGR (Retinitis Pigmentosa GTPase Regulator) mutations are a leading cause of X-linked retinitis pigmentosa. Multiple clinical trials are evaluating AAV-mediated gene replacement therapies for *RPGR*-associated RP [13]. Early results have shown some gains in visual function and safety, although long-term efficacy is still being assessed [14].

CEP290 mutations are the most common cause of LCA. Efforts to treat *CEP290* include both gene augmentation and antisense oligonucleotide approaches [14]. Notably, antisense therapy (such as sepofarsen) aims to correct splicing defects, and clinical trials have shown some improvement in vision in treated patients [14].

CRB1 mutations cause severe early-onset retinal dystrophies, including LCA and RP [14]. Preclinical studies and early-phase research trials are currently testing AAV-based gene replacement strategies for *CRB1*-related diseases [14].

Additional gene therapy trials are also happening for genes such as *CHM* (choroideremia), *USH2A* (Usher syndrome), *ABCA4* (Stargardt disease), and *RS1* (X-linked retinoschisis) [15]. Many of these therapies use AAV vectors, but alternative delivery systems and gene-editing approaches (such as CRISPR/Cas9) are also being looked into for genes with large coding sequences or dominant negative effects [15].

While challenges still remain for these therapies, as previously mentioned, precision medicine is a promising field of healthcare that could help better address the complications and complexities seen in IRDs and how individualized the condition is due to both its clinical and genetic heterogeneity seen among patients [15]. A summary of existing gene therapy preclinical and clinical trials is in Table 1.

Table 1. Clinical and Preclinical Trials for Gene Therapies in Inherited Retinal Diseases.

Trial/Program	Condition	Gene Target	Stage/Status	Organization/ Scientists	Trial/Literature Reference
AV-RPE65 reclinical roof-of-concept 3riard dog)	RPE65-associated Leber congenital amaurosis/ inherited retinal degeneration	*RPE65*	Preclinical large-animal proof-of-concept; supported human translation	University of Pennsylvania/Cornell investigators	Acland et al., Nat Genet 2001 [16]
:PE65 Phase I ene transfer	RPE65-associated LCA/inherited retinal degeneration	*RPE65*	Completed Phase 1	NEI/University of Pennsylvania/CHOP and collaborators	NCT00481546; NCT00516477
uxturna voretigene eparvovec-rzyl; AV2-hRPE65v2)	Biallelic RPE65 mutation-associated inherited retinal disease	*RPE65*	FDA approved Dec. 2017; pivotal Phase 3 completed	Spark Therapeutics	NCT00999609; Russell et al., Lancet 2017 [17]
'oretigene eparvovec ong-term ollow-up	Prior recipients of AAV2-hRPE65v2	*RPE65*	Long-term observational follow-up	Spark Therapeutics/Novartis	NCT03602820; NCT03597399
:PGRORF15 anine roof-of-concept	X-linked retinitis pigmentosa model	*RPGR*	Preclinical large-animal rescue study	University of Pennsylvania/collaborators	Beltran et al., PNAS 2012 [18]
:odon-optimized AV8-RPGR	X-linked retinitis pigmentosa models	*RPGR*	Preclinical mouse-model optimization	University of Oxford/collaborators	Fischer et al., Mol Ther 2017 [19]

https://doi.org/10.3390/jpm16060292

Table 1. *Cont.*

Trial/Program	Condition	Gene Target	Stage/Status	Organization/ Scientists	Trial/Literature Reference
AAV5-RPGR/botaretigene sparoparvovec Phase 1/2	RPGR-associated X-linked retinitis pigmentosa	*RPGR*	Completed Phase 1/2; safety and efficacy signals reported	MeiraGTx/Janssen	NCT03252847; Michaelides et al., Am J Ophthalmol 2024 [20]
BIIB112/cotoretigene toliparvovec Phase 1/2	RPGR-associated X-linked retinitis pigmentosa	*RPGR*	Completed Phase 1/2	Nightstar/Biogen	NCT03116113
LUMEOS Phase 3	RPGR-associated X-linked retinitis pigmentosa	*RPGR*	Phase 3; did not meet primary endpoint reported in 2025	Janssen/MeiraGTx	NCT04671433
AGTC-501/laruparetigene zovaparvovec Phase 1/2 (SKYLINE)	RPGR-associated X-linked retinitis pigmentosa	*RPGR*	Phase 1/2 clinical data published	AGTC/Beacon Therapeutics	NCT03316560; Yang et al., Am J Ophthalmol 2025 [21]
VISTA pivotal trial of AGTC-501/laruzova	RPGR-associated X-linked retinitis pigmentosa	*RPGR*	Randomized pivotal/registrational trial	Beacon Therapeutics	NCT04850118
LANDSCAPE bilateral-administration study	RPGR-associated X-linked retinitis pigmentosa	*RPGR*	Phase 2 open-label bilateral-treatment study	Beacon Therapeutics	NCT07174726
Sepofarsen/QR-110/AON-3 Phase 1b/2	CEP290-associated LCA10 due to c.2991+1655A>G (p.Cys998X)	CEP290	Completed Phase 1b/2 antisense oligonucleotide study	ProQR/Laboratoires Thea/Sepul Bio	NCT03140969; Russell et al., Nat Med 2022 [17]
ILLUMINATE sepofarsen Phase 2/3	CEP290-associated LCA10	*CEP290*	Completed Phase 2/3	ProQR	NCT03913143
HYPERION sepofarsen Phase 3	CEP290-associated LCA10	*CEP290*	Phase 3; first participant dosed reported in 2025	Sepul Bio/ Laboratoires Thea	NCT06891443
EDIT-101 BRILLIANCE	LCA10 due to CEP290 c.2991+1655A>G/ IVS26 mutation	*CEP290*	Completed Phase 1/2 in vivo CRISPR-Cas9 editing trial	Editas Medicine	NCT03872479; Pierce et al., N Engl J Med 2024 [22]
AAV2-REP1 first-in-human choroideremia gene therapy	Choroideremia	*CHM/REP1*	Completed Phase 1/2 dose-escalation	University of Oxford/Nightstar	NCT01461213; MacLaren et al., Lancet 2014 [23]
STAR: BIIB111/AAV2-REP1/timrepigene emparvovec	Choroideremia	*CHM/REP1*	Completed Phase 3; primary endpoint not met	Nightstar/Biogen	NCT03496012; Bergland et al., Nat Med 2023 [24]
BIIB111 bilateral-administration safety study	Choroideremia	*CHM/REP1*	Completed safety study	Nightstar/Biogen	NCT03507686
BIIB111 long-term follow-up	Prior BIIB111-treated choroideremia participants	*CHM/REP1*	Long-term safety and efficacy follow-up	Biogen	NCT03584165

Table 1. *Cont.*

Trial/Program	Condition	Gene Target	Stage/Status	Organization/ Scientists	Trial/Literature Reference
D-110 intravitreal HM gene therapy	Choroideremia	*CHM/REP1*	Phase 1 dose-escalation	Four-dimensional Molecular Therapeutics/Roche	NCT04483440
TELLAR: QR-21a/ultevursen	Usher syndrome type 2A/nonsyn-dromic RP due to USH2A exon 13 mutations	*USH2A*	Completed Phase 1/2 RNA exon-skipping trial	ProQR	NCT03780257
IRIUS: ultevursen	Advanced RP due to USH2A exon 13 mutations	*USH2A*	Phase 2/3; termi-nated/transitioned after program changes	ProQR	NCT05158296
ELESTE: ltevursen	Early-to-moderate RP due to USH2A exon 13 mutations	*USH2A*	Phase 2/3; termi-nated/transitioned after program changes	ProQR	NCT05176717
UNA: ultevursen	RP due to USH2A exon 13 mutations	*USH2A*	Recruiting Phase 2b, randomized sham-controlled	Sepul Bio/ Laboratoires Thea	NCT06627179
AR422459/EIAV-BCA4	ABCA4-associated Stargardt disease	*ABCA4*	Completed Phase 1/2a lentiviral gene therapy	Sanofi/Oxford BioMedica/OHSU/ Quinze-Vingts	NCT01367444; Parker et al., Am J Ophthalmol 2022 [25]
STRA: SB-007 ual-AAV rotein-splicing ıerapy	ABCA4-associated Stargardt disease	*ABCA4*	Ongoing Phase 1/2; dose-expansion initiated	SpliceBio	NCT06942572
ELESTE: AVB-039 ual-AAV ABCA4 ıerapy	ABCA4-associated Stargardt disease	*ABCA4*	Phase 1/2, multicenter open-label dose-escalation	AAVantgarde Bio	NCT07161544
G801 mRNA rans-splicing gene herapy	ABCA4 mutation-associated recessive retinal dystrophy/ Stargardt disease	*ABCA4*	Phase 1/2 first-in-human dose-exploration	VeonGen/ViGeneron	NCT07002398
CU410ST/AAV5-RORA modifier ene therapy	Stargardt disease/ABCA4-associated retinopathy	*ABCA4* pathway modifier, not ABCA4 replacement	Phase 2/3 pivotal modifier-gene trial	Ocugen	NCT05956626
AV8-RS1 ocular ene transfer	X-linked retinoschisis	*RS1*	Completed Phase 1/2a intravitreal trial; safety/ tolerability focus	National Eye Institute	NCT02317887; Cukras et al., Mol Ther 2018 [26]
AAV2tYF-CB-RS1	X-linked retinoschisis	*RS1*	Completed Phase 1/2 intravitreal trial; no measurable treatment effect	AGTC/OHSU and collaborators	NCT02416622; Pennesi et al., Ophthalmol Retina 2022 [27]
AV2/4-RS1	X-linked retinoschisis model	*RS1*	Preclinical Rs1-KO mouse rescue study	University of Florida/collaborators	Scruggs et al., Mol Ther Methods Clin Dev 2022 [28]

Table 1. *Cont.*

Trial/Program	Condition	Gene Target	Stage/Status	Organization/ Scientists	Trial/Literature Reference
LIGHTHOUSE: ATSN-201	RS1-associated X-linked retinoschisis	*RS1*	Phase 1/2/3; pivotal Phase 3 cohort underway in 2026	Atsena Therapeutics	NCT05878860
PIONEER: GS030-DP/ChrimsonR optogenetic therapy	Advanced nonsyndromic retinitis pigmentosa	Mutation-independent optogenetics; retinal ganglion-cell ChrimsonR	Phase 1/2a; first reported partial functional recovery	GenSight Biologics/ Institut de la Vision	NCT03326336; Sahel et al., Nat Med 2021 [29]
ChR2 optogenetic preclinical studies	Rodent/canine retinal degeneration models	Mutation-independent optogenetics; *ChR2*	Preclinical proof-of-concept	Multiple academic groups	Gaub et al., PNAS 2014 [30]
ChrimsonR nonhuman-primate proof-of-concept	Late-stage retinal degeneration platform development	Mutation-independent optogenetics; ChrimsonR/ ChrimsonR-tdT	Preclinical nonhuman-primate safety and functional-expression study	GenSight/Sorbonne/ Institut de la Vision collaborators	Gauvain et al., Commun Biol 2021 [31]
RESTORE/MCO-010 optogenetic therapy	Advanced retinitis pigmentosa	Mutation-independent optogenetics; bipolar-cell MCO	Phase 2b randomized sham-controlled study; positive durability reports	Nanoscope Therapeutics	NCT04945772; Lam et al., Nat Med/PMC 2025 [32]

5. Patient Selection

Clinically using gene therapy in IRDs requires a balance of eligibility and ethical considerations [33]. Precision medicine begins with patient selection protocols that are both biologically and ethically justified, all while managing patients and their families regarding the complexity, limitations and implications of therapy [33].

Eligibility for gene therapy requires, first, a genetic confirmation of disease etiology, primarily in the form of biallelic pathogenic variants in a causative gene [33]. As previously discussed, treatment with Luxturna requires two disease-causing mutations in the RPE65 gene, as established by FDA and EMA criteria [34]. Diagnoses often utilize NGS gene panels due to their efficiency and broad coverage across the genetic spectrum of IRDs [33]. The American Academy of Ophthalmology (AAO) recommends the inclusion of syndromic genes in all IRD panels, given the possibility of delayed systemic involvement, which further leverages the strength of NGS [33]. To reiterate, panels of patients with nonsyndromic presentations also include testing for syndromic genes, as systemic features such as hearing loss in Usher syndrome may emerge only later in life [33]. Furthermore, the accurate interpretation of results, especially in VUS, depends on the analytic sensitivity, quality of the reference database, and expert interpretation, underscoring the importance of collaboration among ophthalmologists, molecular laboratories, and certified genetic counsellors [35].

In addition to the presence of relevant genetic mutations, candidates may also need to demonstrate some level of preserved retinal architecture, as gene therapy cannot regenerate lost photoreceptors [36]. At this stage of testing, optical coherence tomography (OCT) is used to evaluate retinal structure, specifically assessing the continuity of the ellipsoid zone and central retinal thickness [36]. These measures are surrogates for photoreceptor

https://doi.org/10.3390/jpm1606029

viability and have been correlated with improved visual outcomes following subretinal gene delivery [37]. Full-field electroretinography (ERG) is also used to assess the function of rods and cones, supporting diagnosis and disease staging [37]. The quantitative readout provided by full-field ERG is crucial in confirming retinal involvement, especially in conditions such as LCA and RP [33]. This is an especially sensitive and vital test: even in patients with localized macular involvement, full-field ERG can detect subclinical, widespread degeneration that may affect outcomes and eligibility [33]. Furthermore, kinetic and static visual field testing can be used to help determine disease severity and baseline function, identifying patients who fall within regulatory or trial criteria, such as thresholds for legal blindness [33]. This can also serve as a measure of functional outcomes in trials [33]. Finally, fundus autofluorescence (FAF) and infrared reflectance imaging may support the identification of metabolically active RPE; however, FAF should be used with caution in macular dystrophies such as Stargardt disease, where short-wavelength exposure poses a theoretical risk of light toxicity [38].

Due to the progressive and irreversible loss of photoreceptors in IRD, treatment timing is critical, and regulatory approvals provide age-specific frameworks [38]. As explored earlier, Luxturna is currently intended for patients 12 months of age and older [39]. This is based on Phase 3 trial data and long-term follow-up studies, which indicate better visual outcomes in younger patients with less advanced disease [39]. Most ongoing trials in IRDs set age limits to account for the reliability of the test, disease progression and surgical risk [39]. For pediatric candidates, additional considerations include the feasibility of sedated imaging and ERG, as well as the challenges in assessing visual acuity and fields [39]. Clinical trials of different gene therapies may apply more stringent inclusion criteria [39]. The ongoing EDIT-101 trials for CEP290-related Leber congenital amaurosis (LCA10) include only individuals with a certain margin of residual retinal structure, as assessed by OCT [40]. Similarly, clinical trials targeting *RPGR*, *CRB1*, and *CHM* genes may also incorporate additional requirements, such as visual acuity thresholds, preservation of macular function, or exclusion of individuals who have undergone prior ocular surgeries [40].

Beyond initial selection, patients who are candidates for gene therapy require structured long-term follow-ups to assess safety, functional outcomes and disease progression [33]. Retinal imaging, ERF and visual field testing are periodically repeated to monitor the effect of treatment and detect late-onset complications [33]. These can include inflammation and subretinal fibrosis [33]. Clinicians, then, should prepare patients for immediate procedure and a lifelong trajectory of follow-up, re-evaluation and emotional adaptation [33].

This leads to a final, and perhaps most important, aspect of patient selection: comprehensive genetic counselling [33]. The importance of genetic counselling cannot be overstated as an essential and ethical part of patient selection [33]. In both trials and clinical use, patients express both hope and anxiety regarding gene therapy decisions [33]. As such, patients and families may assume curative outcomes. Instead, counselling helps reframe expectations towards stabilization or modest improvement [33]. For instance, in the Luxturna trials, although improved functional vision was observed in many patients, outcomes varied depending on age, disease stage, and baseline function [41]. Genetic counselling is especially vital in IRD, where VUS are frequently encountered and more than 80 genes can contribute to overlapping phenotypes [41]. Here, results require careful and nuanced interpretation and explanation to avoid inappropriate exclusion of false hope [41]. The AAO recommends that post-test counselling be conducted by clinicians or geneticists familiar with ocular genomics and ideally be reoffered throughout life as new therapies and variant classifications evolve [33]. Counselling must address psychosocial dynamics that

https://doi.org/10.3390/jpm16060292

patients and patient families often grapple with, such as feelings of hope, fear, guilt, and grief [33]. These may emerge both pre- and post-therapy, especially in families navigating decisions for children or those living with a progressive disability [33]. Support must not end with the disclosure of test results, and longitudinal counselling (and re-counselling) align with the best ethical practices to support informed and supported autonomy [33].

6. Barriers

Although gene therapy holds promising advancements for IRDs, several barriers must be overcome before it can be widely implemented [33]. These barriers span economic, infrastructure, technical and informational aspects [33].

6.1. Economic

Firstly, the high cost of gene therapy presents a significant barrier to access [42]. In the United States, Luxturna is priced at approximately $850,000 for both eyes, posing challenges at both the system and patient levels [42]. From the insurers' perspective, health technology assessments are complicated by the high upfront cost coupled with uncertain outcomes [42]. These problematize payers' coverage and affect access to gene therapy [43]. However, even when insurance is available, IRD patients often face restrictive costs, especially within the broader scope of the economic burden associated with IRDs [43]. Children with IRDs have 40% higher health expenses than their peers, owing mainly to increased outpatient eye care and psychiatric services [44]. The lifetime cost per person with IRD was estimated at $5.2 million in Australia, with 87% of the cost arising from societal costs, including loss of income for both patients and their caregivers [45]. Unfortunately, such financial burdens and patterns often persist into adulthood for those with IRDs as well [45]. While employment rates for adults with IRDs in Singapore are similar to those of the general population, the income for those with IRDs remains significantly lower [46]. In Canada, individuals with IRDs are 24% less likely to hold paid employment compared to the national average [47]. Furthermore, the estimated per-person societal costs associated with IRDs in Canada range from US$16,470 to over US$275,000 annually [47]. Lost productivity, diminished quality of life, and informal caregiving responsibilities contribute to up to 98% of these costs [48]. Thus, financial inaccessibility encompasses not only the high price of treatment but also the broader economic vulnerability experienced by individuals living with IRDs [48].

6.2. Infrastructural

Furthermore, the actual availability and distribution of centres and trained professionals vary globally and influence accessibility [49]. In Portugal, for example, genetic testing was found to be only available in 54.5% of centres, and of the 26 centres studied, only four actually used the national IRD registry [49]. Moreover, 83.4% of IRD patients experienced a turnaround time of 4 to 9 months for genetic test results [49]. Similarly, in Italy, patients with RPE65-related IRDs often consulted up to 10 healthcare professionals before finding an appropriate specialized centre [49]. This highlights that even when a centre is available, in the absence of a well-organized referral network, barriers to diagnosis and treatment persist [50]. Such a trend is also prevalent in Canada, where a study of 408 patients and caregivers found challenges in accessing genetic testing and specialized care, with many patients reporting delays in diagnosis and treatment [51]. While there are more specialized centres for IRD gene therapy in the United States, access remains uneven [51]. Centres such as the Bascom Palmer Eye Institute and the Massachusetts Eye and Ear Infirmary are concentrated in specific regions, which may lead to disparities in access for patients residing in rural or underserved areas [51].

https://doi.org/10.3390/jpm1606029

6.3. Technical

Even once a centre is located, certain barriers persist [52]. The success of gene therapy in IRDs is dependent on the precise delivery and sustained expression of the therapeutic gene. As touched on briefly, variability in vector transduction efficiency, potential immune response and need for viable target cells can complicate treatment outcomes [52]. For example, the efficiency of AAV vectors can be affected by the presence of pre-existing neutralizing antibodies that can vary among individuals [52]. In some cases, the introduction of viral vectors can activate the immune response and cause inflammation, leading to a potential reduction in efficacy [52]. In the context of IRDs, these immune reactions can exacerbate retinal degeneration and present as gene therapy-associated uveitis (GTU), which has been reported in clinical trials [53]. In regard to the aspect of viable target cells, identifying patients early is crucial for the effective implementation of therapy. Leber congenital amaurosis and achromatopsia, for example, present preserved retinal structure for extended periods and are more ideal candidates for gene therapy when compared to an IRD such as retinitis pigmentosa, which presents with rapid retinal degeneration [54–56].

Informational

On a broader level, a lack of awareness and a clear understanding of gene therapy among patients and healthcare providers can further impede its implementation [57]. Misconceptions and limited access to accurate information may lead to barriers at a societal and mental level [57]. An Australian survey by Mack et al. probing the perspectives of individuals with IRDs found that only 28.3% of participants agreed they have good knowledge of gene therapy [57]. Though 86.9% were able to differentiate between an experimental treatment and an approved therapy, 52.9% incorrectly believed that gene therapy and stem cell therapy are the same. In a study with similar themes by Britten-Jones et al., only 37% of participants correctly responded that gene therapy for the eye is not suitable for all stages of the disease, and only 48% knew that the primary goal of the therapy is to slow the progression of the disease [58]. Such knowledge gaps are also observed in healthcare providers themselves [58]. A survey of optometrists in Australia and New Zealand found that only 38% of participants correctly identified the primary goal of gene therapy (slowing the progression of disease), and 81% indicated a lack of clarity on referral pathways as a key barrier [59].

Knowing this, efforts to address informational gaps are crucial for supporting decision-making and improving the implementation of gene therapy [58]. Britten-Jones et al. also found that individuals who self-reported good knowledge of genetic therapy were approximately three times more likely to feel confident in managing their own or their dependent's eye care following testing [58]. One resource to enhance patient education is the Foundation Fighting Blindness annual VISION conference for patients and families [47]. The conference offers a place to connect with the community, learn about the latest research and treatments and explore new clinical trials and products within a supportive environment [47].

7. Future Directions

Gene therapy, as an emerging technology, still faces some degree of limitations—whether that be immunogenicity, restricted vector capacity or concerns about long-term efficacy—and so fosters a centre for further innovation. CRISPR-Cas9 gene editing, antisense oligonucleotides (ASOs), optogenetics and multi-omics approaches all hold potential, with each technology harbouring its own advantages and challenges, a few of which are discussed below [60].

https://doi.org/10.3390/jpm16060292

7.1. CRISPR-Cas9

CRISPR-Cas9 is a two-component genome-editing system founded on a single-guide RNA (sgRNA) directing a Cas9 endonuclease to specific DNA sequences in order to generate a site-specific double-strand break (DSB) [60]. This break is then repaired by the cell and results in targeted insertions, deletions or precise replacements [60].

Applying CRISPR-Cas9 to IRDs has accelerated, originally beginning with using animal models with relevant mutations to aid in developing therapeutics that can edit photoreceptor or RPE cells in vivo [61]. A landmark preclinical study by Maeder et al. explored EDIT-101, an AAV-delivered CRISPR-Cas9 system aiming to edit the mutation responsible for LCA10 [61]. EDIT-101 achieved sustained editing rates, even exceeding the presumed therapeutic threshold and restoring regular transcript expression for photoreceptor structure and function [61].

Since then, a Phase ½ clinical trial (BRILLIANCE) has been evaluating the safety and tolerability of subretinally delivered EDIT-101 in LCA10 patients [22]. Early interim data thus far have indicated on-target editing in patient-derived retinal cells and no serious adverse events. Though final data is pending, these findings support the feasibility of CRISPR-Cas9 therapeutics in the field of IRDs [22].

At its ideal, CRISPR-Cas9 for IRDs can include the potential for permanent correction of recessive or dominant-negative mutations with a single intervention, standing to eliminate the need for repeat dosing [62]. Furthermore, the programmable nature of sgRNAs offers precise targeting of mutations across diverse IRD-implicated genes [62]. However, off-target cleavage remains a concern: unintended DSBS can cause changes in nontarget loci with variable downstream effects [62]. Preexisting or induced immune responses against the bacterial Cas9 protein could also reduce efficacy and lead to retinal inflammation [62]. Finally, efficient delivery to photoreceptors or RPE cells requires optimized vectors, and the current usage of AAV introduces constraints for the inclusion of larger Cas9 orthologs [63].

That being said, CRISPR-Cas9 editing in other genetic diseases, such as sickle cell disease, has demonstrated reliable on-target gene correction and clinical benefit [64]. For applicable translation to IRDs, general improvements in the CRISPR field can also be applied, such as engineering high-fidelity Cas9 variants, smaller Cas9 orthologs with AAV and the development of non-viral delivery methods [65].

7.2. ASOs

Antisense oligonucleotides, or ASOs, are short synthetic strands of nucleic acids that can hybridize with specific pre-mRNA sequences to modulate splicing [66]. In IRDs, ASOs aim to bind to mutated exons and induce exon skipping, allowing the synthesis of a truncated but partially functional protein [66]. Dulla et al. demonstrated that an intravitreal delivery of ASOs in a murine retinitis pigmentosa model successfully skipped the mutated exon [66]. This resulted in a 35–45% restoration of full-length transcription and partial preservation of photoreceptor function [66].

Several ASO candidates for *CEP290*-related LCA are in the early stages of clinical development [67]. AON-3, now formulated as QR-110 or sepofarsen, targets the c.2991+1655A>G *CEP29*-mutation and was found to restore normal *CEP290* mRNA in patient-derived retinal organoids [67]. Based on these findings, a first-in-human trial is evaluating safety and tolerability in *LCA10* patients [67]. Interim data describe dose-dependent editing in patient-derived retinal cells and no serious adverse events attributable to Cas9 editing [17].

ASOs offer high specificity, and they can be designed with single-nucleotide precision [17,67]. Unlike permanent gene editing, the effects of ASO are reversible; ASO gradually degrades over weeks, allowing for dosing adjustments if adverse effects arise [17,67]. On the flip side of the same coin, however, ASO therapy requires repeated intravitreal

https://doi.org/10.3390/jpm1606029

injections to maintain therapeutic levels, leading to increased procedural burden and risks [17,67]. It is also worth noting that exon skipping often yields retention of only partial function, and off-target splicing effects are also possible [17,67]. However, in IRDs, even partial preservation could maintain functional vision for years, and thus, ASOs present a compelling intermediate between gene supplementation and permanent editing [17,67].

7.3. *Optogenetics*

Optogenetics aims to repurpose surviving inner retinal neurons (typically bipolar or ganglion cells) into light detectors by using microbial opsin genes [29]. Sahel et al. report a successful case [29]. A patient presenting with retinitis pigmentosa received an intravitreal injection with an *AAV2* vector encoding a red-shifted channelrhodopsin, ChrimsonR, under a bipolar-cell-specific promoter [29]. When the patient then wore specifically designed amber-filtered goggles, he was able to locate and count objects, detect moving people, and recognize high-contrast shapes, regaining abilities he had lost prior to treatment [29]. These abilities persisted at six months without significant inflammation or adverse events [29].

Preclinical work in nonhuman primates has confirmed that bipolar-cell-specific expression of ChrimsonR via *AAV2* can yield stable mutation-independent photoreception [68]. A canine model of progressive rod-cone degeneration found that intravitreal delivery of AAV2-ChR2 restored light-driven pupillary reflexes and coordination to moving stimuli [68].

It is worth noting that while intravitreal injection is less invasive than subretinal surgery, visual acuity remains low, and bulky goggles are required to deliver sufficiently intense, wavelength-specific light [29,68]. Device calibration and patient training can take several weeks to achieve reliable performance [29,68]. However, optogenetics offers one of the few viable near-term options for patients lacking residual photoreceptor functions and could be combined with future cell-replacement or gene-correction approaches [29,68].

7.4. *Multi-Omics*

Multi-omics integrates multiple molecular layers (genome, transcriptome, proteome, metabolome and epigenome) to build a comprehensive molecular picture of disease [69]. In IRDs, multi-omics has been employed to elucidate complex genotype-phenotype relationships and identify novel biomarkers for diagnosis and stratification [69]. Liang et al. generated a single-nucleus multi-omics atlas of adult human retinas, combining transcriptomics and chromatin accessibility profiles from more than 250,000 nuclei [69]. Integrating this data revealed a core module of IRD-associated genes, including photoreceptor-specific transcription factors and metabolic enzymes, which had not been apparent from genetics alone [69]. Similarly, Lei et al. applied proteomic and metabolomic profiling to the vitreous samples of RP patients to identify elevated oxidative stress markers and dysregulated lipid pathways, suggesting potential targets for neuroprotection [70].

Advantages of multi-omics include the sensitive detection of subclinical disease stages, the refinement of patient subgroups for clinical trials, and the discovery of drug-target pathways [69,70]. However, this approach is resource-intensive, comprising sample collection, high-throughput sequencing, mass spectrometry, and computational integration [69,70]. From a patient's perspective, multi-omics can yield personalized prognoses and inform the tailoring of future therapies [69,70]. However, broad implementation hinges on developing streamlined and cost-effective assays [69,70]. In practice, multi-omics is thus an emerging, realistic adjunct to genetic testing, with the power to accelerate the diagnosis of unsolved IRDs and prioritize patients for mutation-specific interventions [69,70].

Lastly, prior to implementing precision medicine in IRD therapeutic strategies, safety and procedural risks should be explored and addressed [71]. A recent systematic review

https://doi.org/10.3390/jpm16060292

and meta-analysis found that AAV ocular gene therapy had a cumulative serious adverse event incidence of 8%, with most adverse events attributable to the surgical procedure used to deliver the vector [71]. Ocular inflammation related to high-dose ocular gene therapies was found to be generally transient and resolved upon administration of corticosteroids [71]. Despite these findings, adverse event reporting in ocular gene therapy trials is inconsistent, suggesting that adverse events may occur at a higher rate than reported [71]. Future trials should investigate methods for safe dose selection and optimal delivery, such as intraoperative assistance with optical coherence tomography, to avoid off-target exposure, inflammation, and mechanical injury to the retina [71].

8. Conclusions

Over the past decade, precision medicine has transformed the IRD landscape: NGS panels and complementary imaging modalities now enable genetic diagnoses in the majority of patients, and multi-omics approaches and functional assays deepen our understanding of variant pathogenicity. Informed patient-selection protocols have already yielded tangible clinical benefits, and treatments are increasingly emerging and becoming available.

Despite these advancements, certain challenges persist. A marked subset of IRD cases remains genetically unresolved due to the presence of deep-intronic, structural, or non-coding variants that elude standard assays. Long-term safety and efficacy data for gene-based intervention are still maturing, and high costs, bioinformatic needs and regional disparities continue to limit broad, equitable access.

To bridge these gaps, the field must develop efficient and effective technology pipelines, in addition to forging international consortia to harmonize patient registries, trial eligibility, and post-market surveillance. Sustaining collaboration among geneticists, clinicians, health economists, patient advocates, and policymakers, the promise of precision medicine can be leveraged to translate into durable, accessible treatment; ultimately, to give the gift of sight to as many IRD patients as possible.

Author Contributions: Conceptualization, T.D. and F.R.B.; methodology, T.D. and F.R.B.; validation, T.D., F.R.B. and K.G.; formal analysis, T.D. and F.R.B.; investigation, T.D. and F.R.B.; resources, T.D. and F.R.B.; data curation, T.D. and F.R.B.; writing—original draft preparation, T.D., F.R.B., K.G., K.D., K.S., V.D. and F.A.; writing—review and editing, B.K.T., M.B., I.D. and A.B.; supervision, B.K.T., M.B., I.D. and A.B. All authors have read and agreed to the published version of the manuscript.

Funding: This research received no external funding.

Institutional Review Board Statement: Not applicable.

Informed Consent Statement: Not applicable.

Data Availability Statement: No new data were created or analyzed in this study. Data sharing is not applicable to this article.

Conflicts of Interest: The authors declare no conflicts of interest.

Abbreviations

The following abbreviations are used in this manuscript:

Abbreviation	Full Term
AAV	Adeno-associated virus
ABCA4	ATP Binding Cassette Subfamily A Member 4
AON	Antisense oligonucleotide
ASO	Antisense oligonucleotide
BEST1	Bestrophin 1
CEP290	Centrosomal Protein 290

https://doi.org/10.3390/jpm1606029

CHM	Choroideremia
CRB1	Crumbs Cell Polarity Complex Component 1
CRISPR	Clustered Regularly Interspaced Short Palindromic Repeats
DNA	Deoxyribonucleic acid
ERG	Electroretinography
FAF	Fundus autofluorescence
FDA	Food and Drug Administration
GUCY2D	Guanylate Cyclase 2D
IRDs	Inherited retinal diseases
LCA	Leber congenital amaurosis
NGS	Next-generation sequencing
OCT	Optical coherence tomography
PROM1	Prominin 1
RNA	Ribonucleic acid
RP	Retinitis pigmentosa
RPE65	Retinal pigment epithelium-specific 65 kDa protein
RPGR	Retinitis Pigmentosa GTPase Regulator
RS1	Retinoschisin 1
STGD	Stargardt disease
USH2A	Usherin
VUS	Variants of uncertain significance
WES	Whole exome sequencing
WGS	Whole genome sequencing

eferences

Ben-Yosef, T. Inherited Retinal Diseases. *Int. J. Mol. Sci.* **2022**, *23*, 13467. [CrossRef]

Naithani, N.; Sinha, S.; Misra, P.; Vasudevan, B.; Sahu, R. Precision medicine: Concept and tools. *Med. J. Armed Forces India* **2021**, *77*, 249–257. [CrossRef]

Bravo-Gil, N.; González-Del Pozo, M.; Martín-Sánchez, M.; Méndez-Vidal, C.; Rodríguez-de la Rúa, E.; Borrego, S.; Antiñolo, G. Unravelling the genetic basis of simplex Retinitis Pigmentosa cases. *Sci. Rep.* **2017**, *7*, 41937. [CrossRef]

Huang, C.H.; Yang, C.M.; Yang, C.H.; Hou, Y.C.; Chen, T.C. Leber's Congenital Amaurosis: Current Concepts of Genotype-Phenotype Correlations. *Genes* **2021**, *12*, 1261. [CrossRef] [PubMed]

Tanna, P.; Strauss, R.W.; Fujinami, K.; Michaelides, M. Stargardt disease: Clinical features, molecular genetics, animal models and therapeutic options. *Br. J. Ophthalmol.* **2017**, *101*, 25–30. [CrossRef]

Cremers, F.P.M.; Lee, W.; Collin, R.W.J.; Allikmets, R. Clinical spectrum, genetic complexity and therapeutic approaches for retinal disease caused by ABCA4 mutations. *Prog. Retin. Eye Res.* **2020**, *79*, 100861. [CrossRef]

Christensen, K.D.; Dukhovny, D.; Siebert, U.; Green, R.C. Assessing the Costs and Cost-Effectiveness of Genomic Sequencing. *J. Pers. Med.* **2015**, *5*, 470–486. [CrossRef]

Chen, Z.J.; Lin, K.H.; Lee, S.H.; Shen, R.J.; Feng, Z.K.; Wang, X.F.; Huang, X.F.; Huang, Z.Q.; Jin, Z.B. Mutation spectrum and genotype-phenotype correlation of inherited retinal dystrophy in Taiwan. *Clin. Exp. Ophthalmol.* **2020**, *48*, 486–499. [CrossRef]

Fan, X.; Li, Z.; Sha, L.; Sheng, X.; Rong, W. Genotype-phenotype correlations for 17 Chinese families with inherited retinal dystrophies due to homozygous variants. *Sci. Rep.* **2025**, *15*, 3043. [CrossRef] [PubMed]

Gopinath, C.; Rompicherla, R.; Mathias, G.P.; Patil, R.; Poornachandra, B.; Vinekar, A.; Mochi, T.B.; Braganza, S.; Shetty, K.B.; Kumaramanickavel, G.; et al. Inherited retinal disorders: A genotype-phenotype correlation in an Indian cohort and the importance of genetic testing and genetic counselling. *Graefes Arch. Clin. Exp. Ophthalmol.* **2023**, *261*, 2003–2017. [CrossRef] [PubMed]

Trapani, I.; Auricchio, A. Seeing the Light after 25 Years of Retinal Gene Therapy. *Trends Mol. Med.* **2018**, *24*, 669–681. [CrossRef]

Shaberman, B. A Retinal Research Nonprofit Paves the Way for Commercializing Gene Therapies. *Hum. Gene Ther.* **2017**, *28*, 1118–1121. [CrossRef]

MedlinePlus. Leber Congenital Amaurosis. 2022. Available online: https://medlineplus.gov/genetics/condition/leber-congenital-amaurosis/ (accessed on 5 September 2025).

Alyea, G.; Francis, P.; Mansfield, B.; Focus, H.I. Leber Congenital Amaurosis. Available online: https://rarediseases.org/rare-diseases/leber-congenital-amaurosis/ (accessed on 5 September 2025).

https://doi.org/10.3390/jpm16060292

15. Ameri, H.; Kesavamoorthy, N.; Bruce, D.N. Frequency and Pattern of Gene Therapy Clinical Trials for Inherited Retinal Disease *Adv. Exp. Med. Biol.* **2025**, *1468*, 89–93. [CrossRef]
16. Acland, G.M.; Aguirre, G.D.; Ray, J.; Zhang, Q.; Aleman, T.S.; Cideciyan, A.V.; Pearce-Kelling, S.E.; Anand, V.; Zeng, Y.; Maguir A.M.; et al. Gene therapy restores vision in a canine model of childhood blindness. *Nat. Genet.* **2001**, *28*, 92–95. [CrossRe [PubMed]
17. Russell, S.R.; Drack, A.V.; Cideciyan, A.V.; Jacobson, S.G.; Leroy, B.P.; Van Cauwenbergh, C.; Ho, A.C.; Dumitrescu, A.V.; Ha I.C.; Martin, M.; et al. Intravitreal antisense oligonucleotide sepofarsen in Leber congenital amaurosis type 10: A phase 1b/2 tri *Nat. Med.* **2022**, *28*, 1014–1021. [CrossRef]
18. Beltran, W.A.; Cideciyan, A.V.; Lewin, A.S.; Iwabe, S.; Khanna, H.; Sumaroka, A.; Chiodo, V.A.; Fajardo, D.S.; Román, A.J.; Den W.-T.; et al. Gene therapy rescues photoreceptor blindness in dogs and paves the way for treating human X-linked retinit pigmentosa. *Proc. Natl. Acad. Sci. USA* **2012**, *109*, 2132–2137. [CrossRef]
19. Fischer, M.D.; McClements, M.E.; Martinez-Fernandez de la Camara, C.; Bellingrath, J.S.; Dauletbekov, D.; Ramsden, S.C.; Hicke D.G.; Barnard, A.R.; MacLaren, R.E. Codon-Optimized RPGR Improves Stability and Efficacy of AAV8 Gene Therapy in Tw Mouse Models of X-Linked Retinitis Pigmentosa. *Mol. Ther.* **2017**, *25*, 1854–1865. [CrossRef]
20. Michaelides, M.; Besirli, C.G.; Yang, Y.; TAC, D.E.G.; Wong, S.C.; Huckfeldt, R.M.; Comander, J.I.; Sahel, J.A.; Shah, S.M.; Te J.J.L.; et al. Phase 1/2 AAV5-hRKp.RPGR (Botaretigene Sparoparvovec) Gene Therapy: Safety and Efficacy in RPGR-Associate X-Linked Retinitis Pigmentosa. *Am. J. Ophthalmol.* **2024**, *267*, 122–134. [CrossRef] [PubMed]
21. Yang, P.; Birch, D.; Lauer, A.; Sisk, R.; Anand, R.; Pennesi, M.E.; Iannaccone, A.; Yaghy, A.; Scaria, A.; Jung, J.A.; et al. Subretina Gene Therapy Drug AGTC-501 for XLRP Phase 1/2 Multicenter Study (HORIZON): 24-Month Safety and Efficacy Results. *Am. Ophthalmol.* **2025**, *271*, 268–285. [CrossRef] [PubMed]
22. Pierce, E.A.; Aleman, T.S.; Jayasundera, K.T.; Ashimatey, B.S.; Kim, K.; Rashid, A.; Jaskolka, M.C.; Myers, R.L.; Lam, B.L.; Baile S.T.; et al. Gene Editing for CEP290-Associated Retinal Degeneration. *N. Engl. J. Med.* **2024**, *390*, 1972–1984. [CrossRef]
23. MacLaren, R.E.; Groppe, M.; Barnard, A.R.; Cottriall, C.L.; Tolmachova, T.; Seymour, L.; Clark, K.R.; During, M.J.; Cremers, F. Black, G.C.; et al. Retinal gene therapy in patients with choroideremia: Initial findings from a phase 1/2 clinical trial. *Lancet* **201** *383*, 1129–1137. [CrossRef] [PubMed]
24. Bergland, H.; Burlakov, E.; Wyller, J. The Dynamics of Pasture-Herbivores-Carnivores with Sigmoidal Density Depende Harvesting. *Bull. Math. Biol.* **2023**, *85*, 104. [CrossRef]
25. Parker, M.A.; Erker, L.R.; Audo, I.; Choi, D.; Mohand-Said, S.; Sestakauskas, K.; Benoit, P.; Appelqvist, T.; Krahmer, M.; Ségau Prévost, C.; et al. Three-Year Safety Results of SAR422459 (EIAV-ABCA4) Gene Therapy in Patients with ABCA4-Associate Stargardt Disease: An Open-Label Dose-Escalation Phase I/IIa Clinical Trial, Cohorts 1-5. *Am. J. Ophthalmol.* **2022**, *240*, 285–30 [CrossRef]
26. Cukras, C.; Wiley, H.E.; Jeffrey, B.G.; Sen, H.N.; Turriff, A.; Zeng, Y.; Vijayasarathy, C.; Marangoni, D.; Ziccardi, L.; Kjellstro S.; et al. Retinal AAV8-RS1 Gene Therapy for X-Linked Retinoschisis: Initial Findings from a Phase I/IIa Trial by Intravitre Delivery. *Mol. Ther.* **2018**, *26*, 2282–2294. [CrossRef] [PubMed]
27. Pennesi, M.E.; Yang, P.; Birch, D.G.; Weng, C.Y.; Moore, A.T.; Iannaccone, A.; Comander, J.I.; Jayasundera, T.; Chulay, J. Intravitre Delivery of rAAV2tYF-CB-hRS1 Vector for Gene Augmentation Therapy in Patients with X-Linked Retinoschisis: 1-Year Clinica Results. *Ophthalmol. Retin.* **2022**, *6*, 1130–1144. [CrossRef]
28. Scruggs, B.A.; Bhattarai, S.; Helms, M.; Cherascu, I.; Salesevic, A.; Stalter, E.; Laird, J.; Baker, S.A.; Drack, A.V. AAV2/4-RS1 gen therapy in the retinoschisin knockout mouse model of X-linked retinoschisis. *PLoS ONE* **2022**, *17*, e0276298. [CrossRef]
29. Sahel, J.-A.; Boulanger-Scemama, E.; Pagot, C.; Arleo, A.; Galluppi, F.; Martel, J.N.; Esposti, S.D.; Delaux, A.; de Saint Auber J.-B.; de Montleau, C.; et al. Partial recovery of visual function in a blind patient after optogenetic therapy. *Nat. Med.* **2021**, *2* 1223–1229. [CrossRef]
30. Gaub, B.M.; Berry, M.H.; Holt, A.E.; Reiner, A.; Kienzler, M.A.; Dolgova, N.; Nikonov, S.; Aguirre, G.D.; Beltran, W.A.; Flanner J.G.; et al. Restoration of visual function by expression of a light-gated mammalian ion channel in retinal ganglion cells o ON-bipolar cells. *Proc. Natl. Acad. Sci. USA* **2014**, *111*, E5574–E5583. [CrossRef]
31. Gauvain, G.; Akolkar, H.; Chaffiol, A.; Arcizet, F.; Khoei, M.A.; Desrosiers, M.; Jaillard, C.; Caplette, R.; Marre, O.; Bertin, S et al. Optogenetic therapy: High spatiotemporal resolution and pattern discrimination compatible with vision restoration i non-human primates. *Commun. Biol.* **2021**, *4*, 125. [CrossRef]
32. Lam, B.L.; Zak, V.; Gonzalez, V.H.; Gregori, N.Z.; Chavala, S.H.; Batabyal, S.; Carlson, M.; Kim, S.; Ayyagari, A.; Chang, J.; et a Safety and efficacy of MCO-010 optogenetic therapy in patients with Stargardt disease in USA (STARLIGHT): An open-labe multi-center Ph2 trial. *eClinicalMedicine* **2025**, *87*, 103430. [CrossRef] [PubMed]
33. Duncan, J.L.; Branham, K.; Birch, D.G.; Daiger, S.P.; Ferris, F.L., III; Fishman, G.A.; Heon, E.; Hufnagel, R.B.; Pennesi, M.E Sahel, J.-A.; et al. Guidelines on Clinical Assessment of Patients with Inherited Retinal Degenerations—2022. Availabl online: https://www.aao.org/education/clinical-statement/guidelines-on-clinical-assessment-of-patients-with (accessed on September 2025).

Lyons, B. The First Targeted Gene Therapy Approved in North America: Luxturna Faculty of Medicine, Centre for Blood Research: The University of British Columbia. 2018. Available online: https://cbr.ubc.ca/the-first-targeted-gene-therapy-approved-in-north-america-luxturna/ (accessed on 5 September 2025).
Burke, W.; Parens, E.; Chung, W.K.; Berger, S.M.; Appelbaum, P.S. The Challenge of Genetic Variants of Uncertain Clinical Significance: A Narrative Review. *Ann. Intern. Med.* **2022**, *175*, 994–1000. [CrossRef]
Botto, C.; Rucli, M.; Tekinsoy, M.D.; Pulman, J.; Sahel, J.A.; Dalkara, D. Early and late stage gene therapy interventions for inherited retinal degenerations. *Prog. Retin. Eye Res.* **2022**, *86*, 100975. [CrossRef]
Murthy, R.K.; Haji, S.; Sambhav, K.; Grover, S.; Chalam, K.V. Clinical applications of spectral domain optical coherence tomography in retinal diseases. *Biomed. J.* **2016**, *39*, 107–120. [CrossRef]
Strauss, R.W.; Kong, X.; Ho, A.; Jha, A.; West, S.; Ip, M.; Bernstein, P.S.; Birch, D.G.; Cideciyan, A.V.; Michaelides, M.; et al. Progression of Stargardt Disease as Determined by Fundus Autofluorescence Over a 12-Month Period: ProgStar Report No. 11. *JAMA Ophthalmol.* **2019**, *137*, 1134–1145. [CrossRef]
Health CAfDaTi. Clinical Review Report: Voretigene Neparvovec (Luxturna): (Novartis Pharmaceuticals Canada Inc.): Indication: Vision Loss, Inherited Retinal Dystrophy [Internet]: National Library of Medicine. 2021. Available online: https://www.ncbi.nlm.nih.gov/books/NBK569037/ (accessed on 5 September 2025).
Open-Label, Single Ascending Dose Study to Evaluate the Safety, Tolerability, and Efficacy of EDIT-101 in Adult and Pediatric Participants with Leber Congenital Amaurosis Type 10 (LCA10), with Centrosomal Protein 290 (CEP290)-Related Retinal Degeneration Caused by a Compound Heterozygous or Homozygous Mutation Involving c.2991+1655A>G in Intron 26 (IVS26) of the CEP290 Gene ("LCA10-IVS26") [Internet]. 2018. Available online: https://clinicaltrials.gov/study/NCT03872479 (accessed on 5 September 2025).
Deng, C.; Zhao, P.Y.; Branham, K.; Schlegel, D.; Fahim, A.T.; Jayasundera, T.K.; Khan, N.; Besirli, C.G. Real-world outcomes of voretigene neparvovec treatment in pediatric patients with RPE65-associated Leber congenital amaurosis. *Graefes Arch. Clin. Exp. Ophthalmol.* **2022**, *260*, 1543–1550. [CrossRef]
Darrow, J.J. Luxturna: FDA documents reveal the value of a costly gene therapy. *Drug Discov. Today* **2019**, *24*, 949–954. [CrossRef]
Hitch, J.; Denee, T.; Brassel, S.; Lee, J.; Michaelides, M.; Petersen, J.; Alulis, S.; Steuten, L. Challenges in Value Assessment for One-Time Gene Therapies for Inherited Retinal Diseases: Are We Turning a Blind Eye? *Value Health* **2025**, *28*, 116–124. [CrossRef] [PubMed]
Kessel, L.; Kjellberg, J.; Ibsen, R.; Rasmussen, A.; Nissen, K.R.; la Cour, M. Longitudinal analysis of health care costs in patients with childhood onset inherited retinal dystrophies compared to healthy controls. *BMC Ophthalmol.* **2022**, *22*, 466. [CrossRef]
Schofield, D.; Kraindler, J.; Tan, O.; Shrestha, R.N.; West, S.; Hart, N.; Tan, L.; Ma, A.; Grigg, J.R.; Jamieson, R.V. The health care and societal costs of inherited retinal diseases in Australia: A microsimulation modelling study. *Med. J. Aust.* **2023**, *219*, 70–76. [CrossRef] [PubMed]
Chay, J.; Tang, R.W.C.; Tan, T.E.; Chan, C.M.; Mathur, R.; Lee, B.J.H.; Chan, H.H.; Sim, S.; Farooqui, S.; Teo, K.Y.C.; et al. The economic burden of inherited retinal disease in Singapore: A prevalence-based cost-of-illness study. *Eye* **2023**, *37*, 3827–3833. [CrossRef] [PubMed]
Blindness, F.F. Inherited Retinal Diseases Cost the US and Canadian Economies up to $33 Billion Annually. Available online: https://www.fightingblindness.org/news/inherited-retinal-diseases-cost-the-us-and-canadian-economies-up-to-33-billion-annually-201?gad_source=1&gad_campaignid=23197030064&gbraid=0AAAAAD_ZajF9_BNSx0y7m_VPLhXNs43jp&gclid=Cj0KCQjwve7NBhC-ARIsALZy9HV_cVma2SbCBAc8HFsToY2Ne3u41mbVy50TMGazCZ_TwAl3U6y7sP8aAlPHEALw_wcB (accessed on 5 September 2025).
Ng, Q.X.; Ong, C.; Yaow, C.Y.L.; Chan, H.W.; Thumboo, J.; Wang, Y.; Koh, G.C.H. Cost-of-illness studies of inherited retinal diseases: A systematic review. *Orphanet J. Rare Dis.* **2024**, *19*, 93. [CrossRef]
Marques, J.P.; Ferreira, N.; Moreno, N.; Marta, A.; Vaz-Pereira, S.; Estrela-Silva, S.; Costa, J.; Cardoso, A.R.; Neves, P.; Duarte, L.; et al. Current management of inherited retinal degenerations in Portugal (IRD-PT survey). *Sci. Rep.* **2024**, *14*, 21473. [CrossRef] [PubMed]
Simonelli, F.; Sodi, A.; Falsini, B.; Bacci, G.; Iarossi, G.; Di Iorio, V.; Giorgio, D.; Placidi, G.; Andrao, A.; Reale, L.; et al. Care Pathway of RPE65-Related Inherited Retinal Disorders from Early Symptoms to Genetic Counseling: A Multicenter Narrative Medicine Project in Italy. *Clin. Ophthalmol.* **2021**, *15*, 4591–4605. [CrossRef] [PubMed]
Kherani, I.Z.; Andrews, C.; Pereira, J.A.; Moniz, L.S.; Qian, C.X. Impact of inherited retinal diseases on Canadian patients and families: A mixed-methods study. *Can. J. Ophthalmol.* **2023**, *58*, 532–538. [CrossRef]
Ail, D.; Malki, H.; Zin, E.A.; Dalkara, D. Adeno-Associated Virus (AAV)—Based Gene Therapies for Retinal Diseases: Where are We? *Appl. Clin. Genet.* **2023**, *16*, 111–130. [CrossRef]
Yang, P.; Mustafi, D.; Pepple, K.L. Immunology of Retinitis Pigmentosa and Gene Therapy-Associated Uveitis. *Cold Spring Harb. Perspect. Med.* **2024**, *14*, a041305. [CrossRef]

https://doi.org/10.3390/jpm16060292

54. Hufnagel, R.B.; Ahmed, Z.M.; Corrêa, Z.M.; Sisk, R.A. Gene therapy for Leber congenital amaurosis: Advances and futu directions. *Graefes Arch. Clin. Exp. Ophthalmol.* **2012**, *250*, 1117–1128. [CrossRef] [PubMed]
55. Colella, P.; Auricchio, A. Gene therapy of inherited retinopathies: A long and successful road from viral vectors to patients. *Hu Gene Ther.* **2012**, *23*, 796–807. [CrossRef]
56. Liu, Y.; Zong, X.; Cao, W.; Zhang, W.; Zhang, N.; Yang, N. Gene Therapy for Retinitis Pigmentosa: Current Challenges and Ne Progress. *Biomolecules* **2024**, *14*, 903. [CrossRef]
57. Mack, H.G.; Britten-Jones, A.C.; McGuinness, M.B.; Chen, F.K.; Grigg, J.R.; Jamieson, R.V.; Edwards, T.L.; De Roach, J.; O'Hare, Martin, K.R.; et al. Survey of perspectives of people with inherited retinal diseases on ocular gene therapy in Australia. *Gene Th* **2023**, *30*, 336–346. [CrossRef]
58. Britten-Jones, A.C.; Schultz, J.; Mack, H.G.; Kearns, L.S.; Huq, A.J.; Ruddle, J.B.; Mackey, D.A.; Hewitt, A.W.; Edwards, T.I Ayton, L.N. Patient experiences and perceived value of genetic testing in inherited retinal diseases: A cross-sectional survey. *S Rep.* **2024**, *14*, 5403. [CrossRef]
59. Britten-Jones, A.C.; Mack, H.G.; Vincent, A.L.; Hill, L.J.; Edwards, T.L.; Ayton, L.N. Genetic testing and gene therapy in retin diseases: Knowledge and perceptions of optometrists in Australia and New Zealand. *Clin. Genet.* **2024**, *105*, 34–43. [CrossRef]
60. Jinek, M.; Chylinski, K.; Fonfara, I.; Hauer, M.; Doudna, J.A.; Charpentier, E. A programmable dual-RNA-guided DN endonuclease in adaptive bacterial immunity. *Science* **2012**, *337*, 816–821. [CrossRef]
61. Maeder, M.L.; Stefanidakis, M.; Wilson, C.J.; Baral, R.; Barrera, L.A.; Bounoutas, G.S.; Bumcrot, D.; Chao, H.; Ciulla, D.M.; DaSilv J.A.; et al. Development of a gene-editing approach to restore vision loss in Leber congenital amaurosis type 10. *Nat. Med.* **201** *25*, 229–233. [CrossRef]
62. Pulman, J.; Sahel, J.A.; Dalkara, D. New Editing Tools for Gene Therapy in Inherited Retinal Dystrophies. *Cris. J.* **2022**, *5*, 377–38 [CrossRef] [PubMed]
63. Quinn, J.; Musa, A.; Kantor, A.; McClements, M.E.; Cehajic-Kapetanovic, J.; MacLaren, R.E.; Xue, K. Genome-Editing Strategie for Treating Human Retinal Degenerations. *Hum. Gene Ther.* **2021**, *32*, 247–259. [CrossRef]
64. Park, S.H.; Bao, G. CRISPR/Cas9 gene editing for curing sickle cell disease. *Transfus. Apher. Sci.* **2021**, *60*, 103060. [CrossRef]
65. Yan, A.L.; Du, S.W.; Palczewski, K. Genome editing, a superior therapy for inherited retinal diseases. *Vision. Res.* **2023**, *206*, 10819 [CrossRef] [PubMed]
66. Dulla, K.; Slijkerman, R.; van Diepen, H.C.; Albert, S.; Dona, M.; Beumer, W.; Turunen, J.J.; Chan, H.L.; Schulkens, I.A.; Vorthore L.; et al. Antisense oligonucleotide-based treatment of retinitis pigmentosa caused by USH2A exon 13 mutations. *Mol. Ther.* **202** *29*, 2441–2455. [CrossRef]
67. Garanto, A.; Chung, D.C.; Duijkers, L.; Corral-Serrano, J.C.; Messchaert, M.; Xiao, R.; Bennett, J.; Vandenberghe, L.H.; Colli R.W. In vitro and in vivo rescue of aberrant splicing in CEP290-associated LCA by antisense oligonucleotide delivery. *Hum. M Genet.* **2016**, *25*, 2552–2563. [CrossRef] [PubMed]
68. Nikonov, S.; Aravand, P.; Lyubarsky, A.; Nikonov, R.; Luo, A.J.; Wei, Z.; Maguire, A.M.; Phelps, N.T.; Shpylchak, I.; Willett, K et al. Restoration of Vision and Retinal Responses After Adeno-Associated Virus-Mediated Optogenetic Therapy in Blind Dog *Transl. Vis. Sci. Technol.* **2022**, *11*, 24. [CrossRef] [PubMed]
69. Liang, Q.; Cheng, X.; Wang, J.; Owen, L.; Shakoor, A.; Lillvis, J.L.; Zhang, C.; Farkas, M.; Kim, I.K.; Li, Y.; et al. A multi-omics atla of the human retina at single-cell resolution. *Cell Genom.* **2023**, *3*, 100298. [CrossRef] [PubMed]
70. Li, X.; Cai, S.; He, Z.; Reilly, J.; Zeng, Z.; Strang, N.; Shu, X. Metabolomics in Retinal Diseases: An Update. *Biology* **2021**, *10*, 94 [CrossRef]
71. Sobh, M.; Lagali, P.S.; Ghiasi, M.; Montroy, J.; Dollin, M.; Hurley, B.; Leonard, B.C.; Dimopoulos, I.; Lafreniere, M.; Fergusso D.A.; et al. Safety and Efficacy of Adeno-Associated Viral Gene Therapy in Patients With Retinal Degeneration: A Systemati Review and Meta-Analysis. *Transl. Vis. Sci. Technol.* **2023**, *12*, 24. [CrossRef] [PubMed]

Journal of
Personalized Medicine

MDPI

ticle

Genomic Medicine Among Ophthalmologists: Knowledge, Current Practice, and Barriers

alaa Bakhamees [1,2], Hend Alsafran [1,3], Hani Basher ALBalawi [4,*], Naif M. Alali [4], Yousef A. Alotaibi [5] d Moustafa S. Magliyah [1]

1 Vitreoretinal and Uveitis Division, King Khaled Eye Specialist Hospital, Riyadh 11462, Saudi Arabia; wbakhamees@uj.edu.sa (W.B.); hend_alsafran@hotmail.com (H.A.); mussam8@yahoo.com (M.S.M.)
2 Division of Ophthalmology, Department of Surgery, College of Medicine, University of Jeddah, Jeddah 21589, Saudi Arabia
3 Mohamad Al Dakhan Eye Center, AL-Amiri Hospital, Ministry of Health, Kuwait City 13110, Kuwait
4 Division of Ophthalmology, Department of Surgery, Faculty of Medicine, University of Tabuk, Tabuk 71491, Saudi Arabia; nmalali@ut.edu.sa
5 Department of Ophthalmology, College of Medicine, King Khalid University, Abha 61421, Saudi Arabia; yalotaibi@kku.edu.sa
* Correspondence: hb.albalawi@ut.edu.sa

Abstract

Background/Objectives: To assess the knowledge, attitudes, and practices of ophthalmologists in Saudi Arabia towards genomic medicine and genetic testing, in light of the growing significance of genomics in ophthalmology and the national transition towards precision medicine. **Methods**: A cross-sectional, questionnaire-based survey was conducted among ophthalmologists, including consultants, specialists, fellows, and residents, across Saudi Arabia. The questionnaire included four domains: demographics, knowledge of genomic principles and gene therapy, self-rated confidence in genetic tasks (scored 1–10), and attitudes toward genetic testing. Data were analyzed using descriptive and inferential statistics, with subgroup comparisons performed using chi-square tests and *t*-tests/ANOVA. **Results**: A total of 115 ophthalmologists participated (46% male, 54% female; mean age 34 years; mean post-board experience 4 years). Most were consultants (40%) and practiced in Riyadh (52%). Knowledge was variable: 92% correctly identified human chromosome count, and 99% recognized autosomal recessive inheritance, but only 9% answered DNA base-pairing correctly, and 54% recognized mitochondrial inheritance. Confidence was highest for referral to specialists (mean 7.3/10) and lowest for test selection and counseling (4.7/10). The internet was the primary knowledge source among our sample (65%). The majority of individuals had positive attitudes towards genomic medicine: 90% believed testing was beneficial, 89% considered it enhanced health outcomes, and 89% indicated they would undergo testing themselves. On the other hand, 77% indicated difficulty in access, 91% strongly concurred on the significance of privacy and confidentiality, and more than half expressed concerns regarding misuse and bias. **Conclusions**: Ophthalmologists in Saudi Arabia acknowledge the importance of genetics. Yet, there are substantial gaps in knowledge and familiarity with genomic medicine and genetic testing. To overcome these challenges, it is essential to integrate genetics into ophthalmology curricula.

Keywords: knowledge; attitude; practices; genomic medicine; ophthalmologists

1. Introduction

Genomic medicine is an evolving part of healthcare today and integrates genetic and molecular data into clinical decision-making to improve disease prevention, diagnosis, and treatment. In ophthalmology, genomic medicine improves diagnostic accuracy and facilitates the adoption of a personalized approach for numerous diseases that have a genetic basis, such as retinal dystrophies, congenital glaucoma, and hereditary corneal disorders. Despite these developments in the medical field, research from different countries continues to show significant gaps in the understanding of this field amongst healthcare professionals [1–4]. Such gaps in understanding genomic medicine might affect patient care through delayed referrals to ophthalmic genetic services, delayed genetic testing, and absent or deficient counseling for family members against consanguinity. Surveys of medical students and physicians in the Arab countries revealed predominantly favorable opinions towards genomic medicine, although they highlighted a lack of formal education and practical training. In these studies, healthcare professionals recognized insufficient training and interpretative abilities as significant obstacles in integrating genomics in their practice [5]. Research in Saudi Arabia has demonstrated similar observations; pharmacists and physicians have shown positive attitudes about genetic medicine, but exhibited confusion regarding the application of test results in clinical practice [6,7]. In ophthalmology, genetic testing and gene-based therapies are rapidly evolving, making it critical that physicians in these specialties have a good background and understanding of this rapidly evolving field. Ophthalmologists need to be aware that gene therapy is transforming the treatment of various ophthalmic conditions by addressing the root causes of debilitating diseases like inherited retinal dystrophies [8]. In addition, ophthalmology is one of the leading specialties in the clinical applications of gene therapy, and appropriate referral by ophthalmologists for genetic testing directly impacts eligibility for emerging treatments. In a country with high rates of consanguinity like Saudi Arabia, the accessibility to ophthalmic genetic services and the availability of genetic testing with meaningful interpretation might reflect positively on medical care for affected patients, as well as for other family members through early prevention and premarital genetic counseling. Ethical, legal, and societal issues—such as the proper use of genetic information, possible discrimination, and patient confidentiality—however, remain important considerations [9,10]. In the era of personalised medicine, identification of gaps in the knowledge and understanding of genomic medicine among physicians and ophthalmologists facilitates the transition to personalised medicine. The availability of more genomic information and molecular mechanisms of inherited diseases leads to a better understanding of disease and higher-quality care provided to patients. Improving the practices and applications of genomic medicine among ophthalmologists through proper identification of patients, utilization of genetic testing to yield comprehensive genomic information, and appropriate patient referral represent integral steps towards personalised patient care. Our study aims to evaluate the knowledge, attitudes, and practices of ophthalmologists in Saudi Arabia towards genomic medicine and genetic testing, given the evolving significance of genomics in ocular care. It also assesses demographic factors, understanding of genetics and gene therapy, self-reported trust in genetic counseling and testing, and perspectives on the clinical and ethical aspects of genetic medicine.

2. Materials and Methods

This study was a cross-sectional, questionnaire-based study among ophthalmologists in Saudi Arabia. Eligible participants were ophthalmology consultants, specialists, fellows, and residents. The survey was distributed electronically to ensure accessibility across all regions of the Kingdom. The study was approved by IRB at KKESH as the Saudi Ophthal-

https://doi.org/10.3390/jpm1605026

mology Society (SOS) has no IRB. The SOS has ophthalmologists' contacts, not the collected data, because data collection was performed based on the response from ophthalmologists in this study. The questionnaire (Table S1) was modified from recognized questionnaires used to evaluate knowledge, attitudes, and practices in genomic medicine and tailored for the ophthalmology domain. It consisted of four domains: (1) demographics, (2) understanding of genetic principles, inheritance mechanisms, and gene therapy, (3) self-rated confidence in performing genomics-related tasks such as family history assessment, test interpretation, and counseling, and (4) attitudes and perceptions regarding genomic testing, its availability, benefits, and ethical concerns. To test the understanding of genetic principles, inheritance mechanisms, and gene therapy, questions were modified from a survey that was provided for healthcare professionals [11]. To test self-rated confidence to perform genomics-related tasks, questions were modified from a survey that was provided for primary care physicians [12]. Both sets of questions were modified to more appropriately address ophthalmologists. The face validity of the survey was assessed by ten ophthalmologists to ensure the clarity and the premise of each question. The survey was then piloted for content, design, readability, and comprehension by ten different ophthalmologists. The required amendments were made based on the feedback to develop the final survey. The survey was distributed using professional ophthalmology email lists and contacts between June and August 2025. All ophthalmologists who had active memberships in the Saudi Ophthalmology Society (SOS) were invited to participate in the study. Ophthalmologists who did not have active SOS memberships were excluded. The total number of ophthalmologists who were invited was 429 ophthalmologists. Informed consent was obtained electronically prior to survey completion. The data extraction from the responses was performed electronically through predefined variables and was then transferred to the IBM Statistical Package for Social Sciences (SPSS). The SPSS version 30.0.0 was used to perform the statistical analysis. Descriptive statistics were generated for categorical variables (frequencies, percentages) and continuous variables (means, standard deviations, medians, ranges). Knowledge questions were analyzed for correctness; confidence scores are summarized as mean $\pm$ SD. Attitudinal responses are reported as proportions.

3. Results

A total of 115 ophthalmologists participated in our study, and the response rate was 26.8%. Of these, 53 (46.1%) were male, and 62 (53.9%) were female (Figure 1). The mean age of respondents was 34.4 years (SD $\pm$ 7.6; range: 26–60), with a median of 32 years. The mean post-residency clinical experience was 4.3 years (SD $\pm$ 5.6; range: 0–30), with a median of 2 years. In terms of professional grade, 45 respondents (39.8%) were consultants, 11 (9.7%) specialists, 35 (31.0%) fellows, and 24 (21.2%) residents (Figure 2). The majority of participants had their ophthalmology practice based in Riyadh (52%), followed by Jeddah (9.6%), Alkhobar (7.8%), Dammam (7.0%), and Dhahran (7.0%).

Knowledge questions revealed variable levels of accuracy. Almost all participants correctly identified that humans do not have 50 chromosomes (92%), and 99% recognized misconceptions in statements about autosomal recessive inheritance. In addition, 86% recognized misconceptions in statements about autosomal dominant inheritance. Similarly, 85% understood that not all genetic variants cause disease. Importantly, 85% of ophthalmologists confirmed that gene therapy is no longer confined to research purposes only (85%). However, only 9% correctly answered the DNA base pairing question, and 54% recognized the maternal inheritance pattern of mitochondrial diseases. Sources of information were primarily through the internet (65%), followed by books (14%) and medical school (12%).

https://doi.org/10.3390/jpm16050267

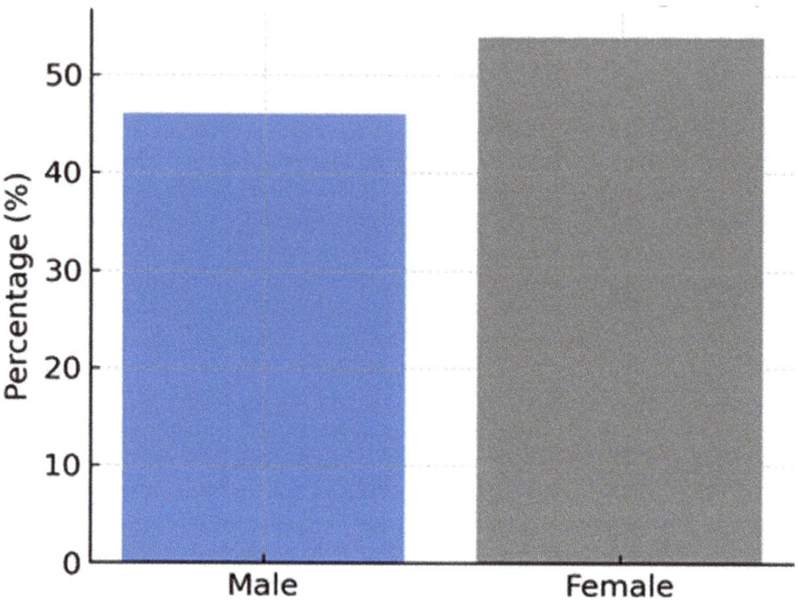

Figure 1. Gender distribution among respondents.

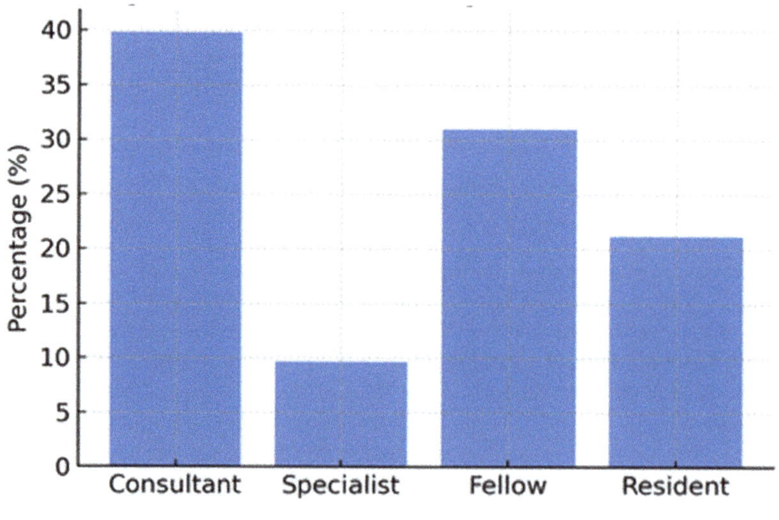

Figure 2. Professional grades of ophthalmologists who responded to the survey.

Confidence scores indicated moderate overall confidence. The highest mean scores were reported for referral to specialists (mean 7.3 $\pm$ 2.3) and obtaining family history (mean 6.6 $\pm$ 2.3). Clinical evaluation scored moderately (mean 5.5 $\pm$ 2.3). In contrast, confidence in deciding appropriate genetic tests (mean 4.7 $\pm$ 2.8), discussing prenatal diagnosis (mean 4.8 $\pm$ 2.8), and providing detailed counselling was low. This pattern highlights the reliance on referral networks rather than independent genetic decision-making).

The majority of participants considered genetic testing to be beneficial (90%) and reported that it has a favorable impact on health and well-being (89%). A substantial proportion (89%) were in favor of having genetic evaluations if recommended. Nonethe-

https://doi.org/10.3390/jpm1605026

less, 77% believed that testing is not readily accessible to the public. Ninety-one percent displayed great agreement with the importance of confidentiality and privacy. Forty-nine percent of individuals expressed concern regarding the potential misuse of genetic data, while 51% indicated apprehension about the possibility of genetic data resulting in discrimination in employment, insurance, or healthcare. Most participants (89%) predicted that genetic testing would become more prevalent in the future. Figure 3 illustrates that individuals exhibited the highest confidence in recommending someone to an expert, while they demonstrated the lowest confidence in selecting a test or providing advice. Figure 4 illustrates that the majority of individuals perceived testing as beneficial; nonetheless, numerous concerns around privacy, accessibility, and potential misuse were prevalent.

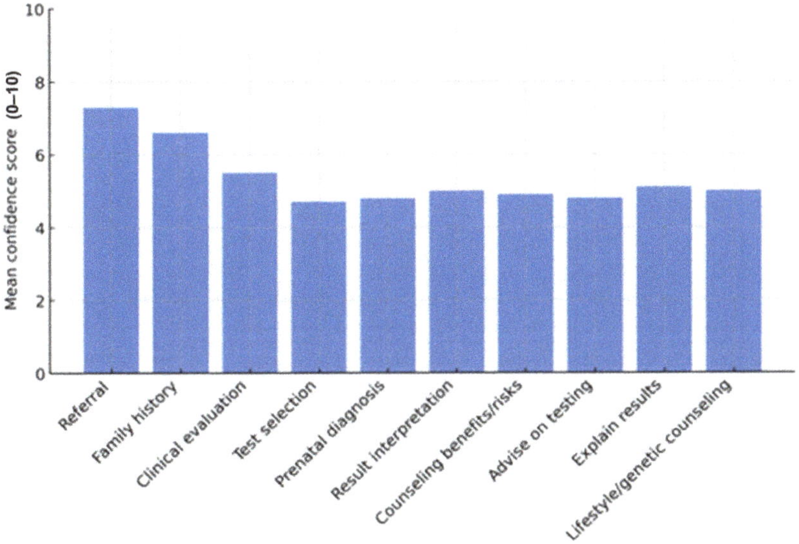

Figure 3. Self-rated confidence in performing clinical tasks that are related to the genomic medicine practice.

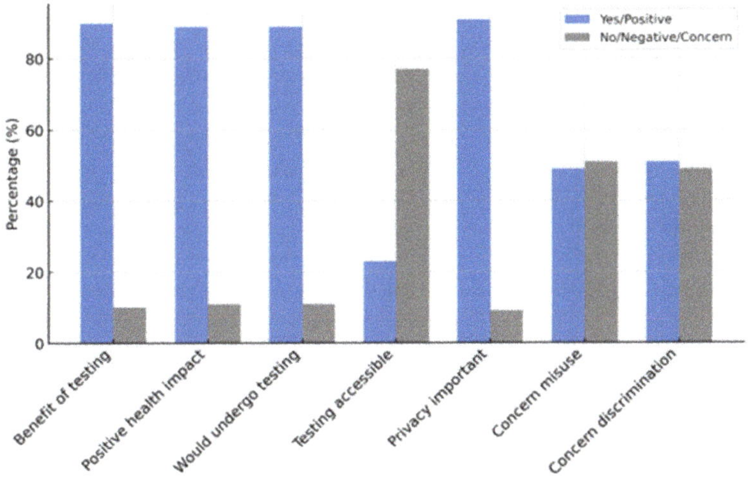

Figure 4. Attitudes and perceptions of ophthalmologists towards genetic testing.

https://doi.org/10.3390/jpm16050267

4. Discussion

This study explored the knowledge, attitudes, and practices of ophthalmologists in Saudi Arabia regarding genomic medicine and genetic testing. To the best of our knowledge, this is the first study to address the gap in understanding genomic medicine and genetic testing in the field of ophthalmology in our region. Based on our survey analysis, our findings indicate significant deficiencies in knowledge, limited confidence in clinical application, and generally positive attitudes toward genetic ophthalmic illnesses. These results, when applied in the context of regional and global data across various medical specialties, suggest the need for comprehensive training, improved infrastructure, and amendments to medical school curricula to enable the effective integration of genetics into ophthalmic service and care.

Despite the advancements in the Human Genome Project [2] and the expanding global understanding and application of genomic medicine [1], our findings reveal ongoing knowledge gaps among ophthalmologists. Participants demonstrated a good understanding of inheritance patterns; yet, some errors related to molecular genetics were found, such as DNA base pairing and mitochondrial inheritance mechanisms. These results support the previous findings highlighting similar deficiencies in knowledge among medical students and pharmacists in Saudi Arabia, as well as physicians who demonstrated uncertainty in the application of pharmacogenomics despite acknowledging its clinical relevance [6,7]. These results also show that while ophthalmologists retained certain background information about human genetics, they were not exposed to more sophisticated material in molecular genetics and special types of inheritance. As only a minority (12%) retained their information from medical school, more in-depth exposure to genomic medicine during medical school, and more importantly, at later stages of their careers, is needed to expand the knowledge of ophthalmologists about genomic medicine.

The consequences of deficient knowledge about genomic medicine are particularly relevant in ophthalmology more than in other specialties. The abundance of inherited retinal diseases, which are associated with an increasing number of genetic variants in disease-causing genes [3], makes the knowledge about genomic medicine and ophthalmic genetics essential for appropriate diagnosis and referrals. The emergence of gene-based therapies further emphasizes the critical importance of early diagnosis and referrals for centers that provide genetic therapy trials.

Notably, our findings were in alignment with international studies demonstrating that non-genetic specialists in other medical specialties—including cardiologists, oncologists, and neurologists—report inadequate training and poor preparedness for genomic applications in clinical practice [13–15]. A comprehensive survey in Australia confirmed that while clinicians recognize genomic relevance, most feel unprepared to implement these tools without substantial additional training [15]. The low correct response rate for the DNA base pairing (9%) in our study, in contrast to the high correct responses for the numbers of chromosomes and the modes of inheritance, reflects the lack of depth in knowledge about genomic medicine despite the good understanding of the general concepts of the subject.

Confidence levels among our participants varied significantly across different genomic medicine applications. Participants expressed the highest confidence in referring patients to genetics specialists but expressed lower confidence in ordering tests independently, interpreting results, and providing genetic counseling. Similar patterns of resorting to referral pathways rather than developing one's own genomic competencies have been widely reported in the literature [15–17]. Similar findings were found among cardiology and oncology studies, where clinicians admitted to avoiding direct genomic decision-making due to a lack of confidence [14]. These patterns have been observed throughout Middle Eastern and Arab countries, where clinicians might lack the appropriate exposure

https://doi.org/10.3390/jpm1605026

to genomic medicine during training and require improvements in genetic services [6,16]. Although referring patients to genetic specialists might be an appropriate decision when dealing with patients with inherited eye diseases, the referral to ophthalmic geneticists might not be easy for some patients who resort to performing genetic testing in the most accessible facility. Ophthalmologists who are confident in interpreting genetic testing might make a difference in the management of these patients through careful monitoring of patients with syndromic or nonsyndromic pathological myopia or appropriate referrals for other specialties for syndromes that involve multiple organs, like Usher syndrome and Bardet–Biedl syndrome [18]. The National Genomic Initiative might need to address these gaps in knowledge and confidence through continuous medical education activities and workshops for ophthalmologists.

Our results highlight that informal educational resources, which include online materials and presentations, served as primary sources of genomic knowledge. These findings indicate broader learning patterns among health care professionals that extend beyond structured, comprehensive education [5–7,16]. Such reliance on informal learning might contribute to incomplete and insufficient understanding and reinforces the critical need for specialty-specific genomic curricula.

The majority of participating ophthalmologists demonstrated positive attitudes toward genetic testing, with nearly 90% expressing willingness to undergo testing themselves if clinically advised. This optimism is supported by the recent advances and the introduction of precision medicine and individualized patient care [1,4,19]. However, participants identified substantial barriers to implementation, including limited service availability, high costs, and insufficient institutional readiness. These concerns align with issues raised throughout the Middle East [6] and persist even in Western countries where limitations in infrastructure and challenges in reimbursement remain significant obstacles [11,19].

Participants expressed significant concerns regarding data confidentiality, genetic discrimination, and the potential for misuse of genetic information. These ethical challenges were not confined to Saudi Arabia, as similar apprehensions were expressed across Canada, the United States, and Europe [10,19]. DuBois et al. specifically reported that both patients and clinicians emphasize the fundamental importance of trust, privacy safeguards, and comprehensive informed consent in the implementation of genomic medicine [19]. Knoppers and Beauvais similarly argued that ethical considerations are inseparable from successful clinical integration of genomic medicine [9].

Our findings suggest that ophthalmologists in Saudi Arabia are not yet adequately prepared for the integration of genomic medicine into their routine practice, despite recognizing its substantial clinical value. This readiness gap is particularly concerning given that precision medicine has been designated as a national health priority, with Saudi Arabia making significant investments in genomics infrastructure and workforce development [17]. For ophthalmology specifically, strengthening genomic literacy is essential to support effective integration of genomic medicine in clinical practice and optimal uptake of emerging therapies for inherited eye diseases today and in the future.

This study is the first study assessing the genetic competencies of ophthalmologists in Saudi Arabia, which provides specialty-specific evidence to the regional literature. In addition, it provides a foundation for educational and policy reforms that could enhance public preparedness for genomics. Limitations of this study include dependence on self-reported data, which may inadequately represent actual competencies, and the cross-sectional design, which restricts causal inference. About half of the study participants were from Riyadh, and this might have resulted in overestimation or underestimation of knowledge and confidence. In addition, this geographical distribution might limit the generalizability of results and might have resulted in a sampling bias. The relatively small

https://doi.org/10.3390/jpm16050267

sample size and unknown response rate further affect representativeness. Additionally, the cross-sectional design might limit the causal inference. This design cannot determine whether increased training would directly improve confidence or practice.

5. Conclusions

This study demonstrates that while ophthalmologists in Saudi Arabia generally recognize the importance of genomic medicine and express positive attitudes toward its use, significant knowledge gaps, limited confidence in clinical application, and systemic barriers hinder its integration into practice. These findings mirror international trends and emphasize the urgent need for structured genomic education, improved infrastructure, and clear legislative frameworks to ensure safe and effective implementation. Strengthening genomic knowledge and confidence among ophthalmologists might be critical not only for accurate diagnosis and timely referral but also for enabling the successful adoption of emerging gene-based therapies and advancing precision medicine in Saudi Arabia. Concrete steps that support this direction include higher exposure for ophthalmic genetics among ophthalmology residents, establishing multidisciplinary clinics with genetic counselors, and developing national guidelines for genetic testing in ophthalmology.

Supplementary Materials: The following supporting information can be downloaded at: https://www.mdpi.com/article/10.3390/jpm16050267/s1, Table S1: Knowledge, Attitude and Practices towards Genomic Medicine among Ophthalmologists in Saudi Arabia.

Author Contributions: Conceptualization, W.B.; Methodology, W.B. and H.A.; Software, H.B.A. and N.M.A.; Formal analysis, W.B., N.M.A. and Y.A.A.; Data curation, M.S.M.; Writing—original draft, W.B. and H.B.A.; Writing—review & editing, W.B., H.A., H.B.A., N.M.A., Y.A.A. and M.S.M.; Visualization, W.B. and H.A.; Supervision, W.B., H.A. and H.B.A.; Project administration, W.B. All authors have read and agreed to the published version of the manuscript.

Funding: This research received no external funding.

Institutional Review Board Statement: The study was conducted in accordance with the Declaration of Helsinki and approved by the Institutional Review Board of King Khaled Eye Specialist Hospital (KKESH); reference: 45148-P. 3/11/2024.

Informed Consent Statement: Informed consent was obtained electronically from the participants after explaining the aims of the study.

Data Availability Statement: All the data presented in this manuscript are available on request.

Conflicts of Interest: The authors declare no conflicts of interest.

Abbreviations

The following abbreviations are used in this manuscript:

KAP	knowledge, attitudes, and practices

References

1. Collins, F.S.; Morgan, M.; Patrinos, A. The Human Genome Project: Lessons from large-scale biology. *Science* **2003**, *300*, 286–29 [CrossRef]
2. Daiger, S.P.; Sullivan, L.S.; Bowne, S.J. Genes and mutations causing retinitis pigmentosa. *Clin. Genet.* **2013**, *84*, 132–141. [CrossRe
3. Haga, S.B.; O'Daniel, J.M.; Tindall, G.M.; Lipkus, I.R.; Agans, R. Survey of US public attitudes toward pharmacogenetic testin *Pharmacogenom. J.* **2012**, *12*, 197–204. [CrossRef]
4. Olwi, D.; Merdad, L.; Ramadan, E. Knowledge of Genetics and Attitudes toward Genetic Testing among College Students i Saudi Arabia. *Public Health Genom.* **2016**, *19*, 260–268. [CrossRef] [PubMed]

https://doi.org/10.3390/jpm1605026

Alzoubi, A.; Kanaan, H.; Alhazaimeh, D.; Gharaibeh, S.; Mukattash, T.L.; Kheirallah, K. Knowledge, attitude, future expectations, and perceived barriers of medical students and physicians regarding pharmacogenomics in Jordan. *Int. J. Clin. Pract.* **2020**, *75*, e13658. [CrossRef]

Alrabiah, Z.; Syed, W.; Babelghaith, S.D.; Al Arifi, M.N. Clinical Knowledge, Attitude, and Perceptions of Community Pharmacists Towards Pharmacogenomics—A Cross-Sectional Study from Saudi Arabia. *Pharmacogenom. Pers. Med.* **2023**, *16*, 433–441. [CrossRef] [PubMed] [PubMed Central]

Alsanosi, S.M.; Al Eissa, M.M. Awareness of pharmacogenomic capabilities among physicians and pharmacists in Saudi Arabia within current clinical practice. *J. Umm Al-Qura Univ. Med. Sci.* **2025**, *11*, 1. [CrossRef]

AlEissa, M.M.; Alhawsawi, A.A.; Alonazi, R.; Magharbil, E.; Aljahdali, A.; AlBalawi, H.B.; Alali, N.M.; Hameed, S.; Abu-Amero, K.K.; Magliyah, M.S. Advances in Precision Therapeutics and Gene Therapy Applications for Retinal Diseases: Impact and Future Directions. *Genes* **2025**, *16*, 847. [CrossRef]

Knoppers, B.M.; Beauvais, M.J.S. Three decades of genetic privacy: A metaphoric journey. *Hum. Mol. Genet.* **2021**, *30*, R156–R160. [CrossRef] [PubMed] [PubMed Central]

Manolio, T.A.; Chisholm, R.L.; Ozenberger, B.; Roden, D.M.; Williams, M.S.; Wilson, R.; Bick, D.; Bottinger, E.P.; Brilliant, M.H.; Eng, C.; et al. Implementing genomic medicine in the clinic: The future is here. *Genet. Med.* **2013**, *15*, 258–267. [CrossRef]

AlRasheed, M.M.; AlAli, H.; Alsuwaid, A.F.; Khalaf, S.; Ata, S.I.; BinDhim, N.F.; Bakheet, D.; Khurshid, F.; Alhawassi, T.M. Gene Therapy Knowledge and Attitude Among Healthcare Professionals: A Cross-Sectional Study. *Front. Public Health* **2021**, *9*, 773175. [CrossRef] [PubMed] [PubMed Central]

Yu, M.W.C.; Fung, J.L.F.; Ng, A.P.P.; Li, Z.; Lan, W.; Chung, C.C.Y.; Li, Y.; Liu, Y.; Chung, B.H.Y.; Wong, W.C.W. Preparing for the genomic revolution: Attitudes, clinical practice, and training needs in delivering genetic counseling in primary care in Hong Kong and Shenzhen, China. *Mol. Genet. Genom. Med.* **2021**, *9*, e1702. [CrossRef] [PubMed] [PubMed Central]

Chow-White, P.A.; Ha, D.; Laskin, J. Knowledge, attitudes, and values among physicians working with clinical genomics: A survey of medical oncologists. *Hum. Resour. Health* **2017**, *15*, 42. [CrossRef]

Christensen, K.D.; Vassy, J.L.; Jamal, L.; Lehmann, L.S.; Slashinski, M.J.; Perry, D.L.; Robinson, J.; Blumenthal-Barby, J.; Feuerman, L.; Murray, M. Are physicians prepared for whole genome sequencing? A qualitative analysis. *Clin. Genet.* **2016**, *89*, 228–234. [CrossRef]

Haga, S.B.; Kim, E.; Myers, R.A.; Ginsburg, G.S. Primary care physicians' knowledge, attitudes, and experience with personal genetic testing. *J. Pers. Med.* **2019**, *9*, 29. [CrossRef] [PubMed]

Mawkili, W.A. The future of personalized medicine in Saudi Arabia: Opportunities and challenges. *Saudi Med. J.* **2025**, *46*, 19–25. [CrossRef]

AlEissa, M.M.; Alhawsawi, A.A.; Milibari, D.; Schatz, P.; AlBalawi, H.B.; Alali, N.M.; Abu-Amero, K.K.; Hameed, S.; Magliyah, M.S. Genetics and Clinical Findings Associated with Early-Onset Myopia and Retinal Detachment in Saudi Arabia. *Genes* **2025**, *16*, 848. [CrossRef] [PubMed]

DuBois, J.M.; Callier, S.L.; Garrison, N.A.; James, C.A.; Henderson, G.E. Attitudes and expectations toward genomics and precision medicine: Perspectives from medical professionals and patients. *BMC Med. Ethics* **2021**, *22*, 41.

Katsanis, S.H.; Katsanis, N. Molecular genetic testing and the future of clinical genomics. *Nat. Rev. Genet.* **2013**, *14*, 415–426. [CrossRef] [PubMed]

https://doi.org/10.3390/jpm16050267

Journal of
Personalized Medicine

MDPI

Article

Intravitreal Aflibercept for the Treatment of Diabetic Retinopathy Among Patients Who Completed PANORAMA: 1-Year Outcomes from the VOYAGE Extension Study

Avery W. Zhou [1,†], Gail M. Teagle [1,†], Liisa M. Baumann [1], Jessica A. Cao [1], Andres Emanuelli [2], Allen Y. Hu [3], Adam S. Berger [4], James C. Major, Jr. [1], Seong Y. Lee [5], Stephen M. Huddleston [6], Victor H. Gonzalez [7], W. Lloyd Clark [8], David S. Liao [9], Ronald M. Kingsley [10], Howard S. Lazarus [11], John F. Payne [12], Eric G. Feinstein [13], Annal D. Meleth [14], Sagar B. Patel [1], Kenneth C. Fan [1], Alyson J. Berliner [15], Hadi Moini [15], Xiaomeng Niu [15], Michael S. Ip [16], SriniVas R. Sadda [16], Hasenin Al-khersan [1] and Charles C. Wykoff [1,*]

1 Retina Consultants of Texas, Retina Consultants of America, Bellaire, TX 77401, USA; gail.teagle@retinaconsultantstexas.com (G.M.T.); liisa.baumann@retinaconsultantstexas.com (L.M.B.); jessica.cao@utsouthwestern.edu (J.A.C.)
2 Emanuelli Research and Development Center, Arecibo 00612, Puerto Rico
3 Cumberland Valley Retina Consultants, Hagerstown, MD 21740, USA
4 Center for Retina and Macular Disease, Clermont, FL 34711, USA
5 Strategic Clinical Research Group, Willow Park, TX 76087, USA
6 Charles Retina Institute, Germantown, TN 38138, USA; stevehudd@gmail.com
7 Valley Retina Institute, McAllen, TX 78503, USA
8 North Carolina Retina Associates, Retina Consultants of America, Raleigh, NC 27609, USA
9 Retina-Vitreous Associates Medical Group, Los Angeles, CA 90017, USA
10 Dean McGee Eye Institute, Oklahoma City, OK 73104, USA; ronald-kingsley@dmei.org
11 John-Kenyon American Eye Institute, Louisville, KY 40222, USA; hlazarus@johnkenyon.com
12 Palmetto Retina Center, Retina Consultants of America, Columbia, SC 29204, USA
13 Central Florida Retina, Orlando, FL 32806, USA
14 Marietta Eye Clinic, Marietta, GA 30060, USA
15 Regeneron Pharmaceuticals, Inc., Tarrytown, NY 10591, USA
16 Doheny Eye Institute, Pasadena, CA 91103, USA
* Correspondence: charleswykoff@gmail.com; Tel.: +1-713-524-3434
† These authors contributed equally to this work.

Abstract: Background/Objectives: Evaluate outcomes and treatment patterns with 2 mg intravitreal aflibercept injection among patients who completed the phase 3 PANORAMA trial and enrolled in the VOYAGE (ClinicalTrials.gov identifier, NCT04708145; 12 January 2021) long-term extension study. **Methods**: During VOYAGE, patients were evaluated every 16 weeks and treated with 2 mg intravitreal aflibercept injection as needed depending on ophthalmoscopic examination findings. Those with no history of panretinal photocoagulation (PRP) received aflibercept if their clinician-determined diabetic retinopathy severity scale (DRSS) level was $\geq$47, corresponding to moderately severe non-proliferative diabetic retinopathy (NPDR). Patients with a history of PRP received aflibercept if active neovascularization was present. New or worsening diabetic retinopathy (DR) severity prompted more frequent treatment. **Results**: 320 patients (1 eye per patient) from 87 sites completed the PANORAMA trial. Of these, 41 patients (13% of PANORAMA completers) from 14 sites (16%) enrolled in VOYAGE after a mean interim period of 33.7 months, and 35 patients (85%) completed study visits through 1 year. At year 1 in VOYAGE, the mean number of anti-vascular endothelial growth factor (VEGF) injections increased from 1.1 per year during the interim period to 3.4 per year and was associated with stabilization or improvement in DRSS level in 81% (26/32) of patients. Mean best-corrected visual acuity (BCVA) remained relatively stable, and mean central subfield thickness (CST) improved by 24.4 μm to 269.5 μm through year 1 of VOYAGE. There were no unexpected safety events. **Conclusions**: Following a mean of 3 years of routine clinical care with associated declines in DRSS level, CST, and BCVA, stabilization of DRSS level and BCVA with reductions in CST was achieved through year 1 of the VOYAGE extension study, with a concurrent increase in aflibercept dosing frequency.

Keywords: aflibercept; diabetic retinopathy; anti-VEGF; extension study

1. Introduction

Diabetic retinopathy (DR) remains a leading cause of global vision loss and is estimated to affect 9.6 million people in the United States alone [1]. Vision-threatening complications from DR include proliferative DR (PDR) and diabetic macular edema (DME) [2]. Diabetic retinopathy severity can be assessed using structured grading of fundus color images based on the Early Treatment Diabetic Retinopathy Study (ETDRS) severity scale [3]. There are 12 steps within the Diabetic Retinopathy Severity Scale (DRSS): levels 10 and 20 represent no DR and very mild DR, respectively; levels 35 and 43 represent mild and moderate non-proliferative DR (NPDR), respectively; levels 47 and 53 represent moderately severe and severe NPDR, respectively; and levels 60, 61, 65, 71, 75, 81, and 85 represent increasing severities of PDR [3]. A higher level within the NPDR portion of the ETDRS DRSS is highly predictive of progression to PDR [4], a finding confirmed in multiple recent prospective clinical trials [5,6].

Anti-vascular endothelial growth factor (VEGF) pharmacotherapy has demonstrated the ability to slow DR progression, reduce DME and PDR development, and improve DRSS levels in a meaningful proportion of patients [6,7]. The randomized, double-masked, sham-controlled 100-week, phase 3 PANORAMA (NCT02718326) trial evaluated 2 mg intravitreal aflibercept injection in patients with moderately severe to severe NPDR (DRSS levels 47 and 53) [6]. In PANORAMA, 402 patients (1 eye per patient) with best-corrected visual acuity (BCVA) of 20/40 or better were randomized to either sham, aflibercept every 16 weeks following 3 initial monthly doses and one 8-week interval (aflibercept 2q16), or aflibercept every 8 weeks following 5 initial monthly doses with pro re nata (PRN) dosing in year 2 if DRSS level was worse than 35 (aflibercept 2q8/PRN). Findings from PANORAMA revealed a significantly greater proportion of patients in the aflibercept 2q8/PRN and 2q16 groups experienced a $\geq$ 2-step DRSS level improvement from baseline at week 52 compared with those in the sham group (80% and 65% versus 15%, respectively), and these improvements were maintained through week 100. Most clinically relevant, fewer patients treated with aflibercept versus sham experienced development of PDR or DME through week 100.

For many patients, DR and its associated manifestations is a chronic disease, and long-term close monitoring and personalized care are needed to achieve optimal clinical outcomes [8–10]. However, data on long-term outcomes are limited among patients with NPDR without DME receiving anti-VEGF injections. The VOYAGE phase 4 open-label PANORAMA extension study was therefore conducted to evaluate the long-term outcomes of patients who completed PANORAMA after an intervening period of routine clinical care and help contribute to our understanding of the long-term efficacy and safety of anti-VEGF treatment among these patients.

2. Materials and Methods

VOYAGE (ClinicalTrials.gov identifier, NCT04708145; 12 January 2021) was a prospective, phase 4 open-label extension study which included patients who completed the preceding phase 3 PANORAMA trial. The study protocol was approved by the Advarra

Institutional Review Board and Ethics Committee at each participating site, and the study was performed in adherence with the principles of the Declaration of Helsinki and local regulations [11]. All patients provided written informed consent. Data from patients between the end of PANORAMA and VOYAGE enrollment (the interim period) were retrospectively collected to evaluate patterns of treatment and clinical outcomes during this phase. Collected data included demographic information, visit dates, original randomized groups in PANORAMA, anti-VEGF treatments, laser procedures such as panretinal photocoagulation (PRP), phakic status, BCVA, central subfield thickness (CST), DRSS level, and glycosylated hemoglobin (HbA1c) when available.

During VOYAGE, patients were treated with 2 mg intravitreal aflibercept injection PRN depending on ophthalmoscopic examination findings and investigator-determined DRSS level. Based on the presence or absence of prior PRP application at VOYAGE enrollment, patients were categorized into Group 1, eyes without PRP, or Group 2, eyes with PRP.

Patients with study eyes without PRP (Group 1) were evaluated every 16 weeks and treated with 2 mg intravitreal aflibercept injection if the clinician-determined DRSS level was 47 (moderately severe NPDR) or worse; patients with DRSS level < 47 were not treated. The interval between visits was decreased to every 8 weeks if DRSS level was ≥ 53, there was $\geq$2-step DRSS level worsening compared to the last protocol-scheduled 16-week visit, or if the patient developed active PDR. The patient could then be treated with aflibercept every 8 weeks until there was no active PDR and DRSS improved to the level observed at the visit before the patient began being seen at 8-week intervals.

Patients with study eyes with PRP (Group 2) were evaluated every 16 weeks and treated with 2 mg intravitreal aflibercept injection if the neovascular disease process was active and stable. If the neovascular process was determined to be inactive, no treatment was given. If new or worsening neovascular disease was present, patients were treated every 8 weeks until the process became stable or inactive, at which time the interval between visits increased to every 16 weeks.

If high-risk PDR (defined as neovascularization of the disc greater than 1/3 disc area or any neovascularization associated with vitreous or preretinal hemorrhage) developed, PRP therapy could be applied at the investigator's discretion, although PRP was not required, and investigators were allowed to use aflibercept monotherapy for PDR management. If vitreous or preretinal hemorrhage developed, aflibercept could have been given as often as every 4 weeks until hemorrhage improved and was no longer considered vision-threatening. Patients who developed clinically relevant DME (defined as CST > 320 μm on optical coherence tomography [OCT] or clinically worse than baseline with associated vision loss) could have been treated with aflibercept every 4 or 8 weeks at the investigator's discretion until the DME resolved.

At all visits, patients underwent ETDRS BCVA testing at 4 m, slit lamp and dilated ophthalmic examination, and spectral-domain OCT imaging. Ultra-widefield fundus photography was performed every 16 weeks and was used to determine DRSS levels and presence of center-involving DME by a central reading center (Doheny Image Reading Center, Los Angeles, CA, USA). Per the reading center protocol, eyes could be graded as DRSS level < 61 if there were no active PDR signs, regardless of the presence of PRP scars.

The objective of VOYAGE was to assess longitudinal DRSS level changes, and the primary efficacy endpoint was the proportion of patients achieving DRSS level of 43 (moderate NPDR) or better at 1 year. Secondary outcomes were the proportion of patients with stable, worsened, or improved DRSS level; mean and annualized aflibercept injection frequencies; mean change in ETDRS BCVA; mean change in CST; and incidence of ocular and systemic adverse events (AEs).

All analyses used observed data. The denominators for percentages varied depending on the total data available for that variable. Group comparisons were based on two-tailed *t*-tests, paired where applicable, or analysis of variance (ANOVA) for continuous variables, and chi-square tests for categorical variables. Statistical analyses were performed using Microsoft Excel 2016 (Microsoft Corp, Redmond, WA, USA) and GraphPad Prism version 10.6.0 for Windows (GraphPad Software, Boston, MA, USA, www.graphpad.com [accessed on 25 August 2025]).

3. Results

Of the 87 sites that participated in the core PANORAMA phase 3 trial, 14 sites (16%) participated in VOYAGE and enrolled patients in the prospective VOYAGE extension study (full list of participating sites in Table S1). Of the 111 patients completing PANORAMA at these sites who were potentially eligible for enrollment, 41 patients (37%) enrolled into VOYAGE from June 2021 to July 2022, constituting 13% of the total 320 patients who completed PANORAMA (Figure 1). The demographics of the VOYAGE patients were consistent with those of the overall PANORAMA population, with all 3 original randomized arms being approximately equally represented within VOYAGE (Table 1). The total mean (SD) time of follow-up from initial enrollment in PANORAMA to the 1-year endpoint of VOYAGE was 5.7 years (0.4), or approximately 5 years and 8 months.

Table 1. Demographic and ocular characteristics of patients in VOYAGE and PANORAMA.

	Prospective VOYAGE Enrollment *		**PANORAMA Enrollment †**			**Enrollment Baseline Totals**	
	Group 1 (*n* = 35)	**Group 2 § (*n* = 6)**	**Sham (*n* = 11)**	**Q16W ¥ (*n* = 12)**	**Q8W (*n* = 18)**	**VOYAGE ‡ (*n* = 41)**	**PANORAMA (*n* = 402)**
Age, mean (SD), yrs	59.4 (12.0)	59.0 (6.3)	63.4 (8.9)	58.1 (14.7)	57.6 (10.0)	59.3 (11.3)	55.7 (10.5)
Male, *n* (%)	19 (54)	2 (33)	5 (46)	6 (50)	10 (56)	21 (51)	225 (56)
Race, *n* (%)							
White	30 (86)	6 (100)	10 (91)	12 (100)	14 (78)	36 (88)	310 (77)
Black	4 (11)	0	1 (9)	0	3 (17)	4 (10)	41 (10)
Asian	1 (3)	0	0	0	1 (6)	1 (2)	23 (6)
Other	0	0	0	0	0	0	28 (7)
Hispanic or Latino, *n* (%)	19 (54)	1 (17)	7 (64)	6 (50)	7 (39)	20 (49)	Not reported
HbA1c, mean (SD), %	8.6 (2.2)	10.2 (3.0)	8.9 (2.7)	8.4 (2.3)	9.2 (2.3)	8.9 (2.4)	8.5 (1.6)
ETDRS letters, mean (SD)	79.3 (8.7)	65.5 (32.2)	82.2 (6.8)	73.8 (23.8)	76.7 (9.9)	77.3 (14.8)	82.4 (6.0)
Snellen equivalent	20/25	20/50	20/25	20/32	20/32	20/32	20/25
CST, mean (SD), µm	291.9 (67.7)	308.0 (75.4)	279.9 (50.4)	294.9 (42.8)	301.9 (88.4)	293.9 (67.9)	247.4 (34.8)
DRSS level, *n* (%)							
≤43	25 (71)	0	6 (55)	6 (50)	13 (72)	25 (61)	0
47	1 (3)	0	0	1 (8)	0	1 (2)	302 (75)
53	1 (3)	0	0	1 (8)	0	1 (2)	100 (25)
≥60	8 (23)	5 (100)	5 (45)	3 (25)	5 (28)	13 (32)	0

CST = central subfield thickness; DRSS = diabetic retinopathy severity scale; ETDRS = Early Treatment Diabetic Retinopathy Study; HbA1c = glycosylated hemoglobin; SD = standard deviation. * Patients assigned to Group 1 (no history of panretinal photocoagulation) and Group 2 (history of panretinal photocoagulation) during VOYAGE. † Patients initially randomized to the sham, every-16-week (Q16W), and every-8-week (Q8W) arms during PANORAMA. ‡ CST *n* = 40 due to 1 case of vitreous hemorrhage at VOYAGE baseline; DRSS *n* = 40 due to 1 case of DRSS level not measured at VOYAGE baseline. § DRSS *n* = 5 due to 1 case of DRSS level not measured at VOYAGE baseline. ¥ DRSS *n* = 11 due to 1 case of DRSS level not measured at VOYAGE baseline.

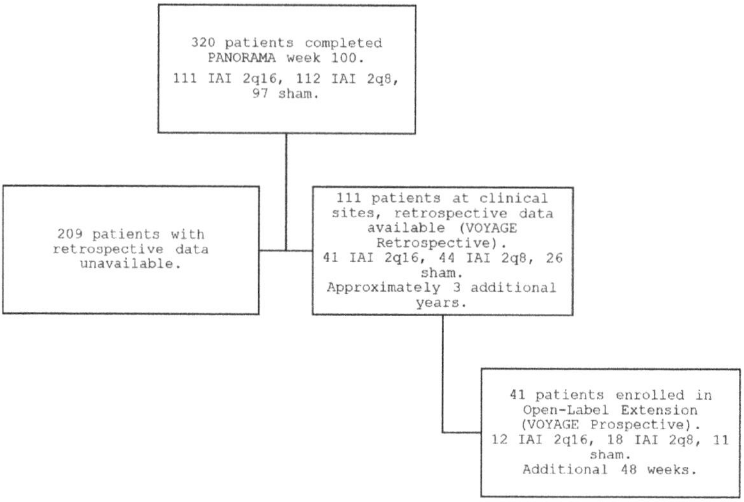

Figure 1. PANORAMA, interim period, and VOYAGE study flow.

3.1. Clinical Course During Interim Period

Among the 41 patients enrolled, the mean length of the interim period from PANORAMA exit to VOYAGE enrollment was 33.7 months (SD 4.8, range 23.9–44.2). During this period, 24 patients (59%, 24/41) received no anti-VEGF injections, while the other 17 patients (41%, 17/41) received a mean of 2.7 anti-VEGF injections per year. Among all patients, a mean of 1.1 injections per year (SD 1.9) were given during the interim period (Figure 2). Patients who had been in the combined aflibercept arms within PANORAMA ($n = 30$) experienced significant decreases in annualized mean anti-VEGF injections from 5.6 injections per year (SD 1.3) during PANORAMA to 1.0 injections per year (SD 1.6) in the interim ($p < 0.001$), whereas sham patients within PANORAMA ($n = 11$) did not have significantly different anti-VEGF injection rates during PANORAMA due to the institution of rescue therapy (2.7 injections per year [SD 3.9]) compared to the interim period (1.4 injections per year [SD 2.6]) ($p = 0.36$).

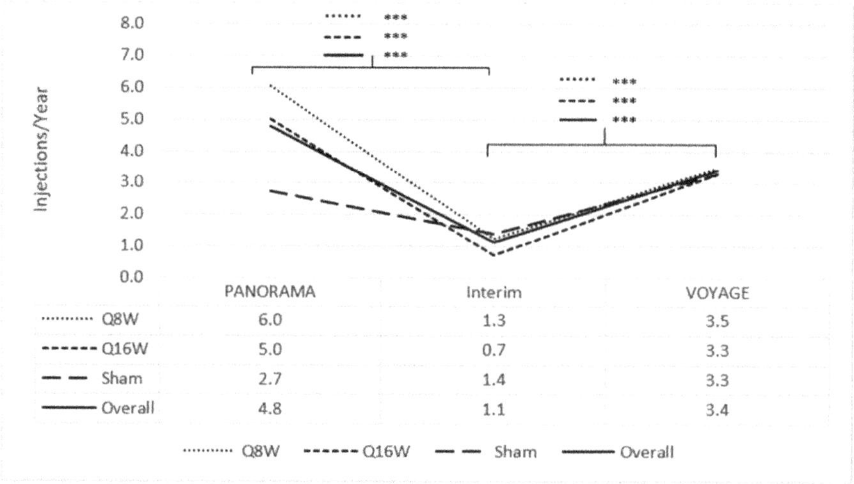

Figure 2. Mean injection frequency from PANORAMA enrollment to VOYAGE 1-year, annualized. The line corresponding to *** signifies statistical significance of <0.001 on a two-tailed t-test.

Three patients (7%, 3/41) received PRP during the interim period. Nine patients (22%, 9/41) received focal macular laser during the interim period. One patient (2%, 1/41) underwent pars plana vitrectomy (PPV) during the interim period for vitreous hemorrhage.

At PANORAMA exit, 73% (8/11) and 89% (24/27) of the sham and combined aflibercept arms had DRSS level $\leq$ 43, respectively. During the interim period, 41% (15/37) of patients worsened, of which 5 patients worsened 1 step and 10 patients worsened $\geq$ 2 steps; 13 patients (35%, 13/37) had stable DRSS levels; and 9 (24%, 9/37) improved by 1 or 2 steps at VOYAGE enrollment compared to PANORAMA exit (Figure 3). Notably, the proportion of patients with PDR (DRSS level $\geq$ 60) increased from 5% (2/38) to 33% (13/40), while the proportion of patients with DRSS level $\leq$ 43 decreased from 84% (32/38) at the beginning of the interim period to 63% (25/40) at the end. Additionally, mean HbA1c remained stable during the interim period (8.9% [SD 1.8] at PANORAMA exit and 8.9% [SD 2.4] at VOYAGE enrollment). Seven patients (18%, 7/39) had center-involving DME by the end of the interim period.

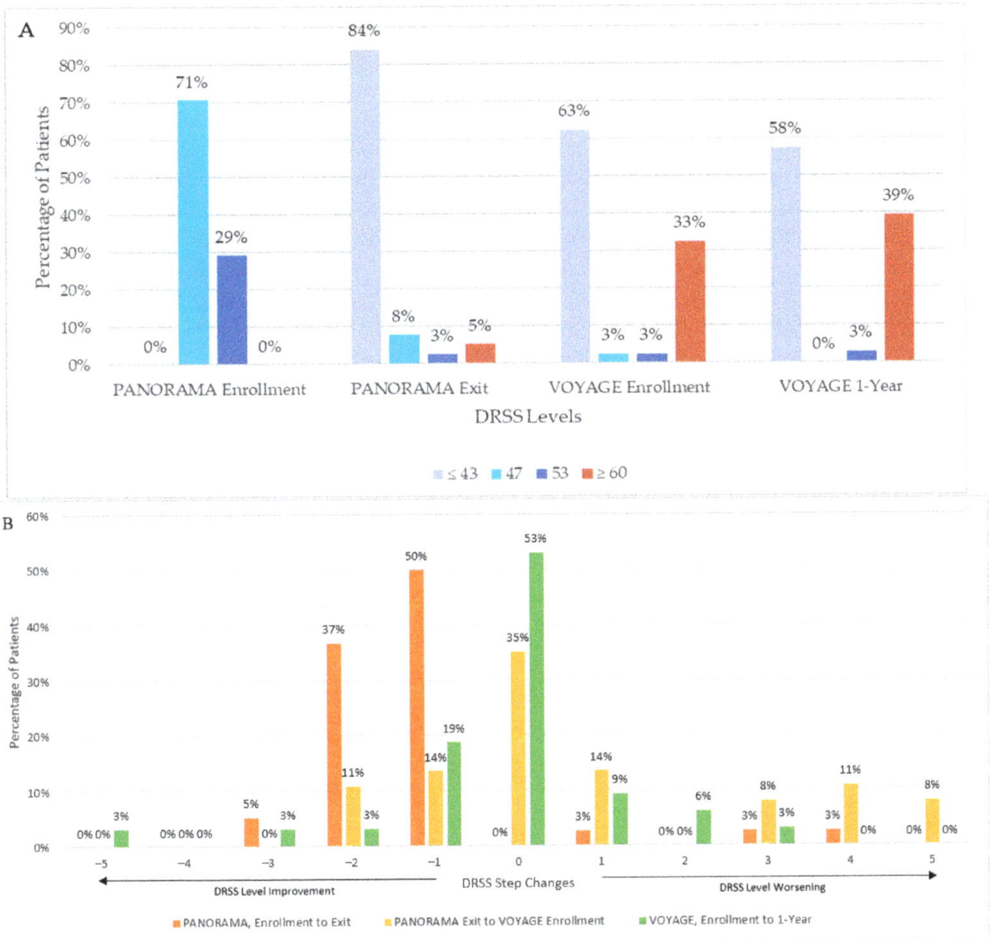

Figure 3. Diabetic Retinopathy Severity Scale (DRSS) levels from PANORAMA enrollment to VOYAGE 1-year. (**A**) Absolute DRSS levels. (**B**) Step changes in DRSS levels; positive values represent DRSS step worsening to a greater severity, and negative values represent DRSS step improvements to a lower severity.

Sub-analysis of the 22 patients (59%, 22/37) who experienced stable or improved DRSS levels during the interim period revealed a roughly equal distribution of patients assigned to PANORAMA Q16W, Q8W, and sham arms (5:10:7); 15 of the 22 patients (68%) had a PANORAMA baseline DRSS level of 47, and the other 7 patients (32%) had a baseline DRSS level of 53. Of the patients with stable or improved DRSS levels during the interim period, 20 patients (91%, 20/22) were in Group 1, and the other 2 patients (9%, 2/22) were in Group 2. This is a similar distribution as that of the 15 patients who experienced worsening DRSS levels during the interim period, with 87% (13/15) in Group 1 and 13% (2/15) in Group 2. There was no meaningful difference in the proportion of patients who improved, remained stable, or worsened during VOYAGE compared with their previous mean anti-VEGF injection frequency during PANORAMA (one-way ANOVA, $p > 0.05$). There were slight differences during the interim period (one-way ANOVA with multiple comparisons, $p = 0.04$): 2.1 greater annual injections for patients who improved compared to remained stable ($p = 0.04$), and 1.8 greater annual injections for patients who improved compared to worsened ($p > 0.05$), while patients who remained stable compared to worsened received approximately the same number of injections ($p > 0.05$).

At PANORAMA exit, mean BCVA was not significantly different between the combined aflibercept and sham arms. Mean BCVA decreased during the interim period from 83.8 letters (SD 6.1) to 77.3 letters (SD 14.8) ($p = 0.009$), representing a mean loss of 6.5 letters (Figure 4A). BCVA losses during the interim period were most notable among patients who had been in the combined aflibercept arms, with combined mean BCVA decreasing by 7.8 mean letters, from 83.3 letters (SD 5.9) at PANORAMA exit to 75.5 letters (SD 16.6) at VOYAGE enrollment ($p = 0.02$). BCVA losses were less among patients previously enrolled in the sham arm (85.2 letters [SD 6.6] to 82.2 letters [SD 6.8]). Patients from all of the PANORAMA arms combined who remained in the NPDR stage ($n = 26$, DRSS level ≤ 53) throughout the interim period also experienced a mean 4.3 letter loss from 85.5 letters (SD 4.2) at PANORAMA exit to 81.2 letters (7.0) at VOYAGE enrollment (paired, $p < 0.001$).

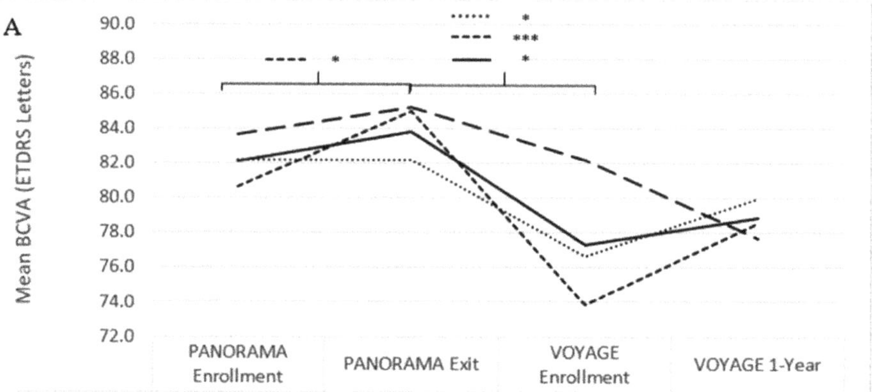

	PANORAMA Enrollment	PANORAMA Exit	VOYAGE Enrollment	VOYAGE 1-Year
Q8W	82.2	82.2	76.7	80.0
Q16W	80.7	85.0	73.8	78.5
Sham	83.6	85.2	82.2	77.7
Overall	82.1	83.8	77.3	78.9

Q8W Q16W Sham Overall

Figure 4. *Cont.*

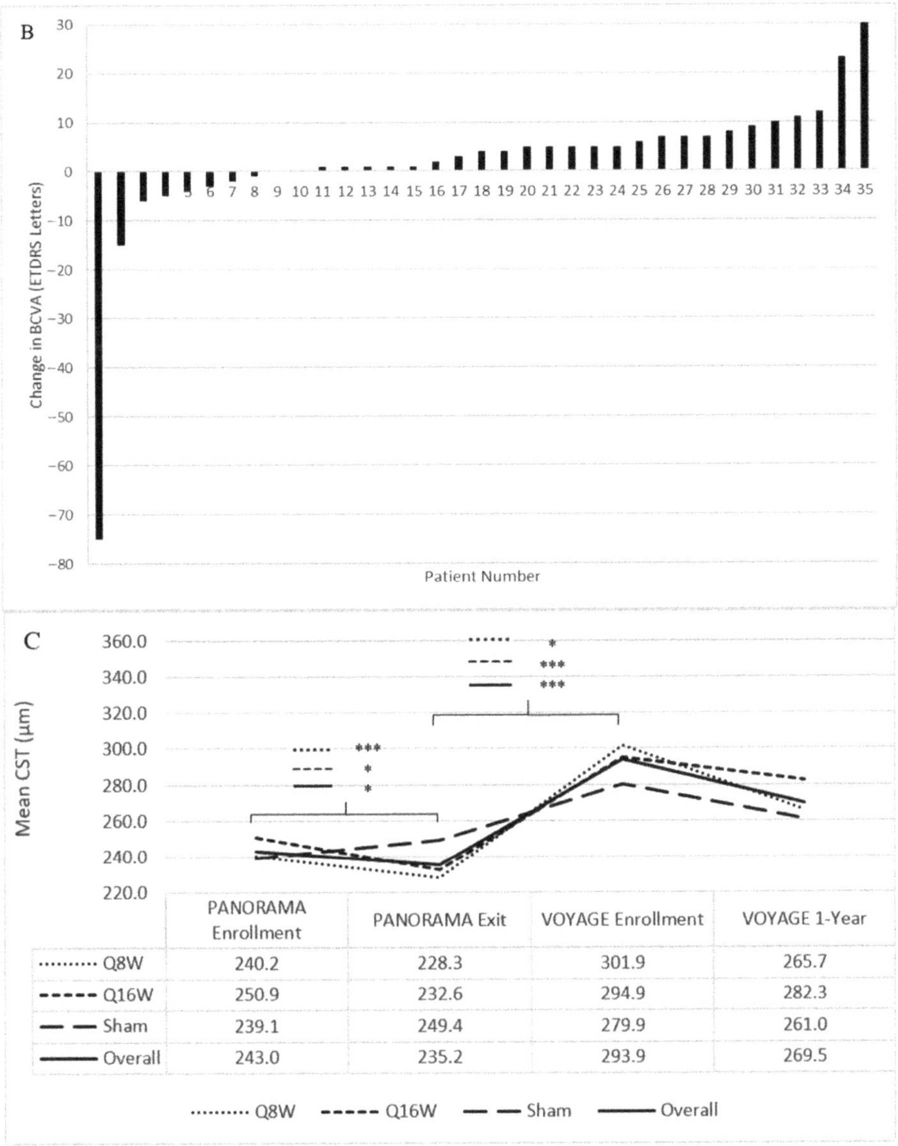

Figure 4. Mean best-corrected visual acuity (BCVA) and central subfield thickness (CST) from PANORAMA enrollment to VOYAGE 1-year. (**A**) Mean BCVA from PANORAMA enrollment to VOYAGE 1-year. (**B**) Change in BCVA from VOYAGE baseline to VOYAGE 1-year for each patient. Notably, patients 1, 2, 29, and 35 had a traumatic cataract resulting in 0 letters read at VOYAGE 1-year, endophthalmitis resulting in a loss of 15 letters by VOYAGE 1-year, cataract extraction resulting in an improvement of 8 letters at VOYAGE 1-year, and vitreous hemorrhage resulting in 0 letters read at VOYAGE baseline, respectively. (**C**) Mean CST from PANORAMA enrollment to VOYAGE 1-year. ETDRS = Early Treatment Diabetic Retinopathy Study. Line-corresponding * signifies statistical significance of $p < 0.05$, and *** signifies statistical significance of $p < 0.001$ on a two-tailed t-test.

At PANORAMA exit, mean CST was not significantly different between the combined aflibercept and sham arms. Mean CST during the interim period increased from 235.2 μm

(SD 39.1) to 293.9 μm (SD 67.9) ($p < 0.001$) (Figure 4C). Changes in CST during the interim period were most notable among patients who had been in the combined aflibercept arms, with combined mean CST increasing by 69.2 μm, from 230.0 μm (SD 32.6) to 299.2 μm (SD 73.5) ($p < 0.001$); patients previously enrolled in the sham arm experienced a smaller increase in mean CST of 30.5 μm, from 249.4 μm (SD 52.4) to 279.9 μm (SD 50.4).

3.2. *Clinical Course During VOYAGE*

Thirty-five patients (85%, 35/41) completed the VOYAGE 1-year primary endpoint; 2 patients died (due to myocardial infarction (MI) and unknown cause), 2 were lost to follow-up, and 2 withdrew consent at week 16 and 48 due to hospitalization following a cerebrovascular accident (CVA) and patient preference, respectively. Of the 164 possible visits among all patients through the first year, 14 visits (9%) were missed.

Through 1 year of VOYAGE, 7 patients (17%, 7/41) received no 2 mg intravitreal aflibercept injections and the remaining 34 (83%, 34/41) received a mean of 3.5 injections (range 1–9 injections); among the entire population, mean injection frequency increased from 1.1 injections per year (SD 1.9) during the interim period to 3.4 injections per year (SD 2.6) during VOYAGE ($p < 0.001$) (Figure 2). Of the patients who had been in the combined aflibercept arms, 2 mg intravitreal aflibercept injection frequency increased from 1.0 injection per year (SD 1.6) during the interim to 3.4 injections per year (SD 2.7) during VOYAGE ($p < 0.001$); patients who had been in the sham arm did not experience a significant change in 2 mg intravitreal aflibercept injection frequency from the interim period (1.4 injections per year [SD 2.6]) to VOYAGE (3.3 injections per year [SD 2.2]) ($p = 0.09$).

There were no meaningful differences in the annualized mean injection frequencies between Groups 1 (3.3 injections per year [SD 2.4]) and 2 (3.7 injections per year [SD 3.5]), or among patients previously assigned to the sham, Q16W, and Q8W arms (mean of 3.3 injections per year [SD 2.2], 3.3 injections per year [SD 3.3], and 3.5 injections per year [SD 2.3], respectively) during VOYAGE. One patient (2%, 1/41) received PRP during year 1 of VOYAGE, and 1 patient (2%, 1/41) received PPV for vitreous hemorrhage.

Mean HbA1c decreased from 8.9% (SD 2.4) at VOYAGE enrollment to 8.1% (SD 1.9) at VOYAGE 1 year. Eleven patients (27%, 11/41) were on glucagon-like peptide-1 receptor agonists during VOYAGE, with no apparent meaningful differences in baseline or 1-year outcomes between these patients and the rest of the VOYAGE cohort.

3.2.1. Diabetic Retinopathy Severity Scale Levels

Overall, DRSS levels appeared relatively stable through 1 year of VOYAGE; 53% (17/32) did not change DRSS level, while 28% (9/32) improved and 19% (6/32) worsened (Figure 3). The proportion of patients with DRSS level ≤ 43 decreased from 63% (25/40) to 58% (19/33), and the proportion of patients with DRSS level ≥ 60 increased from 33% (13/40) to 39% (13/33) from VOYAGE enrollment to year 1.

Of the patients who had PDR (DRSS level ≥ 60; 33%, 13/40) at VOYAGE enrollment, 42% (5/12) improved, 42% (5/12) remained stable, and 17% (2/12) worsened through 1 year. Of the patients who had NPDR (68%, 27/40) at VOYAGE enrollment, 20% (4/20) improved, 60% (12/20) remained stable, and 20% (4/20) worsened through 1 year. One of the patients (5%, 1/20) with NPDR progressed to PDR at 1 year. Four (20%, 4/20) of the patients with NPDR improved by at least 1 step by VOYAGE 1-year. Only 1 patient (3%, 1/32) developed new center-involving DME through VOYAGE 1-year.

The 6 patients (19%, 6/32) with worse DRSS levels through 1 year had mild to moderate NPDR (67%, 4/6) or inactive PDR (33%, 2/6) at VOYAGE baseline. In comparison, 26 patients (81%, 26/32) experienced DRSS level stability or improvement throughout 1 year of VOYAGE, with 23 patients (72%, 23/32) in Group 1 and 3 (9%, 3/32) in Group 2.

There were no meaningful differences ($p > 0.05$) in mean HbA1c at VOYAGE initiation or 1 year, mean 2 mg intravitreal aflibercept injections received in VOYAGE at 1 year, or cumulative mean 2 mg intravitreal aflibercept injections per year since PANORAMA initiation between patients who improved or worsened in DRSS levels at VOYAGE 1-year.

3.2.2. Best-Corrected Visual Acuity and Central Subfield Thickness

Mean BCVA remained stable from VOYAGE baseline (77.3 letters [SD 14.8]) to 1 year (78.9 letters [SD 17.7]) (Figure 4A). In total, 27 patients (77%, 27/35) had stable or improved BCVA through 1 year. At VOYAGE baseline, 1 patient (2%, 1/41) had a vitreous hemorrhage, resulting in 0 letters read (Figure 4B). One patient (3%, 1/35) received cataract surgery while enrolled in VOYAGE and subsequently experienced an 8-letter improvement at 1 year. At VOYAGE 1-year, 1 patient (3%, 1/35) had a traumatic cataract resulting in 0 letters read. Five patients (14%, 5/35) gained at least 10 letters from VOYAGE baseline through 1 year, and 1 patient (3%, 1/35) lost 15 letters following endophthalmitis.

At VOYAGE 1-year, mean CST decreased from 293.9 μm (SD 67.9) to 269.5 μm (SD 34.5) ($p = 0.06$) (Figure 4C). Twenty-one patients (64%, 21/33) had improved CST through 1 year. There was no significant difference in CST decrease among patients who had PDR (46.2 μm [SD 105.3]) versus NPDR at VOYAGE baseline (10.6 μm [SD 40.0]), or between Group 1 (22.3 μm [SD 71.3]) and Group 2 (32.3 μm [SD 84.0]) patients. Patients previously assigned to sham, Q16W, and Q8W during PANORAMA had mean decreases in CST of 13.8 μm (SD 36.1), 13.7 μm (SD 62.4), and 36.8 μm (SD 93.6), respectively, which also did not significantly differ from one another.

3.2.3. Adverse Events

Through 1 year of VOYAGE, treatment-emergent AEs occurred in 28 patients (68%, 28/41), none of which were determined to be related to aflibercept. There was 1 case of traumatic cataract related to the injection procedure at week 48 out of 119 total injections (incidence of 0.8%), which included 72 injections in phakic eyes (incidence of 1% of phakic injections), during the prospective component of VOYAGE. Inflammatory events were reported in 2 patients (5%, 2/41), with 1 case of concurrent anterior chamber cells and vitreous haze, which were reportedly related to keratoconjunctivitis sicca and active PDR, respectively, and did not require treatment, and 1 case of endophthalmitis (incidence of 1/119 injections, or 0.8%) reported as related to the injection procedure. Reported serious AEs included 1 vascular death from a fatal MI (2%, 1/41), 1 death of unknown cause (2%, 1/41), and 1 nonfatal CVA (2%, 1/41).

4. Discussion

Results from the prospective VOYAGE study, which enrolled a subset of patients who completed the PANORAMA phase 3 trial, indicate that during an approximate 3-year period of routine clinical care, DRSS level, CST, and BCVA all appeared to numerically worsen, particularly among patients who had been randomized to receive 2 mg intravitreal aflibercept injection during PANORAMA. Concurrently, there was a decrease in intravitreal anti-VEGF injections administered during the interim period. Then, following initiation of aflibercept therapy for pre-defined DR activity thresholds during VOYAGE, overall mean BCVA and CST increased by 1.8 letters and decreased by 24.4 μm, respectively. Relevant to this reversal, patients received intravitreal anti-VEGF injections more than 4 times as frequently during PANORAMA (4.8 injections per year) and almost 3 times as frequently during VOYAGE (3.4 injections per year) compared to the interim period (1.1 injections per year).

From PANORAMA baseline to the VOYAGE 1-year timepoint, DRSS levels worsened for many patients, with 39% (13/33) of patients developing PDR. This DRSS level worsening occurred predominantly during the interim period, when less frequent anti-VEGF treatment was utilized, and DRSS levels predominantly stabilized with more frequent treatment during VOYAGE. More frequent anti-VEGF dosing may have been needed to achieve maximal DRSS level improvement. Furthermore, the ability to improve DRSS levels may be at least partially dependent on initial disease severity; specifically, in some datasets, DRSS level improvements have been less robust among patients with PDR compared to those with NPDR [12,13]. For example, in CLARITY, 78% of patients treated with a mean of 4.4 aflibercept injections through 1 year did not improve to NPDR [12]; VOYAGE seemed to produce similar results, with 11 of the patients (92%, 11/12) with PDR not returning to NPDR following 1 year of aflibercept treatment. Additionally, there were no meaningful differences in mean HbA1c at VOYAGE baseline or 1 year between patients who experienced improved or worsened DRSS levels at VOYAGE 1-year. Larger studies with longer follow-up time are needed to better identify patient-level factors that may influence who benefits most from sustained aflibercept therapy.

Considering BCVA and CST longitudinally, although both appeared relatively stable between PANORAMA baseline and the VOYAGE 1-year timepoint, there were periods of substantial fluctuation throughout the 5.7 years in between. These changes appear to have been driven by the meaningfully different approaches to clinical care utilized during these 3 time periods. Specifically, during the interim period when patients received routine care outside of a rigid prospective protocol, VA and CST temporarily worsened by over 6 ETDRS letters and 58 μm, respectively. Of note, fluctuations in specific DME biomarkers have been reported to be associated with worse visual outcomes. For example, greater CST fluctuations have been associated with worse VA outcomes at 1 and 2 years among DME patients in retrospective analyses [14,15]. While the visit-to-visit granularity of CST fluctuations is beyond the scope of the current work, overall data suggests that in order to maximize clinical outcomes, it may be worthwhile to consider a personalized approach with more consistent intervention in order to minimize disease fluctuations.

During the interim period, when less structured follow-ups and less consistent anti-VEGF dosing were utilized, clinical characteristics appeared to worsen. According to the 2024 American Society of Retina Specialists Preferences and Trends Survey, inconsistent or insufficient office visits were found to be the factor that has the greatest negative impact on all patient outcomes in the United States [16]. However, providing consistent anti-VEGF therapy to patients in a real-world setting is challenging due to a multitude of factors [17]. Additionally, intravitreal injections carry risk as evidenced by the cases of infectious endophthalmitis and traumatic cataract observed in the current series. In order to address these meaningful hurdles to optimal outcomes and care delivery, multiple therapeutic approaches currently under investigation seek to provide consistent, longitudinal ocular-specific treatment for DR and other chronic, exudative retinal diseases. These include anti-VEGF port delivery systems [18], extended durability agents such as tyrosine kinase inhibitors [19,20], and anti-VEGF gene therapies such as RGX-314 and ADVM-022, both of which have demonstrated durable intraocular anti-VEGF protein production and exudative disease control following subretinal and intravitreal delivery, respectively [21–23]. For any potential more durable therapy, the risks and benefits will need to be considered in the clinical context of each patient.

Limitations of the current work include that of the 320 patients across 5 countries who completed PANORAMA, only 41 patients (13% of PANORAMA completers) enrolled in VOYAGE, and all patients were from United States sites, which may limit the generalizability of the results. The underlying reasons for this are likely multifactorial, including study-site operational limitations, patients lost to follow-up, and the additional significant time commitment after having already participated in PANORAMA. While this low VOYAGE enrollment number raises concerns about selection bias and whether this cohort accurately reflects the entire PANORAMA patient population, no meaningful differences were observed in PANORAMA baseline characteristics between the subset that enrolled in VOYAGE and the full PANORAMA cohort. Additionally, although there were no apparent outcome differences between Group 1 and Group 2 patients, the cohort of patients in Group 2 was small (n = 6), which limited the overall ability to meaningfully compare these groups.

Additionally, a key challenge when assessing aflibercept efficacy and durability are the specific criteria used to determine when and how often to treat. VOYAGE treatment criteria were designed to allow physicians to use clinical judgment as to the necessity of retreatment in cases of DME. While this better reflects a real-world approach, it also generates greater variability in treatment decisions and therefore may have influenced variability in outcomes. Future studies using standardized treatment criteria may reduce this variability and improve consistency among outcomes. Another interesting result from this real-world approach was the observation that, on an individual-patient basis, clinician-determined DRSS levels and reading center-determined DRSS levels sometimes disagreed; whereas investigators' scores were distributed more evenly across all NPDR severity levels, the reading center leaned heavily toward mild NPDR scores. Across all patients enrolled, comparing investigator to reading center scores did not change the results, particularly regarding the number of PDR patients. This discrepancy may be due to various factors, such as access to information or time constraints in the clinic setting.

Another key limitation is that because the treatment regimens during the interim period varied considerably, it is challenging to compare how much of the observed anatomic and functional decline was attributable to undertreatment versus disease progression. Additionally, all analyses utilized observed data, so meaningful outliers may have impacted mean values. For example, true mean BCVA improvement may have been underestimated due to the inclusion of 1 case (3%, 1/35) of 0 letters read at 1 year due to traumatic cataract, resulting in an apparent 75 letter loss from VOYAGE baseline through 1 year. Outliers were described when results were meaningfully impacted.

In summary, the observed changes in ocular characteristics across the mean 5.7 years from PANORAMA enrollment through the VOYAGE 1-year endpoint appeared to correlate with anti-VEGF dosing frequency. Patients who received less frequent 2 mg intravitreal aflibercept injections after PANORAMA exit experienced a trend toward worsening of DRSS level, BCVA, and CST at VOYAGE enrollment, trends which appeared to stabilize or improve after re-initiating regular 2 mg intravitreal aflibercept injections during VOYAGE. More data on long-term outcomes are needed from larger patient populations with NPDR to assess the sustainability of these treatment effects and to adequately inform clinical management of this common, chronic condition. Finally, new, safe therapeutics which meaningfully reduce treatment burden may be valuable for personalized, long-term DR management.

Supplementary Materials: The following supporting information can be downloaded at: https://www.mdpi.com/article/10.3390/jpm15110555/s1, Table S1. Participating sites in PANORAMA and VOYAGE.

Author Contributions: Conceptualization, H.M., S.R.S. and C.C.W.; methodology, A.J.B., H.M., S.R.S. and C.C.W.; formal analysis, A.W.Z., G.M.T., L.M.B., J.A.C., X.N., M.S.I., S.R.S. and C.C.W.; investigation, A.E., A.Y.H., A.S.B., J.C.M.J., S.Y.L., S.M.H., V.H.G., W.L.C., D.S.L., R.M.K., H.S.L., J.F.P., E.G.F., A.D.M., S.B.P., K.C.F. and C.C.W.; resources, A.E., A.Y.H., A.S.B., J.C.M.J., S.Y.L., S.M.H., V.H.G., W.L.C., D.S.L., R.M.K., H.S.L., J.F.P., E.G.F., A.D.M., S.B.P., K.C.F., M.S.I., S.R.S., H.A.-k. and C.C.W.; data curation, A.W.Z., G.M.T., L.M.B., J.A.C., X.N., M.S.I., S.R.S. and C.C.W.; writing—original draft preparation, A.W.Z., G.M.T., L.M.B., J.A.C. and C.C.W.; writing—review and editing, A.W.Z., G.M.T.,

L.M.B., J.A.C., A.E., A.Y.H., A.S.B., J.C.M.J., S.Y.L., S.M.H., V.H.G., W.L.C., D.S.L., R.M.K., H.S.L., J.F.P., E.G.F., A.D.M., S.B.P., K.C.F., A.J.B., H.M., X.N., M.S.I., S.R.S., H.A.-k. and C.C.W.; visualization, A.W.Z., G.M.T., L.M.B., J.A.C., H.A.-k. and C.C.W.; supervision, M.S.I., S.R.S., H.A.-k. and C.C.W.; project administration, H.M. and C.C.W.; funding acquisition, S.R.S. and C.C.W. All authors have read and agreed to the published version of the manuscript.

Funding: This research was primarily supported by Regeneron Pharmaceuticals, support provided primarily by Regeneron Pharmaceuticals, Inc., Tarrytown, New York. Funding was also provided in part by the Texas Retina Research Foundation (TRRF), Houston, Texas.

Institutional Review Board Statement: The study was conducted in accordance with the Declaration of Helsinki and approved by the Advarra Institutional Review Board (Columbia, MD, United States) on 31 March 2021 (IRB approval Pro00044668). The study's clinical trial registration number is identifier NCT04708145 registered with ClinicalTrials.gov on 12 January 2021.

Informed Consent Statement: Informed consent was obtained from all patients involved in the study.

Data Availability Statement: The data collected in the course of this study is not publicly available due to it containing information that could compromise the privacy of research patients. Further inquiries can be directed to the corresponding author.

Conflicts of Interest: Andres Emanuelli, M.D., has received research support from Regeneron. Allen Hu, M.D., has received research support from Regeneron; has been a consultant for Regeneron; and has received payment or honoraria for lectures, presentations, speakers bureaus, manuscript writing, or educational events from Regeneron. Stephen Huddleston, M.D., has received research support from Regeneron. W. Lloyd Clark, M.D., has received research support from Regeneron; has been a consultant for Regeneron; and has received payment or honoraria for lectures, presentations, speakers bureaus, manuscript writing, or educational events from Regeneron. David Liao, M.D., has received research support from Regeneron. Sagar B. Patel, M.D., has been a consultant for Regeneron. Alyson J. Berliner, M.D., Ph.D., has been an employee of Regeneron and owns stock or stock options in Regeneron. Hadi Moini, Ph.D., has been an employee of Regeneron, has received research support from Regeneron, has received support for attending meetings and/or travel from Regeneron, and owns stock or stock options in Regeneron. Michael Ip, M.D., has received research support from Regeneron and has been a consultant for Regeneron. SriniVas R. Sadda, M.D., has been a consultant for Regeneron and a participant on a Data Safety Monitoring Board or Advisory Board for Regeneron. Hasenin Al-khersan, M.D., has been a consultant for Regeneron. Charles C. Wykoff, M.D., Ph.D., has received research support from Regeneron and has been a consultant for Regeneron. Regeneron Pharmaceuticals participated in the design of the study; in the collection, analyses, and interpretation of data; in the writing of the manuscript; and in the decision to publish the results.

Abbreviations

The following abbreviations are used in this manuscript:

AE	Adverse event
ANOVA	Analysis of variance
BCVA	Best-corrected visual acuity
CST	Central subfield thickness
CVA	Cerebrovascular accident
DME	Diabetic macular edema
DR	Diabetic retinopathy
DRSS	Diabetic retinopathy severity scale
ETDRS	Early treatment diabetic retinopathy study
HbA1c	Glycosylated hemoglobin
MI	Myocardial infarction
NPDR	Non-proliferative diabetic retinopathy
OCT	Optical coherence tomography
PDR	Proliferative diabetic retinopathy

PPV	Pars plana vitrectomy
PRN	Pro re nata (as needed)
PRP	Panretinal photocoagulation
Q16W	Every-16-week aflibercept following 3 initial monthly doses and one 8-week interval through 2 years
Q8W	Every-8-week aflibercept following 5 initial monthly doses with pro re nata dosing in year 2 if diabetic retinopathy severity scale level was worse than 35
SD	Standard deviation
VA	Visual acuity
VEGF	Vascular endothelial growth factor

eferences

Lundeen, E.A.; Burke-Conte, Z.; Rein, D.B.; Wittenborn, J.S.; Saaddine, J.; Lee, A.Y.; Flaxman, A.D. Prevalence of Diabetic Retinopathy in the US in 2021. *JAMA Ophthalmol.* **2023**, *141*, 747–754. [CrossRef]

Wang, W.; Lo, A.C.Y. Diabetic Retinopathy: Pathophysiology and Treatments. *Int. J. Mol. Sci.* **2018**, *19*, 1816. [CrossRef]

Early Treatment Diabetic Retinopathy Study Research Group. Fundus Photographic Risk Factors for Progression of Diabetic Retinopathy: ETDRS Report Number 12. *Ophthalmology* **1991**, *98*, 823–833. [CrossRef]

Klein, R.; Klein, B.E.K.; Moss, S.E. How Many Steps of Progression of Diabetic Retinopathy Are Meaningful?The Wisconsin Epidemiologic Study of Diabetic Retinopathy. *Arch. Ophthalmol.* **2001**, *119*, 547–553. [CrossRef] [PubMed]

Maturi, R.K.; Glassman, A.R.; Josic, K.; Baker, C.W.; Gerstenblith, A.T.; Jampol, L.M.; Meleth, A.; Martin, D.F.; Melia, M.; Punjabi, O.S.; et al. Four-Year Visual Outcomes in the Protocol W Randomized Trial of Intravitreous Aflibercept for Prevention of Vision-Threatening Complications of Diabetic Retinopathy. *JAMA* **2023**, *329*, 376–385. [CrossRef] [PubMed]

Brown, D.M.; Wykoff, C.C.; Boyer, D.; Heier, J.S.; Clark, W.L.; Emanuelli, A.; Higgins, P.M.; Singer, M.; Weinreich, D.M.; Yancopoulos, G.D.; et al. Evaluation of Intravitreal Aflibercept for the Treatment of Severe Nonproliferative Diabetic Retinopathy: Results From the PANORAMA Randomized Clinical Trial. *JAMA Ophthalmol.* **2021**, *139*, 946–955. [CrossRef] [PubMed]

Korobelnik, J.F.; Do, D.V.; Schmidt-Erfurth, U.; Boyer, D.S.; Holz, F.G.; Heier, J.S.; Midena, E.; Kaiser, P.K.; Terasaki, H.; Marcus, D.M.; et al. Intravitreal Aflibercept for Diabetic Macular Edema. *Ophthalmology* **2014**, *121*, 2247–2254. [CrossRef]

Gross, J.G.; Glassman, A.R.; Liu, D.; Sun, J.K.; Antoszyk, A.N.; Baker, C.W.; Bressler, N.M.; Elman, M.J.; Ferris, F.L.; Gardner, T.W.; et al. Five-Year Outcomes of Panretinal Photocoagulation vs Intravitreous Ranibizumab for Proliferative Diabetic Retinopathy: A Randomized Clinical Trial. *JAMA Ophthalmol.* **2018**, *136*, 1138–1148. [CrossRef]

Boyer, D.S.; Nguyen, Q.D.; Brown, D.M.; Basu, K.; Ehrlich, J.S. Outcomes with As-Needed Ranibizumab after Initial Monthly Therapy: Long-Term Outcomes of the Phase III RIDE and RISE Trials. *Ophthalmology* **2015**, *122*, 2504–2513.e1. [CrossRef]

Wykoff, C.C.; Ou, W.C.; Khurana, R.N.; Brown, D.M.; Lloyd Clark, W.; Boyer, D.S. Long-term outcomes with as-needed aflibercept in diabetic macular oedema: 2-year outcomes of the ENDURANCE extension study. *Br. J. Ophthalmol.* **2018**, *102*, 631–636. [CrossRef]

World Medical Association. World Medical Association Declaration of Helsinki: Ethical Principles for Medical Research Involving Human Subjects. *JAMA* **2013**, *310*, 2191–2194. [CrossRef]

Sivaprasad, S.; Prevost, A.T.; Vasconcelos, J.C.; Riddell, A.; Murphy, C.; Kelly, J.; Bainbridge, J.; Tudor-Edwards, R.; Hopkins, D.; Hykin, P.; et al. Clinical efficacy of intravitreal aflibercept versus panretinal photocoagulation for best corrected visual acuity in patients with proliferative diabetic retinopathy at 52 weeks (CLARITY): A multicentre, single-blinded, randomised, controlled, phase 2b, non-inferiority trial. *Lancet* **2017**, *389*, 2193–2203. [CrossRef] [PubMed]

Wykoff, C.C.; Eichenbaum, D.A.; Roth, D.B.; Hill, L.; Fung, A.E.; Haskova, Z. Ranibizumab Induces Regression of Diabetic Retinopathy in Most Patients at High Risk of Progression to Proliferative Diabetic Retinopathy. *Ophthalmol. Retina.* **2018**, *2*, 997–1009. [CrossRef] [PubMed]

Starr, M.R.; Salabati, M.; Mahmoudzadeh, R.; Patel, L.G.; Ammar, M.J.; Hsu, J.; Garg, S.; Ho, A.C.; Kuriyan, A.E. Fluctuations in Central Subfield Thickness Associated With Worse Visual Outcomes in Patients with Diabetic Macular Edema in Clinical Trial Setting. *Am. J. Ophthalmol.* **2021**, *232*, 90–97. [CrossRef] [PubMed]

Wang, V.Y.; Kuo, B.L.; Chen, A.X.; Wang, K.; Greenlee, T.E.; Conti, T.F.; Singh, R.P. Fluctuations in macular thickness in patients with diabetic macular oedema treated with anti-vascular endothelial growth factor agents. *Eye* **2022**, *36*, 1461–1467. [CrossRef]

Hahn, P.; Garg, S.J. (Eds.) *2024 Global Trends in Retina Survey*; American Society of Retina Specialists: Chicago, IL, USA, 2024.

Suresh, R.; Yu, H.J.; Thoveson, A.; Swisher, J.; Apolinario, M.; Zhou, B.; Shah, A.R.; Fish, R.H.; Wykoff, C.C. Loss to Follow-Up Among Patients With Proliferative Diabetic Retinopathy in Clinical Practice. *Am. J. Ophthalmol.* **2020**, *215*, 66–71. [CrossRef]

18. Emanuelli, A.; Holekamp, N.M.; Latkany, P.; Hu, A.Y.; Suñer, I.J.; Wykoff, C.C.; Brittain, C.; Howard, D.; Quezada-Ruiz, C Santhanakrishnan, A.; et al. Port delivery system with ranibizumab in the treatment of diabetic retinopathy without cent involved diabetic macular edema: Primary analysis results of the phase 3 Pavilion trial. *Invest. Ophthalmol. Vis. Sci.* **202** *64*, 3754.
19. Study to Evaluate the Safety, Tolerability, and Efficacy of OTX-TKI in Subjects With Moderately Severe to Severe No Proliferative Diabetic Retinopathy. ClinicalTrials.gov Identifier: NCT05695417. Updated 8 December 2023. Available onlir https://clinicaltrials.gov/study/NCT05695417 (accessed on 25 July 2024).
20. Eichenbaum, D.A.; Hershberger, V.; Patel, S.S.; Abbey, A.M.; Bridges, W.Z.; Khanani, A.M.; Ruggiero, S.; Roy, M.; Duker, J. Paggiarino, D.A.; et al. The DAVIO 2 trial: A phase 2, randomized, double-masked, controlled multicenter study of EYP-1901 v aflibercept in previously treated wet age-related macular degeneration. *Investig. Ophthalmol. Vis. Sci.* **2024**, *65*, 4401.
21. Campochiaro, P.A.; Avery, R.; Brown, D.M.; Heier, J.S.; Ho, A.C.; Huddleston, S.M.; Jaffe, G.J.; Khanani, A.M.; Pakola, S.; Pierami D.J.; et al. Gene therapy for neovascular age-related macular degeneration by subretinal delivery of RGX-314: A phase 1/ dose-escalation study. *Lancet* **2024**, *403*, 1563–1573. [CrossRef]
22. Gelfman, C.M.; Grishanin, R.; Bender, K.O.; Nguyen, A.; Greengard, J.; Sharma, P.; Nieves, J.; Kiss, S.; Gasmi, M. Comprehensi Preclinical Assessment of ADVM-022, an Intravitreal Anti-VEGF Gene Therapy for the Treatment of Neovascular AMD an Diabetic Macular Edema. *J. Ocul. Pharmacol. Ther.* **2021**, *37*, 181–190. [CrossRef]
23. Rowe, L.W.; Ciulla, T.A. Gene Therapy for Non-Hereditary Retinal Disease: Age-Related Macular Degeneration, Diabet Retinopathy, and Beyond. *Genes* **2024**, *15*, 720. [CrossRef]

Journal of
Personalized Medicine

MDPI

ticle

rom Screening to Therapy: A Personalized Approach to ROP in National NICU Setting

ylianos Christodoulou [1,*], Fedonas Herodotou [2], Annalisa Quattrocchi [3], Theodoros Potamitis [4] d Vivi Choleva [1]

1 Ophthalmology Department Makarios Hospital, Nicosia 2011, Cyprus; vivi.choleva@gmail.com
2 Medical School, University of Cyprus, Nicosia 2029, Cyprus; fedonascom@gmail.com
3 Department of Primary Care and Population Health, University of Nicosia Medical School, Nicosia 2408, Cyprus; quattrocchi.a@unic.ac.cy
4 Pantheo Eye Centre, Limassol 3076, Cyprus; theodoros@cytanet.com.cy
* Correspondence: stelioschl3@gmail.com

Abstract: Aim: We aimed to investigate the incidence, treatment patterns, and associated risk factors of type 1 retinopathy of prematurity (ROP) in the only tertiary-level Neonatal Intensive Care Unit (NICU) in Cyprus. **Methods**: This retrospective study included all infants screened for ROP between January and December 2023. Data were collected from standardized NICU discharge summaries and included gestational age (GA), birth weight (BW), multiple birth, systemic infection, blood transfusion, oxygen therapy, surgical interventions, and ROP outcomes. Infants were categorized into non-ROP, non-type 1 ROP, and type 1 ROP groups. Statistical analysis was performed to identify differences in risk factor distribution. **Results**: Among 183 infants, 33 (18.0%) developed ROP, with 11 (6.0%) requiring treatment for type 1 ROP. All infants with type 1 ROP were born at ≤28 weeks GA and weighed <1501 g. Type 1 ROP was significantly associated with lower GA, lower BW, systemic infection, surgery, and prolonged oxygen support ($p < 0.05$). Six infants were treated with laser and three with intravitreal bevacizumab. No recurrence was observed in the anti-VEGF group during 18 months of follow-up. Two infants with aggressive ROP died before treatment. **Conclusions**: Type 1 ROP in Cyprus occurred exclusively in extremely preterm infants, associated with the cumulative effect of multiple risk factors. Laser remained the primary treatment, while anti-VEGF was used selectively with favorable outcomes. This study emphasizes the importance of tailoring ROP screening and treatment strategies based on individual neonatal risk profiles, supporting a personalized approach to neonatal ophthalmic care.

Keywords: type 1 ROP; Cyprus; anti-VEGF; laser photocoagulation; prematurity; neonatal risk factors; ROP screening

1. Introduction

Retinopathy of prematurity (ROP) is a worldwide leading cause of childhood blindness, resulting from disrupted retinal vascular development in preterm infants. As neonatal care advances globally, the survival of extremely premature infants has improved, yet this has also contributed to a rising incidence of severe forms of ROP. The pathophysiology of ROP involves two distinct phases. In the first phase, hyperoxia due to preterm birth suppresses vascular endothelial growth factor (VEGF), halting retinal vessel growth. The subsequent hypoxic phase leads to VEGF overexpression, triggering abnormal fibrovascular proliferation and potentially progressing to tractional retinal detachment if untreated [1,2].

Type 1 ROP represents the threshold at which treatment is clinically indicated and is defined by the Early Treatment for ROP (ETROP) criteria as stage 3 ROP in zone I or II with plus disease, or any stage ROP in zone I with plus disease. This classification reflects an aggressive disease course with a high risk of progression, requiring prompt intervention. Management strategies for type 1 ROP have evolved significantly in recent decades. Laser photocoagulation, once the mainstay of treatment, ablates avascular peripheral retina to reduce VEGF production and stabilize neovascularization. However, this technique compromises peripheral visual fields and increases the risk of high myopia [3].

In recent years, anti-VEGF agents like bevacizumab, ranibizumab, and aflibercept have emerged as alternatives or adjuncts to laser therapy. These agents target VEGF more selectively, allowing for continued peripheral retinal vascularization and resulting in less refractive error. Studies demonstrate their efficacy, particularly for aggressive ROP (A-ROP), though concerns remain about potential systemic effects due to VEGF's role in organogenesis and neurodevelopment [2,4,5].

Despite these advancements, the management of type 1 ROP remains complex, influenced by disease severity, anatomical location, and patient-specific factors. Both modalities have demonstrated efficacy, but they carry unique risks and benefits. Laser therapy is associated with greater structural stability in the long term, whereas anti-VEGF agents require careful follow-up due to the risk of late reactivation [6,7].

In Cyprus, neonatal care is centralized in a single tertiary Neonatal Intensive Care Unit (NICU), providing a unique opportunity to examine national ROP trends. To date, no comprehensive epidemiological data exist on the incidence, risk factors, and treatment outcomes of type 1 ROP in this setting. This study addresses this gap by investigating the characteristics and therapeutic patterns of ROP in Cyprus, with a particular emphasis on infants who required treatment for type 1 disease. Our findings aim to inform future clinical guidelines and support the development of personalized screening strategies in similar healthcare environments.

There is a growing recognition that neonatal care, particularly in managing ROP, benefits significantly from personalized medicine. Individual variability in gestational maturity and systemic comorbidities necessitate a tailored approach to screening frequency and therapeutic interventions. This study contributes to the understanding of how personalized neonatal care can optimize outcomes in a real-world NICU setting.

2. Methods

2.1. Study Design and Data Collection

This study was a single-center, retrospective cohort study conducted at the NICU in Makarios Hospital. This study included all infants who underwent ROP screening between 1 January and 31 December 2023.

This centralized setting allowed us to capture a comprehensive national cohort of preterm infants at risk of ROP, minimizing selection bias and ensuring population-level relevance.

2.2. ROP Screening Criteria

ROP screening was conducted according to institutional guidelines based on the UK Royal College of Ophthalmologists and Royal College of Paediatrics and Child Health (2008) recommendations [8]. Although updated UK guidelines were released in 2022, our institution's screening protocol during the study period was still based on the 2008 recommendations, which were in active use throughout 2023. The inclusion criteria for screening were

- Gestational age (GA) at birth <32 weeks;
- Birth weight (BW) < 1501 g.

Additionally, neonatologists could refer infants with GA $\geq$ 32 weeks or BW $\geq$ 1501 g for screening based on clinical concerns.

All examinations were performed by a single experienced pediatric ophthalmologist (VC), ensuring consistency in the diagnostic classification and reducing inter-observer variability.

2.3. Data Collection

Data were extracted from standardized NICU discharge summaries and electronic medical records. These documents provided structured information on demographics, perinatal risk factors, systemic complications, and ROP screening outcomes.

Collected variables included the following:

- Gestational age (in weeks) and birth weight (in grams);
- Type of pregnancy (singleton vs. multiple birth);
- Ethnic background;
- Systemic infections (defined as laboratory-confirmed sepsis);
- Blood transfusions;
- Surgeries (under general anesthesia);
- Duration of oxygen therapy (total hours on supplemental oxygen via mechanical ventilation, CPAP, or nasal cannula);
- ROP outcomes, including zone, stage, presence of plus disease, and treatment modality.

To ensure consistency, two independent investigators extracted data, and discrepancies were resolved through consensus with a third reviewer.

2.4. Classification of ROP and Treatment Protocol

The ROP classification followed the International Classification of ROP (ICROP) and UK screening and treatment guidelines updated in 2022 [9]. Infants were divided into three categories based on the most severe form of ROP observed during the screening period:

- Non-ROP;
- Non-type 1 ROP (defined as the presence of any type of ROP not requiring treatment);
- Type 1 ROP (defined as per ETROP criteria: zone I any stage with plus, zone I stage 3, or zone II stage 2 or 3 with plus disease).

Treatment decisions were made based on the anatomical location and severity of disease:

Laser photocoagulation was the first-line treatment for zone II stage 2 or 3 with plus disease. Treatment was performed using transpupillary green 532 nm laser photocoagulation (Visulas) in a near-confluent pattern.

Intravitreal anti-VEGF injection (bevacizumab 0.625 mg/0.025 mL) was used selectively for aggressive ROP (A-ROP) in cases involving zone I.

No other anti-VEGF agents were available in Cyprus during the study period.

Follow-up after treatment was individualized, with increased frequency during the first 3 months and extended follow-up beyond 18 months for anti-VEGF-treated infants, consistent with UK and international recommendations.

2.5. Statistical Analysis

Numerical variables were expressed as means $\pm$ standard deviation (SD) and categorical variables as percentages. Categorical variables were created for gestational age at birth (GA): group with GA $\leq$ 31 weeks + 6 days and group with GA > 32 weeks.

The study participants were divided into three subgroups based on the outcome: infants diagnosed with non-ROP, non-type 1 ROP, and type 1 ROP.

The incidence and the course of ROP in different GA categories were described by descriptive statistics.

Chi-square or Fisher's exact test for categorical variables and one-way ANOVA for continuous variables were used to compare differences between the groups.

All analyses were conducted using Stata version 18 (StataCorp, College Station, TX 77845, USA). Statistical significance was defined as a p-value < 0.05.

2.6. Ethical Approval

The current study has been registered and was approved by the National Bioethics Committee in Cyprus (n. 2023.01.143), and it was conducted according to the principles of the Declaration of Helsinki. The data were collected anonymously.

3. Results

In total, 183 patients were included in this study with a mean gestational age (GA) of 30.2 ± 2.7 weeks and a mean birth weight (BW) of 1382.5 ± 423.0 g. The incidence of ROP was 18.0% (N = 33). At a mean postmenstrual age of 34.3 ± 2.3 weeks, 22 infants developed non-type 1 ROP (66.6%) and 11 (33.3%) developed type 1 ROP and required treatment bilaterally. Sadly, two infants with type 1 ROP passed away before receiving treatment.

In the three subcategories, the mean GA in weeks was 31.0 ± 2.1 for non-ROP, 27.2 ± 2.4 for non-type 1 ROP, and 25.4 ± 1.5 for type 1 ROP. Additionally, the mean BW in grams was 1493.5 ± 353.8 for non-ROP, 966.4 ± 372.9 for non-type 1 ROP, and 701.6 ± 47.0 for type 1 ROP (Table 1).

Table 1. Patients' characteristics and risk factors' distribution among non-ROP, non-type 1 ROP, and type 1 ROP.

Patients' Characteristics	Non-ROP N = 150	Non-Type 1 ROP N = 22	Type 1 ROP N = 11	p-Trend *
	n (%)	n (%)	n (%)	
Birth weight in grams (mean ± SD)	1493.5 ± 353.8	966.4 ± 372.9	701.6 ± 47.0	**<0.001**
Birth weight < 1501 g				
No	64 (42.7)	2 (9.1)	0 (0)	**<0.001**
Yes	86 (57.3)	20 (90.9)	11 (100)	
Gestational week (mean ± SD)	31.0 ± 2.1	27.2 ± 2.4	25.4 ± 1.5	**<0.001**
Gestational week ≤ 31 + 6 days				
No	70 (46.7)	1 (4.5)	0 (0)	<0.001
Yes	80 (53.3)	21 (95.5)	11 (100)	
Multiple births				
No	94 (82.5)	15 (68.2)	6 (54.5)	0.743
Yes	56 (82.4)	7 (31.8)	5 (45.5)	
Race				
African	13 (8.7)	1 (4.5)	1 (9.1)	0.804
Asian	9 (6.0)	2 (9.1)	1 (9.1)	
Caucasian	128 (85.3)	19 (86.4)	9 (81.8)	

Table 1. *Cont.*

Patients' Characteristics	Non-ROP N = 150	Non-Type 1 ROP N = 22	Type 1 ROP N = 11	*p*-Trend *
Infection				
No	96 (95.0)	4 (18.2)	1 (9.1)	**<0.001**
Yes	54 (65.9)	18 (81.8)	10 (90.9)	
Blood transfusion				
No	30 (96.8)	1 (4.5)	0 (0)	0.081
Yes	120 (79.0)	21 (95.5)	11 (100)	
Surgery				
No	141 (83.9)	19 (86.4)	8 (72.7)	**0.021**
Yes	9 (60.0)	3 (13.6)	3 (27.3)	
Oxygen support				
No	9 (100)	0 (0.0)	0 (0.0)	0.777
Yes	141 (81.0)	22 (94.0)	11 (100)	
)xygen duration in hours (mean ± SD)	362.9 ± 380.3	1513.4 ± 743.9	1844.0 ± 1549.7	**<0.001**

* values in bold font indicate statistical significance ($p < 0.05$).

There was a statistical difference between the three groups for BW < 1501 g, GA ≤ 31 weeks + 6 days, infections, surgery, and prolonged use of oxygen ($p < 0.05$).

As Figure 1 illustrates, the incidence and severity of ROP decrease sharply with increasing gestational age, with treatment-requiring ROP (type 1 ROP) confined almost entirely to infants born at ≤28 weeks, with the highest proportion at 24 weeks, where it accounts for nearly 80.0% of cases.

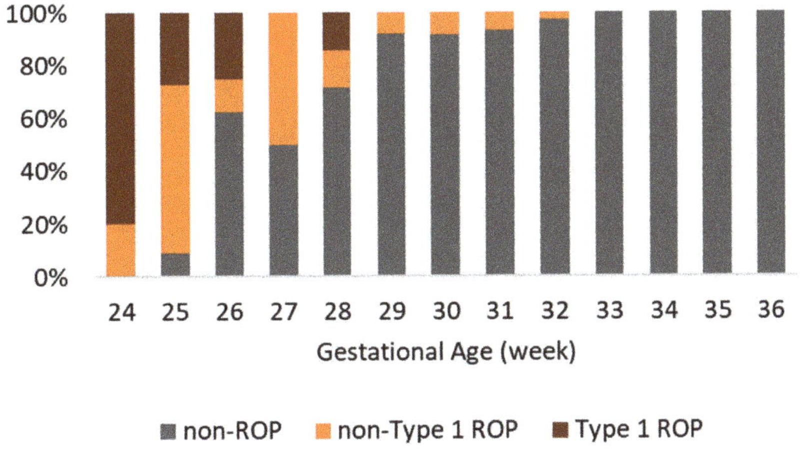

Figure 1. ROP severity trends across gestational ages at birth.

Among the eleven infants diagnosed with type 1 ROP, six received laser photocoagulation, for stage 3 with plus disease in zone 2, three were treated with intravitreal anti-VEGF injections for aggressive ROP, and two with aggressive ROP unfortunately passed away prior to receiving treatment.

For the laser-treated group, the mean postmenstrual age at ROP onset was 34.33 ± 1.03 weeks (range: 33–36 weeks), and the mean age at treatment was 41.00 ± 3.22 weeks (range:

37–46 weeks). Five cases had only one course of laser treatment, and one had additional laser treatment within 2 weeks from the first treatment.

The three infants who received anti-VEGF injections had a mean ROP onset at 34.00 ± 1.00 weeks (range: 33–35 weeks), and treatment was administered at a mean of 36.00 ± 0.00 weeks. The two deceased infants were diagnosed with aggressive posterior ROP at 34 and 38 weeks postmenstrual age, respectively. All three infants who received intravitreal bevacizumab injections showed no recurrence of ROP over the subsequent 18 months. Retinal vascularization was completed after several months, with a mean time of 8.17 ± 0.76 months.

Furthermore, the statistical difference amongst the three groups for BW, GA, and duration of oxygen support can be seen in Figure 2 (all p-values < 0.001).

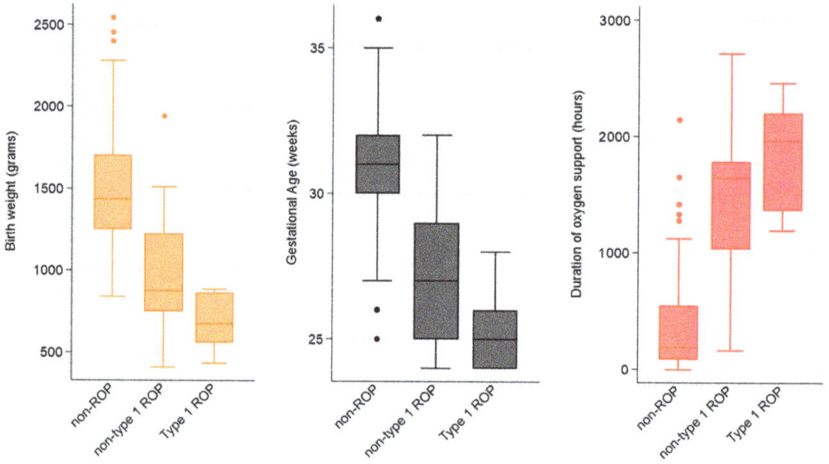

Figure 2. Distribution and comparison of birth weight (orange), gestational age (grey), and duration of oxygen support (red) by ROP category.

However, when non-type 1 ROP cases were compared with type 1 ROP cases, the only statistical difference was found for mean BW (966.4 ± 372.9 vs. 701.6 ± 47.0; $p = 0.032$) and mean GA (27.2 ± 2.4 vs. 25.4 ± 1.5; $p = 0.024$).

It is also noteworthy that, in our cohort, 12 infants had severe intrauterine growth retardation and low postnatal weight gain. Among them, three developed type 1 ROP and required treatment, while another four developed ROP but did not require treatment.

4. Discussion

This study offers valuable epidemiological data on type 1 ROP in Cyprus, focusing on the prevalence, treatment outcomes, and associated risk factors in the country's only tertiary NICU. Among 183 screened babies, the incidence of any ROP was 18.0% and of type 1 ROP was 6.0%. These figures align closely with those from developed nations such as the USA, Spain, and the UK. For instance, the G-ROP study reported a 12.4% treatment rate for type 1 ROP, while Spanish and UK studies documented treatment incidences of 14.6% and 13.8%, respectively [10–12].

Large-scale analyses confirm that almost all treatment-requiring ROP cases occur in the smallest and most premature infants. In the G-ROP cohort, only 0.7% of severe ROP cases were in infants with a birth weight >1251 g, supporting the selective but vigilant screening of high-risk neonates [12]. Our finding that all type 1 ROP cases occurred in

≤28-week infants mirrors other national datasets, where gestational age and birth weight remain the strongest predictors of severe disease [10].

In our study, two treatment modalities were utilized: laser photocoagulation and intravitreal bevacizumab. Laser photocoagulation, the standard treatment for stage 3 ROP in zones 2 and 3, was the predominant choice. Laser is a well-established treatment with a low complication rate and proven safety profile [13,14].

Intravitreal bevacizumab was reserved for aggressive ROP (A-ROP), a rapidly progressing condition. Bevacizumab-treated infants in our cohort demonstrated complete retinal vascularization without recurrence in a 18-month follow-up, similar to findings from Spain, where anti-VEGF therapy showed low recurrence rates and favorable outcomes [1,10,15]. In this one-year review, there was ratio of one case of intravitreal injection to two laser treatments.

Due to the risk of late ROP reactivation and serious visual consequences, extended and diligent follow-up is essential after anti-VEGF therapy. Many experts recommend monitoring infants beyond traditional screening timelines (frequent follow-up to 18 months after treatment and then 6-monthly or annually up to the age of 5 years according to UK ROP treatment guidelines), ensuring that reactivation is caught early before irreversible damage occurs. It is a quick procedure, and selected cases respond well with a high safety profile compared to laser. However, it significantly increases the follow-up workload. As infants grow older, it also becomes increasingly difficult to examine the far retinal periphery [13,14].

Recent studies provide interesting insights into treatment approaches. For instance, Sen et al. (2021) introduced the outcomes of combining anti-VEGF injection and laser photocoagulation in type 1 ROP, concluding that this strategy was effective and safe, potentially reducing the need for the strict long-term follow-up often required with monotherapy [16]. In parallel, Tung et al. (2024) provide additional longitudinal insights, reporting that while ranibizumab-treated eyes showed a myopic shift and longer axial lengths at age three compared with bevacizumab, these differences diminished by age six due to emmetropization [17]. This indicates that early biometric disparities may not translate into long-term refractive disadvantages, though vigilant refractive monitoring remains warranted [17]. Furthermore, a meta-analysis of neurodevelopmental outcomes reported no statistically significant increase in severe neurodevelopmental impairment after intravitreal bevacizumab compared with laser or untreated controls; however, it did reveal a small reduction in Bayley-III motor scores, underscoring the importance of long-term multidisciplinary follow-up [18]. Given the ongoing discussion regarding the systemic effects of anti-VEGF agents like bevacizumab, the inclusion of long-term neurodevelopmental follow-up would be valuable in future studies to assess potential implications on overall infant development.

In our study, risk factor analysis identified low gestational age, low birth weight, and prolonged oxygen therapy as significant contributors to ROP development and progression. These findings are consistent with international studies, which emphasize gestational age and birth weight as dominant risk factors. The G-ROP study reported that infants with gestational ages ≤24 weeks or birth weights ≤500 g had the highest odds of developing type 1 ROP [12], similarly to our cohort, of which the group comprising 24 weeks of gestational age infants has the highest risk of ROP type 1. Consistent with our results, Gaber et al. (2021) identified low gestational age, low birth weight, and prolonged oxygen supplementation as independent predictors of type 1 ROP [19]. Interestingly, this study found an overall incidence of ROP of 34.1%, with type 1 ROP occurring in 26.3% of infants, and additionally suggested apnea and thrombocytopenia as significant associated factors. These results reinforce the multifactorial nature of disease pathogenesis, where both hypoxic–ischemic and inflammatory pathways are implicated [19]. Importantly, moving beyond these well-established clinical parameters, recent attention has shifted towards novel biomarkers. In particular, thrombocytopenia at birth ($<181 \times 10^9$/L) and a characteristic pre-treatment platelet "spike" have been linked to an increased risk of type 1 ROP. Incorporating such laboratory markers into predictive algorithms could substantially enhance screening specificity and support the personalized scheduling of follow-up examinations [20].

Our findings further suggest that the cumulative presence of multiple risk factors exacerbates disease severity, particularly in cases of type 1 ROP. The Spanish study identified late-onset sepsis, mechanical ventilation, and weight at 28 days as independent predictors of ROP progression [10]. Other additional risk factors, for which their role needs to be elucidated further, are maternal pre-eclampsia and gestational diabetes [21], maternal age and emotional stress [22], premature rupture of membranes and chorioamnionitis, higher level of oxygen and fluctuation of oxygen levels, necrotizing enterocolitis, intraventricular hemorrhage, and poor postnatal weight. Some of these results seem to be contradictory in clinical studies due either to different and heterogenous preterm infant populations or different neonatal care across the world. In addition to biological and neonatal factors, broader determinants such as maternal health and socioeconomic status—although not included in our analysis—may also influence ROP development. These aspects, typically managed within neonatal care systems, warrant further investigation in future interdisciplinary research. This study has some limitations. Its retrospective design and relatively small sample size, especially for treated cases, limit the generalizability of the findings. The lack of long-term follow-up data, particularly for infants treated with anti-VEGF therapy, precludes definitive conclusions about treatment safety and durability. Nonetheless, this study establishes a strong foundation for understanding type 1 ROP trends in Cyprus and highlights areas for future research and clinical improvements. Moreover, future studies conducted under the updated 2022 UK guidelines may yield different screening outcomes, particularly with regard to inclusion criteria and follow-up recommendations.

5. Conclusions

This one-year review of type 1 retinopathy of prematurity in Cyprus provides the first national insight into the epidemiology, treatment patterns, and risk factors associated with type 1 ROP in a centralized tertiary NICU setting.

This study confirms that lower gestational age and birth weight are the strongest predictors of ROP severity, with type 1 ROP occurring exclusively in infants born at $\leq$28 weeks. Additional significant associations were found with systemic infections, prior surgeries, and the need for prolonged oxygen support. The findings also highlight the cumulative effect of multiple risk factors, reinforcing the importance of comprehensive neonatal care and early screening.

Laser photocoagulation remained the most frequently used treatment modality, while anti-VEGF was reserved for aggressive ROP cases. Both treatments were effective in halting disease progression, with no recurrence observed during an 18-month follow-up in the anti-VEGF group.

These findings support the ongoing need for tailored screening strategies, resource allocation, and long-term monitoring to optimize outcomes for preterm infants in Cyprus.

Our findings have several practical implications for neonatal ophthalmic care. Type 1 ROP developed exclusively in extremely preterm infants with additional systemic risk factors highlights the value of risk-adapted screening protocols beyond gestational age or birth weight alone. The favorable outcomes observed with both laser and anti-VEGF therapy support their continued use, with anti-VEGF reserved for selected cases where laser is less suitable. Given the extended follow-up required after anti-VEGF treatment, structured post-treatment monitoring is essential. The recent approval of aflibercept for ROP treatment in Cyprus' General Health System as an alternative to bevacizumab introduces new opportunities for individualized treatment, outcome comparisons, and future clinical audits. Finally, the centralized care model in Cyprus offers a strong basis for developing a national ROP registry, which could support quality improvement and personalized screening strategies.

In conclusion, this study provides a comprehensive understanding of type 1 ROP in Cyprus, serving as a foundation for future research and local healthcare improvements.

This study underscores the relevance of personalized medicine in neonatal ophthalmology, advocating for risk-based screening and tailored treatment protocols to improve ROP outcomes in diverse populations.

Author Contributions: Conceptualization, S.C. and V.C.; Methodology, S.C., A.Q. and V.C.; Formal analysis, A.Q.; Data curation, S.C., F.H. and A.Q.; Writing—original draft, S.C. and V.C.; Writing—review & editing, S.C., T.P. and V.C.; Supervision, V.C.; Project administration, S.C. All authors have read and agreed to the published version of the manuscript.

Funding: This research received no external funding.

Institutional Review Board Statement: The current study has been registered and approved by the National Bioethics Committee in Cyprus (n. 2023.01.143, approved on 8 June 2023) and was conducted according to the principles of the Declaration of Helsinki. The data were anonymously collected from the discharged letters of the included patients.

Informed Consent Statement: Informed consent for participation was not required under local legislation, as this was a retrospective study using anonymized data (Cyprus Law 125(I)/2018, European GDPR Regulation (EU) 2016/679: https://eur-lex.europa.eu/eli/reg/2016/679/oj/eng (accessed on 13 August 2025)).

Data Availability Statement: The data supporting the findings of this study are available from the corresponding author upon reasonable request.

Conflicts of Interest: The authors declare no conflicts of interest.

eferences

Wang, S.D.; Zhang, G.M.; Shenzhen Screening for Retinopathy of Prematurity Cooperative Group. Laser therapy versus intravitreal injection of anti-VEGF agents in monotherapy of ROP: A Meta-analysis. *Int. J. Ophthalmol.* **2020**, *13*, 806–815. [CrossRef] [PubMed]

VanderVeen, D.K.; Melia, M.; Yang, M.B.; Hutchinson, A.K.; Wilson, L.B.; Lambert, S.R. Anti-Vascular Endothelial Growth Factor Therapy for Primary Treatment of Type 1 Retinopathy of Prematurity. *Ophthalmology* **2017**, *124*, 619–633. [CrossRef] [PubMed]

Tsiropoulos, G.N.; Seliniotaki, A.K.; Haidich, A.B.; Ziakas, N.; Mataftsi, A. Comparison of adverse events between intravitreal anti-VEGF and laser photocoagulation for treatment-requiring retinopathy of prematurity: A systematic review. *Int. Ophthalmol.* **2022**, *43*, 1027–1062. [CrossRef] [PubMed]

Taher, N.O.; Ghaddaf, A.A.; Al-Ghamdi, S.A.; Homsi, J.J.; Al-Harbi, B.J.; Alomari, L.K.; Almarzouki, H.S. Intravitreal Anti-vascular Endothelial Growth Factor Injection for Retinopathy of Prematurity: A Systematic Review and Meta-Analysis. *Front. Med.* **2022**, *9*, 884608. [CrossRef] [PubMed]

Wiecek, E.; Akula, J.D.; Vanderveen, D.K.; Mantagos, I.S.; Wu, C.; Curran, A.L.; De Bruyn, H.; Peterson, B.; Fulton, A.B. Longitudinal Change of Refractive Error in Retinopathy of Prematurity Treated with Intravitreal Bevacizumab or Laser Photocoagulation. *Am. J. Ophthalmol.* **2022**, *240*, 252–259. [CrossRef] [PubMed]

Zhang, D.L.; Yoon, H.H.; Raye-Ann, O.D.; Arzu, J.; Rahmani, S. Postnatal Growth Trajectories and Neurodevelopmental Outcomes Following Bevacizumab Treatment for Retinopathy of Prematurity. *Clin. Ophthalmol.* **2022**, *16*, 2713–2722. [CrossRef] [PubMed]

Tan, H.; Blasco, P.; Lewis, T.; Ostmo, S.; Chiang, M.F.; Campbell, J.P. Neurodevelopmental outcomes in preterm infants with retinopathy of prematurity. *Surv. Ophthalmol.* **2021**, *66*, 877–891. [CrossRef] [PubMed]

Royal College of Paediatrics and Child Health, Royal College of Ophthalmologists & British Association of Perinatal Medicine. 2008. Available online: https://curriculum.rcophth.ac.uk/wp-content/uploads/2014/12/2008-SCI-021-Guidelines-Retinopathy-of-Prematurity.pdf (accessed on 13 August 2025).

9. The Royal College of Ophthalmologists. Treating Retinopathy of Prematurity in the UK. Clinical Guidelines. March 202 Available online: https://www.rcophth.ac.uk (accessed on 13 August 2025).
10. de las Rivas Ramírez, N.; Luque Aranda, G.; Rius Diaz, F.; Perez Frias, F.J.; Sánchez Tamayo, T. Risk factors associated wi Retinopathy of Prematurity development and progression. *Sci. Rep.* **2022**, *12*, 21977. [CrossRef] [PubMed]
11. Tavassoli, S.; Wach, R.; Haynes, R.; Markham, R.; Williams, C. Estimate of incidence of ROP requiring treatment in extrem preterms and impact on service—7 year review in tertiary unit. *Eye* **2019**, *33*, 845–849. [CrossRef] [PubMed]
12. Ying, G.S.; Bell, E.F.; Donohue, P.; Tomlinson, L.A.; Binenbaum, G.; G-ROP research group. Perinatal Risk Factors for th Retinopathy of Prematurity in Postnatal Growth and Rop Study. *Ophthalmic Epidemiol.* **2019**, *26*, 270–278. [CrossRef] [PubMed
13. Yasin, A.; Sinha, S.; Smith, R.; Jain, S.F.; Hejkal, T.; Rychwalski, P. Reactivation of retinopathy of prematurity six years aft intravitreal injection of bevacizumab. *J. Am. Assoc. Pediatr. Ophthalmol. Strabismus* **2023**, *27*, 236–239. [CrossRef] [PubMed]
14. Taylor, K.; Ghergherehchi, L.; Rao, P.; Harper III, C.A.; Chang, E. Very late-onset reactivation of retinopathy of prematurity po anti-VEGF bevacizumab treatment for type 1 ROP: A case report. *J. Am. Assoc. Pediatr. Ophthalmol. Strabismus* **2021**, *25*, 180–18 [CrossRef] [PubMed]
15. Ortiz-Seller, A.; Martorell, P.; Barranco, H.; Pascual-Camps, I.; Morcillo, E.; Ortiz, J.L. Comparison of different agents and doses anti-vascular endothelial growth factors (aflibercept, bevacizumab, conbercept, ranibizumab) versus laser for retinopathy prematurity: A network meta-analysis. *Surv. Ophthalmol.* **2024**, *69*, 585–605. [CrossRef] [PubMed]
16. Sen, P.; Agarwal, A.A.K.; Bhende, P.; Ganesan, S. Treatment outcomes of combination of anti-vascular endothelial growth fact injection and laser photocoagulation in Type 1 ROP and APROP. *Int. Ophthalmol.* **2022**, *42*, 95–101. [CrossRef] [PubMed]
17. Tung, H.F.; Chen, Y.L.; Chen, Y.C.; Chiu, S.L.; Chen, S.N. Six years follow-up of type 1 retinopathy of prematurity (ROP) treate with intravitreal injection of ranibizumab and bevacizumab: Long-Term Outcomes of intravitreal injection in Type 1 ROP. *Medicir* **2024**, *103*, e39251. [CrossRef] [PubMed]
18. Tsai, C.Y.; Yeh, P.T.; Tsao, P.N.; Chung, Y.C.E.; Chang, Y.S.; Lai, T.T. Neurodevelopmental Outcomes after Bevacizumab Treatmer for Retinopathy of Prematurity. *Ophthalmology* **2021**, *128*, 877–888. [CrossRef] [PubMed]
19. Gaber, R.; Sorour, O.A.; Sharaf, A.F.; Saad, H.A. Incidence and Risk Factors for Retinopathy of Prematurity (ROP) in Bigges Neonatal Intensive Care Unit in Itay Elbaroud City, Behera Province, Egypt. *Clin. Ophthalmol.* **2021**, *15*, 3467–3471. [CrossRe [PubMed]
20. Parrozzani, R.; Marchione, G.; Fantin, A.; Frizziero, L.; Salvadori, S.; Nardo, D.; Midena, G. Thrombocytopenia as Type 1 RO Biomarker: A Longitudinal Study. *J. Pers. Med.* **2021**, *11*, 1120. [CrossRef] [PubMed]
21. Kim, S.J.; Port, A.D.; Swan, R.; Campbell, J.P.; Chan, R.P.; Chiang, M.F. Retinopathy of prematurity: A review of risk factors an their clinical significance. *Surv. Ophthalmol.* **2018**, *63*, 618–637. [CrossRef] [PubMed]
22. Stylianou-Riga, P.; Kouis, P.; Kinni, P.; Rigas, A.; Papadouri, T.; Yiallouros, P.K.; Theodorou, M. Maternal socioeconomic factor and the risk of premature birth and low birth weight in Cyprus: A case–control study. *Reprod Health* **2018**, *15*, 157. [CrossRe [PubMed]

Journal of
Personalized Medicine

MDPI

ticle

wo Machine Learning Models to Economize Glaucoma creening Programs: An Approach Based on Neural Nets

olfgang Hitzl [1,2,*], Markus Lenzhofer [1,2], Melchior Hohensinn [1,2] and Herbert Anton Reitsamer [1,2]

[1] Department of Ophthalmology and Optometry, Paracelsus Medical University, University Hospital Salzburg, Muellner Hauptstrasse 48, 5020 Salzburg, Austria; m.lenzhofer@salk.at (M.L.); m.hohensinn@salk.at (M.H.); h.reitsamer@salk.at (H.A.R.)
[2] Research Program Experimental Ophthalmology and Glaucoma Research, Paracelsus Medical University, Muellner Hauptstrasse 48, 5020 Salzburg, Austria
* Correspondence: w.hitzl@salk.at; Tel.: +43-676-8997-24290

Abstract: Background: In glaucoma screening programs, a large proportion of patients remain free of open-angle glaucoma (OAG) or have no need of intraocular eye pressure (IOP)-lowering therapy within 10 years of follow-up. Is it possible to identify a large proportion of patients already at the initial examination and, thus, to safely exclude them already at this point? **Methods**: A total of 6889 subjects received a complete ophthalmological examination, including objective optic nerve head and quantitative disc measurements at the initial examination, and after an average follow-up period of 11.1 years, complete data were available of 585 individuals. Two neural network models were trained and extensively tested. To allow the models to refuse to make a prediction in doubtful cases, a reject option was included. **Results**: A prediction for the first endpoint, 'remaining OAG-free and no IOP-lowering therapy within 10 years', was rejected in 57% of cases, and in the remaining cases (43%), 253/253 (=100%) received a correct prediction. The second prediction model for the second endpoint 'remaining OAG-free within 10 years' refused to make a prediction for 46.4% of all subjects. In the remaining cases (53.6%), 271/271 (=100%) were correctly predicted. **Conclusions**: Most importantly, no eye was predicted false-negatively or false-positively. Overall, 43% all eyes can safely be excluded from a glaucoma screening program for up to 10 years to be certain that the eye remains OAG-free and will not need IOP-lowering therapy. The corresponding model significantly reduces the screening performed by and work load of ophthalmologists. In the future, better predictors and models may increase the number of patients with a safe prediction, further economizing time and healthcare budgets in glaucoma screening.

Keywords: glaucoma; machine learning; neural network; screening; prediction

1. Introduction

Glaucoma is a leading cause of irreversible blindness [1]. Worldwide, it is estimated that about 66.8 million people have visual impairment caused by glaucoma, with 6.7 million suffering from blindness. Intraocular pressure (IOP) is the most important—because it is modifiable—risk factor for the development and progression of this disease [2]. Glaucoma is mostly asymptomatic until late in its course, when visual problems arise [3]. However, with early treatment, it is often possible to protect the eyes against serious vision loss [2]. Therefore, early diagnosis should be targeted. Due to the lack of symptoms in the early disease stage of glaucoma in most patients, this can only be achieved through screening programs. The most common subgroup of glaucoma in Europe is open-angle glaucoma

(OAG). It is well known in glaucoma research that age, IOP, PEX, and topographic disc parameter are univariable risk factors for predicting OAG.

A major goal in glaucoma research is to combine these risk factors in a multivariable fashion and to make predictions on a personalized level. Machine learning algorithms such as neural networks can personalize diagnosis for patients on an individual level, although several issues remain unresolved [4–6]. Because no such tools are currently in use that predict 10-year occurrence of OAG, we investigated to what extent a reliable prediction is feasible.

Several univariable risk factors for developing OAG are well known, such as age [4], increased IOP [2], PEX [7–9], and topographic disc parameters such the cup-to-disc ratio (C/D) [10,11]. Increased age, IOP, and cup-to-disc ratio, as well as PEX, are positively related to an increased risk of OAG. For example, age is an important risk factor for developing OAG; however, it is still unclear precisely how it affects the progression of OAG over time, particularly in relation to and in combination with other risk factors. Even if all these univariable risk factors are identifiable through a single examination at one point in time, it is difficult to diagnose OAG in certain cases, so why should we even consider attempting to make a prediction over a long period of 10 years?

There are mainly three reasons why models with a reject option should be used: (1) It is well known that patients with no or a small number of risk factors are highly likely to remain OAG-free over a long period. For example, subjects aged ≤ 50 years old with an IOP $\leq$ 18mmHg and a cup-to-disc ratio (C/D) ≤ 0.2 are highly likely to remain OAG-free over many years [3,10,11]. Thus, the basic idea is to identify a—hopefully as large as possible—subpopulation at the initial examination that will remain OAG-free at the 10-year follow-up point. (2) Studies have demonstrated that 10-year OAG incidence is quite low, ranging from 0.7 to 2.2% [12,13]. Hence, most patients remain OAG-free over 10 years, which makes predicting OAG freeness easier compared to incidences around 50%. (3) The third, and by far the most important, reason is related to the so called 'reject option' of the model. It is definitely not necessary to identify every single eye that remains stable. Usually, one expects that a model will make a prediction for every single patient. However, to reduce the screening time, it is sufficient to identify a preferably large subpopulation of patients with eyes that remain stable. If the prediction is too difficult and the accuracy of the prediction model is 'in doubt', it is still better to refuse to make a prediction instead of making a false-positive or false-negative prediction. Patients who do not receive a prediction are sent to the glaucoma specialist as usual. This so-called 'reject option' is crucial and a highly desirable advantage, because the models are not 'forced to make a prediction'. In other words, if the model has enough evidence, then it makes a prediction; otherwise, it refuses to make a prediction and asks the glaucoma expert to make the final decision (or to make no prediction at all). There is a cost to developing this model, because we have to accept that a large number of eyes do not receive a prediction. On the other hand, the reject option substantially increases the accuracy of the model for those patients who receive a prediction. This allows for identifying a large number of patients for whom the corresponding eye can safely be excluded, and, thus, much time and effort in screening studies can be saved. All definitions, endpoints, methods, and results refer to right eyes, as machine learning algorithms are expected to clearly distinguish between right and left eyes. New models for left eyes can be trained and tested using the same methods.

This study will answer the following questions by considering the principle of very high accuracy: (1) Which of these endpoints shows reasonable results? (2) How good are the performances of the neural network models in terms of accuracy? How many patients receive a false-negative or false-positive prediction? (3) To what extent do these models help to reduce daily work load, i.e., how many eyes receive a prediction, and in how many cases is the algorithm in doubt? (4) How can these approaches be improved in the future?

2. Materials and Methods

The Salzburg-Moorfields-Collaborative-Glaucoma Study (SMCGS) began in 1996 and is part of a large 25-year glaucoma blindness prevention program in Austria, Europe. The SMCGS is a retrospective monocentric population-based longitudinal cohort study. This study mainly provides information for and identifies glaucoma suspects, offering timely and adequate treatment in clear-cut cases of glaucoma.

2.1. Definition of Definite OAG

We defined glaucoma as a progressive optic neuropathy leading to the loss of retinal nerve fibers and glia cells, with characteristic alterations on the optic nerve head and with or without corresponding functional alterations in visual field examination [14]. The following parameters were used here: (a) Optic nerve head (ONH)—notching, rimming, arbitrary chosen subjective cup-to-disk (C/D) ratio of 0.45 or more, or C/D asymmetry between the two eyes >0.3 not explainable through other diseases. (b) Visual field—glaucomatous visual field defects corresponding to optic disc changes. (c) Open anterior chamber angle [14]. Inclusion criteria: age $\geq$ 40 years, no OAG or other type of glaucoma, best spectacle-corrected visual acuity >6/9, refractive range ranging from -6.00 to $+4.00$ diopters with a difference in refraction between both eyes <3.00 diopters. Exclusion criteria: pseudophakia, IOP-lowering therapy at the initial examination, and eye diseases potentially leading to visual field defects or secondary increases in intraocular pressure, contraindication against beta blockers, systemic corticosteroid therapy, or pregnancy.

During the study's duration of more than 27 years, up to 24 ophthalmologists and 7 ophthalmic assists specially trained in using the study protocol performed ophthalmic examinations and graded each patient. SMCGS data collection started on the 1st December 1996. Baseline: The ophthalmic assistants were responsible for oral education and SMCGS, questionnaire interviews, best corrected visual acuity (BCVA) measurements with the Early Treatment Diabetic Retinopathy Study (EDTRS) chart, subjective refraction, visual field examination (VF; Motion-Sensitivity Test (MST), Humphrey Frequency Doubling Technology Perimetry (FDT, Humphrey FDT matrix, Humphrey Instruments Inc., San Leandro, CA, USA), Humphrey Field Analyzer II or II-I [HFA, Humphrey Instruments Inc., San Leandro, CA, USA]), central corneal thickness (CCT) with ultrasound pachymetry (Pocket II, Quantel Medical, Cournon d'Auvergne Cedex, France) and structural imaging (confocal scanning laser ophthalmoscopy was carried out using TopSS® (Fa. LDT, San Diego, CA, USA)), which refers to a scanning laser tomography technique for analyzing the eye, specifically the optic nerve head. This method uses scanning laser tomography to depict the top surface of the optic nerve, allowing for detailed analysis of structural changes. Subsequently, all subjects underwent a standardized eye examination with intraocular pressure (IOP) assessment in miosis and mydriasis through Goldmann applanation tonometry (Haag Streit, Koeniz, Switzerland), gonioscopy (to exclude angle-closure), slit lamp anterior segment examination, and dilated fundus slit lamp biomicroscopy for optic disc assessment using a Volk 90 D lens, including subjective C/D. PEX was diagnosed during the initial clinical examination in the glaucoma screening ambulance using a slit lamp. Recorded TopSS® values included the C/D ratio, total contour area, effective area, neuroretinal rim area, half-depth area, half-depth volume, and volume below. If results were abnormal or inconclusive during the VF-examination at baseline, a second confirmation test was performed for clarification.

2.2. Definition of Endpoints

We defined two different endpoints: E1—composite endpoint, i.e., freeness of OAG and no IOP-lowering therapy; E2: freeness of OAG (with or without IOP-lowering therapy).

If a patient (1) still wants to join the screening program, (2) agrees to receive IOP-lowering therapy if necessary, and (3) is only interested in determining whether OAG will develop, then E2 is best. E1 is suitable for informing and safely excluding the patient from a screening program. Here, we want to show that for E1 and E2, ocular hypertension (OHT) might develop (in the case of E2, with a possibly necessary IOP-lowering treatment), but OAG will not develop.

Age, IOP [2], PEX [7–9], and 8 optic nerve head parameters (TopSS®) were used as continuous predictors for E1 and E2.

2.2.1. Years Follow-Up

Patients free of glaucoma (OAG or another type of glaucoma) at the baseline visit received follow-up only. All examinations were carried out the same manner as at the baseline examination. According to the results of the baseline examination, patients were also scheduled for interim visits in the first decade. Complete data for the baseline visit and the 10-year visit were used to train and validate the machine learning models.

2.3. *Statistical Methods and Model Development*

Data were cleaned for inaccurate or missing data, resulting in data for 585 patients, with full records of each predictor and the outcome variable. Univariable logistic regression models were used to estimate the odds ratios of each individual predictor with 95% confidence intervals.

2.4. *Machine Learning Algorithms, Training and Testing*

Multilayer perceptron neural networks, nearest-neighbor classifiers, Bayes classifiers, random forest models, logistic regression models, and support vector machines were trained and tested.

2.5. *Data for Model Training and Testing*

The full sample (n = 585) was randomly split into a training sample (n = 486) and a test sample (n = 117). No data from the test sample were used for model training. All neural networks were first trained and 10-fold cross-validated in a training sample (n = 468) and finally tested in an independent randomly selected test sample (n = 117) to ensure generalization to new, previously unseen eyes.

2.6. *Methods for Model Training*

2.6.1. Neural Nets

Adaptive moment estimation was used as a stochastic gradient descent method. To mitigate overfitting, an early stopping approach and 10-fold cross-validation were used. L2-regularization techniques were also used. Additionally, early stopping, batch normalization layers, and L2-regularization techniques were used. The batch size was 64 and the maximal number of training rounds was 5000 (Table S1). The network architecture is illustrated in Figure S1.

2.6.2. Other Models

All other models were trained according to the default settings of MATHEMATICA [15].

2.7. *Feature Selection*

Potential risk factors were selected as input variables, which are listed in Table 1. Although some of these risk factors were not significant, after applying a genetic algorithm and the reject option (as described in the next subsection), these predictors were still useful for limiting the number of rejected cases.

Table 1. Univariable odds ratios and descriptive statistics of various predictors for composite endpoint E1: freeness of. OAG and having no IOP-lowering therapy within 10 yrs.

	OAG-Free and no IOP Lowering Therapy 10 yr FU (n = 544)		OAG or IOP-Lowering Therapy at 10 yr FU (n = 41)			
	Mean	**Std**	**Mean**	**Std**	**Odds Ratio**	***p*-Value**
Age (yrs)	58.84	7.96	60.7	7.29	1.02 (0.99–1.08)	0.16 [1]
IOP (mmHg)	15.1	2.83	18.5	4.27	1.33 (1.21–1.46)	<0.0001 [1,*]
PEX	12/532	2.2%	3/38	7.3%	3.5 (0.6–13.7)	0.027 [2,*]
Effective Area (mm^2)	0.95	0.40	1.08	0.32	2.37 (1.02–5.5)	0.042 [1,*]
Neuroretinal Rim Area (mm^2)	1.29	0.32	1.19	0.18	0.38 (0.13–1.09)	0.07 [1]
Half Depth Area (mm^2)	0.37	0.21	0.44	0.20	4.0 (1.01–15.8)	0.047 [1,*]
Half Depth Volume (mm^3)	−0.06	0.06	−0.07	0.05	0.08 (0.008–7.09)	0.26 [1]
Volume Below (mm^3)	−0.25	0.18	−0.31	0.20	0.23 (0.05–0.996)	0.047 [1,*]
Cup-To-Disc Ratio/0.1 unit change	0.42	0.14	0.48	0.12	1.46 (1.11–1.92)	0.006 [1,*]

[1] Independent t-test [2] Fisher's Exact test (one sided), odds ratios are based on univariable logistic regression models, *: indicates statistical significance.

2.8. Reject Option

From a clinical point of view, most importantly, we wanted to avoid making false-negative predictions for both endpoints. This means that E2 would predict that the patient will not suffer from OAG within 10 years, even though they may develop OAG within this period. For E2, a false-negative prediction may lead to irreversible eye damage or even blindness. For E1, the same scenario would occur, and no medication would be administered, which could also result in OAG or blindness. The predictors, however, did not have enough predictive power to achieve this goal for the whole cohort. Thus, it was reasonable to allow the algorithms to apply a 'reject option' in doubtful cases [16]. This means that 2 cut-offs for the posterior probabilities, instead of 1 cut-off, were first chosen in the training sample and then applied and tested in the test sample. Finally, to assess model performances, the percentages of predicted subjects and total correct predicted cases were computed in the training and test samples and compared to determine whether the networks generalized well to new, previously unseen data.

The advantage of this approach was that it minimized the number of false-negative and false-positive predictions. This important advantage came at a cost, as a large number of cases did not receive a prediction. We recommend that patients who do not receive a prediction should still join a glaucoma screening program to benefit from expert medical knowledge.

All analyses were carried out using STATISTICA 13 [17] and MATHEMATICA 13, developed by Wolfram Research, Inc., Champaign, IL (2023) [15].

3. Results

In the original screening study, 6889 subjects were screened and 976 subjects were examined ten years later. Finally, after applying all inclusion and exclusion criteria and removing all missing data, 585 right eyes with complete data were included.

3.1. Demographic Data at Baseline

An overview is given in (Table 2).

Table 2. Overview of baseline demographic data of n = 585 subjects with complete data at baseline and 10 year follow-up [1].

	Mean	SD	−95% CI	+95% CI
Age (y)	58.9	8.1	58.8	59.6
Follow-up (years)	11.1	1.1	10.99	11.2
IOP (mmHg)	15.3	3.2	15.1	15.6
Total Contour Area (mm^2)	2.23	0.44	2.20	2.27
Effective Area (mm^2)	0.96	0.39	0.93	0.99
Neuroretinal Rim Area (mm^2)	1.28	0.33	1.25	1.31
Half Depth Area (mm^2)	0.38	0.21	0.36	0.40
Half Depth Volume (mm^3)	−0.06	0.057	−0.066	−0.057
Volume Below (mm^3)	−0.26	0.19	−0.27	−0.24
Cup-To-Disc Ratio	0.42	0.14	0.41	0.43
	N	**Percentage**	**−95% CI**	**95% CI**
Endpoint E1: OAG [2] at 10-year FU or IOP lowering therapy within 10 years	41/585	7%	5.1%	9.4%
Endpoint E2: OAG [2] at 10-year FU	21/585	3.6%	2.23%	5.43%

[1] All results refer to right eyes. [2] OAGs included 6 primary open angle glaucoma (1.03%), 3 pseudoexfoliation glaucoma (0.51%), 0 pigmentary glaucoma (0%), and 12 normal tension glaucoma (2.05%).

3.2. Overview of Demographic Data at 10-Year Follow-Up

Within our dataset, OAGs included 6 primary open-angle glaucoma (1.03%) cases, 3 pseudoexfoliation glaucoma (0.51%) cases, 0 pigmentary glaucoma (0%) cases, and 12 normal tension glaucoma (2.05%) cases. A total of 41 of 585 eyes had OAG or received at least one or more types of IOP-lowering eye therapy within 10 years (E1), corresponding to an average 10-year incidence of 7% (5.1–9.4%). Differences between those who fulfilled E1 or not and the corresponding univariable prediction power (odds ratios) levels of possible candidate predictors are given in Table 1.

An overview of the performance accuracies of the machine learning models is given in Table 3, while the advantages and disadvantages of using the selected neural network models with both E1 and E2 are given in Table 4. The neural network models had the smallest percentage of unpredicted patients compared to the classical machine learning algorithm. An overview of the model performance with various combinations of cut-offs for endpoint E1 is given in Table S2. The logistic regression model (classical approach) also achieved 100% NPV; however, the number of unpredicted patients was considerably larger at 69.2%. The models M1 and M2 demonstrated excellent results, with a sufficiently large proportion of eyes receiving a prediction. Most importantly, no eye was predicted false-negatively or false-positively.

Table 3. Results of six machine learning algorithms to predict endpoint E1 based on accuracy. Results are given before application of the reject option and are based on the 10-fold cross-validation. Similar results were found for endpoint E2.

Model Performance	Support Vector Machine	Nearest Neighbors	Random Forest	Bayes Classifier	Neural Network
(NPV/PPV)%	93.2/92.3%	93.2/92.3%	93.2/92.4%	90.4/85.5%	93.5/93.2%

After application of the reject option, the best neuronal network model achieved a NPV of 100%, but rejected 314 of 585 (53.6%) patients in the overall sample and similar results were found for endpoint E2 (Table 4).

Table 4. Overview performance, advantages and disadvantages of two predictive neural network models with endpoints E1 [1] and E2 [2].

Endpoint	Percentage of Eyes Filtered Out/Received a Prediction (%)	Performances of the Models [3] (n/%)	Advantages	Disadvantages	Remarks
E1 [2]	57%/43%	253/253 (100%)	In total, 43% of all eyes can safely be excluded from a glaucoma screening program for up to 10 years if one wants to be certain that the eye remains OAG-free and will not require IOP-lowering therapy. This also significantly reduces the screening amount.	57% did not receive a prediction.	Eyes can safely be excluded from the OAG screening program, especially if the patient wants to leave the screening program.
E2 [1]	53.6%/46.4%	271/271 (100%)	Overall, 46.4% of all eyes can safely be excluded from a glaucoma screening program for up to 10 years if one wants to be certain that the eye remains OAG-free. This significantly reduces the screening workload of ophthalmologists.	Overall, 53.6% did not receive a prediction. Eyes receiving IOP-lowering therapy were not filtered out.	This model is designed for patients in a glaucoma screening setting within a hospital, assuming these patients want to remain within the screening program and continue with IOP-lowering therapy.

[1] Endpoint 1 (E1): remaining OAG-free within 10 years. [2] Endpoint 2 (E2) composite endpoint: remaining OAG-free + no IOP-lowering therapy within 10 years of FU. [3] Performances measured in the training and test sample based on neural networks.

3.3. Illustration of the Models Using Real Data

To better illustrate the models, typical data used in a glaucoma screening setting are provided at the initial examination, illustrating the predictions, decisions, and observations made by M1 for E1 (Table 5). On the left side, we see the predictors evaluated during the initial examination: age, IOP, effective area, neuroretinal rim area, volume below, half-depth area, half-depth volume, C/D, and PEX. On the right side, we see the predictions for M1 for E1 during the initial examination and corresponding observations of both endpoints made at the 10-year follow-up. Eyes highlighted in green were identified via the prediction model, and every single eye was correctly predicted. Eyes highlighted in gray did not receive a prediction, because the algorithm believed that their status was 'in doubt' and refused to make a prediction (i.e., the corresponding eye was 'filtered out'). For E1, 332 eyes (57%) were filtered out and did not receive a prediction, while 253 (43%) of all eyes received a prediction. In summary, all 253 eyes were correctly predicted (100%), meaning that no eye was predicted false-negatively or false-positively.

Table 5. Illustration of prediction model for endpoint E1 based on real data at the initial exam, predicted and observed endpoints at. 10-year follow-up. Identified eyes (green) received a prediction by the model and can safely be excluded from the screening program. Eyes without a prediction (gray) should be send to a glaucoma expert. Patients who suffered of OAG or needed IOP lowering therapy are highlighted in red. No predictions were done in these cases. 332 eyes (57%) were filtered out and did not receive a prediction, 253 (43%) of all eyes received a prediction. 253 out of 253 eyes were correctly predicted (100%). Most importantly, no eye was predicted false-negatively.

Initial Exam									Predictions of Endpoint E1 Made at Initial Exam	Observed Endpoint E1 at the 10 yr FU
Age	IOP [1]	EA [2]	NR [3]	VB [4]	HDA [5]	HD [6]	C/D [7]	PEX [8]		
62	12	0.85	1.22	−0.15	0.19	−0.02	0.41	No	No prediction	OAG-free/no IOP low. therapy
63	14	0.66	1.46	−0.15	0.24	−0.03	0.31	No	OAG-free/no IOP low. therapy	OAG-free/no IOP low. therapy
56	15	1.49	1.18	−0.35	0.60	−0.07	0.56	No	OAG-free/no IOP low. therapy	OAG-free/no IOP low. therapy
61	15	1.22	0.76	−0.52	0.48	−0.11	0.62	No	No prediction	OAG
66	14	1.41	1.10	−0.34	0.50	−0.09	0.56	No	OAG-free/no IOP low. therapy	OAG-free/no IOP low. therapy
42	17	0.51	1.73	−0.10	0.19	−0.03	0.23	No	OAG-free/no IOP low. therapy	OAG-free/no IOP low. therapy
54	14	0.85	0.91	−0.13	0.32	−0.02	0.49	No	No prediction	OAG
69	13	0.96	1.14	−0.18	0.39	−0.05	0.46	No	OAG-free/no IOP low. therapy	OAG-free/no IOP low. therapy
66	14	1.13	1.21	−0.31	0.34	−0.06	0.48	No	OAG-free/no IOP low. therapy	OAG-free/no IOP low. therapy
70	14	1.09	1.44	−0.17	0.27	−0.028	0.43	Yes	No prediction	IOP low. therapy
59	18	0.83	1.18	−0.21	0.22	−0.04	0.41	No	OAG-free/no IOP low. therapy	OAG-free/no IOP low. therapy
62	15	0.99	1.21	−0.45	0.39	−0.12	0.45	No	No prediction	OAG-free/no IOP low. therapy
57	12	0.50	1.39	−0.06	0.20	−0.01	0.27	No	OAG-free/no IOP low. therapy	OAG-free/no IOP low. therapy
58	13	1.16	0.97	−0.65	0.66	−0.22	0.54	No	No prediction	OAG-free/no IOP low. therapy
57	16	1.25	0.94	−0.41	0.69	−0.12	0.57	No	No prediction	OAG-free/no IOP low. therapy
62	12	1.21	1.25	−0.64	0.70	−0.19	0.49	No	No prediction	OAG-free/no IOP low. therapy

[1] Intraocular eye pressure (mmHg), [2] effective area (mm^2), [3] neuroretinal rim area (mm^2), [4] volume below (mm^3), [5] half depth area (mm^2), [6] half depth volume (mm^3), [7] cup-to-disc area, [8] pseudoexfoliation syndrome.

3.4. Illustration for the Need for a Reject Option

To better understand both why a large number of eyes were filtered out and the difficulty of predicting E1, we provide deeper insights how close both data clouds (E1, yes/no) closely stick together and illustrate the overlap between both data distributions (Figure 1). As indicated, there is a large overlap between both distributions, indicating the difficulty of identifying eyes for which accurate predictions can be made and eyes that must be rejected during the initial examination for making predictions for the future.

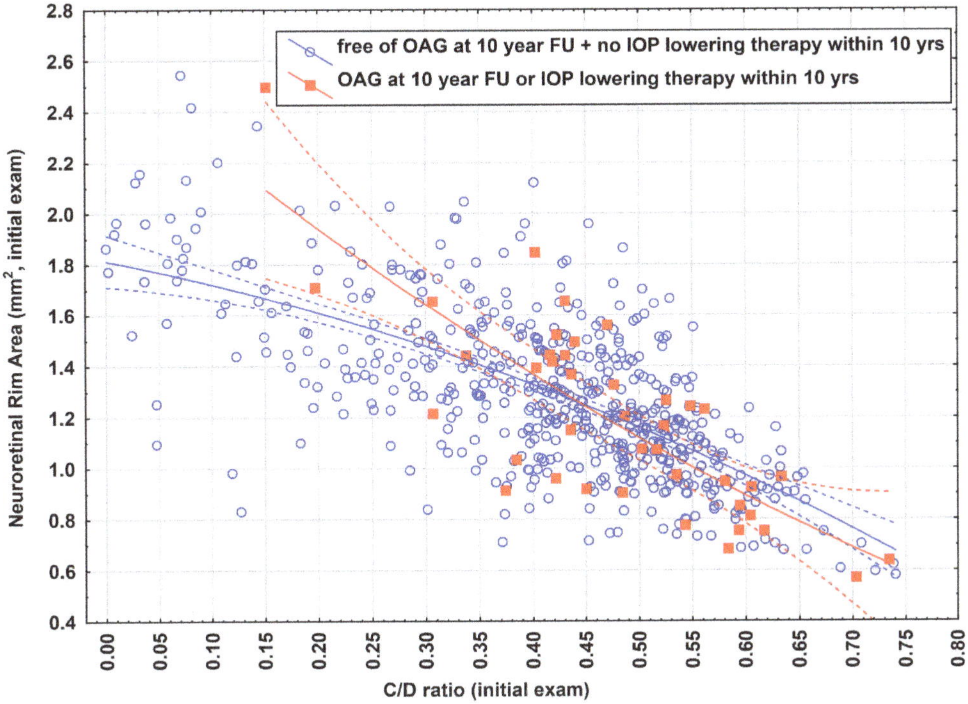

Figure 1. Scatterplot of C/D ratio and neuroretinal rim area (mm^2) of 585 eyes suggesting the need of a reject option. All eyes were OAG-free without receiving IOP-lowering eye therapy at the initial exam. Red dots indicate eyes fulfilling endpoint E1 (freeness of OAG + no IOP-lowering therapy within 10 years of FU) at the 10-year FU, blue dots indicate eyes which do not fulfill endpoint E1 at the 10 yr FU. Eyes with values in the left part of the figure ('low risk region') are very likely to remain OAG-free and having no IOP-lowering therapy within 10 years whilst eyes in the right region ('high risk region') are at high risk for developing a OAG or will receive an IOP-lowering therapy within 10 years of FU. It is precisely the main task of neural networks to identify regions of low risk in the space of all input variables (including age, IOP, optic nerve head parameters and PEX), simultaneously.

4. Discussion

This study provides a completely new and safe approach for identifying a large subpopulation of eyes remaining free of open-angle glaucoma without needing IOP-lowering therapy within 10 years. The most important benefit of M1 is that 43% of the eyes in the screening population could safely be excluded already at the initial examination, i.e., no predicted eye received a false-positive or false-negative prediction. It is important to emphasize that this accuracy could only be achieved by allowing the algorithm to refuse to make a prediction, occurring in 57% of eyes. Therefore, there is no need to further examine eyes that receive a OAG screening prediction within the next 10 years, saving corresponding time, effort, and costs. This implies that these eyes are no longer within a screening program and, thus, will not receive IOP-lowering therapy. This was a key point and crucial for explaining not only why E1 focuses on OAG but also why these eyes do not receive IOP-lowering therapy.

4.1. Discussion of Model M1

In this model, the patient will receive a positive response if they not only remain OAG-free over 10 years but also do not require IOP-lowering therapy, which is an important form of subjective relief for the person.

4.2. Discussion of Model M2

The patient receives a positive response if they remain OAG-free over 10 years. This model is the right choice for patients who are willing to remain in a glaucoma screening program. In this case, the eye may still receive IOP-lowering therapy if necessary. Therefore, E2 was defined as remaining OAG-free (with adequate IOP-lowering therapy if ocular hypertension arises). IOP-lowering therapy was not included compared to E2. A detailed overview of the clinical pathway used to guide the patient workflow is given in Figure 2.

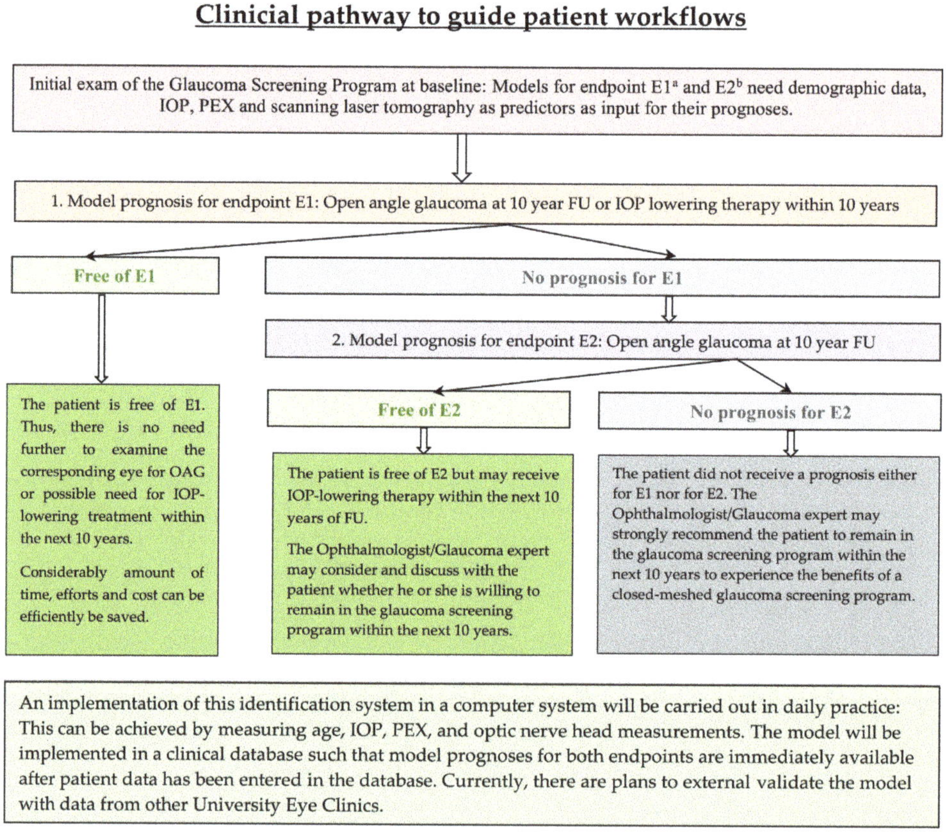

Figure 2. Clinicial pathway to guide patient workflows. a: Endpoint 1; b: Endpoint 2.

4.3. PEX as Risk Factor and How It Was Handled by the Models

Additionally, we analyzed how the models handled patients with PEX. There were 570 eyes without PEX, and 44% received a prediction. All predictions were correct. A total of 15 eyes had PEX, and the algorithms refused to make a prediction in all 15 eyes. This suggests that PEX is a risk factor that deserves special attention from glaucoma experts.

4.4. Implication for Practical Purposes

This identification system can be implemented in a computer system in daily practice: This can be carried out by measuring age, IOP, PEX, and optic nerve head measurements. The models can be implemented in a clinical database so that model prognoses for both endpoints are immediately available after patient data have been entered in the database. Currently, we plan to externally validate the model with other University Eye Clinics. Creating an open access form of the model is currently under discussion.

Of course, we do not screen for all known sight-threatening diseases but for one major cause of visual impairment. Therefore, we also consider personal responsibility and suggest that subjects should be screened anyway due to the risk of contracting other eye-threatening diseases. We suggest that the remaining patients without a prediction should be screened more closely.

4.5. Outlook and Further Developments

We have many ideas for further improving the models in the future: First, we plan to test and analyze more candidate predictor variables based on image data, e.g., GDx®, OCT®, HRT II®, or other structural imaging methods. Modern deep learning methods based on convolutional neural networks (CNNs), such as Inception net, VGGNet, ResNet, R-CNN+LSTM models, or classification maps, have already demonstrated utility for assessing various disease processes, including cataracts, glaucoma, age-related macular degeneration, and diabetic retinopathy [4,18–22]. Of course, these methods should also be applied, especially in combination with clinical data, for predicting the above-addressed endpoints.

Another option is to establish prediction models for subgroups of OAG or related diseases. Moreover, we could ask ourselves if we should increase or decrease the follow-up time (e.g., to 5 or 15 years). Here, we provide models for assessing the development of the most common sub-form of glaucoma (OAG), which is only one of the major reasons for the irreversible impairment of visual function and blindness worldwide. Applying our approach to the other subgroups of glaucoma and other major diseases causing irreversible impairment may reduce the burden of routine screenings tremendously.

4.6. Strengths and Limitations of This Study

4.6.1. Strengths

The most important strength of this study is that it provides methods for safely excluding 43% of all eyes during the initial examination and correctly predicting OAG freeness and freeness from IOP-lowering therapy for 10 years. This significantly decreases the practical screening workload in daily work. Another strength is that the models are not only theoretical concepts/ideas/suggestions, but they can also easily be implemented in any database and then be applied in daily practice. The large sample size of about 600 eyes is also an important strength of this study. A large sample size is important for creating with statistically sound models, as emphasized in mathematical statistics and machine learning theory. It is important to train and independently validate the models with large samples to avoid overlearning and to provide accurate predictions when the models are confronted with new, previously unseen data (generalization). Another strength of this study concerns the sample: right and left eyes were carefully distinguished and were not merged. This would artificially increase the sample size, but in that case, data independence may be undermined. In this case, prediction models may struggle to predict new, previously unseen data.

4.6.2. Limitations

There might be a possible imbalance between positive and negative groups in terms of predictive performance. This might be due to the fact that optic nerve head measurements were made using TopSS® (Fa. LDT, San Diego, CA, USA), which is outdated. We think that using predictors with higher predictive power (e.g., genetic markers) or using modern topographic measurements of the optic nerve head might improve predictions. Additionally, we recommend conducting follow-up studies with larger samples and evaluating the model with external independent data. However, for this study with such a long FU over 10 years, it was necessary to use this method to achieve a sufficiently large sample size. As described in the Materials and Methods section, visual field examinations were carried out using various different methods. In large-cohort studies such as ours, this is a common drawback over a long study period of more than 20 years, which implies that no uniform data source for the visual field was available. We strongly support using the above procedure for only examining cases where a shallow chamber is observed, as the vast majority of ophthalmologists in practice perform gonioscopy only in cases of a suspected configuration of the anterior segment. When comparing the results of different glaucoma screening programs, it is important to consider to which population the results finally refer. It is important to point out that data for these models were sampled from a European sample. It is well known that ethnicity and race are risk factors for glaucoma, and, therefore, we suggest applying these models in Caucasian patients only.

5. Conclusions

Overall, 43% of all eyes can safely be excluded from a glaucoma screening program for up to 10 years while remaining certain that the eyes remain OAG-free and will not need IOP-lowering therapy. We suggest applying this model to inform patients of their future eye health 10 years ahead and to safely exclude the identified eye from further screening within this period. This has a positive impact on reducing the enormous working and screening workloads of ophthalmologists. We suggest applying these neural network models for screening purposes to decide which eyes can be safely excluded and which eyes should be followed-up more closely and sent to a glaucoma expert. This filtering system and identification method will reduce the time and healthcare budgets required for glaucoma screening in the future.

Supplementary Materials: The following supporting information can be downloaded at: https://www.mdpi.com/article/10.3390/jpm15080361/s1, Figure S1: An illustration of the network architecture with all layers and activation functions; Table S1: An overview about pre-processing, model training, split of data into training, validation and test sample, training stop criteria, selection of thresholds for the reject option and final test of the models based on neural networks; Table S2: Overview of model performances with various combinations of cut-offs for the neural network model with endpoint E1.

Author Contributions: Conceptualization, W.H. and M.L.; methodology, W.H.; software, W.H.; validation, W.H.; formal analysis, W.H.; investigation, W.H., M.L., M.H., H.A.R.; resources, W.H., M.L., M.H., H.A.R.; data curation, W.H.; writing—original draft preparation, W.H., M.L., M.H., H.A.R.; writing—review and editing, W.H., M.L., M.H., H.A.R.; visualization, W.H.; supervision, H.A.R.; project administration, H.A.R.; funding acquisition, H.A.R. All authors have read and agreed to the published version of the manuscript. All authors have not published or submitted any related papers from the same study elsewhere. All authors meet all four criteria for authorship in the ICMJE recommendations. This original manuscript or parts of it has not been published before. The manuscript was neither previously rejected nor evaluated in any form by another journal. We hereby declare that we had full access to all the data in the study and take responsibility for the integrity of the data and the accuracy of the data analysis as well as the decision to submit the publication.

Funding: This study was supported financially by the Government of Salzburg (grant number: 9/1-60,712/1-1996), Austria.

Institutional Review Board Statement: The study was supported and approved by the Health administration council of the Federal State of Salzburg and conforms to the provisions of the Declaration of Helsinki in 1995. The study was approved by a local ethic committee (No 1120/2024). This study follows the CONSORT-AI Extension guidelines and the SPIRIT-AI guidelines.

Informed Consent Statement: Patient consent was waived by the Ethics Committee due to the retrospective nature.

Data Availability Statement: Data are available on request due to legal restrictions.

Conflicts of Interest: H.A.R. and M.L. are consultants of Allergan Plc., W.H. and M.H. have nothing to disclose. There is no conflict of the authors in regard to collection of data, design of the study, in the collection, analyses or interpretation of data, in the writing of the manuscript or in the decision to publish the results.

eferences

Vision Loss Expert Group of the Global Burden of Disease Study; GBD 2019 Blindness and Vision Impairment Collaborators. Prevalence of Vision Loss in High-Income Countries and in Eastern and Central Europe in 2020: Magnitude and Temporal Trends. *Ophthalmic Epidemiol.* **2025**, 1–14, *ahead of print*.

Johns, K.L.; Faralli, J.A.; Filla, M.S.; Shah, N.S.; Sun, Y.Y.; Keller, K.E.; Peters, D.M. Age-Related Dysregulation of $\alpha 5\beta 1$ and $\alpha v\beta 3$ Integrin Activity Alters Contractile Properties of Trabecular Meshwork Cells. *Investig. Ophthalmol. Vis. Sci.* **2025**, *66*, 31. [CrossRef] [PubMed]

Adelpour, M.; Moghimi, S.; Nishida, T.; Meller, L.; Du, K.H.; Kamalipour, A.; Tansuebchueasai, N.; Mahmoudinezhad, G.; Zangwill, L.M.; Weinreb, R.N. Short-Term Rates of Visual Field Change Predict Glaucoma Progression. *Ophthalmol. Glaucoma* **2025**, *ahead of print*. [CrossRef] [PubMed]

Tonti, E.; Tonti, S.; Mancini, F.; Bonini, C.; Spadea, L.; D'Esposito, F.; Gagliano, C.; Musa, M.; Zeppieri, M. Artificial Intelligence and Advanced Technology in Glaucoma: A Review. *J. Pers. Med.* **2024**, *14*, 1062. [CrossRef] [PubMed]

Wu, J.H.; Lin, S.; Moghimi, S. Application of artificial intelligence in glaucoma care: An updated review. *Taiwan J. Ophthalmol.* **2024**, *14*, 340–351. [CrossRef]

Ravindranath, R.; Stein, J.D.; Hernandez-Boussard, T.; Fisher, A.C.; Wang, S.Y.; SOURCE Consortium. The Impact of Race, Ethnicity, and Sex on Fairness in Artificial Intelligence for Glaucoma Prediction Models. *Ophthalmol. Sci.* **2024**, *5*, 100596. [CrossRef] [PubMed]

Shan, S.; Wu, J.; Cao, J.; Feng, Y.; Zhou, J.; Luo, Z.; Song, P.; Rudan, I.; Global Health Epidemiology Research Group (GHERG). Global incidence and risk factors for glaucoma: A systematic review and meta-analysis of prospective studies. *J. Glob. Health* **2024**, *14*, 04252. [CrossRef] [PubMed]

Mastronikolis, S.; Pagkalou, M.; Baroutas, G.; Kyriakopoulou, K.; Makri, O.E.; Georgakopoulos, C.D. Pseudoexfoliation syndrome: The critical role of the extracellular matrix in pathogenesis and treatment. *IUBMB Life* **2022**, *74*, 995–1002. [CrossRef] [PubMed]

Ghaffari Sharaf, M.; Damji, K.F.; Unsworth, L.D. Recent advances in risk factors associated with ocular exfoliation syndrome. *Acta Ophthalmol.* **2020**, *98*, 113–120. [CrossRef] [PubMed]

Qiao, C.Y.; Wang, S.Y. Standardizing the diagnosis and treatment of ocular hypertension based on evidence-based medicine. *Chin. Med. J.* **2024**, *104*, 2195–2199.

Svedberg, E.; Ekström, C. Distribution of cup-disc ratio in a Swedish population. *Upsala J. Med. Sci.* **2023**, *128*, 10-48101. [CrossRef] [PubMed]

Ekström, C.; Carlsson, C. Incidence of blindness in open-angle glaucoma in Sweden: A long-term follow-up study. *Upsala J. Med. Sci.* **2024**, *129*, 10-48101. [CrossRef] [PubMed]

Wang, Y.X.; Yang, H.; Wei, C.C.; Xu, L.; Wei, W.B.; Jonas, J.B. High myopia as risk factor for the 10-year incidence of open-angle glaucoma in the Beijing Eye Study. *Br. J. Ophthalmol.* **2023**, *107*, 935–940. [CrossRef] [PubMed]

Spaeth, G.L. European Glaucoma Society Terminology and Guidelines for Glaucoma, 5th edition. *Br. J. Ophthalmol.* **2021**, *105*, 1–169. [CrossRef]

Wolfram Research, Inc. *Mathematica*, version 13.3; Wolfram Research: Champaign, IL, USA, 2023.

Franc, V.; Prusa, D.; Voracek, V. Optimal strategies for reject option classifiers. *J. Mach. Learn. Res.* **2023**, *24*, 1–49.

Cloud Software Group, Inc. *Spotfire*, version 14, Data Science Workbench. Cloud Software Group: Fort Lauderdale, FL, USA, 2023. Available online: https://www.spotfire.com/ (accessed on 28 October 2024).

18. Lan, C.H.; Chiu, T.H.; Yen, W.T.; Lu, D.W. Artificial Intelligence in Glaucoma: Advances in Diagnosis, Progression Forecastin and Surgical Outcome Prediction. *Int. J. Mol. Sci.* **2025**, *26*, 4473. [CrossRef]
19. Carlà, M.M.; Gambini, G.; Giannuzzi, F.; Boselli, F.; De Luca, L.; Rizzo, S. Testing the Reliability of ChatGPT Assistance fo Surgical Choices in Challenging Glaucoma Cases. *J. Pers. Med.* **2025**, *15*, 97. [CrossRef]
20. Wąż, P.; Zorena, K.; Murawska, A.; Bielińska-Wąż, D. Classification Maps: A New Mathematical Tool Supporting the Diagnosis Age-Related Macular Degeneration. *J. Pers. Med.* **2023**, *13*, 1074. [CrossRef] [PubMed]
21. Demir, F.; Burak, T. An Effective and Robust Approach Based on R-CNN+LSTM Model and NCAR Feature Selection fo Ophthalmological Disease Detection from Fundus Images. *J. Pers. Med.* **2021**, *11*, 1276. [CrossRef] [PubMed]
22. Govindaiah, A.; Baten, A.; Smith, R.T.; Balasubramanian, S.; Bhuiyan, A. Optimized Prediction Models from Fundus Imaging an Genetics for Late Age-Related Macular Degeneration. *J. Pers. Med.* **2021**, *11*, 1127. [CrossRef] [PubMed]

Journal of
Personalized Medicine

MDPI

ticle

uccess of Strabismus Surgery in Intermittent Exotropia

dro Lino [1,2,3,4,5,*], Pedro Vargues de Aguiar [1] and João Paulo Cunha [6,7]

1 NOVA National School of Public Health, Public Health Research Centre, Comprehensive Health Research Center, CHRC, LA-REAL, CCAL, NOVA University Lisbon, 1649-004 Lisbon, Portugal; pedroaguiar@ensp.unl.pt
2 Santa Maria Local Health Unit, 1649-028 Lisbon, Portugal
3 CUF Cascais Hospital, 2750-663 Cascais, Portugal
4 CUF Tejo Hospital, 1350-352 Lisbon, Portugal
5 Higher School of Technology and Health of Lisbon, Polytechnic Institute of Lisbon, 1990-096 Lisbon, Portugal
6 Ophthalmology Unit, CUF Cascais Hospital, 2750-663 Cascais, Portugal; joao.cunha@estesl.ipl.pt
7 Department of Morpho-Functional Sciences, Higher School of Technology and Health of Lisbon, Polytechnic Institute of Lisbon, 1990-096 Lisbon, Portugal
* Correspondence: pedro.lino@estesl.ipl.pt

Abstract: Introduction: Intermittent exotropia (IXT) is the most common form of childhood divergent strabismus. Surgery remains the primary approach to control ocular deviation and preserve binocular function. Although previous studies report a success rate of approximately 75%, factors influencing surgical outcomes remain insufficiently explored. This study evaluates the effectiveness of strabismus surgery in children with IXT and identifies predictors of postoperative alignment stability. **Methods**: This retrospective study included 258 children with basic-type IXT or divergence excess who underwent bilateral lateral rectus recession. Clinical records and surgical data were analyzed to determine the overall success rate and identify associated predictive factors. **Results**: The sample included 166 females (64.3%) and 92 males (35.7%), with a mean age of 11.19 ± 3.73 years. Surgical success was achieved in 238 patients (92.2%). Success rates were similar across sexes (92.8% in females vs. 91.3% in males). No significant associations were found between surgical success and sex, age, preoperative occlusion therapy, binocular function, or IXT subtype. However, patients with moderate preoperative deviations had higher success rates. A statistically significant difference was observed in the preoperative deviation angle between successful (31 ± 7.08Δ) and unsuccessful (42 ± 7.27Δ) cases. A lower AC/A ratio was also associated with better outcomes, although it was not the main predictor. **Discussion**: The high success rate (92.2%) suggests a limited impact of demographic or preoperative variables. The preoperative deviation angle emerged as the strongest predictor of success, with smaller angles correlating with more favorable surgical outcomes. These findings underscore the importance of accurate preoperative assessment in surgical planning for IXT.

Keywords: intermittent exotropia; surgery; surgical success; recurrence

1. Introduction

Intermittent exotropia (IXT) is the most common type of divergent strabismus in children. It is defined as a deviation that is present intermittently and alternates with periods of orthotropia [1–3]. The deviation usually appears during early childhood (between 1 and 5 years of age) and typically becomes more frequent over time. It often manifests during distance fixation or in situations of fatigue, distraction, or illness. As the child grows, the deviation may also appear at near fixation and can eventually progress to constant

 https://doi.org/10.3390/jpm15080333

exotropia (XT) [1]. The development of amblyopia is rare and usually occurs only when the condition becomes constant at an early age or when it coexists with other amblyogenic factors, such as uncorrected refractive errors [1].

Typically, during periods of ocular alignment, individuals exhibit binocular vision and stereopsis. When the deviation is present, anomalous retinal correspondence (ARC) may occur. Depending on the patient's age and the maturity of the visual system, suppression or diplopia may develop [1–5].

According to Duane's classification, IXT can be divided into four types: divergence excess, basic type, convergence insufficiency, and pseudo-divergence excess [1,5].

There is currently no universally accepted first-line treatment for IXT [1]. Treatment options include medical approaches, such as occlusion therapy and the use of minus lenses to stimulate convergence, and orthoptic therapy, consisting of fusion exercises, which remain controversial due to ongoing debate regarding their effectiveness and their potential negative impact on surgical outcomes. Orthoptic therapy may be useful only in cases of convergence insufficiency, as it can promote fixation and improve fusion. Therefore, surgical intervention is the mainstay of treatment for most IXT cases. Surgery typically yields satisfactory results, although undercorrection or overcorrection may occur in the immediate postoperative period. Over time, XT may recur, and additional surgery may be required [1,4–7]. Surgery for IXT has reported success rates of 70–80%, but recurrence can occur in up to 50% of cases within three years. Several prognostic factors strongly influence outcomes [8–14]. A smaller preoperative deviation angle is associated with better surgical success and a reduced need for reoperation [5,8,10,15]. Younger age at the time of surgery, particularly between 3 and <5 years, is also linked to higher success rates [8,14]. The type of exotropia is another important factor: the pseudo-divergence excess subtype is associated with better alignment and lower recurrence [14–16]. Postoperative alignment during the first week is a strong predictor of long-term success, especially in adults. In cases with large deviation angles (>60 PD), the likelihood of achieving orthophoria is high, although binocular success may be limited [5,9]. A family history of strabismus surgery does not appear to significantly influence surgical outcomes [4].

This study aims to evaluate the effectiveness of bilateral lateral rectus recession surgery in children with intermittent exotropia (IXT), with a particular focus on identifying predictive factors for long-term alignment stability. In contrast to previous studies, this research provides a comprehensive analysis of a large pediatric cohort in Portugal, applying a personalized medicine approach to stratify surgical outcomes based on clinical profiles such as preoperative deviation angle and AC/A ratio.

2. Methodology

This was a retrospective study [17].of patients treated at CUF Cascais Hospital, involving a cohort of children who underwent strabismus surgery for intermittent exotropia. The procedure performed was classic bilateral lateral rectus recession under general anesthesia. All surgeries were conducted by the same surgeon, and the surgical dose was determined based on the distance deviation angle using Park's formula (Table 1).

Inclusion criteria: Children aged 4 to 18 years with a confirmed diagnosis of intermittent exotropia who underwent surgical correction. Only patients with complete medical records—including preoperative data, surgical reports, and postoperative follow-up—were included. All participants had normal visual acuity (i.e., no amblyopia) and no associated ocular or systemic conditions that could influence the evaluation of surgical outcomes.

Table 1. Parks' formula for exotropia surgery.

Exotropia Angle in PD	Amount of Recession/Resection in Mm	
Two muscles	BLRc	LRc + MRs (R&R)
15	4.0	4.0 + 3.0
20	5.0	5.0 + 4.0
25	6.0	6.0 + 4.0
30	7.0	7.0 + 5.5
35	7.5	7.5 + 5.5
40	8.0	8.0 + 5.5
45	8.5	8.5 + 6.0
50	9.0	9.0 + 6.5
60	10	9.0 + 7.0

Legend: PD, prismatic diopters. BLRc, bilateral lateral rectus recession. LRc, lateral rectus recession. MRs: medial rectus resection.

Exclusion criteria: Patients were excluded if they presented other ocular or systemic pathologies, unilateral or bilateral amblyopia, chromosomal abnormalities or systemic diseases (e.g., congenital anomalies or neurological disorders), paralytic or restrictive exotropia, dissociated vertical deviation or alphabet patterns, constant exotropia, or other types of divergent strabismus such as consecutive or sensory exotropia.

The following parameters were documented and analyzed: sex, age, age at surgery, refractive error (spherical equivalent), distance deviation in prism diopters (PD) before surgery, preoperative sensory status, type of surgical procedure performed, postoperative deviation in PD at six months, and sensory function at six months. A six-month follow-up was chosen because ocular alignment is generally more stable after this period, allowing for a more accurate assessment of residual deviation. This timeframe also permits evaluation of sensory adaptation (e.g., binocular fusion), identification of relapses or overcorrections, and assessment of symptoms and quality of life. Moreover, it is a commonly used interval in scientific literature, facilitating comparison with other studies.

In all patients, deviations were measured using the alternate cover test with prisms for both near (33 cm) and distance (6 m) fixation. To differentiate between true divergence excess and pseudo-divergence excess, measurements were repeated after occlusion (1 h) of the non-dominant eye. The AC/A ratio was calculated using the gradient method, with the addition of −2.00 D lenses.

Sensory status was evaluated using fusion (Worth 4-dot test) and stereopsis (Wirt test for near, Vectograph for distance).

Definition of surgical success: Residual ocular deviation $\leq$10 PD at distance fixation six months after surgery (whether eso- or exotropic), with the presence of sensory fusion and stereopsis of 80 arcseconds or better, as assessed by either near (Wirt) or distance (Vectograph) stereotests. This combined motor and sensory criterion aligns with prior literature and enables a comprehensive evaluation of functional surgical outcomes.

Statistical analysis [18,19]: Data were entered into a custom SPSS® version 29 database and analyzed using univariate, bivariate, and multivariate statistical methods. Variables were classified according to their characteristics and categorized accordingly.

Qualitative sociodemographic and clinical variables were analyzed using descriptive statistics, and quantitative variables were summarized using measures of central tendency and dispersion. Logistic regression was used to identify factors associated with stable post-operative alignment, including both crude and adjusted models. Variables included in the model were selected based on clinical relevance and statistical significance in bivariate analysis, and multicollinearity was assessed to ensure model robustness. A significance level of 5% was adopted, and p-values below this threshold were considered statistically significant.

All stages of the research complied with ethical and regulatory standards for Good Practice in Health Research and were approved by the Ethics Committee of the CUF Group—Health Services (approval number: 2024/488).

3. Results

The sample included 258 participants: 166 females (64.3%) and 92 males (35.7%). The participants' ages ranged from 5 to 18 years, with a mean age of 11.19 ± 3.73 years.

The mean age at the time of surgery was 8.75 ± 12.19 years, with a minimum of 4 years and a maximum of 17 years.

Out of the total sample, 238 patients (92.2%) achieved surgical success, defined as a residual eso- or exodeviation ≤10 PD and stereopsis better than 80 arcseconds. The remaining 20 patients (7.8%) did not meet the criteria for success. In the success group, the mean refractive error (spherical equivalent) was −0.63 ± 1.424 D, while in the no-success group, it was −0.63 ± 1.134 D.

Ophthalmologic characteristics: Table 2 shows the associations between each of the characteristics studied in each of the groups (success vs. non-success).

Table 2. Association between exposures and outcome.

Exposure	Group: Success	Group: No Success	OR	p-Value	95% Confidence Interval
Gender					
Female (reference)	154 (92.8%)	12 (7.2%)			
Male	84 (91.3%)	8 (8.7%)	0.818	0.673	0.322; 2.080
Age	11.22 ± 3.589	12.20 ± 5.414	1.031	0.627	0.911; 1.168
Surgical Age	8.76 ± 12.617	9.80 ± 5.519	1.001	0.954	0.962; 1.042
Prior occlusive treatment					
Yes	196 (91.2%)	19 (8.8%)			
No (reference)	42 (97.7%)	1 (2.3%)	0.246	0.177	0.032; 1.886
XTI type					
DET	51 (89.5%)	6 (10.5%)			
BT (reference)	187 (93%)	14(7%)	0.636	0.378	0.233; 1.739
Moderate preoperative deviation					
Yes	76 (100%)	0(0%)			
No (reference)	162 (89%)	20 (11%)	9.259 *	0.01	1.648; 196.3
Magnitude of preoperative deviation	31 ± 7.080	42 ± 7.270	0.837	<0.001	0.777; 0.901
AC/A ratio	7.09 ± 3.735	11.27 ± 9.035	0.920	0.013	0.861; 0.983
Binocular Preoperative					
Yes	233 (92.5%)	19 (7.5%)			
No (reference)	5 (83.3%)	1 (16.7%)	2.453	0.424	0.272; 22.077
Surgical Dose (mm)	13.65 ± 2.5	15.33 ± 3.395	0.817	0.025	0.685; 0.975

* For this calculation, the authors do a direct substitution of 0 by 1 OR (odds ratio).

- Preoperative occlusive treatment: 196 patients (91.2%) underwent occlusion therapy as an anti-suppression exercise.
- Binocular function before surgery: 233 patients (92.5%) had binocular function prior to surgery. The odds ratio (OR) for surgical success in patients with binocular vision was 2.453 ($p = 0.424$).
- IXT type: 187 patients (93%) had basic-type intermittent exotropia, and 51 patients (89.5%) had divergence excess type. The OR for surgical success in patients with basic-type IXT was 0.636 ($p = 0.378$).
- Preoperative deviation angle: The mean deviation at distance was 31 $\pm$ 7.08Δ in the success group and 42 $\pm$ 7.27Δ in the no-success group. Patients with moderate deviation had a significantly higher chance of surgical success.
- AC/A ratio: The mean AC/A ratio was 7.09 $\pm$ 3.735 in the success group and 11.27 $\pm$ 9.035 in the no-success group. A statistically significant difference was found (OR = 0.920; $p = 0.013$), suggesting that a higher AC/A ratio is associated with lower surgical success.
- Total surgical dose: The mean total amount of recession (bilateral) was 13.65 $\pm$ 2.5 mm in the success group and 15.33 $\pm$ 3.395 mm in the no-success group. Although there was no statistically significant difference between larger setbacks ($t = 1.891$; $p = 0.078$), logistic regression showed a significant association ($p = 0.025$).
- Sex: Surgical success was achieved in 154 females (92.8%) and 84 males (91.3%). Although females tended to have a slightly higher success rate, the difference was not statistically significant (OR = 0.818; $p = 0.673$).
- Age and age at surgery: The mean age in the success group was 11.22 $\pm$ 3.589 years, compared to 12.20 $\pm$ 5.414 years in the no-success group. The mean age at surgery was 8.76 $\pm$ 12.617 years in the success group and 9.80 $\pm$ 5.519 years in the no-success group. There was no significant association between these variables and surgical success, although younger patients tended to have better outcomes (OR = 1.031; $p = 0.627$ for age; OR = 1.001; $p = 0.954$ for surgical age).

By further analyzing associations and interactions between variables using binary logistic regression, it was found that the preoperative deviation angle was the only exposure significantly influencing surgical outcome.

In the optimized logistic regression model (which included variables with $p < 0.2$ and excluded those with adjusted $p > 0.05$ after testing for collinearity), the only statistically significant predictor of surgical success was the preoperative deviation angle: patients with smaller deviation angles had a significantly higher probability of successful outcomes (OR = 0.837; $p < 0.001$).

4. Discussion

The primary objective of surgical intervention in intermittent exotropia (IXT) is to improve ocular alignment while preserving or enhancing binocular function. Therefore, surgical decisions are generally based on the clinical characteristics and functional impact of the strabismus. Large-angle exodeviations associated with reduced fusional amplitudes and a tendency toward loss of binocularity are typical indications for surgery.

4.1. Surgical Outcomes and Success Rates:

This study included 258 patients—166 females (64.3%) and 92 males (35.7%)—with ages ranging from 5 to 18 years (mean: 11.19 $\pm$ 3.73 years). The mean age at the time of surgery was 8.75 $\pm$ 12.19 years, with a minimum of 4 years and a maximum of 17 years. Surgical success was achieved in 238 patients (92.2%), while 20 patients (7.8%) did not achieve the defined criteria for success.

The overall surgical success rate in this study—exceeding 90%—is higher than what has been reported in several previous studies. For example, Donahue et al. reported a success rate of approximately 70% in a cohort of 197 patients in Florida [20]. This study represents the first publication from Portugal addressing bilateral surgery for IXT. Although a previous study with a small sample size reported a 100% success rate [4], our findings are based on a larger and more representative cohort. Reported success rates in the literature vary depending on the follow-up period. Kopmann et al. reported a success rate of 83.8% on the first postoperative day [5], while Thorisdottir et al. reported an 80% success rate at two months postoperatively [21]. In this context, our success rate at six months supports the high efficacy of bilateral lateral rectus muscle recession for IXT.

4.2. Factors Influencing Surgical Outcomes:

- Preoperative deviation angle: Statistical analysis showed that a smaller preoperative deviation angle was associated with higher surgical success. The mean angle in the success group was 31 ± 7.08Δ, compared to 42 ± 7.27Δ in the no-success group. Patients with moderate deviations were significantly more likely to achieve success (OR = 9.259; $p = 0.01$). Quantitative analysis further confirmed the protective role of a smaller angle (OR = 0.837; $p < 0.001$), indicating that each additional prism diopter increased the risk of failure by approximately 16%. These results are consistent with previous findings, including those of Kopmann et al. (2024) [5], Tibrewal (2017) [22], and Thorisdottir (2022) [21], all of which suggest that patients with smaller preoperative angles have better outcomes.
- Age at surgery: The mean age in the success group was 11.22 ± 3.59 years, compared to 12.20 ± 5.41 years in the no-success group. The mean surgical age was 8.76 ± 12.62 years in the success group and 9.80 ± 5.52 years in the no-success group. Although no statistically significant association was found ($p = 0.627$ for age; $p = 0.954$ for surgical age), there was a tendency toward better results in younger patients. This is in agreement with Issaho et al. (2017) [11], although some authors, such as Jiménez-Romo (2023), argue that age is not a significant predictor of surgical success [23].
- Binocular function: Preoperative binocular function was present in 233 patients (92.5%). Although a tendency toward better outcomes in these patients was observed (OR = 2.453; $p = 0.424$), the association was not statistically significant. This suggests that surgery may either preserve or restore binocular function, depending on the preoperative status.
- AC/A ratio: The mean AC/A ratio was 7.09 ± 3.73 in the success group and 11.27 ± 9.04 in the no-success group. A higher AC/A ratio was significantly associated with lower surgical success (OR = 0.920; $p = 0.013$), indicating that patients with greater accommodative convergence relative to accommodation are less likely to benefit from surgery [24].
- Gender: Surgical success was achieved in 154 female patients (92.8%) and 84 male patients (91.3%). Although there was a slight trend toward higher success in females (OR = 0.818; $p = 0.673$), the difference was not statistically significant and may be due to chance.
- Preoperative occlusion therapy: Occlusion therapy was performed in 196 patients (91.2%). While it appeared to be a potential protective factor (OR = 0.246; $p = 0.177$), the association was not statistically significant. This finding is in line with the anterior works [14], who suggested that children undergoing occlusion therapy before surgery may have better outcomes.
- Surgical dose: The mean bilateral recession was 13.65 ± 2.5 mm in the success group and 15.33 ± 3.39 mm in the no-success group. Although the direct comparison did not

reach statistical significance ($p = 0.078$), logistic regression revealed a significant negative association between larger recession amounts and surgical success (OR = 0.817; $p = 0.025$), indicating that higher surgical doses may be associated with a lower likelihood of favorable outcomes.

4.3. Study Limitations:

This study has several limitations, primarily related to its retrospective design. Patients were not randomly assigned to treatment protocols; instead, the surgical approach was based on the clinical judgment and experience of the operating surgeon. This may introduce selection bias and limit the generalizability of our findings. Nevertheless, the large sample size and comprehensive analysis strengthen the conclusions and provide meaningful insights into the factors influencing surgical success in IXT.

5. Conclusions

Children diagnosed with the basic type of intermittent exotropia tended to achieve more favorable surgical outcomes. After adjusting for potential confounding variables, a statistically significant association was found between smaller preoperative deviation angles and a greater likelihood of surgical success.

Although younger age at the time of surgery and the presence of preoperative binocular function did not reach statistical significance, these factors may still hold clinical relevance and should be considered during surgical planning and decision-making.

Author Contributions: P.L., P.V.d.A. and J.P.C. designed the study. P.L. collected the data under the supervision of P.V.d.A. and J.P.C. P.L. analyzed the data with statistical guidance from P.V.d.A. and scientific input from J.P.C. All authors have read and agreed to the published version of the manuscript.

Funding: This research was funded by Fundação para a Ciência e Tecnologia (FCT, Portugal) through national funds to the Associated Laboratory in Translation and Innovation Towards Global Health REAL (LA/P/0117/2020).

Institutional Review Board Statement: The study was reviewed and approved by the Ethics Committee of Grupo CUF Saude (approval number 2024/488, approval date: 10 October 2024).

Informed Consent Statement: The authors have given their consent for the publication of this manuscript. As this was a retrospective study with a positive opinion from the ethics committee, the requirement for informed consent was waived.

Data Availability Statement: The raw data supporting the conclusions of this article will be made available by the authors on request.

Conflicts of Interest: The authors declare that they have no competing interests.

eferences

Tejedor, J.Y.C. *Strabismus and Amblyopia*, 1st ed.; McGraw-Hill Interamericana de España S.L.: Madrid, Spain, 2022.
Jeanrot, N.; Ducret, V. *Manuel de Strabologie: Aspects Cliniques et Thérapeutiques*; Elsevier-Masson: Issy-les-Moulineaux, France, 2018.
von Noorden, G.K.; Campos, E. *Binocular Vision and Ocular Motility*, 6th ed.; Mosby: Maryland Heights, MO, USA, 2022.
Cristóvão, D.; Seldon, R.; De, M.; Vieira, L. Exotropia intermitente: From surgical success to long-term need for reoperation. *Oftalmologia* **2013**, *37*, 259. (In Portuguese)
Kopmann, S.; Grenzebach, U.; Ehrt, O.; Biermann, J. Effectiveness of strabismus surgery in intermittent exotropia and factors influencing outcome. *J. Clin. Med.* **2024**, *13*, 1031. [CrossRef] [PubMed]
Anand, K.; Krishnan, A.; Kumar, P.; Bharadwaj, A.; Dutta, P.; Rastogi, A.; Hariani, A. Comparative Study of Bilateral Versus Unilateral Strabismus Surgery in the Management of Lateral Incomitance in Intermittent Exotropia. *J. Pediatr. Ophthalmol. Strabismus* **2023**, *60*, 277–281. [CrossRef] [PubMed]
Yildirim, C.; Mutlu, F.M.; Chen, Y.; Altinsoy, H.I. Assessment of central and peripheral fusion and near and distance stereoacuity in intermittent exotropic patients before and after strabismus surgery. *Am. J. Ophthalmol.* **1999**, *128*, 222–230. [CrossRef] [PubMed]

8. Rajavi, Z.; Hafezian, S.F.; Yaseri, M.; Sheibani, K. Early postoperative alignment as a predictor of 6-month alignment aft intermittent exotropia surgery. *J. Pediatr. Ophthalmol. Strabismus* **2014**, *51*, 274–282. [CrossRef] [PubMed]
9. Huh, J.; Ha, S.G.; Kim, S.H. Recovery From Suppression with Successful Motor Alignment After Surgery for Intermitte Exotropia. *J. Pediatr. Ophthalmol. Strabismus* **2020**, *57*, 21–26. [CrossRef] [PubMed]
10. Maruo, T.; Kubota, N.; Sakaue, T.; Usui, C. Intermittent exotropia surgery in children: Long term outcome regarding changes binocular alignment. A study of 666 cases. *Binocul. Vis. Strabismus Q.* **2001**, *16*, 265–270. [PubMed]
11. Issaho, D.C.; Wang, S.X.; Weakley, D.R. Intermittent exotropia surgery: Results in different age groups. *Arq. Bras. Oftalmol.* **201** *80*, 355–358. [CrossRef] [PubMed]
12. Xu, M.; Zheng, F.; Peng, Y.; Wang, C.; Lou, J.; Yu, H.; Wang, Y.; Yu, X. Effects of orthoptic therapy in children with intermitte exotropia after surgery: Study protocol for a randomized controlled trial. *Trials* **2022**, *23*, 1123. [CrossRef] [PubMed]
13. Farid, M.F.; Abdelbaset, E.A. Surgical outcomes of three different surgical techniques for treatment of convergence insufficienc intermittent exotropia. *Eye* **2018**, *32*, 693–700. [CrossRef] [PubMed]
14. Bae, G.H.; Bae, S.H.; Choi, D.G. Surgical outcomes of intermittent exotropia according to exotropia type based on distance/ne differences. *PLoS ONE* **2019**, *14*, e0214478. [CrossRef] [PubMed]
15. Hong, S.; Ha, S.; Seo, Y.; Kim, S. Analysis of Postoperative Outcomes in Patients with Intermittent Exotropia According t Preoperative Change of Angle of Deviation. *Korean J. Ophthalmol. KJO* **2021**, *35*, 130–135. [CrossRef] [PubMed]
16. Lavrich, J.B. Intermittent exotropia: Continued controversies and current management. *Curr. Opin. Ophthalmol.* **2015**, *26*, 375–38 [CrossRef] [PubMed]
17. Fortin, M.F. *Fundamentos E Etapas no Processo de Investigação*; Lusodidacta: Sintra, Portugal, 2009.
18. Oliveira, A. *Bioestatística Descodificada*, 2nd ed.; LIDEL—Edições Técnicas, Lda.: Lisboa, Portugal, 2014; Volume 1.
19. Vicente, V.; Aguiar, P. *Practical Epidemiology with GLM*; Editora d'Ideias: Coimbra, Portugal, 2023.
20. Donahue, S.P.; Chandler, D.L.; Wu, R.; Marsh, J.D.; Law, C.; Areaux, R.G., Jr.; Ghasia, F.F.; Li, Z.; Kraker, R.T.; Cotter, S.A.; et a Eight-Year Outcomes of Bilateral Lateral Rectus Recessions versus Unilateral Recession-Resection in Childhood Basic-Typ Intermittent Exotropia. *Ophthalmology* **2024**, *131*, 98–106. [CrossRef] [PubMed]
21. Thorisdottir, R.; Malmsjö, M.; Tenland, K.; Blohmé, J.; Hesgaard, H. The success of unilateral surgery for constant and intermitte exotropia and factors affecting it in a large Scandinavian case series. *J. Pediatr. Ophthalmol. Strabismus* **2021**, *58*, 34–41. [CrossRe [PubMed]
22. Tibrewal, S.; Singh, N.; Bhuiyan, M.; Ganesh, S. Factors affecting residual exotropia after two muscle surgery for intermitter exotropia. *Int. J. Ophthalmol.* **2017**, *10*, 1120–1125. [CrossRef] [PubMed]
23. Jiménez-Romo, C.A.; Rangel-Padilla, A.; Páez-Garza, J.H. Timely Surgery in Intermittent Exotropia. *J. Binocul. Vis. Ocul. Mot* **2023**, *73*, 21–27. [CrossRef] [PubMed]
24. Brodsky, M.C.; Horwood, A.M.; Riddell, P.M. Intermittent exotropia: Are we underminusing by not overminusing? *J. AAPO* **2015**, *19*, 397–398. [CrossRef] [PubMed]

Journal of
Personalized Medicine

MDPI

ticle

ffect of Prior Laser-Assisted In Situ Keratomileusis on the 'alibration Accuracy of Extended Depth of Focus Intraocular enses: A Direct Comparative Study

Iung Lin [1,2,3,4], Chen-Cheng Chao [1,4] and Chao-Kai Chang [1,5,*]

1 Nobel Eye Institute, Taipei 100008, Taiwan; petercard@gmail.com (I.-H.L.); aachengachen@gmail.com (C.-C.C.)
2 Graduate Institute of Clinical Medicine, College of Medicine, National Taiwan University, Taipei 100225, Taiwan
3 Department of Ophthalmology, Taipei Medical University Hospital, Taipei 110301, Taiwan
4 Department of Optometry, MacKay Junior College of Medicine, Nursing and Management, Taipei 112021, Taiwan
5 Department of Optometry, Da-Yeh University, Chunghua 515006, Taiwan
* Correspondence: chaokai@ms17.hinet.net; Tel.: +886-2-2370-5666

Abstract: Background: Personalized precision medicine has become a prevailing trend and applies to the selection of intraocular lenses (IOLs) for cataract surgery based on the unique corneal morphology of each person. The choice of presbyopia-correcting IOLs for post-laser-assisted in situ keratomileusis (LASIK) cataract surgery is a significant concern. However, few direct comparison studies exist between eyes with and without LASIK history. We analyzed the performance of extended depth of focus (EDOF) IOL implantation in these two groups. **Methods:** In this retrospective single-center study, we included patients with or without previous LASIK who underwent cataract surgery and EDOF Symfony IOL implantation, with ≥1 follow up. All patients underwent optical biometry using the IOLMaster. IOL power was calculated using the Sanders Retzslaff Kraff/theoretical and Haigis-L formulas for patients without and with LASIK, respectively. Uncorrected distance visual acuity (UDVA), uncorrected near visual acuity (UNVA), refraction, and corneal tomography were recorded. The prediction error was the absolute difference between the postoperative sphere and target refraction. The right eyes of patients who met the inclusion criteria were selected for analysis. **Results:** Among the 321 recruited eyes, 18 underwent previous LASIK. After 1:3 age/sex matching, 17 LASIK and 49 non-LASIK eyes from 66 patients were analyzed. No significant preoperative differences existed in target refraction, spherical equivalent, or best-corrected visual acuity. All surgical procedures were uneventful. LASIK exhibited non-inferiority to non-LASIK for predictive refraction error and UNVA. An age/sex-matched regression analysis indicated no UDVA superiority between the two groups. **Conclusions:** Previous LASIK may have no discernible effect on the visual performance of presbyopia-correcting EDOF IOLs with respect to the absolute refractive error, UNVA, and UDVA. Longer follow-up and larger-scale studies are required to further validate these results.

Keywords: laser in situ keratomileusis; cataract; extended depth of focus; absolute prediction error

1. Introduction

Laser-assisted in situ keratomileusis (LASIK) is a widely utilized refractive surgery for correcting myopia and astigmatism by reshaping the corneal stroma with an excimer laser. This reshaping allows the focal point of incoming light to be realigned onto the retina, thereby improving visual acuity [1]. While LASIK is highly effective in reducing the dependence on corrective lenses, it can also alter corneal biomechanics and induce higher-order aberrations, such as coma and spherical aberration. These optical changes may influence visual quality, although their impact on contrast sensitivity remains debated [2].

With the aging of LASIK-treated individuals, an increasing number of these patients are now undergoing cataract surgery. Nowadays, personalized precision medicine has become a prevailing trend. The same applies to the selection of intraocular lenses (IOLs) for cataract surgery. We should choose the most suitable IOL based on the unique corneal morphology of each individual. The selection of an appropriate intraocular lens (IOL) for post-LASIK eyes presents unique challenges due to the altered corneal biomechanics and shape, which affects the accuracy of IOL power calculations. Traditional IOL calculation formulas often yield suboptimal refractive outcomes in post-LASIK eyes, necessitating specialized formulas or newer technologies to enhance predictability. Among various IOL options, multifocal and extended depth of focus (EDOF) IOLs have been proposed as potential solutions for presbyopia correction in these patients. However, concerns remain regarding their performance in eyes with previous LASIK, particularly in terms of visual quality, dysphotopsia, and contrast sensitivity.

Although some studies have suggested that multifocal IOLs can be successfully implanted in post-LASIK eyes under specific conditions—such as the presence of regular corneal astigmatism and the use of optimized IOL power calculation methods [3,4]—comparative data between post-LASIK and non-LASIK eyes remain limited. In particular, direct assessments of EDOF IOL performance in post-LASIK patients are scarce. Given the growing number of patients seeking spectacle independence after cataract surgery, a clearer understanding of how EDOF IOLs function in post-LASIK eyes is essential for optimizing surgical outcomes and patient satisfaction.

Against this background, this study aims to provide a comparative analysis of EDOF IOL implantation outcomes in patients with and without a history of LASIK. By evaluating the postoperative visual performance, we seek to determine whether EDOF IOLs are a viable option for individuals who have previously undergone LASIK.

2. Materials and Methods

2.1. Study Design and Ethical Approval

Patients who visited the Taipei Nobel Eye Clinic from 2022 to 2023 were consecutively enrolled. This study was approved by the Ethics Committee of the National Changhua University of Education (Changhua, Taiwan) and registered on ClinicalTrials.gov (identifier NCT06165796).

2.2. Patients

The inclusion criteria comprised the following: (1) the presence of cataracts in both eyes, (2) age between 50 and 80 years, and (3) a corrected distance visual acuity (CDVA) under 20/40 in both eyes. Phacoemulsification cataract surgery was performed in all patients with or without previous myopic LASIK surgery. The exclusion criteria included the following: (1) complicated cataracts, (2) corneal opacities or irregularities, (3) corneal astigmatism > 1.50 diopters, (4) dry eye (Schirmer's test I $\leq$ 5 mm), (5) amblyopia, (6) anisometropia, (7) surgical complications such as posterior capsular bag rupture or vitreous loss, (8) IOL tilt or decentration, (9) coexisting ocular pathologies, (10) glaucoma, (11) non-dilating pupil, (12) history of intraocular surgery or retinopathy, (14) optic nerve or macular diseases, and (15) refusal or inability to maintain follow-up. Patients with optic zone decentration or irregular astigmatism in the LASIK group were excluded. Among patients who visited the Taipei Nobel Eye Clinic between 2022 and 2023, 331 eyes of 186 patients were recruited for this study.

2.3. Surgery

Clear corneal phacoemulsification and IOL implantation were performed by the same surgeon (Chao-Kai Chang). The surgical procedure involved the application of topical anesthesia, a three-step clear corneal incision (2.25 mm) at 180° (temporal in both eyes), a 5.0 mm continuous curvilinear capsulorhexis, phacoemulsification using the stop-and-chop technique, IOL implantation with an injector, IOL centration, and sutureless incisions. We exclusively used EDOF Symfony IOLs (Johnson & Johnson, Santa Ana, CA, USA).

2.4. Ophthalmic Examinations

The patients underwent comprehensive preoperative examinations and were subsequently assessed at 1 d, 1 week, and 1 month postoperatively. Each ophthalmological examination included tests for uncorrected distance visual acuity (UDVA) and CDVA at far and near distances, manifest refraction, biomicroscopy, and applanation tonometry. Corneal curvature values were exported from a Pentacam machine (Pentacam HR; Oculus GmbH, Wetzlar, Germany) using a Scheimpflug keratometry system. Fundus examinations were performed preoperatively. Preoperatively, all patients underwent optical biometry using the IOLMaster (IOLMaster 500, Carl Zeiss Meditec AG, Jena, Germany). The IOL power was calculated using the Sanders Retzlaff Kraff/theoretical (SRK/T) formula for patients without LASIK and the Haigis-L formula for patients with LASIK. The postoperative refraction target was emmetropia. This means that based on the post-IOL implantation refraction degree predicted by the IOLMaster, we chose an IOL as close to 0 degrees as possible for the IOL implantation, and that degree was defined as target refraction. Postoperatively, the IOL concentration was additionally evaluated using retro-illumination.

2.5. Statistical Analysis

The main post-surgery measurements used to compare the performance between patients with and without LASIK included the following: (i) ophthalmic examinations assessing UDVA, CDVA, and uncorrected near visual acuity (UNVA) at 40 cm and (ii) prediction error, defined as the absolute difference between the postoperative manifest sphere and target refraction. By using a model of generalized estimating equations (GEE), the regression analysis was adjusted for the following covariates: age, sex, axial length, anterior chamber depth (ACD), corneal curvature (K), IOL power, and preoperative sphere.

Non-inferiority tests [5] were conducted to assess whether the LASIK group's performance was not inferior to that of the non-LASIK group with respect to three post-cataract surgery outcomes: absolute predictive error, UDVA, and UNVA. The null hypothesis posits that the difference in the group mean is not less than the inferiority margin, in contrast to the alternative hypothesis that the difference in the group mean is less than the inferiority margin. To assess the non-inferiority of the LASIK group compared with the non-LASIK group, a 95% confidence interval of the difference in the means of target refraction between the groups was constructed [5].

If the upper limit of the interval does not exceed the predefined non-inferiority margin of 0.5 diopters (D) in the prediction error, non-inferiority is confirmed. Similarly, for UNVA and UDVA, the predefined non-inferiority margins are both a 0.1 logarithm of the minimum angle of resolution (logMAR) [6,7].

3. Results

Among the 321 recruited eyes, 18 had undergone previous LASIK, while the remaining 303 had not. After 1:3 matching for age and sex, the analysis included a final sample of

17 LASIK eyes and 49 non-LASIK eyes from 66 patients. All the 17 LASIK eyes had received LASIK surgery at ages 20 to 50. Table 1 presents the demographic characteristics of the patients and preoperative visual acuity data. No significant preoperative differences were observed in the target refraction, spherical equivalent, or best-corrected visual acuity. The LASIK eyes exhibited longer axial lengths (27.57 ± 1.43 mm) compared with the non-LASIK eyes (25.63 ± 1.80 mm), and the ACD was also deeper in LASIK eyes (3.57 ± 0.36 mm) than in non-LASIK eyes (3.34 ± 0.37 mm). A corneal topography revealed flatter K1 and K2 values (38.07 ± 2.18 and 38.82 ± 2.17, respectively) in the LASIK eyes in comparison with the non-LASIK eyes (43.13 ± 1.55 and 44.46 ± 1.81, respectively) (Table 1). All surgical procedures were performed smoothly, and all IOLs were positioned within the capsular bag.

Table 1. Demographic and clinical characteristics of patients with and without LASIK in the original and propensity-matched cohorts.

	Original Data		
Previous LASIK	**LASIK (18 Eyes)**	**Non-LASIK (303 Eyes)**	
	Mean ± SD	**Mean ± SD**	***p* Value**
Preop CDVA (logMAR)	0.44 ± 0.27	0.32 ± 0.29	0.0754
Age (years)	50.78 ± 7.14	60.95 ± 8.34	<0.0001 *
Sex (M/F)	7/11	114/189	0.914
Target refraction (D)	−0.59 ± 0.38	−0.57 ± 0.30	0.8403
AXL (mm)	24.73 ± 1.66	27.60 ± 1.39	<0.0001 *
ACD (mm)	3.55 ± 0.35	3.18 ± 0.43	0.0005 *
Sphere (D)	−6.07 ± 5.35	−2.08 ± 4.76	0.0007 *
Cylinder(D)	−1.11 ± 0.8	−1.2 ± 0.90	0.6894
Flat K (D)	37.97 ± 2.15	43.44 ± 1.40	<0.0001 *
Steep K (D)	38.71 ± 2.16	44.33 ± 1.50	<0.0001 *
IOL power (D)	20.08 ± 2.85	18.39 ± 4.80	0.0289
	Matched Data		
Previous LASIK	**LASIK (17 Eyes)**	**Non-LASIK (49 Eyes)**	
	Mean ± SD	**Mean ± SD**	***p* Value**
Preop CDVA (logMAR)	0.45 ± 0.27	0.34 ± 0.29	0.1879
Age (years)	51.47 ± 6.71	52.08 ± 6.26	0.7345
Sex (M/F)	7/10	21/28	0.9038
Target refraction (D)	−0.66 ± 0.26	−0.55 ± 0.29	0.2065
AXL (mm)	27.57 ± 1.43	25.63 ± 1.8	0.0001 *
ACD (mm)	3.57 ± 0.36	3.34 ± 0.37	0.0307 *
Sphere (D)	−6.28 ± 5.44	−4.82 ± 4.88	0.3063
Cylinder (D)	−1.12 ± 0.83	−1.38 ± 1.11	0.3715
Flat K (D)	38.07 ± 2.18	43.13 ± 1.55	<0.0001 *
Steep K (D)	38.82 ± 2.17	44.46 ± 1.81	<0.0001 *
IOL power (D)	20.09 ± 2.93	15.83 ± 4.83	<0.0001 *

* p value < 0.05; CDVA, corrected distance visual acuity; logMAR, logarithm of the minimum angle of resolution; AXL, axial length; ACD, anterior chamber depth; LASIK, Laser Assisted In Situ Keratomileusis; M, male; F, female; D, diopter; K, keratometry: the measurement of the corneal curvature/power; SD, standard deviation; IOL, intraocular lens.

Table 2 presents the results of the non-inferiority tests at one month post-operation. For the UNVA, the mean was 0.315 ± 0.305 logMAR in the LASIK group and 0.736 ± 1.307 logMAR in the non-LASIK group. The respective non-inferiority margins exceeded the upper bounds of their corresponding confidence intervals (non-inferiority margins: 0.1; 95% CI: −0.8143, −0.0269), confirming the non-inferiority of the LASIK group compared with the non-LASIK group. For the predictive refraction error, the mean was 0.656 ± 0.264 D in the LASIK group and 0.551 ± 0.287 D in the non-LASIK group. The respective non-inferiority margins exceeded the upper bounds of their corresponding confidence intervals (non-inferiority margins: 0.5; 95% CI: −0.0442, 0.2541), confirming the non-inferiority of the LASIK group compared with the non-LASIK group. In contrast, for the UDVA, the mean was 0.300 ± 0.362 logMAR in the LASIK group and 0.117 ± 0.156 logMAR in the non-LASIK group. The non-inferiority margin fell within the interval, with the mean of the LASIK group being greater than that of the non-LASIK group (non-inferiority margins: 0.1; 95% CI: 0.0033, 0.3585). However, further age- and sex-matched regression analyses did not suggest that either group was significantly superior in terms of the UDVA ($p = 0.063$) (Table 3). It only revealed that the axial length has a significant influence on the UDVA ($p = 0.034$) (Table 3).

Table 2. Non-inferiority tests of predicted refractive errors and postoperative visual acuity between the LASIK and non-LASIK groups at one month post-operation.

	LASIK (SD) n = 17	Non-LASIK (SD) n = 49	Non-Inferiority Margin	95% CI	Outcome
UNVA (logMAR)	0.315 (0.305)	0.736 (1.307)	0.1	−0.8143, −0.0269	Not inferior
UDVA (logMAR)	0.300 (0.362)	0.117 (0.156)	0.1	0.0033, 0.3585	Non-LASIK is inferior to LASIK
Prediction error (D)	0.656 (0.264)	0.551 (0.287)	0.5	−0.0442, 0.2541	Not inferior

UDVA, uncorrected distance visual acuity; UNVA, uncorrected near visual acuity; logMAR, logarithm of the minimum angle of resolution; CI, confidence interval; LASIK, Laser Assisted In Situ Keratomileusis; D, diopter; SD, standard deviation.

Table 3. Age- and sex-matched regression analysis by using the model of generalized estimating equations (GEEs), showing no significant superiority between the LASIK and non-LASIK groups at one month post-operation.

Dependent Variable: PostopUDVA							
Parameter	Level	Est.	SE	95% CI		Z	*p* Value
Intercept		3.4494	2.2501	−0.961	7.860	1.53	0.1253
AXL		−0.1076	0.0508	−0.207	−0.008	−2.12	0.0341
Previous LASIK	1 (yes)	0.1770	0.0952	−0.010	0.364	1.86	0.0631
ACD		0.1443	0.1278	−0.106	0.395	1.13	0.2590
Sphere		0.0140	0.0119	−0.009	0.037	1.17	0.2413
Steep K		−0.0221	0.0290	−0.079	0.035	−0.76	0.4451

UDVA, uncorrected distance visual acuity; AXL, axial length; ACD, anterior chamber depth; CI, confidence interval LASIK, Laser Assisted In Situ Keratomileusis; K, keratometry: the measurement of the corneal curvature/power; Z, z-score; SE, standard error; Est., estimates.

4. Discussion

In this retrospective single-center study, we compared the performance of EDOF IOLs after cataract surgery between eyes with and without a history of prior LASIK for myopia correction. The non-inferiority tests showed that the LASIK group was not inferior to the non-LASIK group for both the absolute predictive refractive error and the UNVA. Specifically, the upper bounds of the 95% confidence intervals for the mean differences were below the pre-defined non-inferiority margins of 0.5 D for refractive error and 0.1 logMAR for the UNVA. For the UDVA, while the non-inferiority test suggested that the LASIK group was superior, the subsequent age- and sex-matched regression analysis did not find a statistically significant difference between the two groups after adjusting for potential confounders, such as the axial length and ACD. Our data indicate that previous LASIK did not negatively impact the visual outcomes of the EDOF IOLs in terms of predictive refractive error, UNVA, and UDVA when compared with the non-LASIK eyes in this cohort.

IOL power formulas use biometric measurements to predict the refractive outcomes of different IOLs. Measurement methods can be classified as vergence, ray tracing, artificial intelligence, or a combination of these methods [8]. These methods have been employed to predict the postoperative effective lens position and anticipate refractive outcomes, with the aim of minimizing predictive errors [9]. The traditional power calculation model relies on the axial length, corneal K value with only the anterior radius, and ACD for prediction [10]. Current IOL formulas include not only the three variables mentioned above but also lens thickness, central corneal thickness, and white-to-white corneal diameter. For example, the SRK/T formula is one of the most widely used methods for calculating the IOL [8]. In a study by Ota et al., which used the SRK/T formula to calculate the same type of EDOF IOL used in our study, 38–61% of the eyes were within 0.3 D of the prediction error. The discrepancy observed between this study and ours may be attributable to variations in the axial length between Ota et al.'s series (mean: 24.0 ± 1.3 mm, 25.4 ± 1.8 mm) and our dataset (mean: 25.6 ± 1.8 mm) [11]. In an investigation by Jeon et al., which used the SRK/T formula alongside newer formulas such as Barrett Universal II, Kane, and Olsen to calculate the Vivity EDOF IOLs (Alcon, Fort Worth, TX, USA) in patients with a mean axial length of 23.53 mm, a mean absolute prediction error of approximately 0.3 D was reported across all formulas, with the SRK/T formula exhibiting a larger standard deviation [12]. Despite the larger standard deviation, the SRK/T formula remains a reliable choice for calculating the EDOF IOL.

The consideration of not using presbyopia-correcting IOLs in patients with cataract who have a history of LASIK has been discussed in a previous review [13]. This discussion arises from the potential for greater residual refractive errors due to less predictable IOL power calculations compared with non-LASIK eyes. Such unpredictability can lead to unsatisfactory visual outcomes or necessitate re-enhancement procedures [13]. To address inaccuracies in corneal radius and keratometric measurements following refractive surgery procedures, several specialized IOL power calculation formulas have been introduced. Among these, the Haigis-L formula has gained popularity because it does not require previous refractive surgery data [14]. In the study by Abulafia et al., which examined patients with a history of LASIK or photorefractive keratectomy, the mean absolute prediction error was 0.68 ± 0.45 D via the Haigis-L method, 0.63 ± 0.48 D via the Shammas method, and 0.52 ± 0.43 D using the Barrett true-K formula [4]. These values were similar to the 0.65 ± 0.26 D observed in our study, which used the Haigis-L formula.

An interesting observation from our results pertains to the uncorrected distance visual acuity (UDVA) outcomes. Specifically, the LASIK group exhibited a mean UDVA of 0.300 ± 0.362 logMAR, which was notably worse than the 0.117 ± 0.156 logMAR observed in the non-LASIK group. The 95% confidence interval for the difference (0.0033 to 0.3585) encompassed the non-inferiority margin of 0.1 logMAR, indicating that the LASIK group could not be confirmed as non-inferior to the non-LASIK group in this parameter. While the regression analysis did not reveal a statistically significant difference between the groups after adjusting for confounders, this finding raises important considerations. One possible explanation is the presence of subtle corneal irregularities or higher-order aberrations (HOAs) induced by prior LASIK, which may impact the distance vision quality despite acceptable refractive outcomes. LASIK surgery, especially when performed years prior with older technologies, can result in postoperative corneal asphericity and induction of coma aberrations, both of which can degrade the image quality under scotopic conditions and reduce the UDVA even when refraction is close to plano [15,16]. In contrast, non-LASIK eyes typically preserve a more regular corneal shape, which may contribute to sharper unaided distance vision following the EDOF IOL implantation. Additionally, the significantly longer axial lengths and flatter corneal curvatures seen in the LASIK group could have influenced the effective lens position (ELP) or created minor defocus, leading to slight reductions in the UDVA. Previous studies have shown that small prediction errors in ELP estimation can have a disproportionate impact on the UDVA, particularly in eyes with long axial lengths [17]. It was consistent with our study: in the regression analysis, after adjusting for confounders, the LASIK and non-LASIK groups had no difference in terms of UDVA, but the axial length had a significant influence on the UDVA. Our study also revealed that the LASIK group may have a better UNVA and a greater prediction error compared with the non-LASIK group, which could be proof that small prediction errors in the ELP estimation could cause more minor defocus toward the minus degree of refraction, which mimics mild myopic eyes and therefore cause lower UDVA and better UNVA in the LASIK group.

Our study has some limitations. First, our samples were retrospectively selected, presenting a limitation regarding sample size. The relatively small sample size, particularly in the LASIK group, may limit the generalizability of the results. Moreover, after matching the groups based on age and sex, most of the data could not be used. Second, differences in the preoperative demographics and clinical characteristics, including the axial length and ACD, between the groups could introduce potential errors in data interpretation. Third, the follow-up period of one month after surgery may be short for EDOF IOLs because EDOF IOLs may have better visual outcome after a longer follow-up period. Fourth, additional parameters that are important measures of visual quality and satisfaction, such as contrast sensitivity, wavefront aberration, and subjective questionnaires for photic phenomena, such as halo and glare, were excluded. Fifth, the SRK/T formula is a reliable choice for calculating the EDOF IOL; however, it is an early-generation formula. Now, we have more modern formulas which can improve the refraction prediction accuracy, such as the Barrett True-K formula. Due to the retrospective nature of the study, we could not assess the result by utilizing these modern formulas. Further prospective studies with larger cohorts, longer follow-up periods, modern formulas, and comprehensive assessments are warranted to validate our findings.

5. Conclusions

In conclusion, our study demonstrated that previous LASIK may have no discernible effect on the visual performance of presbyopia-correcting EDOF IOLs with respect to the absolute refractive error, UNVA, and UDVA. For further validation, longer follow-up and larger-scale or multicenter studies are required to ensure the robustness and generalizability of our results in diverse clinical settings.

Author Contributions: Conceptualization, C.-C.C. and I.-H.L.; methodology, C.-C.C.; software, C.-C.C.; validation, I.-H.L. and C.-K.C.; formal analysis, C.-C.C.; investigation, I.-H.L.; resources, C.-K.C.; data curation, C.-C.C.; writing—original draft preparation, C.-C.C. and I.-H.L.; writing—review and editing, I.-H.L.; visualization, C.-K.C.; supervision, C.-K.C.; project administration, C.-K.C.; All authors have read and agreed to the published version of the manuscript.

Funding: This research received no external funding.

Institutional Review Board Statement: The study was conducted in accordance with the Declaration of Helsinki, and approved by the Ethics Committee of NATIONAL CHANGHUA UNIVERSITY OF EDUCATION (NCUEREC-111-085, approved on 16 November 2022).

Informed Consent Statement: Patient consent was waived owing to the retrospective nature of the study.

Data Availability Statement: The original contributions presented in this study are included in the article. Further inquiries can be directed to the corresponding author.

Conflicts of Interest: The authors declare no conflicts of interest.

Abbreviations

The following abbreviations are used in this manuscript:

ACD	Anterior chamber depth
CDVA	Corrected distance visual acuity
D	Diopter
EDOF	Extended depth of focus
IOLs	Intraocular lenses
K	Corneal curvature
LASIK	Laser-assisted in situ keratomileusis
logMAR	Logarithm of the minimum angle of resolution
SE	Spherical equivalent
SRK/T	Sanders Retzlaff Kraff/theoretical
UDVA	Uncorrected distance visual acuity
UNVA	Uncorrected near visual acuity

References

1. Kim, T.I.; Del Barrio, J.L.A.; Wilkins, M.; Cochener, B.; Ang, M. Refractive surgery. *Lancet* **2019**, *393*, 2085–2098. [CrossRe [PubMed]
2. Mai, E.L.; Chang, C.-K.; Lee, C.-Y.; Lian, I.-B.; Chao, C.-C. Higher-order aberrations of topography-guided LASIK and wavefron optimized LASIK in high- and low-myopic eyes: A non-randomized controlled trial. *J. Pers. Med.* **2023**, *13*, 399. [CrossRe [PubMed]
3. Yeu, E.; Cuozzo, S. Matching the patient to the intraocular lens: Preoperative considerations to optimize surgical outcome *Ophthalmology* **2021**, *128*, e132–e141. [CrossRef] [PubMed]
4. Abulafia, A.; Hill, W.E.; Koch, D.D.; Wang, L.; Barrett, G.D. Accuracy of the Barrett True-K formula for intraocular lens powe prediction after laser in situ keratomileusis or photorefractive keratectomy for myopia. *J. Cataract. Refract. Surg.* **2016**, *42*, 363–36 [CrossRef] [PubMed]
5. Walker, J. Non-inferiority statistics and equivalence studies. *BJA Educ.* **2019**, *19*, 267–271. [CrossRef] [PubMed]
6. Ang, M.; Tan, D.; Mehta, J.S. Small incision lenticule extraction (SMILE) versus laser in-situ keratomileusis (LASIK): Stud protocol for a randomized, non-inferiority trial. *Trials* **2012**, *13*, 75. [CrossRef] [PubMed]
7. Day, A.C.; Burr, J.M.; Bunce, C.; Doré, C.J.; Sylvestre, Y.; Wormald, R.P.L.; Round, J.; McCudden, V.; Rubin, G.; Wilkins, M. Randomised, single-masked non-inferiority trial of femtosecond laser-assisted versus manual phacoemulsification catara surgery for adults with visually significant cataract: The FACT trial protocol. *BMJ Open* **2015**, *5*, e010381. [CrossRef] [PubMed
8. Kane, J.X.; Chang, D.F. Intraocular lens power formulas, biometry, and intraoperative aberrometry: A review. *Ophthalmology* **202** *128*, e94–e114. [CrossRef] [PubMed]
9. Shajari, M.; Sonntag, R.; Niermann, T.; Holland, D.; Kohnen, T.; Priglinger, S.; Mayer, W.J. Determining and comparing th effective lens position and refractive outcome of a novel rhexis-fixated lens to established lens designs. *Am. J. Ophthalmol.* **202** *213*, 62–68. [CrossRef] [PubMed]
10. Simpson, M.J. Pre-clinical estimation of the intraocular lens A-constant, and its relationship to power, shape factor, and asphericit *Appl. Opt.* **2021**, *60*, 5662–5668. [CrossRef] [PubMed]
11. Ota, Y.; Bissen-Miyajima, H.; Nakamura, K.; Hirasawa, M.; Minami, K. Binocular visual function after staged implantation c extended-depth-of-focus intraocular lens targeting emmetropia and -0.5 diopter: A prospective comparison. *PLoS ONE* **202** *15*, e0238135. [CrossRef] [PubMed]
12. Jeon, S.; Taroni, L.; Lupardi, E.; Hoffer, K.J.; Fontana, L.; Schiano-Lomoriello, D.; Kwon, H.; Savini, G. Accuracy of nine formula to calculate the powers of an extended depth-of-focus IOL using two SS-OCT biometers. *J. Refract. Surg.* **2023**, *39*, 158–16 [CrossRef] [PubMed]

. Khor, W.B.; Afshari, N.A. The role of presbyopia-correcting intraocular lenses after laser in situ keratomileusis. *Curr. Opin. Ophthalmol.* **2013**, *24*, 35–40. [CrossRef] [PubMed]
. Chen, X.; Yuan, F.; Wu, L. Metaanalysis of intraocular lens power calculation after laser refractive surgery in myopic eyes. *J. Cataract. Refract. Surg.* **2016**, *42*, 163–170. [CrossRef] [PubMed]
. Marcos, S.; Barbero, S.; Llorente, L.; Merayo-Lloves, J. Optical response to LASIK surgery for myopia from total and corneal aberration measurements. *Investig. Ophthalmol. Vis. Sci.* **2001**, *42*, 3349–3356. [PubMed]
. Feng, Z.; Wang, Q.; Du, C.; Yang, F.; Li, X. High-order aberration changes after femtosecond LASIK surgery in patients with high myopia. *Ann. Palliat. Med.* **2021**, *10*, 7689–7696. [CrossRef] [PubMed]
. Yin, S.; Guo, C.; Qiu, K.; Ng, T.K.; Li, Y.; Du, Y.; Chen, B.; Wang, H.; Zhang, M. Assessment of the influence of keratometry on intraocular lens calculation formulas in long axial length eyes. *Int. Ophthalmol.* **2022**, *42*, 3211–3219. [CrossRef] [PubMed]

Journal of
Personalized Medicine

MDPI

Article

Evaluation of the Choroidal Thickness and Retinal Nerve Fiber Layer Thickness in Patients with Vasovagal Syncope

Hasan B. Isleyen [1], Batur G. Kanar [2,*], Guzide Akcay [3], Serdar Demir [4], Hatice S. Kanar [3] and Mehmet V. Yazicioglu [2]

1 Cardiology Department, Istanbul Nişantaşı Üniversitesi, Istanbul 34475, Turkey; isleyenburak44@gmail.com
2 Cardiology Department, School of Medicine, Istinye University, Istanbul 34396, Turkey; mvefik@yahoo.com
3 Ophthalmology Department, Dr Lütfi Kırdar Kartal Eğitim ve Araştırma Hastanesi, Istanbul 34862, Turkey; hselensonmez@hotmail.com (H.S.K.)
4 Cardiology Department, Kartal Koşuyolu High Specialization Training and Research Hospital, Istanbul 34846, Turkey; sdemirmd@gmail.com
* Correspondence: baturkanar@hotmail.com

Abstract: Aim: The aim of this study was to evaluate choroidal and peripapillary retinal nerve fiber layer (RNFL) thicknesses in individuals with vasovagal syncope (VVS). **Method**: A total of 67 consecutive patients with VVS and 61 healthy control subjects were enrolled this study. The choroidal thickness (CT) at the fovea, the nasal to fovea thickness, and the temporal to fovea thickness were measured, alongside pRNLFT measurements assessed by swept-source optical coherence tomography (SS-OCT). **Results**: The mean foveal CT (408.7 ± 92.5 μm vs. 342.1 ± 60.2 μm, $p < 0.01$), the mean nasal CT (385.2 ± 88.3 μm vs. 329.2 ± 47.6 μm, $p < 0.001$), and the mean temporal CT (379.5 ± 51.6 μm vs. 321.48 ± 43.2 μm, $p < 0.03$) were statistically thicker in patients with VVS compared to the healthy controls. There was no statistically significant difference in the global pRNFLT measurements and all quadrants between the study groups. **Conclusions**: The CT in all regions was found to be thicker in patients with VVS compared to the healthy controls, while there were no differences in pRNFLT values. These results suggest that choroidal circulation might be affected by local neurotransmitter alterations in patients with VVS.

Keywords: choroidal thickness; optical coherence tomography; vasovagal syncope

1. Introduction

Syncope is a loss of consciousness defined by a loss of postural tone, amnesia, and rarely, the disruption of smooth muscle tonus, with a short duration and spontaneous complete recovery [1]. Vasovagal syncope (VVS) is a common form of syncope that originates from a sudden failure of the autonomic nervous system to sustain adequate vascular tone under orthostatic stress. It may be a compensatory maneuver to protect the central nervous system and heart from permanent ischemic damage. Even though VVS is commonly benign, repeated episodes could adversely affect quality of life and might increase the risk of major adverse events [2].

In vasovagal syncope, the cardioinhibitory pathway involves parasympathetic hypertonicity, which affects the sinoatrial and atrioventricular nodes and may cause a long asystole or nodal rhythm [3]. On the other hand, the vasodepressor efferent pathway causes a decrease in vascular sympathetic tone, leads to arterial and venous dilation, and results in a reduction in peripheral vascular resistance and arterial blood pressure. Consequently, blood is pooled in the lower extremities and/or in the splanchnic beds, and venous return is reduced. As a result, stroke volume decreases, causing cerebral and systemic hypoperfusion [1,3,4].

As far as recent studies are concerned, the pathophysiology of VVS has still not been clearly clarified. It has been proposed that the development of VVS is associated with changes in hemodynamic parameters that result from variations in the plasma levels of vasoactive substances, such as nitric oxide, catecholamines, endothelin, prostanoids, or vasopressin, as part of the body's response to orthostatic stress [1,5]. Moreover, paradoxical peripheral vasodilation caused by endothelial dysfunction might be important in improper excessive hypotension during orthostatic stress in individuals with VVS. Factors like inflammation and oxidative stress have also been associated with impaired endothelial function in these patients [5,6].

The choroid has a highly vascular structure, and choroidal blood flow is crucial for the health of the retina, supplying oxygen and nutrients to its outer layers [7]. Neurogenic control significantly influences choroidal blood flow through the autonomic nervous system [8]. Various factors, including neurotransmitters and local metabolic signals, modulate these neurogenic controls [9]. This regulation is vital during changes in light conditions or visual tasks, ensuring efficient nutrient delivery and waste removal from retinal tissues. As the use of optical coherence tomography (OCT) technology, especially swept-source optical coherence tomography (SS-OCT) technology, has increased, non-invasive detailed evaluation of choroidal and retinal tissues has become possible [10].

In this study, we aimed to investigate whether dysregulation of the parasympathetic and/or sympathetic nervous system affects ocular structural measurements by evaluating choroidal thickness (CT) and peripapillary retinal nerve fiber layer thickness (pRNFLT) in individuals with VVS.

2. Materials and Methods

2.1. Patient Population

The data used in this study were acquired prospectively. This study was conducted in accordance with the principles outlined in the Declaration of Helsinki and received approval from the institutional ethics committee. Patients aged between 18 and 60 years who exhibited a history of recurrent episodes of apparent syncope, having experienced more than two such occurrences in the past six months, were included in the study. The inclusion criteria included (1) a positive drug-free head-up tilt table test (HUTT), in which syncope was deemed to have reproduced spontaneous symptoms; (2) absence of left ventricular systolic dysfunction and valve insufficiency and/or stenosis over a mild degree (estimated ejection fraction > 50% using transthoracic echocardiography); (3) absence of obesity (body mass index < 30), hematologic or biochemical abnormalities, or use of drugs known to predispose to orthostatic hypotension. The exclusion criteria can be listed as (1) patients not meeting the above criteria; (2) individuals with a history of systemic diseases that might affect CT and pRNFLT, such as systemic arterial hypertension, diabetes mellitus, and rheumatologic diseases based on self-reported medical history; (3) eyes with high myopia (>6D); (4) advanced-level cataracts, age-related macular degeneration, or a history of retinal vascular disease; (5) patients with abnormal intraocular pressure (IOP), glaucoma, or ocular hypertension; (6) patients with a history of intraocular surgery and tachycardia or autonomic dysfunction associated with neurologic disorders including Parkinsonism, autonomic failure, peripheral neuropathy, or postural tachycardia syndrome.

2.2. Head-Up Tilt Table Testing Protocol

All patients stopped taking cardioactive medication for at least five half-lives prior to HUTT. Each patient was gently secured to the tilt table, ensuring appropriate positioning to allow for the use of a footboard for weight bearing. HUTT was performed in the morning after a 12 h overnight fasting period. A minimum 15 min equilibration time, with the patients resting in a supine position in a dark, quiet environment, was allowed before the commencement of baseline recordings for the HUTT procedure. In our standard protocol, there were 15 min of rest followed by 45 min (or until the onset of symptoms) at a 70-degree angle [11]. The predictive value of HUTT was enhanced with sublingual glyceryl trinitrate [11,12]. Systemic arterial blood pressure and heart rate were continuously recorded, automatically calculating all the R-R intervals throughout the test using a non-invasive, beat-by-beat monitor CardioLab® (GE Healthcare, Chicago, IL, USA), and data were collected by a computer that processed them using ad hoc software.

2.3. *Ophthalmic Examinations*

All participants in the study underwent an extensive and thorough ophthalmic assessment, which included a variety of tests designed to evaluate different aspects of visual function and ocular health. The evaluation began with an assessment of best-corrected visual acuity, which was performed using the Snellen chart. Additionally, intraocular pressure was measured employing the Goldmann applanation tonometry technique, a reliable method for gauging the pressure within the eye.

The examination also encompassed slit lamp biomicroscopy, a diagnostic procedure that allows for detailed observation of the anterior segment of the eye, and a dilated fundus examination to facilitate a comprehensive view of the retina and other posterior structures. To measure the axial length of the eye, the IOL Master 500 (manufactured by Carl Zeiss Meditec Inc., based in Jena, Germany) was utilized, providing precise measurements essential for evaluating ocular dimensions.

Furthermore, the choroidal thickness (CT) and the peripapillary retinal nerve fiber layer thickness (pRNFLT) were quantified using the swept-source optical coherence tomography (SS-OCT) system, specifically the Topcon Triton model from Japan. It is worth mentioning that all measurements and assessments were consistently carried out by the same trained technician during similar time frames, specifically between 9:00 a.m. and 12:00 p.m., to minimize potential variabilities. HUTT and OCT procedures were not performed on the same day.

In determining the choroidal thickness, which was defined as the axial distance from the retinal pigment epithelium (RPE) to the outer interface of the choroid/sclera, evaluations were conducted by a single ophthalmologist (H.S.K). When H.S.K performed the OCT evaluation, she did not know whether the patient had VVS or not, and the study was single-blind. The CT measurements were specifically taken in the subfoveal region, as well as at distances of 1500 µm temporally and 1500 µm nasally from the foveal region. For the assessment of the pRNFLT, the measurements were obtained using OCT by employing a circular scan with a diameter of 3.46 mm that was centered on the optic disk.

The resulting data provided pRNFLT values for each of the four quadrants—superior (S), inferior (I), nasal (N), and temporal (T)—as well as the global mean values by using software program. It is important to note that the statistical analyses were conducted using the average values derived from both eyes of each participant, allowing for a comprehensive evaluation of the visual and ocular health indicators across the sample. Figures 1 and 2 demonstrate the OCT and pRNLFT measurements for participants with VVS and a healthy control.

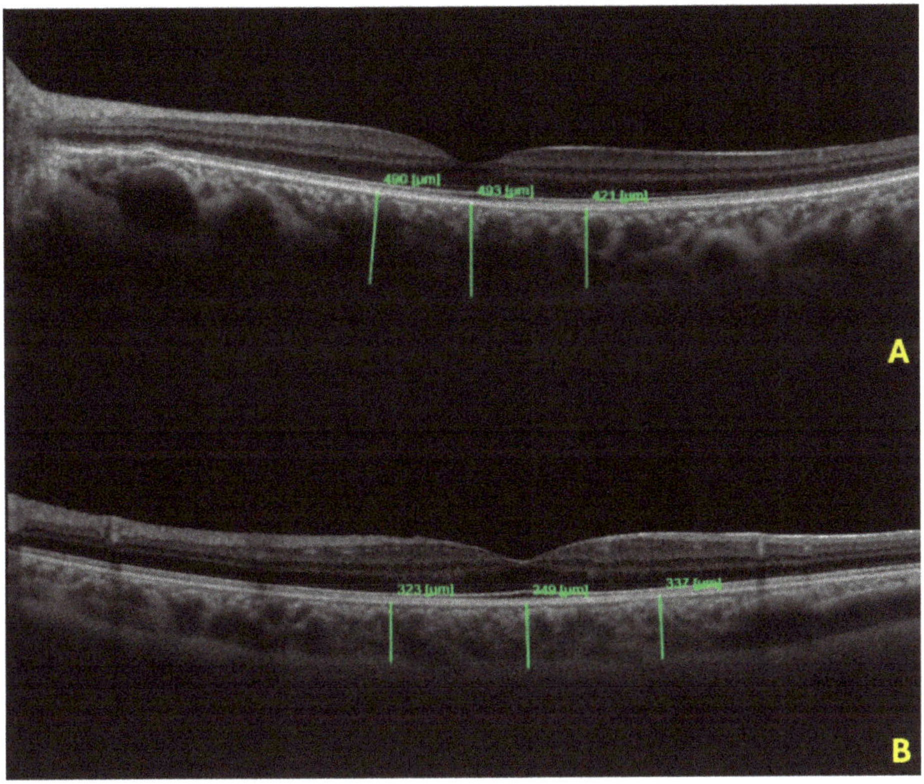

Figure 1. (**A**): Increased CT in the fovea, temporal to fovea, and nasal to fovea regions in a patient with VVS; (**B**): CT in the fovea, temporal to fovea, and nasal to fovea regions in a healthy control.

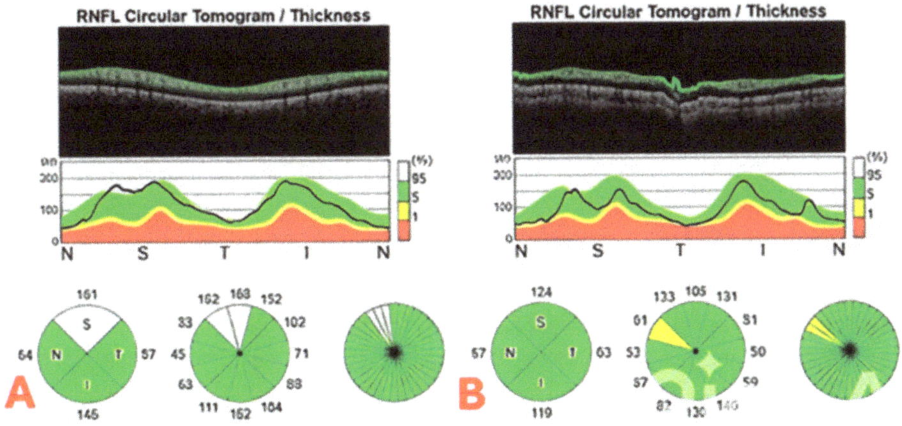

Figure 2. (**A**): pRNFL images of a healthy control; (**B**): pRNFL images of a patient with VVS.

2.4. Statistical Analysis

Statistical analyses were conducted utilizing SPSS software, specifically version 21, provided by SPSS Inc., located in Chicago, IL, USA. Continuous variables in the study were presented as mean values accompanied by their corresponding standard deviation (SD). To ensure the validity of the assumed linear relationships and the principle of homoscedasticity across the datasets, we evaluated these assumptions through the examination of standardized residuals plots. Furthermore, the assumption of normality for the dependent variable was assessed using the Kolmogorov–Smirnov statistical criterion.

In addition, to detect significant differences among categorical variables, the Chi-square test was employed. As all continuous variables demonstrated a normal distribution, statistical comparisons of quantitative data were carried out using the unpaired-sample *t*-test method. It is important to note that differences were regarded as statistically significant when the *p*-value was less than 0.05. This level of significance indicates that we could reject the null hypothesis in favor of the alternative hypothesis, suggesting that there is a meaningful difference worthy of further discussion and analysis.

3. Results

A total of 67 patients with VVS were included in this study, and their data were compared with those of 61 age- and sex-matched healthy controls. The mean age of patients with VVS was 35.2 ± 6.3 years, while that of the control group subjects was 36.3 ± 7.4 years. Demographic and clinical information about the patients and control subjects is summarized in Table 1. No significant differences were noted in the values of intraocular pressure, axial length, systemic arterial blood pressure measurements, smoking status, age, and sex between patients with VVS and the healthy controls.

Table 1. Demographic and clinical data of the study population.

	Patients with VVS (n = 67)	Healthy Controls (n = 61)	p Value
Age (years)	35.2 ± 6.3	36.3 ± 7.4	0.13
Gender (Female%)	42(62.7%)	35(57.4%)	0.08
Body mass index (kg/m^2)	22.4 ± 5.6	21.5 ± 3.9	0.23
Smoking	14(20.9%)	12(19.6%)	0.47
SRE (D)	+0.71 ± 0.2	+0.58 ± 0.3	0.55
Axial length (mm)	23.08 ± 0.4	22.98 ± 0.3	0.67
Intraocular pressure (mm Hg)	16.25 ± 5.3	18.04 ± 4.8	0.25
Systolic BP (mmHg)	108.3 ± 7.2	123.4 ± 9.3	0.22
Diastolic BP (mmHg)	76.7 ± 4.7	79.9 ± 5.9	0.12
Mean BP (mmHg)	86.7 ± 5.5	94.3 ± 6.9	0.19

Note: data are presented as mean ± standard deviation while categorical variables are expressed as percentages. Abbreviations: BP: blood pressure; SRE: spherical refractive error.

In the CT evaluation, a statistically significant difference was noted between patients with VVS and the healthy controls. The mean foveal CT (408.7 ± 92.5 μm vs. 342.1 ± 60.2 μm, $p < 0.001$), mean nasal CT (385.2 ± 88.3 μm vs. 329.2 ± 47.6 μm, $p < 0.001$), and mean temporal CT (379.5 ± 91.6 μm vs. 321.48 ± 43.2 μm, $p < 0.001$) were statistically thicker in patients with VVS compared to the healthy controls. There was no statistically significant difference in pRNFLT measurements between patients with VVS and the healthy controls. Table 2 summarizes the comparison of SS-OCT measurements between the study groups.

Table 2. Summary of statistical analyses for comparison of SFCT, pRNFLT (average), and quadrants of pRNFLT.

	Participants with VVS (n = 67)	Healthy Controls (n = 61)	p Value
Foveal CT (μm)	408.7 ± 92.5	342.1 ± 60.2	**<0.001**
Nasal CT (μm)	385.2 ± 98.3	329.2 ± 47.6	**<0.001**
Temporal CT (μm)	379.5 ± 91.6	321.48 ± 43.2	**<0.001**
Global pRNFLT (μm)	106.7 ± 7.4	108.2 ± 6.2	0.11
Inferior pRNFLT (μm)	128.6 ± 8.3	129.2 ± 8.9	0.41
Superior pRNFLT (μm)	127.6 ± 7.9	129.8 ± 8.4	0.31
Nasal pRNFLT (μm)	86.5 ± 6.7	87.6 ± 6.3	0.24
Temporal pRNFLT (μm)	84.4 ± 6.5	86.2 ± 6.8	0.26

Note: data are presented as mean ± standard deviation. Bold values indicate statistical significance $p < 0.05$. Abbreviations: CT: choroidal thickness; pRNFLT: peripapillary retinal nerve fiber layer thickness; SFCT: subfoveal choroidal thickness; VVS: vasovagal syncope.

4. Discussion

In this study, we evaluated the CTs and pRNFLT in participants with VVS and compared these values with those of healthy controls. The main outcomes of this study are as follows: (1) the mean CT in all regions was significantly thicker in participants with VVS compared to the control group. (2) There were no significant differences in all pRNFLT measurements between study groups.

Both sympathetic and parasympathetic pathways contribute to choroidal blood flow regulation, with sympathetic fibers generally causing vasoconstriction and parasympathetic fibers promoting vasodilation [7]. Parasympathetic stimulation, particularly through acetylcholine release, promotes vasodilation, increasing blood flow to meet the metabolic demands of the retina, especially during high visual activity. In contrast, sympathetic activation, associated with norepinephrine, causes vasoconstriction, reducing blood flow [13]. Various neurotransmitters also influence choroidal blood flow regulation. For example, nitric oxide promotes vasodilation, while other molecules like vasoactive intestinal peptide and substance p additionally modulate vessel diameter [7,13].

The dysregulation of the autonomous nerve system and the alteration of neurotransmitters have crucial roles in VVS pathogenesis. Jardine at el. showed parasympathetic hypertonicity in participants with VVS [14]. Aksu et al. showed that low endothelin-1 levels, which is a pro-inflammatory vasoconstrictor peptide, are associated with a higher risk of VVS. In addition, neuropeptide Y may also play a role in VVS by increasing peripheral vascular resistance and decreasing cardiac output during orthostatic regulation [15]. Liao et al. revealed that neuropeptide Y plasma levels are significantly reduced in individuals with VVS [16]. Gallegos et al. showed that nitric oxide levels are increased in VVS, probably due to high catecholamine plasma levels. Nitric oxide synthase could be activated by $\beta-2$ receptors, increasing the release of nitric oxide from the vascular endothelium and leading to excessive vasodilation [17]. Endothelin-1 was found to be negatively correlated with choroidal blood flow, and endothelin-1 increases vasoconstriction in choroid and retinal blood. [18,19]. Some studies conducted with animals have shown that choroidal vasodilation and choroidal thickness may increase due to increased nitric oxide [20,21]. In this study, we found that the CT in the fovea, nasal to the fovea, and temporal to the fovea regions was statistically significantly thicker than in the healthy controls. Increased CT in participants with VVS might be related to the increase in parasympathetic activity and the change in neurotransmitters.

Thicker CT is linked to several ocular diseases and serves as an important biomarker for diagnosis and management [22,23]. Pachychoroid spectrum diseases, age-related macular degeneration, and some uveitic diseases are among the main diseases in which CT is important [22,24]. Patients with central serous chorioretinopathy have an especially high CT and type A personality traits [25–27]. It is known from previous studies that participants with VVS have stressed personality structures [28,29]. Therefore, participants with VVS may also be prone to ocular diseases such as central serous chorioretinopathy due to their high CT. Further studies may clarify this relationship.

The pRNFL is the region surrounding the optic disk where nerve fibers from the retina converge to form the optic nerve and is supplied by the central retinal artery [30]. This layer consists primarily of the axons of ganglion cells and is essential for transmitting visual information from the retina to the brain. The health of the pRNFL is vital for visual function, as changes in its thickness can indicate various ocular diseases, especially glaucoma [31,32]. Thinning of the pRNFL is often a sign of damage to the optic nerve and progressive loss of ganglion cells, necessitating careful monitoring [31]. We compared the pRNFLT values of participants with VVS with healthy controls, and we did not find any differences between participants with VVS and the healthy controls. It is known that there are distinct differences between choroidal and retinal artery blood flow [33]. Retinal blood flow is tightly regulated by local metabolic demands, allowing it to adjust to the oxygen needs of the inner retina. In contrast, choroidal blood flow is influenced more by systemic factors rather than local needs, leading to less autoregulation [33–35]. For this reason, while we detected changes in CTs in participants with VVS, we may not have detected changes in pRNFLT values, which indicate retinal artery blood flow.

This study has some limitations. For instance, the size of the study groups was relatively small. Moreover, a manual method was used to measure CTs instead of using an automated software program, which is more reliable. We evaluated only choroidal thickness and no other parameters such as the choroidal vascular index [36]. Patients' anxiety status and/or personality evaluation were not recorded. In this study, we did not evaluate the neurotransmitter levels in plasma and/or serum. In the HUTT protocol, we did not use the Vasovagal Syncope International Study (BASIS) criteria for the subgroup analysis of the participants with VVS. The VASIS classification includes the following categories: mixed (VASIS-1), cardioinhibition (VASIS-2A), severe cardioinhibition/asystole (VASIS-2B), and pure vasodepression (VASIS-3). There may be differences in the subgroup analysis of the participants in terms of CT measurements [37].

5. Conclusions

In conclusion, we showed that participants with VVS exhibited greater CT across all measured regions when compared to healthy controls. Conversely, there were no significant variations observed in the thickness of the pRNFL. These findings imply that the choroidal blood flow could be influenced by changes in local neurotransmitter levels in individuals suffering from VVS. This interplay underscores the connection between cardiovascular health and CT alterations, suggesting a need for monitoring in individuals with frequent syncopal episodes to prevent complications and maintain ocular health. Further investigation into these dynamics may yield insights beneficial for clinical practice regarding VVS and ocular health.

Author Contributions: H.B.I.: writing—original draft, software, investigation, formal analysis, data curation, conceptualization. B.G.K.: writing—original draft, validation, formal analysis, data curation, conceptualization. G.A.: writing—original draft, validation, resources, methodology, investigation, formal analysis, data curation. S.D.: writing—original draft, validation, resources, methodology, investigation, formal analysis, data curation. H.S.K.: writing—original draft, validation, formal analysis, data curation, conceptualization. M.V.Y.: data curation, reviewing and editing. All authors have read and agreed to the published version of the manuscript.

Funding: This research received no external funding.

Institutional Review Board Statement: The study was conducted in accordance with the Declaration of Helsinki, and approved by the ethics committee of the Marmara University School of Medicine (protocol code: 11.2023.1269 and date of approval: 11 December 2023).

Informed Consent Statement: Informed consent was obtained from all subjects involved in this study.

Data Availability Statement: Certain confidentiality constraints prevent us from disclosing the underlying database used in this study.

Conflicts of Interest: The authors declare no conflicts of interest.

eferences

Longo, S.; Legramante, J.M.; Rizza, S.; Federici, M. Vasovagal syncope: An overview of pathophysiological mechanisms. *Eur. J. Intern. Med.* **2023**, *112*, 6–14. [CrossRef] [PubMed]

Sandhu, R.K.; Raj, S.R.; Thiruganasambandamoorthy, V.; Kaul, P.; Morillo, C.A.; Krahn, A.D.; Guzman, J.C.; Sheldon, R.S. Canadian Cardiovascular Society Clinical Practice Update on the Assessment and Management of Syncope. *Can. J. Cardiol.* **2020**, *36*, 1167–1177. [CrossRef]

van Dijk, J.G.; van Rossum, I.A.; Thijs, R.D. Timing of Circulatory and Neurological Events in Syncope. *Front. Cardiovasc. Med.* **2020**, *7*, 36. [CrossRef] [PubMed]

van Dijk, J.G.; van Rossum, I.A.; Thijs, R.D. The pathophysiology of vasovagal syncope: Novel insights. *Auton. Neurosci.* **2021**, *236*, 102899. [CrossRef]

Pachon-M, J.C. Neurocardiogenic syncope: Pacemaker or cardioneuroablation? *Heart Rhythm.* **2020**, *17*, 829–830. [CrossRef] [PubMed]

Pietrucha, A.Z. Endothelial function in vasovagal syncope. [published correction appears]. *Expert. Rev. Cardiovasc. Ther.* **2014**, *12*, 1387–1389, Erratum in *Expert Rev. Cardiovasc. Ther.* **2015**, *13*, 455–484. https://doi.org/10.1586/14779072.2015.1024484. [CrossRef]

Reiner, A.; Fitzgerald, M.E.C.; Del Mar, N.; Li, C. Neural control of choroidal blood flow. *Prog. Retin. Eye Res.* **2018**, *64*, 96–130. [CrossRef]

Motamed Shariati, M.; Khazaei, S.; Yaghoobi, M. Choroidal vascularity index in health and systemic diseases: A systematic review. *Int. J. Retin. Vitr.* **2024**, *10*, 87–96. [CrossRef]

Shin, D.Y.; Hong, K.E.; Lee, N.Y.; Park, C.K.; Park, H.Y.L. Association of choroidal blood flow with autonomic dysfunction in patients with normal tension glaucoma. *Sci. Rep.* **2022**, *12*, 5136–5142. [CrossRef]

Singh, S.R.; Vupparaboina, K.K.; Goud, A.; Dansingani, K.K.; Chhablani, J. Choroidal imaging biomarkers. *Surv. Ophthalmol.* **2019**, *64*, 312–333. [CrossRef]

Aponte-Becerra, L.; Novak, P. Tilt Test: A Review. *J. Clin. Neurophysiol.* **2021**, *38*, 279–286. [CrossRef] [PubMed]

van Zanten, S.; Sutton, R.; Hamrefors, V.; Fedorowski, A.; de Lange, F.J. Tilt table testing, methodology and practical insights for the clinic. *Clin. Physiol. Funct. Imaging* **2024**, *44*, 119–130. [CrossRef]

Wei, X.; Balne, P.K.; Meissner, K.E.; Barathi, V.A.; Schmetterer, L.; Agrawal, R. Assessment of flow dynamics in retinal and choroidal microcirculation. *Surv. Ophthalmol.* **2018**, *63*, 646–664. [CrossRef] [PubMed]

Piotrowski, R.; Baran, J.; Sikorska, A.; Krynski, T.; Kulakowski, P. Cardioneuroablation for Reflex Syncope: Efficacy and Effects on Autonomic Cardiac Regulation-A Prospective Randomized Trial. *JACC Clin. Electrophysiol.* **2023**, *9*, 85–95. [CrossRef] [PubMed]

Aksu, T.; Davila, A.; Gupta, D. The "heart brain" and neuromodulation for vasovagal syncope. *Auton. Neurosci.* **2021**, *236*, 102892. [CrossRef]

Liao, Y.; Xu, W.R.; Li, H.X.; Tang, C.S.; Jin, H.F.; Du, J.B. Plasma Neuropeptide Y Levels in Vasovagal Syncope in Children. *Chin. Med. J.* **2017**, *130*, 2778–2784. [CrossRef]

Gallegos, A.; Márquez-Velasco, R.; Allende, R.; Gómez-Flores, J.R.; Cázares-Campos, I.; González-Hermosillo, A.; Bojalil, R.; Cárdenas, M.; Márquez, M.F. Serum concentrations of nitric oxide and soluble tumor necrosis factor receptor 1 (sTNFR1) in vasovagal syncope: Effect of orthostatic challenge. *Int. J. Cardiol.* **2013**, *167*, 2321–2322. [CrossRef]

Hétu, S.; Pouliot, M.; Cordahi, G.; Couture, R.; Vaucher, E. Assessment of retinal and choroidal blood flow changes using laser Doppler flowmetry in rats. *Curr. Eye Res.* **2013**, *38*, 158–167. [CrossRef]

Finzi, A.; Cellini, M.; Strobbe, E.; Campos, E.C. ET-1 plasma levels, choroidal thickness and multifocal electroretinogram in retinitis pigmentosa. *Life Sci.* **2014**, *118*, 386–390. [CrossRef]

20. Li, C.; Fitzgerald, M.E.; Del Mar, N.; Reiner, A. Stimulation of Baroresponsive Parts of the Nucleus of the Solitary Tract Produce Nitric Oxide-mediated Choroidal Vasodilation in Rat Eye. *Front. Neuroanat.* **2016**, *10*, 94. [CrossRef] [PubMed]
21. Erdinest, N.; London, N.; Ovadia, H.; Levinger, N. Nitric Oxide Interaction with the Eye. *Vision* **2021**, *5*, 29. [CrossRef] [PubMed] [PubMed Central]
22. Kim, Y.H.; Oh, J. Choroidal Thickness Profile in Chorioretinal Diseases: Beyond the Macula. *Front. Med.* **2021**, *8*, 79742 [CrossRef]
23. Sinawat, S.; Thongmee, W.; Sanguansak, T.; Laovirojjanakul, W.; Sinawat, S.; Yospaiboon, Y. Oral Spironolactone versus Conservative Treatment for Non-Resolving Central Serous Chorioretinopathy in Real-Life Practice. *Clin. Ophthalmol.* **2020**, *1* 1725–1734. [CrossRef]
24. Steiner, M.; Esteban-Ortega, M.D.M.; Muñoz-Fernández, S. Choroidal and retinal thickness in systemic autoimmune and inflammatory diseases: A review. *Surv. Ophthalmol.* **2019**, *64*, 757–769. [CrossRef] [PubMed]
25. Mathews, R.; Horo, S.; Jose, D.; Kavalakatt, J.A.; J, G.R.; John, S.S. Role of Psychological Stress and Choroidal Thickness in Central Serous Chorioretinopathy. *Nepal. J. Ophthalmol.* **2023**, *15*, 36–46. [CrossRef]
26. Mukherji, S.; Karmakar, S.; Dasgupta, S. Association of Central serous chorioretinopathy with type of personality, anxiety and depression. *Indian. J. Ophthalmol.* **2024**, *72*, S60–S65. [CrossRef] [PubMed]
27. Mansour, A.M.; Koaik, M.; Lima, L.H.; Casella, A.M.B.; Uwaydat, S.H.; Shahin, M.; Tamim, H.; Sanchez-Ruiz, M.J.; Mansour, H.A.; Dodwell, D. Physiologic and Psychologic Risk Factors in Central Serous Chorioretinopathy. *Ophthalmol. Retin.* **2017**, *1*, 497–507. [CrossRef]
28. Abuzainah, B.; Gutlapalli, S.D.; Chaudhuri, D.; Khan, K.I.; Al Shouli, R.; Allakky, A.; Ferguson, A.A.; Khan, A.I.; Hamid, P. Anxiety and Depression as Risk Factors for Vasovagal Syncope and Potential Treatment Targets: A Systematic Review. *Cureus* **2022**, *14*, e32793. [CrossRef]
29. Ng, J.; Sheldon, R.S.; Ritchie, D.; Raj, V.; Raj, S.R. Reduced quality of life and greater psychological distress in vasovagal syncope patients compared to healthy individuals. *Pacing Clin. Electrophysiol.* **2019**, *42*, 180–188. [CrossRef]
30. Zabel, P.; Kałużny, J.J.; Wiłkość-Dębczyńska, M.; Gębska-Tołoczko, M.; Suwała, K.; Kucharski, R.; Araszkiewicz, A. Peripapillary Retinal Nerve Fiber Layer Thickness in Patients with Alzheimer's Disease: A Comparison of Eyes of Patients with Alzheimer's Disease, Primary Open-Angle Glaucoma, and Preperimetric Glaucoma and Healthy Controls. *Med. Sci. Monit.* **2019**, *25*, 1001–1008. [CrossRef] [PubMed] [PubMed Central]
31. Rao, H.L.; Pradhan, Z.S.; Suh, M.H.; Moghimi, S.; Mansouri, K.; Weinreb, R.N. Optical Coherence Tomography Angiography in Glaucoma. *J. Glaucoma* **2020**, *29*, 312–321. [CrossRef] [PubMed] [PubMed Central]
32. Deshpande, G.A.; Gupta, R.; Bawankule, P.; Raje, D.; Chakraborty, M. Evaluation of ganglion cell-inner plexiform layer thickness in the diagnosis of preperimetric glaucoma and comparison to retinal nerve fiber layer. *Indian J. Ophthalmol.* **2021**, *69*, 1113–1119. [CrossRef]
33. Benagiano, V.; Rizzi, A.; Sannace, C.; Alessio, G.; Ribatti, D.; Dammacco, R. Aqueous humor as eye lymph: A crossroad between venous and lymphatic system. *Exp. Eye Res.* **2024**, *243*, 109904. [CrossRef]
34. Brylla, E.; Tscheudschilsuren, G.; Santos, A.N.; Nieber, K.; Spanel-Borowski, K.; Aust, G. Differences between retinal and choroidal microvascular endothelial cells (MVECs) under normal and hypoxic conditions. *Exp. Eye Res.* **2003**, *77*, 527–535. [CrossRef]
35. Vader, M.J.C.; Habani, Y.I.; Schlingemann, R.O.; Klaassen, I. miRNA Levels as a Biomarker for Anti-VEGF Response in Patients with Diabetic Macular Edema. *J. Pers. Med.* **2021**, *11*, 1297. [CrossRef] [PubMed]
36. Hwang, S.; Kang, M.H.; Seong, M.; Cho, H.; Shin, Y.U. Swept-Source OCT Angiography Features in Patients after Macular Hole Surgery. *J. Pers. Med.* **2022**, *12*, 1493. [CrossRef]
37. Sutton, R.; Brignole, M.; Menozzi, C.; Raviele, A.; Alboni, P.; Giani, P.; Moya, A. Dual-chamber pacing in the treatment of neurally mediated tilt-positive cardioinhibitory syncope: Pacemaker versus no therapy: A multicenter randomized study. The Vasovagal Syncope International Study (VASIS) Investigators. *Circulation* **2000**, *102*, 294–299. [CrossRef]

Journal of
Personalized Medicine

MDPI

ticle

iabetic Macular Edema in the Western Part of Romania: creening to Improve Patient Outcomes

riana Ivanescu [1,2], Simona Popescu [1,3,*], Deiana Roman [1], Monica Dragomir [1] and Romulus Timar [1,3]

1 Second Department of Internal Medicine, "Victor Babes" University of Medicine and Pharmacy, 300041 Timisoara, Romania; adriana.ivanescu@umft.ro (A.I.); roman.deiana@umft.ro (D.R.); monica.dragomir@umft.ro (M.D.); timar.romulus@umft.ro (R.T.)

2 Opticlass Ophtalmology Clinic, 300012 Timisoara, Romania

3 Department of Diabetes, "Pius Brinzeu" Emergency Hospital, 300723 Timisoara, Romania

* Correspondence: popescu.simona@umft.ro

Abstract: Background: Diabetes mellitus (DM) is a global healthcare concern with a rising prevalence. Patients with DM have a severely diminished quality of life due to the extensive range of connected complications. One of the most impactful diabetes-associated pathologies is diabetic macular edema (DME), as it is a major cause of blindness globally. Patients with DME present many concomitant diseases that influence their prognosis. The present research seeks to describe the most frequent DME-related comorbidities. **Method**: This study enrolled 105 participants previously diagnosed with type 1 DM (T1DM) or type 2 DM (T2DM) (77 presenting with DME), who were evaluated regarding other associated comorbidities. **Results**: Patients in the DME group presented a median age of 65, with a mean disease duration of 15 years and inadequate glycemic control, reflected by a mean HbA1c of 7.5%. All patients presented at least one comorbidity, with hypertension (100%) and dyslipidemia (62.3%) being the most prevalent. Spearman analysis revealed a statistically significant correlation between DME and diabetes duration ($p = 0.01$), proliferative diabetic retinopathy ($p = 0.004$), and chronic kidney disease ($p = 0.034$). **Conclusions**: Patients with DME often present multiple comorbidities that must be screened for and addressed through a multidisciplinary approach.

Keywords: diabetes mellitus; diabetic macular edema; health status; comorbidities; multidisciplinary; personalized medicine

1. Introduction

Diabetes mellitus (DM) is a chronic metabolic disease characterized by continuous hyperglycemia. According to the International Diabetes Federation's (IDF) 10th edition, the worldwide prevalence of diabetes is rising at an alarming rate, posing a significant challenge to public health [1]. DM is a leading contributor to major health issues, including cardiovascular diseases (CVD) such as acute myocardial infarction and strokes, as well as other severe complications like blindness and chronic kidney disease (CKD) [2].

Diabetic eye disease comprises several pathological changes, which include, among others, diabetic retinopathy (DR), diabetic macular edema (DME), glaucoma, cataracts, and even changes involving the ocular surface [3].

DME, with a continuously rising prevalence, is one of the most serious complications related to DM, as it is one of the leading causes of vision impairment worldwide [4]. DME can occur in any stage of DR, and its presence requires prompt and decisive therapeu-

 https://doi.org/10.3390/jpm15030106

tic intervention in order to prevent progression and irreversible retinal damage while simultaneously lowering the risk of blindness in patients with DM [5].

DME is characterized by retinal thickening, mostly in the outer and inner plexiform layers, mainly determined by a breakdown of the blood–retinal barrier [6]. This abnormal accumulation of fluid, lipids, and proteins involves the macular area and frequently impacts the fovea, directly leading to decreased visual acuity among patients with DM [2].

DME prevalence varies significantly, ranging from 4.2% to 14.3% in individuals with T1DM and from 1.4% to 5.57% in those with T2DM [7,8]. The high prevalence of DME not only severely affects patients' quality of life but also places a heavy economic overload on healthcare systems worldwide [2].

DME has a multifactorial nature, with a wide range of factors involved in its development. Gender, ethnicity, diabetes type/duration, or genetic factors represent unmodifiable factors, while hypertension (HTN), dyslipidemia, obesity, and chronic kidney disease are the most frequent pathologies linked to DME. Last but not least, habits like smoking or alcohol consumption also have a negative impact on DME evolution [9].

It is well known that patients with DM in general, not only those with DME, exhibit a higher risk of associated health problems than those who do not have DM. Approximately 60–70% of individuals with diabetes have at least one comorbidity, while 25–30% already present with more than two comorbidities at the time of their DM diagnosis. However, in everyday clinical practice, when these patients are screened for diabetes-related ocular complications, overall health status might be somewhat disregarded, resulting in overlooking potential factors that impact the development of these complications, especially DME. Many patients with DM, even those recently diagnosed, may already present chronic complications due to the prolonged metabolic dysregulation that often precedes the formal diagnosis of DM. For example, DM has been associated with changes in intraocular pressure (IOP). A recent study found that diabetes progression and altered glycemic control are directly linked to increased IOP before resulting in glaucoma [10]. Therefore, a thorough general and ophthalmologic evaluation is mandatory in all diabetic patients [11].

Regarding the systemic management of DME and other diabetes-related complications, the general consensus among healthcare professionals still involves glycemic control. However, considering the complex health status of patients with DM and the multiple risk factors involved in DME development, additional measures must be taken, such as strict blood pressure control, lowering lipid levels, and the proper management of obesity and renal status [12]. Last but not least, smoking and alcohol consumption cessation must be recommended in all patients with DM, despite the degree of retinal complications. These suggest that improving outcomes for patients with DME may require a broader approach, incorporating the investigation of additional risk factors and innovative treatment strategies beyond glycemic management alone [13].

The aim of this research was to evaluate the general health status of patients with DME, focusing on the diseases most frequently related to both DME and DM, in general, in order to raise awareness regarding the need for more stringent healthcare management of these patients, while also observing which are the most important risk factors implied in the appearance and evolution of DME, in order to more promptly screen and take preventative measures to ensure the prevention of blindness.

2. Materials and Methods

2.1. Study Design and Patient Selection

In this retrospective cross-sectional study, we included patients previously diagnosed with either T1DM or T2DM. All the patients took part in their prescheduled appointments at the Diabetes Care Center within the "Pius Brinzeu" Emergency County Hospital in Timisoara, Romania.

We examined the medical records of 227 patients from the Diabetes Center between 16 July 2024 and 6 August 2024, and we enrolled a total number of 105 patients (55 male and 50 female subjects). 122 patients declined to participate in this research or did not comply with the study's eligibility criteria. The inclusion criteria comprised patients above 18 years of age with a prior DM diagnosis (either T1DM or T2DM). Exclusion criteria included other DM subtypes (gestational and secondary DM), significant cognitive impairment or other neuro-psychiatric disorders that prevented patients from giving informed consent, comorbidities that necessitated hospitalization during our study, institutionalized patients, and patients who presented any ocular pathologies that would interfere with a proper retinal examination (advanced cataracts and significant vitreous hemorrhage). Other retinal diseases that could interfere with an adequate classification of DME and DR by altering the examined retinal structures (severe myopia, detachment of the retina, or significant macular pucker) were also excluded from this research.

The protocol for the present study was approved by the Ethics Committee of the "Pius Brinzeu" Emergency County Hospital, Timisoara, Romania (approval no. 472/15.07.2024), adhering to the principles outlined in the Declaration of Helsinki, revised in 2013, and its subsequent amendments.

2.2. Data Collection and Medical Assessment

The following patient data were retrieved: gender, age, weight and height, diabetes type, disease duration, current medication, comorbidities, and smoking status. Additionally, a complete fundus examination was performed by a trained ophthalmologist, using a Topcon SL-D2 biomicroscope.

The assessment of biological parameters comprised a complete blood panel for all patients during their visit at the Diabetes Care Center. Diagnosis of DM was previously established through the presence of a fasting plasma glucose level > 7.0 mmol/L (126 mg/dL), 2 h post-load plasma glucose > 11.1 mmol/L (200 mg/dL), or HbA1c level above 6.5% (48 mmol/mol). Disease duration refers to the number of years from the initial DM diagnosis to the date of inclusion in the present research. Weight and height were measured for all participants, and the Body Mass Index (BMI) was calculated using the metric system. Following the World Health Organization (WHO) criteria regarding obesity, patients with BMI values above 25 kg/m^2 were considered overweight, while those with BMI equal to or above 30 kg/m^2 were diagnosed with different degrees of obesity. Blood pressure was also evaluated in all patients with the aid of an aneroid sphygmomanometer and hypertension was diagnosed in the presence of a systolic blood pressure value above or equal to 140 mmHg and a diastolic blood pressure above or equal to 90 mmHg. Meanwhile, CVD presence was derived from patients' medical history and referred to either a previous diagnosis of coronary heart disease or cerebrovascular disease. Diabetic neuropathy was evaluated by performing nerve conduction velocity (NCV), with values less than 40 m/s being considered pathological, as well as with the usage of the Michigan Neuropathy Screening Instrument (MNSI) with resulting clinical scores above 2.5, questionnaire scores above 7, or overall scores over 9.5. Chronic kidney disease (CKD) was determined at values below 60 mL/min of the creatinine-based glomerular filtration rate (eGFR) estimate. Dyslipidemia was diagnosed based on lipid panel values. Smoking habits were self-reported.

A board-certified ophthalmologist performed an extensive fundus examination after prior pupil dilation on all patients with a Topcon SL-D2 biomicroscope (Tokyo, Japan). Cataract diagnosis or prior cataract surgery with intraocular lens implantation (IOL) was reported. Retinal structures were examined and DME and DR diagnosis were established according to the Early Treatment Diabetic Retinopathy Study Design (ETDRS) guidelines [14]. DME was considered in the following circumstances: retinal thickening or the presence of hard exudates within 1 disk diameter from the center of the fovea [15].The presence of microaneurysms, hemorrhages, exudates, venous beading, or neovascularization was taken into account in DR staging as follows: non-proliferative diabetic retinopathy (NPDR) with mild, moderate, and severe NPDR stages and proliferative diabetic retinopathy (PDR) [16]. IOP measurement was performed for all patients with a Perkins handheld applanation tonometer (Perkins Mk3 tonometer, Haag-Streit, Koniz, Switzerland). Patients' medical charts were also reported prior to the ophthalmologic treatments, including retinal laser photocoagulation or intravitreal injections with anti-VEGF.

2.3. Statistical Analysis

Statistical analysis was performed using the IBM Statistical Package for Social Sciences software (version 28, Armonk, NY, USA, accessed on 1 August 2024, https://www.ibm.com). The characteristics of the two study subgroups were presented using descriptive statistics, including the median, percentage, and interquartile range (IQR), depending on the variable type. The normality of the data distribution was evaluated using visual tools, such as histograms and probability plots, as well as analytical tests, specifically the Shapiro–Wilk test. Since the data were not normally distributed, numerical variables were reported as medians with the 25th and 75th IQRs, and the Mann–Whitney U test was used for comparisons between groups. Categorical variables were described as frequencies and percentages, with comparisons among groups performed using the Chi-squared or Fisher's exact test, depending on the data. The relationship between DME and the risk factors T1DM and T2DM was assessed using the point-biserial correlation (rpb) for continuous variables and the Phi coefficient (ϕ) for categorical variables. We also conducted a multivariate logistic regression to determine potential risk factors for DME within the study population. A p-value (two-tailed) of less than 0.05 was considered statistically significant.

3. Results

3.1. General Characteristics of the Study Population

The study included 105 participants, divided into two groups based on DME presence (n = 77) or absence (n = 28). The median age of the participants was 66 (IQR: 59–73) years. Those within the DME group were observed to be younger; however, this difference did not present a statistical significance value (p = 0.071). Both groups were similar regarding gender distribution, as seen in Table 1.

A total of 92.4% of the total study population had T2DM, and the rest T1DM. Disease duration was significantly longer in the DME group (median 15 years) compared to the group without DME (median 10 years), as seen in Figure 1. This indicates that patients with diabetes and DME had a longer DM duration than those without DME.

In terms of diabetes management, most of the patients were treated with non-insulin antidiabetic drugs, 30.5% were under treatment with insulin, and 12.4% received a combination of the two. There was no statistically significant difference in the distribution of these treatments between groups (p = 0.219). The current and maximum HbA1c levels were recorded, with the median values were slightly higher in the DME group (current HbA1c: 7.50%, IQR: 6.72–8.27; maximum HbA1c: 10.90%, IQR: 8.95–13) compared to the group without DME (current HbA1c: 6.85%, IQR: 6.42–7.80; maximum HbA1c: 9.45%, IQR: 8.85–10.70). The prevalence of dyslipidemia, HTN, obesity, and CVD comorbidities did not differ notably between the two studied groups. CKD was present only among patients who also presented with DME. Diabetic neuropathy was also more common in patients with an associated diagnosis of DME, though this finding did not reach statistical significance. Still, all patients with DME had HTN in the researched population, 48.1% of them presenting moderate HTN, while dyslipidemia was diagnosed in 62.3% of the same subgroup. Furthermore, almost half of this subgroup presented with at least one other comorbidity (46.8%).

Table 1. General characteristics of the study population.

Variables	Total (n = 105)	DME (−) (n = 28)	DME (+) (n = 77)	p-Value
Age (years)	66 (59, 73)	69.5 (60.2, 74)	65 (58, 71.5)	0.071
Male n (%)	55 (52.4)	14 (50)	41 (53.2)	0.768
T1DM/T2DM n (%)	8 (7.6)/97 (92.4)	1 (3.6)/27 (96.4)	7 (9.1)/70 (90.9)	0.679
Disease duration	15 (8, 20)	10 (6.25, 15)	15 (9, 20)	**0.010**
Diabetes treatment n (%)				0.219
OAD	58 (55.2)	19 (67.9)	39 (50.6)	
INS	32 (30.5)	7 (25)	25 (32.5)	
OAD + INS	13 (12.4)	1 (3.6)	12 (15.6)	
OAD + weekly injection	2 (1.9)	1 (3.6)	1 (1.3)	
Current HbA1c %	7.30 (6.50, 8.07)	6.85 (6.42, 7.80)	7.50 (6.72, 8.27)	0.098
Maximum HbA1c %	10.1 (8.95, 12.55)	9.45 (8.85, 10.70)	10.90 (8.95, 13)	0.102
Dyslipidemia n (%)	70 (66.7)	22 (78.6)	48 (62.3)	0.161
HTN n (%)				0.292
Mild	29.5 (31)	7 (25)	24 (31.2)	
Moderate	48 (45.7)	11 (39.3)	37 (48.1)	
Severe	26 (24.8)	10 (35.7)	16 (20.8)	
Obesity n (%)	31 (29.5)	10 (35.7)	21 (27.3)	0.402
Comorbidities n (%)	42 (40)	15 (53.6)	27 (35.1)	0.087
CKD	11 (10.5)	0 (0)	11 (14.3)	**0.034**
Diabetic neuropathy	13 (12.4)	1 (3.6)	12 (15.6)	0.177
CVD	18 (17.1)	5 (17.9)	13 (16.9)	0.907
Smoking n (%)	22 (21)	3 (10.7)	19 (24.7)	0.120

Mann–Whitney U test and either the Chi-square (χ^2) test, Fisher's exact test, or Bowker's test, as appropriate. Data are expressed as the median, interquartile range (IQR), or percentage (n, %). DME, diabetic macular edema; DM, diabetes mellitus; OAD, oral antidiabetics; INS, insulin; HbA1c, hemoglobin A1c; HTN, hypertension; CKD, chronic kidney disease; CVD, cardiovascular disease. Differences that are statistically significant, defined as those with a value of $p < 0.05$, are highlighted in bold.

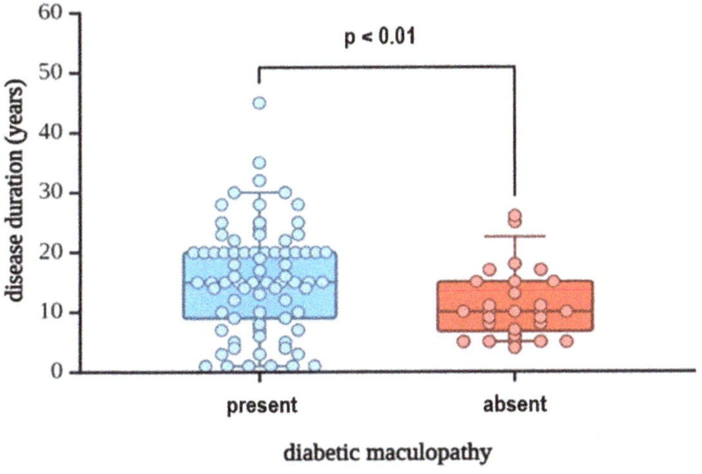

Figure 1. Disease duration and diabetic maculopathy status. Circles represent individual data points. Created with Biorender.com.

3.2. Ophthalmic Findings

Intraocular pressure (IOP) measurements in both the right eye (RE) and left eye (LE) did not vary significantly between groups. DR presence was significantly associated with DME ($p < 0.001$), with a greater proportion of patients in the DME group having PDR, as seen in Table 2. This led to the conclusion that macular edema was not only associated with diabetic retinopathy but also with more severe cases of the disease.

Table 2. Ophthalmologic characteristics of the study population.

Variables	Total (*n* = 105)	DME (−) (*n* = 28)	DME (+) (*n* = 77)	*p*-Value
IOP—RE mmHg	15 (14, 17)	16 (15, 17.7)	15 (13, 17)	0.204
IOP—LE mmHg	16 (14, 18)	16 (15, 18)	16 (13, 18)	0.266
Cataract *n* (%)				
• Absent	15 (14.3)	5 (17.9)	10 (12.9)	0.528
• Present	41 (39)	9 (32.1)	32 (41.6)	0.498
• Pseudophakia	49 (46.7)	14 (50)	35 (45.5)	0.515
Diabetic retinopathy *n* (%)				
• Absent	16 (15.2)	15 (53.5)	0	**<0.001**
• Mild non-proliferative	4 (3.8)	3 (10.7)	2 (2.6)	0.084
• Moderate non-proliferative	9 (8.6)	2 (7.2)	7 (9.1)	1
• Severe non-proliferative	34 (32.4)	6 (21.4)	28 (36.4)	0.166
• Proliferative	42 (40)	2 (7.2)	40 (51.9)	**<0.001**
Intravitreal injections *n* (%)	87 (82.9)	17 (60.7)	70 (90.9)	**<0.001**
Laser photocoagulation *n* (%)	56 (53.3)	6 (21.4)	50 (64.9)	**<0.001**

Mann–Whitney U test and either the Chi-square (χ^2) test or Fisher's exact test, as appropriate. Data are expressed as the median (interquartile range, IQR) or percentage (*n*, %). IOP, intraocular pressure; RE, right eye; LE, left eye; DME, diabetic macular edema. Statistically significant differences, with a $p < 0.05$, are highlighted in bold.

The use of intravitreal injections and laser photocoagulation was significantly more common in the DME group (both $p < 0.001$), indicating the need for more aggressive ophthalmologic intervention in these patients.

3.3. Correlation Analysis of DME with Risk Factors for T1DM and T2DM

Correlation analysis was conducted to assess which demographic or clinical factors correlated with the presence of DME (Table 3). A strong positive correlation was detected with DR ($r_{pb} = 0.643$), while weaker correlations were found with disease duration ($r_{pb} = 0.246$), current HbA1c ($\phi = 0.241$), and CKD ($r_{pb} = 0.206$).

Table 3. Correlation between DME and risk factors in T1DM and T2DM.

	Age	Gender	Disease Duration	Current HbA1c	Dys-Lipidemia	HTN	CKD	Diabetic Neuropathy	Smoking	DR
p-Value	0.070	0.768	**0.011**	**0.014**	0.119	0.117	**0.035**	0.098	0.273	**<0.001**
Correlation coefficient	−0.178	−0.029	0.246	0.241	0.152	−0.153	0.206	0.161	0.107	0.643

Point-biserial correlation (rpb) and Phi coefficient (ϕ), as appropriate. Abbreviations: DME, diabetic macular edema; HbA1c, hemoglobin A1c; HTN, hypertension; CKD, chronic kidney disease; Statistically significant differences, with a $p < 0.05$, are highlighted in bold.

3.4. Association Between DME and Several Demographic and Clinical Factors

In order to obtain more information regarding DME in patients with DM, a multivariate logistic regression analysis was performed, investigating potential factors associated with DME, as shown in Table 4. After adjusting for multiple confounding factors, including risk factors T1DM and T2DM, only PDR remained statistically significant as an independent factor linked to DME occurrence (p = 0.004).

Table 4. Risk factors associated with DME in the study population.

Variables	Model 1		Model 2		Model 3	
	OR (95%CIs)	p-Value	OR (95%CIs)	p-Value	OR (95%CIs)	p-Value
Age	0.887 (0.438, 2.260)	0.802	0.922 (0.343, 2.476)	0.871	1.135 (0.388, 3.322)	0.818
Gender	0.948 (0.894, 1.005)	0.702	0.948 (0.890, 1.010)	0.970	0.954 (0.893, 1.020)	0.169
Disease duration	1.069 (1.005, 1.137)	**0.034**	1.088 (1.014, 1.166)	**0.018**	1.066 (0.990, 1.148)	0.089
Current HbA1C	1.312 (0.852, 2.021)	0.218	1.349 (0.843, 2.160)	0.212	1.088 (0.654, 1.809)	0.744
Severe HTN			0.471 (0.164, 1.351)	0.161	0.385 (0.119, 1.248)	0.112
Dyslipidemia			0.353 (0.113, 1.101)	0.073	0.500 (0.150, 1.674)	0.261
PDR					10.715 (2.16, 52.97)	**0.004**

Model 1 adjusted for: age; gender; disease duration; current HbA1c. Model 2 adjusted for: age; gender; disease duration; severe HTN; dyslipidemia. Model 3 adjusted for: age; gender; disease duration; severe HTN; dyslipidemia; PDR. OR, odds ratio; CI, confidence interval; HbA1c, hemoglobin A1c; HTN, hypertension; PDR, proliferative diabetic retinopathy. Differences that are statistically significant, defined as those with a probability value of $p < 0.05$, are highlighted in bold.

4. Discussion

The global prevalence of DME is increasing. As the number of DM cases rises, a corresponding rise in complications related to diabetes is expected [17]. With the worldwide increase in the aging population [18], the concept of multimorbidity has received significant attention among medical practitioners [19], particularly regarding patients with T2DM, who present a greater risk of having numerous co-occurring conditions [20]. Our research focused on observing DME cases in the western Romanian population with T2DM, which is known to be highly prevalent in this part of the country. Conditions such as arterial hypertension, chronic kidney disease, and obesity have a major impact on ocular complications related to DM, including vision-threatening DME [21].

In our study group, those who suffered from DME had longer DM duration, with a median of 15 years (p = 0.010), data that align with the current literature findings, which report a direct correlation between diabetes duration and the development and progression of ophthalmologic complications such as DME and DR. Notably, patients with T2DM might present DME at the time of DM diagnosis, underlining the importance of screening in both recently diagnosed patients, as well as patients who have been diagnosed for a longer period of time [6,22]. Regarding glycemic control, HbA1c levels were suboptimal in the whole research group but were particularly elevated among patients with DME (median value 7.5%, maximum value 10.9%). Increased HbA1c values are known to be linked to DME occurrence and progression, while conversely, adequate glycemic control positively impacts ocular-related complications. According to DDCT/EDIC, a 10–25% decrease in the risk of DME occurrence can be obtained by only a 1% decrease in HbA1c levels [23].

DR severity is the major risk factor linked to DME. Although DME can be found at any degree of DR, an increase in DR severity has been associated with the rising prevalence of DME [14]. Our research found a strong positive correlation between the presence of DR and DME (p = 0.643). Moreover, PDR was a statistically significant factor involved in DME occurrence (p = 0.004). Intravitreal injections and retinal laser photocoagulation prevailed as treatment strategies among our population, emphasizing the need for a more decisive approach when facing diabetes-related ocular complications. This situation seriously impacts DM patients' quality of life [24]. Even so, treatment outcomes do not always meet the desired results, suggesting other general health factors may have a greater impact on visual outcomes [25].

More than 60% of patients with DM present at least one comorbidity at the time of their DM diagnosis [26]. Our research population aligns with these findings, as the majority of the evaluated patients presented at least one comorbidity, arterial hypertension and dyslipidemia being the most prevalent pathologies among our DME subgroup. All these components lead to the appearance of metabolic syndrome, which in turn increases the risk of cardiovascular complications, one of the most serious ones being atrial fibrillation. Also, DME and metabolic syndrome are closely linked through their shared pathophysiological mechanisms, primarily related to insulin resistance, chronic inflammation, and vascular dysfunction [27]. All DME patients were diagnosed with HTN, with different degrees of severity, presenting a slight predominance towards moderate HTN (48.1%), according to data sustained by a study conducted by Zhang M et al. [28]. On the other hand, HTN presence, regardless of the severity, is linked to an increase in the probability of DME occurrence of 40% [29]. The Wisconsin Epidemiologic Study of Diabetic Retinopathy found that systemic hypertension triples the prevalence of DME. It has been proposed that hypertension serves as a risk factor for the development of macular edema, and its management could provide significant benefits for patients with uncontrolled blood pressure. Sustaining the importance of HTN management, according to UKPDS 69, a reduction of only 10 mmHg in systolic blood pressure reduced the risk of DME development by 15% [30], while the optimal blood pressure values assessment among patients with DM could be represented by a 24 h measurement, due to the more significantly predictive power concerning the evaluation cardiovascular risk in these patients [31].

Previous studies have indicated that dyslipidemia is linked to DME. Furthermore, a global multicenter study found that high triglyceride levels and low HDL cholesterol levels were associated with an increased risk of diabetic microvascular diseases. Dyslipidemia is one of the most frequent comorbidities found in patients with DM [26]. Our research revealed that 66.7% of evaluated patients presented this pathology, 62.3% belonging to the DME subgroup. Treating dyslipidemia should address all cholesterol fractions, yet elevating HDL-cholesterol levels must become a therapeutic target, especially among patients with DME, as it was found to decrease the risk of DME, as stated by Klein et al. and confirmed by another study conducted by Chung et al. [32,33].

Besides HTN and dyslipidemia, 46.8% of the DME subpopulation presented at least one other comorbidity, such as CKD, diabetic polyneuropathy, or CVD. Regarding these comorbidities, we found a statistically significant correlation between CKD and DME ($p = 0.034$). Multiple reports have evaluated the relationship between DME and CKD. Acan et al. reported CKD is a risk factor for DME development [13], while another study from Melbourne observed no associations between GFR and DME in 61 Caucasian patients with DME [34]. In contrast, another population-based study indicated that CKD was significantly associated with incident DME during a 10-year follow-up examination [35]. The positive association between DME and GFR was also sustained by a single-center retrospective observational study involving patients with T2DM in South China [36]. These different results among various studies suggest that although both CKD and DME share a comparable pathology mechanism, microangiopathy, the exact influence of renal factors on DME remains unclear [37].

Lifestyle-related habits are also of great importance when deciding upon a therapeutic approach for a patient with DM and DME [38]. Obesity is known to be especially prevalent in patients with T2DM, and its management becomes mandatory, as lowering body mass is known to have a beneficial effect on visual outcomes post-DME treatment [39]. In our research, 27.3% of DME patients had obesity, results that the relatively small research group might determine. We consider that further research is necessary in this direction, as there are studies that link not only BMI values but also abdominal fat distribution (waist-to-hip ratio) to the development of diabetes-related ocular pathologies [39,40].

Regarding smoking addiction, we have found that 24.7% of patients with DME were active smokers. Since smoking was self-reported, we did not take past or occasional smokers into account, as we considered it would impede result precision. However, we underscore the need for these categories to be included in future research. Data regarding the direct impact of smoking on DME is somewhat inconclusive in the existing literature. Still, smoking cessation should be advised in all patients with DM, as nicotine is known to impair insulin activity and negatively impact glycemic control [41,42].

As shown in existing studies and as we have observed in the present study, most of the patients with DME have multiple associated diseases that facilitate the appearance of macular edema and accelerate its progression. For this reason, it is very important to identify these pathologies as early as possible so that through their correct management, we can try to prevent the occurrence and subsequent progression of DME.

Although somewhat restricted by the relatively small population size, this research accurately reflects the general health status among patients with DM with DME evaluated in hospital settings in the western part of our country, and the baseline health characteristics of the studied cohort are reflected with precision. Furthermore, considering the consecutive patient enrollment in this research, the heterogeneity of the final study group emphasizes the diversity of patients that medical practitioners encounter in daily clinical practice, accentuating the need for a personalized medical approach for each patient.

Our results have shown that patients with DME generally present multiple associated comorbidities. Therefore, a stringent treatment plan is mandatory, which is an objective achieved in Romania for DM patients by regular check-ups every 3 months, while chronic complication screening is usually performed annually. These particular visits also address patient education regarding diabetes and diabetes treatment. Yet, further education is needed concerning the associated general and ocular diseases and their symptoms to better understand the disease and facilitate better treatment adherence among patients. Besides an increase in the degree of health education, as multiple comorbidities threaten each diabetic patient's quality of life, we consider that general and ophthalmologic health status screening should be performed at least every 6 months, as a proper diagnosis timing could lead to the more personalized and effective management of these patients.

Regarding the ophthalmologic evaluation of diabetic patients, while medical settings equipped with optical coherence tomography (OCT) would represent the ideal scenario since it represents the gold standard in the diagnosis of DME and other diabetes-related pathologies, the patients often do not have access to hospitals equipped as such. As such, it is important that screening is performed for all patients with DM, whether at the initial consultation or well into their diagnosis [43]. Still, we emphasize the importance of an extended ophthalmologic examination using fundus photography and OCT for a personalized treatment protocol and a precise follow-up.

Future research perspectives also refer to expanding the study population to a larger and younger demographic group while conducting a multicenter, prospective study for a more accurate representation of diabetes-related ocular complications such as DME and associated comorbidities and their interrelation, the main objective remaining individualized patient management and the subsequent quality of life improvement.

5. Conclusions

This body of research underlines the importance of close monitoring for DME in patients with DM, underlining the risks represented by this complication and the major impact on the quality of life of these patients while simultaneously identifying individuals for which DME is more prevalent. In all evaluated patients associated with at least one other comorbidity, HTN, dyslipidemia, or CKD were more prevalent and are known to be the most significant risk factors involved in DME occurrence.

Considering the continuously growing numbers of people with DM worldwide, the necessity of personalized medicine becomes more and more evident, especially given the multitude of complications that accompany this disease. A personalized approach could translate into early complication detection, better quality of life, and improved morbidity and mortality rates. In this particular case, patients with DM would benefit from early DME detection and subsequent management, guaranteeing sight preservation.

Author Contributions: Conceptualization, A.I., S.P., and R.T.; methodology, R.T.; software, D.R.; validation, S.P. and R.T.; formal analysis, R.T.; investigation, A.I.; data curation, D.R.; writing—original draft preparation, A.I.; writing—review and editing, A.I. and M.D.; visualization, R.T.; supervision, R.T.; project administration, R.T.; funding acquisition, A.I. All authors have read and agreed to the published version of the manuscript.

Funding: We would like to acknowledge "Victor Babes" University of Medicine and Pharmacy Timisoara for their support in covering the costs of publication for this research paper.

Institutional Review Board Statement: This study was conducted according to the Declaration of Helsinki (2013 version) and was approved by the Ethics Committee of the Emergency County Hospital "Pius Brinzeu" Timișoara, Romania (approval no. 472/15.07.2024).

Informed Consent Statement: Informed consent was obtained from all participants involved in the present study.

Data Availability Statement: All available data can be provided upon request to the corresponding author.

Conflicts of Interest: The authors declare no conflicts of interest. The funders had no role in the study design, data collection, analysis, or interpretation nor in writing or publishing the results of the current manuscript.

References

1. Sun, H.; Saeedi, P.; Karuranga, S.; Pinkepank, M.; Ogurtsova, K.; Duncan, B.B.; Stein, C.; Basit, A.; Chan, J.C.N.; Mbanya, J.C et al. IDF Diabetes Atlas: Global, Regional and Country-Level Diabetes Prevalence Estimates for 2021 and Projections for 204 *Diabetes Res. Clin. Pract.* **2022**, *183*, 109119. [CrossRef] [PubMed]
2. Zhang, J.; Zhang, J.; Zhang, C.; Zhang, J.; Gu, L.; Luo, D.; Qiu, Q. Diabetic Macular Edema: Current Understanding, Molecula Mechanisms and Therapeutic Implications. *Cells* **2022**, *11*, 3362. [CrossRef] [PubMed]
3. Mrugacz, M.; Pony-Uram, M.; Bryl, A.; Zorena, K. Current Approach to the Pathogenesis of Diabetic Cataracts. *Int. J. Mol. Sc* **2023**, *24*, 6317. [CrossRef]
4. Shah, J.; Nguyen, V.; Hunt, A.; Mehta, H.; Romero-Nuñez, B.; Zarranz-Ventura, J.; Viola, F.; Bougamha, W.; Barnes, R.; Barthelme D.; et al. Characterization of Poor Visual Outcomes of Diabetic Macular Edema: The Fight Retinal Blindness! Project. *Ophthalmc Retin.* **2022**, *6*, 540–547. [CrossRef]
5. Chew, E.Y.; Davis, M.D.; Danis, R.P.; Lovato, J.F.; Perdue, L.H.; Greven, C.; Genuth, S.; Goff, D.C.; Leiter, L.A.; Ismail-Beigi, F.; et a The Effects of Medical Management on the Progression of Diabetic Retinopathy in Persons with Type 2 Diabetes. *Ophthalmolog* **2014**, *121*, 2443–2451. [CrossRef]
6. Musat, O.; Cernat, C.; Labib, M.; Gheorghe, A.; Toma, O.; Zamfir, M.; Boureanu, A.M. Diabetic Macular Edema. *Rom. J. Ophthalmo* **2015**, *59*, 133–136. [PubMed]
7. Thomas, R.L.; Dunstan, F.D.; Luzio, S.D.; Chowdhury, S.R.; North, R.V.; Hale, S.L.; Gibbins, R.L.; Owens, D.R. Prevalence c Diabetic Retinopathy within a National Diabetic Retinopathy Screening Service. *Br. J. Ophthalmol.* **2015**, *99*, 64–68. [CrossRef]
8. Yau, J.W.Y.; Rogers, S.L.; Kawasaki, R.; Lamoureux, E.L.; Kowalski, J.W.; Bek, T.; Chen, S.-J.; Dekker, J.M.; Fletcher, A.; Grauslunc J.; et al. Global Prevalence and Major Risk Factors of Diabetic Retinopathy. *Diabetes Care* **2012**, *35*, 556–564. [CrossRef] [PubMed
9. Yu, A.J.; Masalkhi, M.; Brown, R.; Chen, B.; Chhablani, J. Racial and Ethnic Distribution in Diabetic Macular Edema Clinical Trial in the United States (2002–2021). *Ophthalmol. Retin.* **2023**, *7*, 1035–1041. [CrossRef]

Braha, A.; Simion, A.; Timar, R.; Timar, B. Factors Associated with Increased Intraocular Pressure in Type 2 Diabetes Patients. *J. Clin. Med.* **2024**, *13*, 676. [CrossRef]

Busch, C.; Katzmann, J.L.; Jochmann, C.; Unterlauft, J.D.; Vollhardt, D.; Wiedemann, P.; Laufs, U.; Rehak, M. General Health of Patients with Diabetic Macular Edema—The LIPSIA Study. *PLoS ONE* **2021**, *16*, e0252321. [CrossRef] [PubMed]

Eleftheriadou, A.; Riley, D.; Zhao, S.S.; Austin, P.; Hernández, G.; Lip, G.Y.H.; Jackson, T.L.; Wilding, J.P.H.; Alam, U. Risk of Diabetic Retinopathy and Diabetic Macular Oedema with Sodium–Glucose Cotransporter 2 Inhibitors and Glucagon-like Peptide 1 Receptor Agonists in Type 2 Diabetes: A Real-World Data Study from a Global Federated Database. *Diabetologia* **2024**, *67*, 1271–1282. [CrossRef] [PubMed]

May, M.; Framke, T.; Junker, B.; Framme, C.; Pielen, A.; Schindler, C. How and Why SGLT2 Inhibitors Should Be Explored as Potential Treatment Option in Diabetic Retinopathy: Clinical Concept and Methodology. *Ther. Adv. Endocrinol.* **2019**, *10*, 204201881989188. [CrossRef]

Early Treatment Diabetic Retinopathy Study Design and Baseline Patient Characteristics. *Ophthalmology* **1991**, *98*, 741–756. [CrossRef] [PubMed]

Gundogan, F.C.; Yolcu, U.; Akay, F.; Ilhan, A.; Ozge, G.; Uzun, S. Diabetic Macular Edema: A Short Review. *Pak. J. Med. Sci.* **2016**, *32*, 505–510. [CrossRef]

Yang, Z.; Tan, T.-E.; Shao, Y.; Wong, T.Y.; Li, X. Classification of Diabetic Retinopathy: Past, Present and Future. *Front. Endocrinol.* **2022**, *13*, 1079217. [CrossRef] [PubMed]

Acan, D.; Calan, M.; Er, D.; Arkan, T.; Kocak, N.; Bayraktar, F.; Kaynak, S. The Prevalence and Systemic Risk Factors of Diabetic Macular Edema: A Cross-Sectional Study from Turkey. *BMC Ophthalmol.* **2018**, *18*, 91. [CrossRef]

Shehan, C.L. (Ed.) *The Wiley Blackwell Encyclopedia of Family Studies*; John Wiley & Sons, Inc.: Chichester, West Sussex, UK, 2016; ISBN 978-1-119-08562-1.

Nicholson, K.; Almirall, J.; Fortin, M. The Measurement of Multimorbidity. *Health Psychol.* **2019**, *38*, 783–790. [CrossRef]

Cicek, M.; Buckley, J.; Pearson-Stuttard, J.; Gregg, E.W. Characterizing Multimorbidity from Type 2 Diabetes. *Endocrinol. Metab. Clin. N. Am.* **2021**, *50*, 531–558. [CrossRef]

Lee, R.; Wong, T.Y.; Sabanayagam, C. Epidemiology of Diabetic Retinopathy, Diabetic Macular Edema and Related Vision Loss. *Eye Vis.* **2015**, *2*, 17. [CrossRef]

Klein, R.; Knudtson, M.D.; Lee, K.E.; Gangnon, R.; Klein, B.E.K. The Wisconsin Epidemiologic Study of Diabetic Retinopathy XXII. *Ophthalmology* **2008**, *115*, 1859–1868. [CrossRef] [PubMed]

Diabetes Control and Complications Trial (DCCT)/Epidemiology of Diabetes Interventions and Complications (EDIC) Study Research Group Intensive Diabetes Treatment and Cardiovascular Outcomes in Type 1 Diabetes: The DCCT/EDIC Study 30-Year Follow-Up. *Diabetes Care* **2016**, *39*, 686–693. [CrossRef]

Fernández-Vigo, J.I.; Contreras, I.; Crespo, M.J.; Beckford, C.; Flores-Moreno, I.; Cobo-Soriano, R.; Pareja, J.; Martín, M.D.; Moreno, L.; Arrevola-Velasco, L. Expert Panel Consensus for Addressing Anti-VEGF Treatment Challenges of Diabetic Macular Edema in Spain. *OPTH* **2022**, *16*, 3097–3106. [CrossRef]

Gurung, R.L.; FitzGerald, L.M.; Liu, E.; McComish, B.J.; Kaidonis, G.; Ridge, B.; Hewitt, A.W.; Vote, B.J.; Verma, N.; Craig, J.E.; et al. Predictive Factors for Treatment Outcomes with Intravitreal Anti-Vascular Endothelial Growth Factor Injections in Diabetic Macular Edema in Clinical Practice. *Int. J. Retin. Vitr.* **2023**, *9*, 23. [CrossRef]

Iglay, K.; Hannachi, H.; Joseph Howie, P.; Xu, J.; Li, X.; Engel, S.S.; Moore, L.M.; Rajpathak, S. Prevalence and Co-Prevalence of Comorbidities among Patients with Type 2 Diabetes Mellitus. *Curr. Med. Res. Opin.* **2016**, *32*, 1243–1252. [CrossRef] [PubMed]

Rosca, C.I.; Lighezan, D.F.; Nisulescu, D.-D.; Sharma, A.; Neagu, M.N.; Nistor, D.; Georgescu, D.; Kundnani, N.R. Metabolic Syndrome: A Strange Companion of Atrial Fibrillation; A Blessing in Disguise from the Neuropsychiatric Point of View. *Biomedicines* **2023**, *11*, 2012. [CrossRef]

Zhang, M.; Wu, J.; Wang, Y.; Wu, J.; Hu, W.; Jia, H.; Sun, X. Associations between Blood Pressure Levels and Diabetic Retinopathy in Patients with Diabetes Mellitus: A Population-Based Study. *Heliyon* **2023**, *9*, e16830. [CrossRef] [PubMed]

Klein, R.; Klein, B.E.; Moss, S.E.; Cruickshanks, K.J. The Wisconsin Epidemiologic Study of Diabetic Retinopathy: XVII. The 14-Year Incidence and Progression of Diabetic Retinopathy and Associated Risk Factors in Type 1 Diabetes. *Ophthalmology* **1998**, *105*, 1801–1815. [CrossRef]

Matthews, D.R.; Stratton, I.M.; Aldington, S.J.; Holman, R.R.; Kohner, E.M.; UK Prospective Diabetes Study Group. Risks of Progression of Retinopathy and Vision Loss Related to Tight Blood Pressure Control in Type 2 Diabetes Mellitus: UKPDS 69. *Arch. Ophthalmol.* **2004**, *122*, 1631–1640. [CrossRef]

O'Brien, E.; Parati, G.; Stergiou, G.; Asmar, R.; Beilin, L.; Bilo, G.; Clement, D.; de la Sierra, A.; de Leeuw, P.; Dolan, E.; et al. European Society of Hypertension Position Paper on Ambulatory Blood Pressure Monitoring. *J. Hypertens.* **2013**, *31*, 1731–1768. [CrossRef]

32. Klein, B.E.K.; Myers, C.E.; Howard, K.P.; Klein, R. Serum Lipids and Proliferative Diabetic Retinopathy and Macular Edema in Persons With Long-Term Type 1 Diabetes Mellitus: The Wisconsin Epidemiologic Study of Diabetic Retinopathy. *JAMA Ophthalmol.* **2015**, *133*, 503–510. [CrossRef] [PubMed]
33. Chung, Y.-R.; Park, S.W.; Choi, S.-Y.; Kim, S.W.; Moon, K.Y.; Kim, J.H.; Lee, K. Association of Statin Use and Hypertriglyceridemia with Diabetic Macular Edema in Patients with Type 2 Diabetes and Diabetic Retinopathy. *Cardiovasc. Diabetol.* **2017**, *16*, [CrossRef] [PubMed]
34. Man, R.E.K.; Sasongko, M.B.; Wang, J.J.; MacIsaac, R.; Wong, T.Y.; Sabanayagam, C.; Lamoureux, E.L. The Association of Estimated Glomerular Filtration Rate With Diabetic Retinopathy and Macular Edema. *Investig. Ophthalmol. Vis. Sci.* **2015**, *5*4810. [CrossRef] [PubMed]
35. Romero-Aroca, P.; Baget-Bernaldiz, M.; Navarro-Gil, R.; Moreno-Ribas, A.; Valls-Mateu, A.; Sagarra-Alamo, R.; Barrot-De La Puente, J.F.; Mundet-Tuduri, X. Glomerular Filtration Rate and/or Ratio of Urine Albumin to Creatinine as Markers for Diabetic Retinopathy: A Ten-Year Follow-Up Study. *J. Diabetes Res.* **2018**, *2018*, 5637130. [CrossRef]
36. Zhuang, X.; Cao, D.; Yang, D.; Zeng, Y.; Yu, H.; Wang, J.; Kuang, J.; Xie, J.; Zhang, S.; Zhang, L. Association of Diabetic Retinopathy and Diabetic Macular Oedema with Renal Function in Southern Chinese Patients with Type 2 Diabetes Mellitus: A Single-Centre Observational Study. *BMJ Open* **2019**, *9*, e031194. [CrossRef]
37. Wang, L.; Jin, L.; Wang, W.; Gong, X.; Li, Y.; Li, W.; Liang, X.; Huang, W.; Liu, Y. Association of Renal Function with Diabetic Retinopathy and Macular Oedema among Chinese Patients with Type 2 Diabetes Mellitus. *Eye* **2023**, *37*, 1538–1544. [CrossRef]
38. Bhattacharjee, H.; Barman, M.; Garg, M. Diabetic Retinopathy and Diabetic Macular Edema: Fighting the Emerging Global Burden. In *Diabetic Macular Edema*; Saxena, S., Cheung, G., Lai, T.Y.Y., Sadda, S.R., Eds.; Springer Nature: Singapore, 2022; pp. 221–227. ISBN 978-981-19730-6-2.
39. Graue-Hernandez, E.O.; Rivera-De-La-Parra, D.; Hernandez-Jimenez, S.; Aguilar-Salinas, C.A.; Kershenobich-Stalnikowitz, D.; Jimenez-Corona, A. Prevalence and Associated Risk Factors of Diabetic Retinopathy and Macular Oedema in Patients Recently Diagnosed with Type 2 Diabetes. *BMJ Open Ophthalmol.* **2020**, *5*, e000304. [CrossRef]
40. Hwang, I.C.; Bae, J.H.; Kim, J.M. Relationship between Body Fat and Diabetic Retinopathy in Patients with Type 2 Diabetes: A Nationwide Survey in Korea. *Eye* **2019**, *33*, 980–987. [CrossRef]
41. Boretsky, A.; Gupta, P.; Tirgan, N.; Liu, R.; Godley, B.F.; Zhang, W.; Tilton, R.G.; Motamedi, M. Nicotine Accelerates Diabetes-Induced Retinal Changes. *Curr. Eye Res.* **2015**, *40*, 368–377. [CrossRef]
42. Cai, X.; Chen, Y.; Yang, W.; Gao, X.; Han, X.; Ji, L. The Association of Smoking and Risk of Diabetic Retinopathy in Patients with Type 1 and Type 2 Diabetes: A Meta-Analysis. *Endocrine* **2018**, *62*, 299–306. [CrossRef]
43. Nicoară, S.D. Spectral Domain Optical Coherence Tomography in the Diagnosis and Monitoring of Diabetic Macular Edema. In *OCT—Applications in Ophthalmology*; Lanza, M., Ed.; InTech: London, UK, 2018; ISBN 978-1-78923-754-2.

Journal of
Personalized Medicine

MDPI

ticle

:orrected Axial Length and Choroidal Thickness: A Correlation .nalysis for Scientific Purposes

arco Gioia [1], Maddalena De Bernardo [1], Ferdinando Cione [1,2,*], Martina De Luca [1] and Nicola Rosa [1]

1 Eye Unit—Department of Medicine, Surgery, Dentistry "Scuola Medica Salernitana", University of Salerno, via S. Allende, 84081 Baronissi, Italy; mgioia@unisa.it (M.G.); mdebernardo@unisa.it (M.D.B.); nrosa@unisa.it (N.R.)
2 AOU San Giovanni di Dio e Ruggi D'Aragona, 84131 Salerno, Italy
* Correspondence: fcione@unisa.it

Abstract: Purpose: Choroidal thickness (ChT) is an important measurement for evaluating eye and systemic disorders, but it is influenced by numerous elements, especially axial length (AL). It is known that the presence of a linear relationship between ChT and AL exists, but recently it has been shown that the AL measurement obtained with the current optical biometry is not very precise and needs to be corrected. This study aimed to verify if a similar correlation also persists with this corrected AL (ALc). **Methods:** All subjects underwent a complete eye examination, including spectral domain optical coherence tomography (OCT) with enhanced depth image (EDI) mode and AL measurement with IOLMaster. After a normality check of the data, the correlations between ChT with AL and ALc were investigated through the Pearson correlation coefficient. p values < 0.05 were considered statistically significant. **Results:** In total, 100 eyes of 50 healthy patients were evaluated. The mean AL was 24.36 ± 1.23 mm and mean ALc was 24.25 ± 1.22 mm. The mean nasal ChT, subfoveal ChT, and temporal ChT were, respectively, 250.57 ± 93.93 μm, 307.18 ± 101.66 μm, and 313.72 ± 88.86 μm. A significant negative linear correlation was found by comparing both AL and ALc to ChT (all $r < -0.500$, all $p < 0.050$). The negative linear correlation was stronger between nasal ChT and both AL and ALc (all $r = -0.581$). **Conclusions:** Through OCT and optical biometry, we confirmed that a statistically significant correlation persists between ALc and ChT, equal to the uncorrected AL. On these bases, in ChT studies or protocols, we recommend stratifying population according to ALc because linear correlation is still present; however, the cut-off values should be changed according to the systematic errors in optical biometry. In addition, both AL and ChT changes should be evaluated according to ALc.

Keywords: axial length; choroidal thickness; corrected axial length; ChT-AL correlation

1. Introduction

Choroid evaluation is becoming an emerging topic in ophthalmology due to its role in the diagnosis and follow-up of several pathologies and conditions [1–3]. Spaide et al., with their pioneering studies, first described a method of obtaining images of the choroid using conventional optical coherence tomography (OCT) with the aim of evaluating choroidal thickness (ChT) measurements using these images [4–6]. In fact, in the last few years, several authors investigated the role of ChT in several systemic and eye diseases, even though the assessment of this choroidal parameter is very difficult because it is affected by several factors, such as body position, axial length (AL), drug intake, and drug withdrawal [1,2]. The relationship between AL and ChT has been studied in detail: in fact, it is known in the scientific literature that a significant relationship exists between AL and ChT [2,3,7–17]. A linear relationship seems to be present between AL and ChT, with short eyes having a thicker choroid, and long eyes having a thinner one [3].

For this reason, in a study evaluating ChT and ChT changes, it essential to stratify subjects according to AL, in order to obtain homogeneous and comparable samples. However, studies that evaluate ChT generally do not consider that AL evaluation, especially in patients affected by cataracts, are more challenging and the risk of bias is really high. In fact, especially in cases of biometry being based on group refractive index (GRI) or when evaluating extremely long eyes, AL measurements need to be corrected [18].

Several authors proposed different AL correcting factors [18–22], but most of them are strictly designed for IOL power calculation [19–22]. Instead, other correcting equations are based on erroneous AL measurements due to lens opacity or GRI-based biometry [18,22], such as the corrected AL (ALc) by De Bernardo et al. [18].

Corrected ALs potentially have a double impact in ChT evaluation studies:

(1) A change in the relationship between AL and ChT measurements could occur;
(2) More important, the choice of AL cut-off values in these types of studies could change accordingly.

Regarding point 1, if we consider that many AL correction factors are generally applied only in specific AL ranges [19–22], they could influence the linear relationship with a "zone of conflict" when passing the cut-off values for adjustment application. For example, Wang–Koch adjustments, which are usually applied in case of long eyes, could modify this linear relationship.

Regarding point 2, the cut-off values of AL in ChT studies become crucial: the choice of the right values is essential for patients' recruitment, samples stratifications, change analysis, and outcome evaluations. To better understand the impact of corrected AL on ChT studies, some examples of AL/ChT studies are reported:

- AL changes related to ChT changes in pharmacological studies [23];
- AL and ChT changes in myopia studies in children and adolescents [24];
- AL and ChT changes in myopia studies in adults [25];
- AL and ChT changes in accommodation studies [14];
- AL stratification in ChT studies [26].

Why do we pay great attention to ChT reliability, and also forget to take AL reliability in choroidal studies into consideration?

We tried to answer this question and so far, to the best of our knowledge, no studies investigated the influence of corrected AL with ChT. Does the relationship between AL and ChT remain unaltered? If not, how should studies evaluating ChT stratify samples? The purpose of this study was to evaluate the correlation between ChT and ALc, because only this latter AL adjustment is not exclusively linked to IOL power calculation accuracy; however, it eliminates systematic error in biometry.

2. Materials and Methods

2.1. Participants

In this study, healthy subjects with no ocular diseases which could influence the AL or OCT measurement, such as cataract or corneal and vitreous opacities, were recruited between September 2022 and January 2023. The exclusion criteria were systemic and ocular diseases, previous eye surgery, age under 18 or over 40 years old, pregnant women and eyes with AL < 21.00 mm or AL > 27.50 mm.

The present study adhered to the ethical principles of the Declaration of Helsinki. All the participants were carefully informed about the purpose of the study and written informed consent was acquired from each subject. Institutional Review Board (IRB) approval was also obtained from the ComEtico Campania Sud (CECS), prot. n°16544.2.2

2.2. Clinical and Instrumental Examination

All patients underwent a complete eye examination consisting of the following:

- slit lamp inspection;
- visual acuity test;
- fundus examination.

All recruited patients had a best corrected visual acuity >20/25 and absence of abnormalities at both slit lamp and fundus examinations. The evaluation also included a spectral domain optical coherence tomography (OCT) evaluation with enhanced depth image (EDI) mode (Spectralis; Heidelberg Engineering; Heidelberg, Germany, version 6.0) and AL measurement with IOLMaster (Carl Zeiss Meditec AG, Jena, Germany, version 5.4.4.0006). The OCT exams were performed without the instillation of mydriatics eye drops, given the related ChT thinning in the temporal sector [23].

2.2.1. OCT Analysis

OCT scans were performed with the Heidelberg Spectralis spectral domain (SD) device. The SD-OCT uses a spectrometer to detect the interference pattern of the light reflected from different tissue layers [27]. SD-OCTs can produce high-speed images of the tissue with high axial resolution, for this reason, they are widely used in ophthalmology to perform the diagnosis and management of several pathologies [27]. The OCT analysis was performed using the OCT software measurement tool (Heidelberg Eye Explorer HEYEX, version 5.3; Heidelberg Engineering). The macular region was evaluated through a horizontal 30° linear OCT B-scan passing through the fovea, with an average of 100 frames for every B-scan. Only scans through the fovea and images with a high signal-to-noise ratio (minimum of 20 dB) were included and used for the ChT evaluation. All subjects were analyzed between 2:00 p.m. and 4:00 p.m. in order to reduce bias related to the diurnal ChT variations.

The ChT assessment was performed at the subfoveal level, at 1500 μm nasally and temporally from the fovea, perpendicularly from the hyper-reflective line of the outer border of the retinal pigment epithelium to the hyper-reflective sclero-choroidal junction centered at the base of the fovea.

2.2.2. AL Measurements

The AL measurements were performed in the routinely used method with an IOL Master 500, which is a GRI-based biometer; it measures AL utilizing partial coherence interferometry (PCI) technology. AL was measured with a semiconductor laser diode that emits a dual beam of infrared light (780 nm). The signal produced by the interference between the light reflected from the tear film and the one reflected by the retinal pigment epithelium is received by the photodetector, which is used to calculate the optical distance between the corneal surface and the retina. This optical distance is used to calculate the geometrical intraocular distances [28]. In addition, IOLMaster 500 measures keratometry values at a 2.5 mm zone on the anterior cornea with six measured points, and it measures anterior chamber depth (ACD) using lateral slit illumination [28]. The AL measurements were taken utilizing the phakic option available on the biometer. The AL values were then corrected utilizing the following formula from De Bernardo et al.:

$$ALc = -0.017 + 0.996 * AL$$

where ALc is the corrected AL, and AL is the AL detected with the optical biometer by utilizing the phakic option [18]. Contrary to many other AL adjustments, ALc should be used independently from a specific AL range, because it is based on the assumption of a systematic error correction in the optical biometer, noting the influence of lens opacity and GRI on the reliability of the AL measurement. For this reason, the AL of all participants was corrected [29].

2.3. Statistical Analysis

Data collection was performed with Microsoft Excel and statistical analysis with IBM SPSS software (International Business Machine Corporation, Armonk, NY, USA, version 26.0). The Kolmogorov–Smirnov Test was performed to assess the normal distribution of the data. The Student T-test was used for pair-wise comparisons of AL and ALc. The correlations between ChT with AL and ALc were investigated using the Pearson correlation coefficient (r) and the Pearson coefficient of determination. Pearson's analysis with bootstrap was also performed in additional evaluation according to eye-side subgroups. In all analyses, p values < 0.05 were considered statistically significant. Additionally, the mean, standard deviation, median, minimum, and maximum were calculated for each data point.

The preliminary sample size was calculated with G*Power software (Version 3.1.9.7, Faul, Erdfelder, Lang, & Buchner, 2020.Available at https://www.gpower.hhu.de, access date: 10 October 2024). Given a conventional effect size q of 0.6, it was estimated that a sample size of 47 eyes for each group (94 eyes in total) would be necessary, with a significance level of 5% and a test power of 80%.

3. Results

In total, 100 eyes of 50 healthy subjects (23 males and 22 females) with a mean age of 27.6 ± 2.3 years (ranging from 24 to 35 years) were evaluated. Both AL measurements and ChT data were normally distributed (all $p > 0.050$). The descriptive statistics of the data are reported in Table 1.

Table 1. Descriptive statistics of uncorrected and corrected axial length and nasal, subfoveal, and temporal choroidal thickness.

Parameter	AL	ALc	ChT Nasal	ChT Subfoveal	ChT Temporal
MEAN	24.36 mm	24.25 mm	250.57 μm	307.18 μm	313.72 μm
SD	1.23 mm	1.22 mm	93.03 μm	101.66 μm	88.86 μm
MEDIAN	24.12 mm	24.00 mm	250.00 μm	299.50 μm	301.00 μm
MIN	21.49 mm	21.39 mm	73.00 μm	75.00 μm	135.00 μm
MAX	27.31 mm	27.18 mm	507.00 μm	504.00 μm	501.00 μm

SD: standard deviation; Min: minimum; Max: maximum; AL: axial length, ALc: corrected axial length according to De Bernardo et al.; ChT: choroidal thickness.

A statistically significant decrease was found with ALc compared to AL: mean difference was −0.11 mm ± 0.06 mm ($p < 0.001$).

Even if a small change in slopes and intercepts in linear relationships analysis was found, as reported in Figures 1–3, a moderate negative correlation persists between both AL and ALc and ChT in different sectors. In detail, the findings were as follows:

- a negative correlation was found between both AL and ALc with subfoveal ChT (r: −0.581, $p < 0.001$);
- a negative correlation was found between both AL and ALc with nasal ChT (r: −0.527, $p < 0.001$);

- a negative correlation was found between both AL and ALc with temporal ChT (r: −0.577, $p < 0.001$).

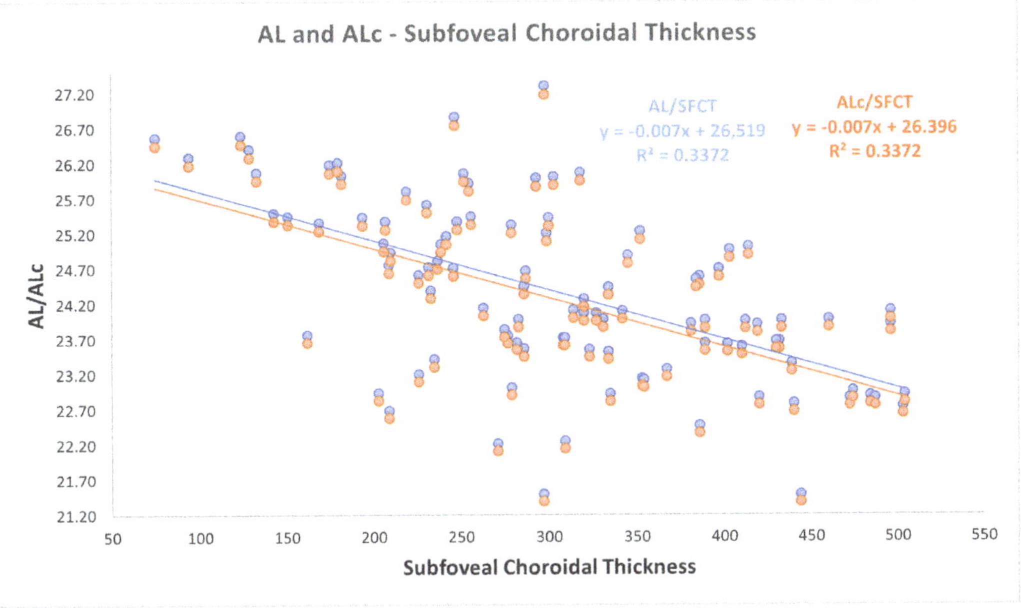

Figure 1. The relationship between both axial length (AL) and corrected AL (ALc) with subfoveal choroidal thickness.

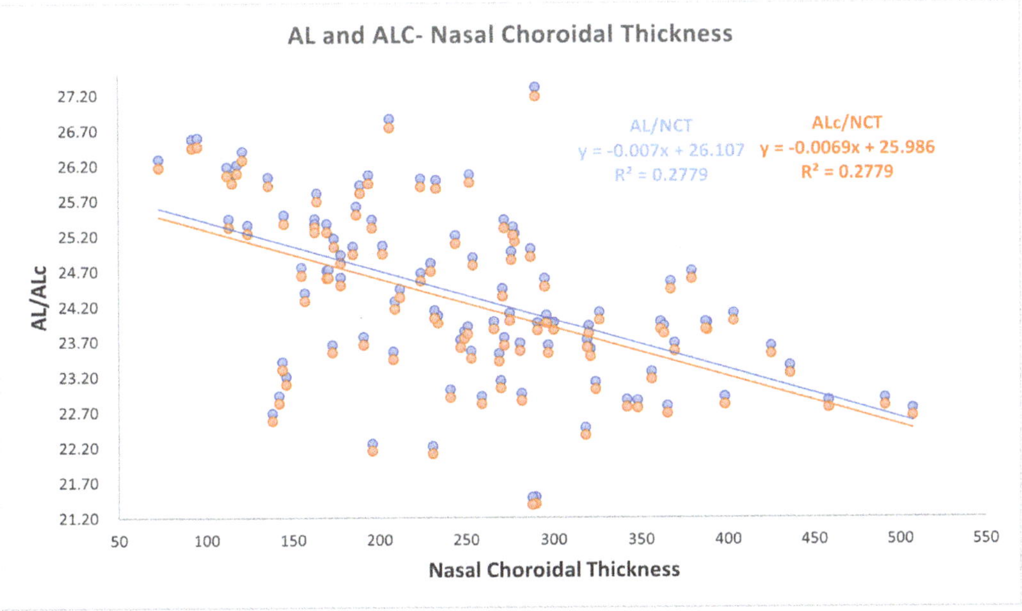

Figure 2. The relationship between both axial length (AL) and corrected AL (ALc) with nasal choroidal thickness.

Correlation analyses between AL and the choroidal parameters also with coefficient of determination according to Pearson are defined in Table 2 and in Figures 1–3.

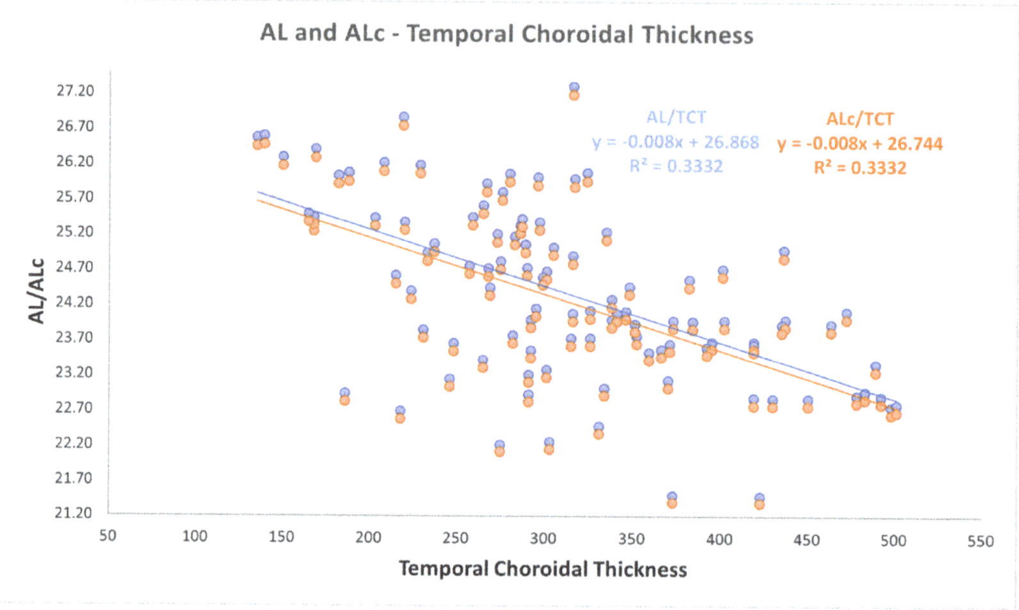

Figure 3. The relationship between both axial length (AL) and corrected AL (ALc) with temporal choroidal thickness.

Table 2. Correlation between uncorrected and corrected axial length and choroidal parameters.

Correlation	r	95% CI	R^2	*p*-Value
AL—Subfoveal ChT	−0.527	−0.669 −0.383	0.3372	0.000
AL—Nasal ChT	−0.581	−0.705 −0.449	0.2779	0.000
AL—Temporal ChT	−0.577	−0.700 −0.451	0.3332	0.000
ALc—Subfoveal ChT	−0.527	−0.669 −0.383	0.3372	0.000
ALc—Nasal ChT	−0.581	−0.705 −0.449	0.2779	0.000
ALc—Temporal ChT	−0.577	−0.700 −0.451	0.3332	0.000

AL: axial length, ALc: corrected axial length according to De Bernardo et al.; ChT: choroidal thickness; r: correlation coefficient according to Pearson correlation analysis; 95% CI: 95% confidence interval around r according to Pearson correlation analysis; R^2: coefficient of determination according to Pearson correlation analysis, *p*-value: level of significance according to Pearson correlation analysis.

Also, subgroups according to eye sides were normally distributed ($p > 0.050$) and the additional evaluation according to eye side subgroups is reported in Table 3.

Table 3. Correlation between uncorrected and corrected axial length and choroidal parameters in right eye and left eye subgroups.

Correlation	r—RE (*p*-Value)	95% CI—RE	r—LE (*p*-Value)	95% CI—LE
AL—Subfoveal ChT	−0.548 (0.000)	−0.727 −0.352	−0.621 (0.000)	−0.774 −0.412
AL—Nasal ChT	−0.546 (0.000)	−0.719 −0.334	−0.507 (0.000)	−0.697 −0.285
AL—Temporal ChT	−0.533 (0.000)	−0.711 −0.312	−0.624 (0.000)	−0.782 −0.421
Alc—Subfoveal ChT	−0.548 (0.000)	−0.727 −0.352	−0.621 (0.000)	−0.774 −0.412
ALc—Nasal ChT	−0.546 (0.000)	−0.719 −0.334	−0.507 (0.000)	−0.697 −0.285
Alc—Temporal ChT	−0.533 (0.000)	−0.712 −0.312	−0.624 (0.000)	−0.782 −0.421

RE: right eyes; LE: left eyes; AL: axial length, ALc: corrected axial length according to De Bernardo et al.; ChT: choroidal thickness; r: correlation coefficient according to Pearson correlation analysis; 95% CI: 95% confidence interval around r according to Pearson correlation analysis; *p*-value: level of significance according to Pearson correlation analysis.

4. Discussion

In the literature, a negative correlation between ChT and AL has been clearly described.

Bulut A et al. studied 53 myopic children's eyes, for SE up to −0.75 diopter, and compared them to 64 emmetropic ones, with SE between −0.50 and +0.50 D. Myopic eyes showed a significantly thinner choroid than the emmetropic control eyes in subfoveal site and in three additional sites carried out every 750 μm temporal (T1, T2 and T3) and nasal (N1, N2 and N3) to the fovea. Furthermore, in the same population including myopic and emmetropic children, ChT was negatively correlated with AL and positively correlated with SE [7].

Gupta P et al. focused on the distribution of choroidal thickness in 448 myopic eyes compared to 116 emmetropic ones and concluded that highly myopic eyes have a significantly thinner peripapillary choroid and showed a different distribution of thickness compared with the controls [8].

Sonoda S et al. examined a large (7500 μm width) choroidal area of 180 right eyes of 180 healthy volunteers with an AL range between 21.9 and 27.7 mm, showing no statistically significant correlation between AL and total choroidal area, luminal area and stromal area. However, the authors found an inverse correlation between AL and the ratio of the luminal to stromal area, thus considering the luminal area to be more affected by reduction than the stromal one [9].

El-Shazly A et al. elaborated on the effect of ocular parameters, such as spherical equivalent (SE) and axial length (AL), on ChT. They assessed the ChT of patients with different degrees of myopia. AL showed a significant positive correlation with SE ($r = 0.90$ and $p < 0.001$) but a negative correlation with subfoveal, 2 mm nasal, temporal, upper and lower ChTs ($r = -0.78, -0.83, -0.75, -0.76$, and -0.69, respectively) ($p < 0.001$). Moreover, they checked if the ChT is affected uniformly throughout the macula or at different rates in different macular regions. In fact, they observed the thinnest choroid in the 2 mm nasal and the thickest choroid in the 2 mm temporal in mild and moderate myopia, in the 2 mm lower in the sever myopia, and in the 2 mm upper in advanced myopia. SE and AL were discovered to be the most important determinants for subfoveal nasal and temporal

ChTs; the SE was the only determining factor for 2 mm upper ChT, while AL was the only determinant for 2 mm lower ChT [10].

Liu B et al. studied adult highly myopic eyes and confirmed AL as the most significant predictor of the sub foveal ChT [11].

All the above-mentioned studies analyzed studies according to AL groups or between specific AL cut-off values. However, these limits could be affected by the reliability of AL measurements. Firstly, authors evaluate AL correction related to IOL power calculation. In fact, to reduce the percentage of eyes with hyperopic refractive outcome, Wang et al. published several preoperative AL correction factors [19–21].

Cooke et al., with the so-called Cooke modified AL (CMAL), instead demonstrated that CMAL can simulate a sum-of-segments AL by using a biometer that works with GRI. In fact, it is well-known that GRI-based biometers give a shorter value of AL in short eyes and longer values of AL in long eyes [22].

Contrary to the Wang–Koch AL-correcting factors [19–22], both ALc and CMAL should be applied not only in long eyes, but in eyes of all AL ranges [18,22,29].

Therefore, ALc was proposed based on the influence of lens opacity and GRI on the reliability of the AL measurement: in this way, a correcting factor applied to preoperative AL could eliminate any systematic error biometry [18]. IOLMaster 500 measures AL by utilizing a GRI, meaning that it uses a mean refractive index to calculate AL [29], so it is not able to internally correct such a systematic error, because it is inherent to the instrument operating principle [18,28,29]. Similarly, ALc should be also applied for all phakic AL measurements for all other GRI-based biometers, independently from both AL acquisition technologies and specific AL ranges [29]. Hence, even if our study found the same relationship between AL with ChT and between ALc with ChT, the cut-off values should be changed with consideration of the reliability of AL. For example, it is known that "High myopia" is defined as the presence of myopic refractive error associated with AL $\geq$ 26.00 mm [30,31], but when performing studies that analyzed ChT in myopic eyes, the cut-off values should be arranged according to the corrected AL.

To sum up, several sources of error could affect the reliability of AL measurement:

- Inaccurate measurement technique: for example, contact ultrasound biometry is known to be unreliable;
- Principle of function of optical biometer: GRI-based biometers are more sensitive to AL measurement error, rather than sum-of-segments biometers;
- Eye length, with less reliable AL values with GRI-based biometers in case of long eyes.
- Lens opacity, that could affect reliability of all types of optical biometers, but especially GRI-based biometers.
- In all these cases, both clinicians and researchers should pay attention in both AL and ChT evaluation.

A bias in these types of studies can be represented by accommodation. In fact, in this scenario, changes in crystalline lens could contribute to AL overestimation [12]. Particularly, Woodman EC et al. observed both AL and ChT changes accompanying accommodation in myopes and emmetropes. At baseline, myopes had an average AL of 24.73 $\pm$ 1.04 mm (n = 33) and emmetropes of 23.37 $\pm$ 0.81 mm (n = 16), with a high significantly difference (p< 0.001) between them. They described choroidal thinning by 9 $\pm$ 18 μm in myopic subjects during accommodation and by 7 $\pm$ 22 μm in emmetropes ones, with a statistically significant difference between the two groups (p < 0.05). Changes in AL and ChT were shown to have a highly significant but weak negative association at analysis of covariance (p < 0.001, r^2 = 0.077, slope b = −0.321) [13].

Kaple D et al. likewise compared AL and ChT changes during accommodation in young adult emmetropes and myopes, especially at peripheral sites. Upon accommodation, the AL changes maximally on-axis (41 ± 17 μm) and minimally at the 20° nasal site (26 ± 17 μm). On the other hand, the overall ChT decreased by 21 ± 7 μm ($F1276 = 23.85$, $p < 0.001$). ChT decreased more in myopes (23 ± 11 μm) than emmetropes (17 ± 8 μm) ($p = 0.02$). The greatest decrease of 30 ± 14 μm occurred on-axis and the lowest one of 14 ± 14 μm occurred at 30° temporally. ChT changes account for about 60% of changes arising for AL: the authors concluded that AL and ChT changes during accommodation are not significantly correlated with any position [14].

This phenomenon could be explained by the action of the ciliary muscle, choroidal non-vascular smooth muscle, and choroidal blood flow. The ciliary muscle is involved in the accommodation process and its contraction could also be transferred to the choroid, causing choroidal drag and scleral circumference reduction. Choroidal smooth muscle and blood flow could change in tone during accommodation, contributing to this event [15–17].

This knowledge highlights the cause and the possible management of eventual refractive errors occurring after measuring AL with optical biometry. It suggests measuring AL immediately following accommodation or during accommodation with an instrument that also provides measurements of lens thickness.

As a vascular tunic of the ocular globe, choroid is richly vascularized and provides the oxygen and nutrients required for the retinal pigment epithelium and of the outer retina. For the same reason, it can be reached by toxins, autoantibodies, and immunocomplexes, and so it can be involved in the pathogenesis of various ocular disorders. Investigating the eventual adaptations of the negative correlation between ChT and AL in various pathologic cohorts can reveal new features of their pathogenesis. For example, De Bernardo M et al. confirmed the existence of a significant correlation between AL and all the choroidal parameters in a celiac group, except for CVI, in a study comparing the subfoveal ChT of celiac patients with healthy controls [2].

It was already proven that ALc played a clinically relevant role in IOL power calculation [18,29], and AL correction is also essential in different fields of biometry. In fact, several reasons can clarify the importance of utilizing ALc in ChT studies:

(1) Ignoring AL correction could introduce bias to the ChT evaluation of patients grouped by AL. It results in an unreliable estimation of ChT of patients with macular edema and subretinal fluid [23] and in a difficult comparison between these patients and their healthy controls. Grading and staging different ocular and systemic pathologies through ChT could be an interesting clinical and therapeutic skill, so its trustworthy use is decisive.
(2) AL correction is essential for both patients with cataracts and subjects that underwent GRI-based biometry, as discussed in previous paragraphs.
(3) Studies concerning myopia progression and ChT [32,33] should be carried out according to ALc. The choice of AL cut-off values should be taken according to corrected AL values.
(4) Not only AL cut-off values, but also evaluation of both AL and ChT changes, should be analyzed according to ALc [14,24,25].
(5) In addition, relationships between ChT and retinal diseases [34] should be analyzed with ALc values.
(6) In conclusion, patients' stratification according to AL should be performed with ALc in ChT studies [26].

It should be noted that ALc by De Bernardo et al. [18] was developed by noting an apparent reduction in AL in post cataract surgery eyes: on this basis, they verified that the refractive index of the human lens could change according to the cataract grade, making AL measurement in GRI-based biometers unreliable [18]. De Bernardo et al. demonstrated the presence of a systematic error in AL measurement in all cataractous eyes, despite the AL range [18]. For this reason, lens thickness was not considered by ALc: this parameter could be unreliable in case of cataract. ALc has more strength in eyes with cataract, therefore it should be considered, especially in case of examination of cataractous eyes. The OCT examinations were performed without any mydriatic eye drops. This should be considered a point of strength of this study. In fact, a significant thinning of the ChT in the temporal sector following the administration of tropicamide + phenylephrine has been demonstrated [23]. Such thinning was not observed in the subfoveal or nasal zone, probably because the presence of the optic nerve in the nasal choroidal side could influence the ChT, or due to an asymmetric choroidal watershed and choroidal vessels in the temporal choroid. For these reasons, the nasal and subfoveal ChT are not affected by mydriatics [23]. Avoiding pharmacological mydriasis has guaranteed the maximum reliability of ChT data, even in the temporal sector.

Since AL measurement with GRI-based biometry is inaccurate because they assume a global refractive index for different structures (cornea, aqueous, lens, vitreous), ChT measurements should not be influenced by GRI, but it was demonstrated that brightness of OCT images can influence the measurements of choroidal parameters. Therefore, ChT should not be corrected but OCT evaluation must be performed by using the same parameters [35]. Furthermore, OCT's light source is also a specific wavelength of light, thus it is also affected by the choroidal refractive index; therefore caution should be taken, especially when comparing different OCT devices in evaluation of choroidal parameters.

This study is affected by some limitations. Firstly, we evaluated both eyes for each subject. In fact, ocular measurements are more alike between fellow eyes. This similarity could cause a compounding of data; therefore, analyzing fellow eyes cannot be treated as if they were independent [36]. To overcome this problem, appropriate statistical analyses could be performed, such as the bootstrap or generalized estimating equations [36]. If the correlation between the left and right eyes of each patient is not accounted for in the statistical analysis, errors may occur in the obtained results: in fact, ignoring inter-eye correlation can lead to smaller p-values when both eyes are in the same group [36]. Another solution could be represented by the choice of using only one eye for each subject [36]. For this reason, we performed an additional analysis with bootstrap by evaluating subgroups based on the eyes' side (Table 3) and similarly a strong negative linear correlation was found both with AL and ALc compared to ChT (all $r < -0.500$, all $p < 0.050$).

In addition, the relationship between CMAL and ChT was not evaluated because the lens thickness (LT) measurement, required for CMAL [22], was not available with IOL Master 500. On the other hand, Wang–Koch adjustments were not analyzed because they were designed specifically to reduce hyperopic refractive error in long eyes [19–21].

A future prospective is represented by confirming the same relationship is also present in the case of "atypical" eyes: for example, it is well-known that refractive surgery causes a keratometry flattening, but also an AL, anterior chamber depth, and central corneal thickness (CCT) decrease [37,38]. Therefore, when the impact of corneal changes on IOL power calculation [37,38] and of CCT reduction on intraocular pressure measurement [39] are well-known, the impact of AL decrease on ChT evaluation is less well-known.

In conclusion, a statistically significant linear correlation persists between ALc and ChT, as in to the uncorrected AL. Due to systematic errors in GRI-based optical biometry, we recommend recruiting and stratifying population according to ALc, in order to apply the correct cut-off values in ChT studies. Therefore, both AL and ChT changes should be evaluated according to ALc.

Author Contributions: Conceptualization, M.G. and F.C.; methodology, M.D.B.; validation, M.D.B. and N.R.; formal analysis, F.C.; investigation and data curation, F.C. and M.D.L.; writing—original draft preparation, M.G. and M.D.L.; writing—review and editing, M.G.; visualization, M.D.L.; supervision, N.R.; project administration, M.D.B. All authors have read and agreed to the published version of the manuscript.

Funding: This research received no external funding.

Institutional Review Board Statement: The study was conducted in accordance with the Decla-ration of Helsinki and approved by the Institutional Review Board of ComEtico Campania Sud (CECS) on 10 March 2017, protocol number 16544.2.2.

Informed Consent Statement: Informed consent was obtained from all subjects involved in the study.

Data Availability Statement: The datasets generated and analyzed during the current study are available from the corresponding author upon reasonable request.

Conflicts of Interest: The authors declare no conflicts of interest.

eferences

de Bernardo, M.; Altieri, V.; Coppola, A.; Gioia, M.; Rosa, N. Choroidal evaluation in patients under alpha-lytic therapy. *Graefe's Arch. Clin. Exp. Ophthalmol.* **2020**, *258*, 2729–2736. [CrossRef] [PubMed]

de Bernardo, M.; Vitiello, L.; Battipaglia, M.; Mascolo, F.; Iovino, C.; Capasso, L.; Ciacci, C.; Rosa, N. Choroidal structural evaluation in celiac disease. *Sci. Rep.* **2020**, *11*, 16398. [CrossRef] [PubMed]

Flores-Moreno, I.; Lugo, F.; Duker, J.S.; Ruiz-Moreno, J.M. The relationship between axial length and choroidal thickness in eyes with high myopia. *Am. J. Ophthalmol.* **2013**, *155*, 314–319. [CrossRef]

Spaide, R.F.; Koizumi, H.; Pozzoni, M.C. Enhanced depth imaging spectral-domain optical coherence tomography. *Am. J. Ophthalmol.* **2008**, *146*, 496–500, Erratum in *Am. J. Ophthalmol.* **2009**, *148*, 325. [CrossRef] [PubMed]

Fujiwara, T.; Imamura, Y.; Margolis, R.; Slakter, J.S.; Spaide, R.F. Enhanced depth imaging optical coherence tomography of the choroid in highly myopic eyes. *Am. J. Ophthalmol.* **2009**, *148*, 445–450. [CrossRef] [PubMed]

Jonas, J.B.; Spaide, R.F.; Ostrin, L.A.; Logan, N.S.; Flitcroft, I.; Panda-Jonas, S. IMI-Nonpathological Human Ocular Tissue Changes With Axial Myopia. *Investig. Ophthalmol. Vis. Sci.* **2023**, *64*, 5. [CrossRef] [PubMed]

Bulut, A.; Oner, V.; Buyuktarakcı, Ş.; Kaim, M. Associations between choroidal thickness, axial length and spherical equivalent in a paediatric population. *Clin. Exp. Optom.* **2016**, *99*, 356–359. [CrossRef]

Gupta, P.; Cheung, C.Y.; Saw, S.M.; Bhargava, M.; Tan, C.S.; Tan, M.; Yang, A.; Tey, F.; Nah, G.; Zhao, P.; et al. Peripapillary choroidal thickness in young Asians with high myopia. *Investig. Ophthalmol. Vis. Sci.* **2015**, *56*, 1475–1481. [CrossRef]

Sonoda, S.; Sakamoto, T.; Yamashita, T.; Uchino, E.; Kawano, H.; Yoshihara, N.; Terasaki, H.; Shirasawa, M.; Tomita, M.; Ishibashi, T. Luminal and stromal areas of choroid determined by binarization method of optical coherence tomographic images. *Am. J. Ophthalmol.* **2015**, *159*, 1123–1131. [CrossRef]

10. El-Shazly, A.A.; Farweez, Y.A.; ElSebaay, M.E.; El-Zawahry, W.M.A. Correlation between choroidal thickness and degree of myopia assessed with enhanced depth imaging optical coherence tomography. *Eur. J. Ophthalmol.* **2017**, *27*, 577–584. [CrossRef] [PubMed]
11. Liu, B.; Wang, Y.; Li, T.; Lin, Y.; Ma, W.; Chen, X.; Lyu, C.; Li, Y.; Lu, L. Correlation of subfoveal choroidal thickness with axial length, refractive error, and age in adult highly myopic eyes. *BMC Ophthalmol.* **2018**, *18*, 127. [CrossRef]
12. Atchison, D.A.; Smith, G. Possible errors in determining axial length changes during accommodation with the IOL Master. *Optom. Cision Sci.* **2004**, *81*, 283–286. [CrossRef] [PubMed]
13. Woodman, E.C.; Read, S.A.; Collins, M.J. Axial length and choroidal thickness changes accompanying prolonged accommodation in myopes and emmetropes. *Vision. Res.* **2012**, *72*, 34–41. [CrossRef] [PubMed]
14. Kaphle, D.; Schmid, K.L.; Suheimat, M.; Read, S.A.; Atchison, D.A. Central and peripheral choroidal thickness and eye length changes during accommodation. *Ophthalmic Physiol. Opt.* **2023**, *43*, 311–318. [CrossRef] [PubMed]
15. Tamm, E.; Lütjen-Drecoll, E.; Jungkunz, W.; Rohen, J.W. Posterior attachment of ciliary muscle in young, accommodating old, presbyopic monkeys. *Investig. Ophthalmol. Vis. Sci.* **1991**, *32*, 1678–1692.
16. Woodman-Pieterse, E.C.; Read, S.A.; Collins, M.J.; Alonso-Caneiro, D. Regional changes in choroidal thickness associated with accommodation. *Investig. Ophthalmol. Vis. Sci.* **2015**, *56*, 6414–6422. [CrossRef] [PubMed]
17. Hoseini-Yazdi, H.; Read, S.A.; Alonso-Caneiro, D.; Collins, M.J. Retinal OFF-pathway overstimulation leads to greater accommodation-induced choroidal thinning. *Investig. Ophthalmol. Vis. Sci.* **2021**, *62*, 5. [CrossRef]

18. de Bernardo, M.; Cione, F.; Capasso, L.; Coppola, A.; Rosa, N. A formula to improve the reliability of optical axial lengt measurement in IOL power calculation. *Sci. Rep.* **2022**, *12*, 18845. [CrossRef]
19. Wang, L.; Shirayama, M.; Ma, X.J.; Kohnen, T.; Koch, D.D. Optimizing intraocular lens power calculations in eyes with axia lengths above 25.0 mm. *J. Cataract. Refract. Surg.* **2011**, *37*, 2018–2027. [CrossRef] [PubMed]
20. Wang, L.; Koch, D.D. Modified axial length adjustment formulas in long eyes. *J. Cataract. Refract. Surg.* **2018**, *44*, 1396–139 [CrossRef] [PubMed]
21. Wang, L.; Holladay, J.T.; Koch, D.D. Wang-Koch axial length adjustment for the Holladay 2 formula in long eyes. *J. Catarac Refract. Surg.* **2019**, *45*, 117. [CrossRef] [PubMed]
22. Cooke, D.L.; Cooke, T.L. Approximating sum-of-segments axial length from a traditional optical low-coherence reflectometr measurement. *J. Cataract. Refract. Surg.* **2019**, *45*, 351–354. [CrossRef] [PubMed]
23. Gioia, M.; de Bernardo, M.; Pagliarulo, S.; Cione, F.; Mottola, F.F.; Marca, A.L.; de Pascale, I.; Albano, G.; Rosa, N. Evaluation o Tropicamide-Phenylephrine Mydriatic Eye Drop Instillation on Choroidal Thickness. *J. Clin. Med.* **2023**, *12*, 6355. [CrossRef]
24. Hansen, M.H.; Kessel, L.; Li, X.Q.; Skovgaard, A.M.; Larsen, M.; Munch, I.C. Axial length change and its relationship wit baseline choroidal thickness—A five-year longitudinal study in Danish adolescents: The CCC2000 eye study. *BMC Ophthalmo* **2020**, *20*, 152. [CrossRef] [PubMed]
25. Ulaganathan, S.; Read, S.A.; Collins, M.J.; Vincent, S.J. Daily axial length and choroidal thickness variations in young adult Associations with light exposure and longitudinal axial length and choroid changes. *Exp. Eye Res.* **2019**, *189*, 107850. [CrossRef [PubMed]
26. Xuan, M.; Wang, D.; Xiao, O.; Guo, X.; Zhang, J.; Yin, Q.; Wang, W.; He, M.; Li, Z. Choroidal Vascularity and Axial Lengt Elongation in Highly Myopic Children: A 2-Year Longitudinal Investigation. *Investig. Ophthalmol. Vis. Sci.* **2024**, *65*, 7. [CrossRef
27. Zeppieri, M.; Marsili, S.; Enaholo, E.S.; Shuaibu, A.O.; Uwagboe, N.; Salati, C.; Spadea, L.; Musa, M. Optical Coherenc Tomography (OCT): A Brief Look at the Uses and Technological Evolution of Ophthalmology. *Medicina* **2023**, *59*, 2114. [CrossRef
28. Pathak, M.; Sahu, V.; Kumar, A.; Kaur, K.; Gurnani, B. Current Concepts and Recent Updates of Optical Biometry—A Compre hensive Review. *Clin. Ophthalmol.* **2024**, *18*, 1191–1206. [CrossRef] [PubMed]
29. Cione, F.; de Bernardo, M.; Di Paola, I.; Caputo, A.; Graziano, M.; Rosa, N. IOL power calculation in long eyes: Selection of th best axial length adjustement factor using the most common formulas. *Heliyon* **2024**, *10*, e36609. [CrossRef] [PubMed]
30. Stopyra, W.; Langenbucher, A.; Grzybowski, A. Intraocular Lens Power Calculation Formulas—A Systematic Review. *Ophthalmo Ther.* **2023**, *12*, 2881–2902. [CrossRef] [PubMed]
31. Voytsekhivskyy, O.; Tutchenko, L. Comparison of the prediction accuracy of 13 formulas in long eyes. *Graefe's Arch. Clin. Exp Ophthalmol.* **2023**, *261*, 2575–2583. [CrossRef] [PubMed]
32. Li, Z.; Cui, D.; Hu, Y.; Ao, S.; Zeng, J.; Yang, X. Choroidal thickness and axial length changes in myopic children treated wit orthokeratology. *Cont. Lens Anterior Eye.* **2017**, *40*, 417–423. [CrossRef] [PubMed]
33. Wang, Z.; Chen, J.; Kang, J.; Niu, T.; Guo, L.; Fan, L. Axial Length Control Is Associated with a Choroidal Thickness Increase ir Myopic Adolescents After Orthokeratology. *Eye Contact Lens.* **2023**, *49*, 512–520. [CrossRef]
34. Sato, M.; Minami, S.; Nagai, N.; Suzuki, M.; Kurihara, T.; Shinojima, A.; Sonobe, H.; Akino, K.; Ban, N.; Watanabe, K.; et a Association between axial length and choroidal thickness in early age-related macular degeneration. *PLoS ONE* **2020**, *15*, e024035 [CrossRef]
35. Rosa, N.; Gioia, M.; Orlando, R.; De Luca, M.; D'Aniello, E.; Fioretto, I.; Sannino, C.; De Bernardo, M. Impact of Brightness or Choroidal Vascularity Index. *J. Clin. Med.* **2024**, *13*, 1020. [CrossRef]
36. Hoffer, K.J.; Aramberri, J.; Haigis, W.; Olsen, T.; Savini, G.; Shammas, H.J.; Bentow, S. Protocols for studies of intraocular lens formula accuracy. *Am. J. Ophthalmol.* **2015**, *160*, 403–405. [CrossRef] [PubMed]
37. Anders, P.; Anders, L.M.; Barbara, A.; Szentmary, N.; Langenbucher, A.; Gatzioufas, Z. Intraocular lens power calculation in eyes with previous corneal refractive surgery. *Ther. Adv. Ophthalmol.* **2022**, *14*, 25158414221118524. [CrossRef] [PubMed]
38. Anter, A.M.; Bleeker, A.R.; Shammas, H.J.; Suraneni, S.; Kingrey, B.; Murphy, D.A.; Leal, S.; Ghalibafan, S.; Tonk, R.S.; Cooke, D.L. et al. Comparison of Legacy and New No-History IOL Power Calculation Formulas in Postmyopic Laser Vision Correction Eyes *Am. J. Ophthalmol.* **2024**, *264*, 44–52. [CrossRef] [PubMed]
39. Albis-Donado, O.; Ramirez-Neria, P.; Rios-Acosta, N.; Stalmans, I. The influence of altitude on the differences between Goldmanr tonometry and Pascal dynamic contour tonometry: An ecological meta-analysis. *Indian. J. Ophthalmol.* **2024**, *72* (Suppl. S3) S398–S403. [CrossRef] [PubMed]

Journal of Personalized Medicine

MDPI

ticle

valuating the Feasibility of a Telescreening Program for .etinopathy of Prematurity (ROP) in Denmark

ıjer A. Al-Abaiji [1,*], Regitze Bangsgaard [1], Mads Kofod [1], Carsten Faber [1,2], Ann-Cathrine Larsen [1], ;nes Galbo Brost [1], Carina Slidsborg [1], Kristian Klemp [1], Morten Breindahl [3], Morten Dornonville de la Cour [1,2] d Line Kessel [1,2]

1 Department of Ophthalmology, Copenhagen University Hospital—Rigshospitalet, 2100 Copenhagen, Denmark
2 Department of Clinical Medicine, University of Copenhagen, 2200 Copenhagen, Denmark
3 Department of Neonatal and Pediatric Intensive Care—Rigshospitalet, 2100 Copenhagen, Denmark
* Correspondence: hala0012@regionh.dk

Abstract: Objectives: This study investigates the feasibility of implementing telescreening for retinopathy of prematurity (ROP) using the ICON GO® widefield camera operated by a non-physician healthcare professional (NPHP). We hypothesized that images captured by an NPHP are adequate to evaluate ROP changes without further examinations. Secondly, the level of agreement between independent ROP graders were evaluated based on the fundus photographs. **Methods**: National ROP screening criteria were gestational age (GA) < 32 weeks or birthweight (BW) < 1500 g. Exclusion criteria were children hospitalized and born outside the Capital Region and examinations not performed by an NPHP. The screenings were performed using the ICON GO®. The NPHP selected the best images for evaluation by an *on*-site ophthalmologist, regarding whether re-examination was necessary and if so, whether the re-examination was beneficial. Lastly, the images were re-evaluated by an independent *off*-site ophthalmologist. **Results**: A total of 415 screening sessions on 165 patients performed by an NPHP were included. Re-examination was necessary in three screening sessions and beneficial in two. The level of agreement between the *on*-site and *off*-site ophthalmologists regarding ROP screening outcome was $k = 0.82$, ROP stage $k = 0.69$, plus disease $k = 0.69$, and lastly ROP zone $k = 0.37$. Of the screened children, ninety-seven (58.8%) had no ROP at any time points, sixty-two (37.6%) had some stage of ROP not requiring treatment, and six (3.6%) received ROP treatment. **Conclusions**: Telemedicine screening for ROP with the ICON GO® camera performed by an NPHP was feasible with an almost-perfect agreement and negligible need for re-examinations. The approach effectively identified children needing treatment, supporting the use of telescreening in ROP management.

Keywords: telescreening; prematurity; retinopathy of prematurity; imaging; non-physician healthcare professional

1. Introduction

Retinopathy of prematurity (ROP) is a vision-threatening retinal disease seen in children born preterm with low birth weight (BW) [1–3]. ROP is caused by a disturbance in the development of the immature eye [4]. In Denmark, screening for ROP has been performed for many years by highly specialized ophthalmologists using binocular indirect ophthalmoscopy (BIO) [5]. Another and more recent ROP screening method is using a camera, where wide-angle retinal photographs are captured. Screening with a camera enables telescreening consultation by recording and sending electronic image files of the patient's eyes [6]. This approach allows the patient's condition to be assessed remotely and at a later timepoint, while simultaneously enabling comparison of disease progression or regression over time. Classification of ROP is based on the current third edition established by the International Classification of Retinopathy of Prematurity (ICROP3) [3]. The latest update of the classification was required in part due to advancements in modern technology. These advancements enable clinicians to observe more detailed retinal changes associated with ROP that need further attention.

Another advantage of telescreening for ROP is that it can be performed by non-physician healthcare professionals (NPHPs) and thus ensure a more efficient use of ophthalmological resources. In addition, screening with a camera may be less stressful for the children compared to BIO and the images can be stored and reviewed to ensure patient safety and enable quality studies and further research [7]. BIO is, however, still considered the gold standard of ROP screening [8,9]. A recently published study, which presented the latest advancements in ROP telemedicine, concluded that telemedicine can be an alternative to BIO [10]. However, it is important to note that there are huge differences in both the incidence and severity of ROP depending on the population studied. Furthermore, ROP telemedicine studies have employed a variety of designs (retrospective, prospective), methods (camera model, BIO as reference, digital BIO), professional performing the exam (ophthalmologist, non-physician), grader (ophthalmologist, non-physician, or AI), and outcome measures (severe ROP, presence of plus disease, ROP classification), where most have focused on the presence of plus disease [9,11–17].

Several original studies and a review have already compared screening outcomes between widefield cameras versus BIO [9,11,18,19]. This study focuses on comparing evaluations from independent ophthalmologists of images captured by an NPHP using exclusively a widefield camera.

The purpose of this study was to evaluate whether an NPHP can achieve reliable image quality in a new telemedicine setup for ROP in the Capital region of Denmark. We analyzed the frequency of re-examinations by an *on*-site ophthalmologist due to insufficient image quality. Additionally, we evaluated the level of agreement between independent ophthalmologists regarding ROP stage, zone, plus disease, and screening outcome.

2. Materials and Methods

2.1. Study Population and Recruitment

At the beginning of the study, the Danish national screening criteria for ROP was gestational age (GA) < 32 weeks or birthweight (BW) < 1500 g. Since April 2023, the national guidelines narrowed to GA < 32 weeks and BW < 1600 g. Screening starts no later than 5 weeks postnatally and at a post-menstrual age (PMA) of at least 31 weeks. The children were recruited as part of the clinical routine by healthcare staff involved in screening for ROP.

Children included in our study were born and hospitalized at one of the four neonatal intensive care units (NICUs) within the Capital region of Denmark. Children were included in the study in a one-year period from 5 September 2022 to 25 September 2023. The screening sessions included were performed by the NPHP using the ICON GO® camera (Phoenix ICON™ trademark of Neolight, LLC, Phoenix, AZ, USA). Exclusion criteria encompassed screening sessions performed using other methods than the ICON GO® or sessions conducted by an ophthalmologist on days when the NPHP was physically absent, such as during holidays or work leave. These exclusions were solely due to the absence of the NPHP, and not due to difficult cases or an inability to perform the screenings. The general condition of the child was always discussed with the team managing the child prior to the ROP screening to ensure that the child was fit for the examination. The ROP screening was postponed in cases where the neonatologists evaluated that the child was too weak, and if the *on*-site ophthalmologist could accept the level of risk by postponing the screening. The NPHP performed the screening sessions three days a week, with one of three *on*-site ophthalmologists available each day.

Fundus pigmentation was noted at the first screening session due to its potential impact on image processing and evaluation. Fundus pigmentation was categorized as defined by the American Academy of Ophthalmology as follows: light (choroidal vessels visible within the macula), medium (choroidal vessels visible outside the arcades, but not within the macula), or dark (choroidal vessels not visible within the macula nor outside the arcades) [20].

2.2. Preparation of the Child Prior to ROP Examination

Local anesthesia was obtained using one drop of 0.4% oxybuprocaine, followed by two instillations with 10 min intervals of either 0.5% tropicamide and 2.5% phenylephrine or cyclomydrile (cyclopentolat hydrochlorid 0.2%/phenylephrin hydrochlorid 1%) applied by the neonatal nurse. After 30–45 min, the eyes were expected to be fully dilated. In cases of minimal effect, the eye drops were re-administered. Prior to inserting the eye speculum, local anesthesia was re-administered. Viscotears (Bausch & Lomb Nordic AB, Stockholm, Sweden) eye gel (2 mg/g carbomer) was administered for two main purposes: to lubricate and protect the cornea, and to serve as a bridge between the camera tip and the cornea.

To minimize the burden of the screening examinations, the children were swaddled and offered sugar water or breast milk, along with a pacifier, to help them stay calm and distracted. Vital signs of the child were monitored by the neonatal nurse assisting with the examination and screening was paused depending on the condition of the child.

2.3. Telescreening Setup

Before the study began, the NPHP completed five months of hands-on training under the supervision of an ROP expert (ophthalmologist). Additionally, the NPHP underwent retinal imaging training conducted by a clinical education specialist, who also reviewed images captured by the NPHP and who could approve the NPHP as a certified imaging technician. The clinical education specialist was from Neolight, Scottsdale, AZ, USA, which is a medical technology company providing solutions for neonatal care, for instance the photography device for ROP imaging as the ICON GO® (www.theneolight.com). The *on-* and *off*-site graders completed a case-based online training in grading ROP at the home page of the American Academy of Ophthalmology [21].

A portable wide-angled ICON GO® camera (Phoenix ICON™ trademark of Neolight, LLC, Phoenix, AZ, USA) was used for obtaining fundus photographs. Prior to each screening session, the ICON GO® was re-calibrated and the automated white balance function was set using a standard white background to ensure the level of brightness was equal to white during the recordings. The bedside setup consisted of an NPHP who was in the room with the child and a neonatal nurse. The dilating effect of the eyedrops was evaluated prior to the screening, and re-dilating drops were given if the pupil of either eye was < 6 mm in diameter. The NPHP recorded a video of the fundus of each eye. The initial video duration was set to a maximum of 90 s per eye. The examination was terminated either when the NPHP was satisfied with the images or when further technical improvement was not possible. From the video, the best frames per eye presenting all four quadrants and the central retina were chosen. The images were digitally exported to the Topcon IMAGEnet i-base V3.23.0 database (Topcon Europe Medical B.V., Capelle Aan De Ijssel, The Netherlands).

The *on*-site ophthalmologist was available at the same time and hospital where the screenings were performed, and reviewed the images outside the screening room. The *on*-site ophthalmologist decided if the image quality was sufficient to plan the screening outcome. The *on*-site ophthalmologist informed the parents on the screening results and outcome. In cases of insufficient images, the *on*-site ophthalmologist decided if the child should be re-examined and by which method (ICON GO® or BIO) to ensure patient safety. All images obtained during the screening session were re-evaluated by an independent *off*-site ophthalmologist within 3 days of the screening session. The *off*-site ophthalmologist worked from a separate office and did not have any direct contact with the patients. The *on*-site and *off*-site ophthalmologist were blinded to each other´s assessment. In cases of disagreement, the *off*-site ophthalmologist´s decision would overrule the *on*-site ophthalmologist. The *off*-site ophthalmologist was also the surgeon who would make the final decision regarding Type 1 ROP treatment. There are no official guidelines regarding treatment for late ROP sequelae, hence these cases were discussed in case of disagreement. Information regarding the child's GA, BW, and PMA on the screening day was available for all ophthalmologists during the image evaluation, as were previously captured images in order to evaluate a possible regression or progression in ROP.

2.4. ROP Classification and Screening Outcome

ROP classification, including stage, zone, and plus disease, was assessed by the ophthalmologists for each eye of every patient according to the third International Classification of ROP [3]. All ophthalmologists used a standard guideline to determine the screening outcome based on the overall ROP evaluation of both eyes, as shown in Table 1. If one eye showed more severe clinical findings, the screening outcome was based on that eye. The ROP treatment criteria for Type 1 were based on the randomized clinical trial titled the Early Treatment for Retinopathy of Prematurity Study (ETROP) [22].

Table 1. Screening outcome depending on ROP classification.

Screening	Treatment
One-week-or-less Follow-up	Type 1 ROP
Zone I: immature vascularization, no ROP	
Zone I: Stage 1 or Stage 2 ROP	Zone I with plus disease
Immature retina extending into posterior Zone II	Zone I Stage 3 without plus
Suspected presence of AP-ROP	Zone II Stage 2 or 3 with plus disease
Stage 3 ROP	
One- to two-week Follow-up	A-ROP
Posterior Zone II: immature vascularization	A-ROP is characterized by the rapid onset of abnormal
Zone II: Stage 2 ROP	neovascularization and severe plus disease, occurring
Zone I: unequivocally regressing ROP	without the chronologic stage progression of ROP
Two-week Follow-up	Hybrid-ROP
Zone II: Stage 1 ROP	
Zone II: no ROP, immature vascularization	Stage 3 including A-ROP characteristics in same eye
Zone II: unequivocally regressing ROP	with plus disease
Two- to three-week Follow-up	
Zone III: Stage 1 or 2 ROP	
Zone III: regressing ROP	
Stop Screening	
PMA > 36 weeks AND no sign of ROP in earlier screenings in Zone I or entire Zone II	
Fully regressed ROP	

Note: Screening and treatment schedule inspired by Fierson et al. (2018) [23]. ROP classification following the current guidelines as defined by ICROP3 [3]. The definition of Hybrid-ROP is as described by Sanghi et al., 2012 [24].

2.5. Data Access and Management

The children's medical files were reviewed prior to each screening session to track where the child was hospitalized and to achieve a status of the general health condition of the child. Information on GA, BW, and PMA was extracted from the medical file. PMA and GA were converted from total days to weeks.

2.6. Statistical Methods

Descriptive statistics for GA, BW, and PMA were tested for normality. Data that were non-parametric or had a small sample size were analyzed using the Mann–Whitney test to assess differences between included and excluded patients. Normally distributed variables were analyzed using the unpaired *t*-test.

The screening outcome was defined as the final conclusion for each session, which included an overall evaluation of both eyes. However, the ROP classification was assessed separately for each eye of every patient by both on-site and off-site ophthalmologists. To simplify the results section, we tested for statistical differences between the eyes. If no significant differences were found between the right and left eyes, we would present the ROP classification for one eye only. Consequently, the kappa statistics were provided for the screening outcome (based on both eyes) and the ROP classification (based on one eye).

The level of agreement regarding the screening outcome and ROP classification (zone, stage, and presence of plus disease) was analyzed by Cohen's kappa. The weighted kappa was presented for each of the three *on*-site ophthalmologists compared with the *off*-site ophthalmologist, as well as for all *on*-site ophthalmologists collectively compared with the *off*-site ophthalmologist. The kappa statistic has a range of k < 0.00 to k = 1, sorted in six categories depending on the value. The strength of the agreement according to the kappa value is graded as poor (k < 0.00), slight (k = 0.00–0.20), fair (k = 0.21–0.40), moderate (k = 0.41–0.60), substantial k = 0.61–0.80), and almost perfect (k = 0.81–1.00) [25]. The *p*-values computed as part of the kappa statistics were not presented, because the assumption of no association was unreasonable [26] (pp. 433–437).

The Chi-square test was performed to analyze the statistical differences between the right and left eyes in the ROP classification (stage, zone, and plus disease) for each of the *on*-site and *off*-site graders. A *p*-value less than 0.05 was considered statistically significant. Data were collected in REDcap (Research Electronic Data Capture, Vanderbilt University, Nashville, TN, USA) and analyzed using Stata 18.5 (StataCorp LLC, College Station, TX, USA).

2.7. Approvals

The Danish Data Protection Agency approved the study (P-2020–1206). Ethical board approval was waived by The Danish National Medical Research Ethics Committee (VMK, decision number VMK-protokol_200921_V1). The legal department at Rigshospitalet decided that the study could be performed by approval from the local head of department.

3. Results

3.1. Study Population Characteristics

A total of 556 screening sessions were performed on 174 patients during the study period. The 141 (25%) screening sessions exclusively performed by an ophthalmologist were excluded from the study. Thus, the study was based on 415 screening sessions (75% of all performed screening sessions) performed by the NPHP on 165 children (53% males). Additionally, nine (5%) patients were exclusively examined by the on-site ophthalmologists, see Figure 1. We examined the data for inclusion bias and found that the excluded patients compared to the included had a significantly higher mean GA (30.9 $\pm$ 0.7 and 28.9 $\pm$ 2.4 weeks, $p = 0.017$), mean BW (1442.6 $\pm$ 176.7 and 1206.9 $\pm$ 394.3 g, $p = 0.04$), and mean PMA at the time of screening (38.01 $\pm$ 4.4 and 36.2 $\pm$ 2.6 weeks, $p = 0.0003$), respectively.

Each child was on average screened 2.5 times by the NPHP during the screening period, ranging from 1 to 12 screening sessions per patient. A total of 97 (58.8%) patients did not develop any ROP (Stage 0), whereas $n = 68$ (41.2%) were graded as having ROP (Stage 1–4A) during the screening period. ROP stage, using the most severe stage encountered for each patient during the screening period, was Stage 1: $n = 3$ (1.8%), Stage 2: $n = 42$ (25.5%), Stage 3: $n = 21$ (12.7%), A-ROP: $n = 1$ (0.6%), Stage 4A: $n = 1$ (0.6%), see Figure 2. The patient evaluated as having ROP Stage 4A was examined using ultrasound in full anesthesia initially before treatment. Here, the surgeon found Stage 3 ROP in all four quadrants but retinal detachment was not observed. No patients were graded as having Stage 4B or 5.

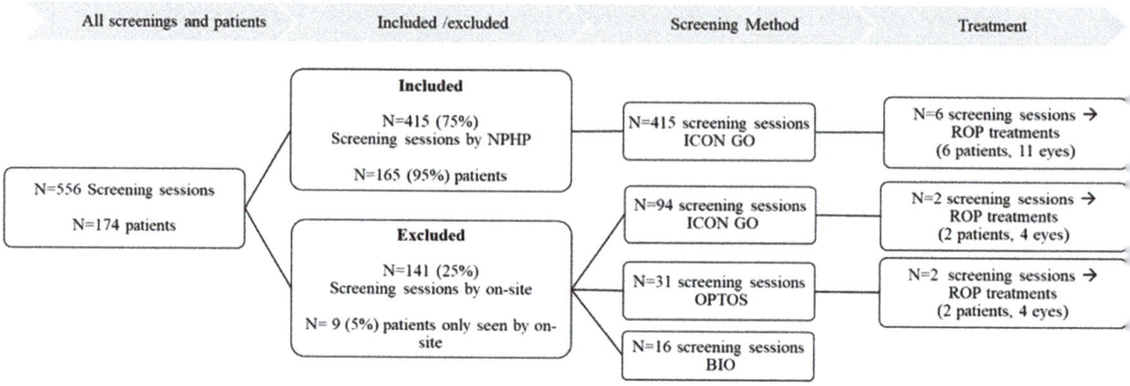

Figure 1. Flowchart of the included patients and screenings during study period. Nine patients received treatment on both eyes, and one patient was treated on the left eye only during the study period. Abbreviations: non-physician healthcare professional (NPHP), binocular indirect ophthalmoscopy (BIO), and retinopathy of prematurity (ROP).

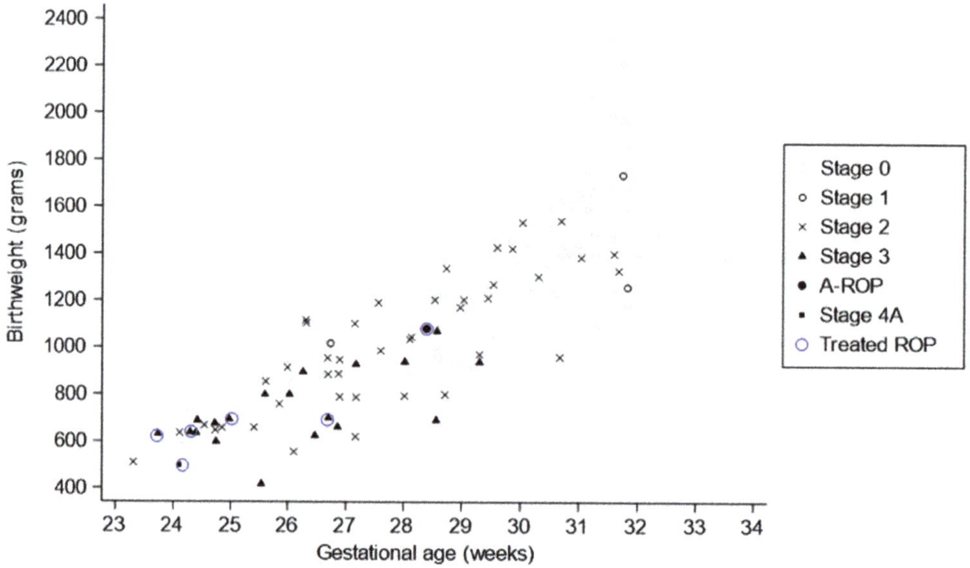

Figure 2. Scatterplot (jitter) of birthweight and gestational age for each patient differentiating the maximum stage of retinopathy of prematurity (ROP) detected during the screening period. Patients receiving treatment for ROP are marked with a blue open circle; the symbol inside the open circle is for the same patient.

Six patients (3.6%) (eleven eyes) included in the study received laser therapy for ROP, see Figure 2. The median PMA at the time of treatment was 36.3 weeks (IQR: 34.9–42.7, range: 33.6–46.7), see Table 2. The decision to treat was based on screening sessions performed by the NPHP, see Figure 1. Four out of six cases were due to Type 1 ROP and A-ROP. The remaining two cases received treatment due to structural changes that did not meet the treatment criteria for Type 1 ROP (e.g., suspicion of retinal traction or fold with or without the presence of hemorrhages or persistent Stage 3 ROP), see Table 3.

Table 2. PMA (weeks) at maximum ROP stage during the study period.

	N (%)	PMA, Median	PMA, (Min–Max)
Any ROP	68 (41.2)	34.6	(31.3–46.7)
Stage 1	3 (1.8)	36.7	(32.1–36.7)
Stage 2	42 (25.5)	34.1	(31.3–39.4)
Stage 3	20 (12.7)	34.9	(31.9–46.7)
A-ROP	1 (0.6)	34.9	(34.9–34.9)
Stage 4A	1 (0.6)	42.7	(42.7–42.7)
Treatment for ROP	6 (3.6)	36.3	(33.6–46.7)

Note: Post-menstrual age (PMA) in weeks tabulated with the maximum stage of retinopathy of prematurity (ROP) during the screening period. No children had re-activated ROP or Stage 4B or 5. PMA at the first treatment for ROP is also presented. Patients who did not develop ROP during the study (n = 97, 58.8%) are not presented in this table.

One patient received treatment on one eye only. Five patients were treated on both eyes; in one of those eyes, the last treatment was performed outside the study period at a PMA of 41 + 4. Additionally, one patient had a maximum Stage 0 seen in Zone II without plus during the study period but received treatment after the end of the study due to progression to post Zone II Stage 3 with plus disease. The screening sessions during the study period but prior to the development of treatment warranting ROP are included in the kappa analyses.

Table 3. Specifications of patients who received treatment for ROP.

ID	GA	BW	ROP Classification and Outcome	Indication	PMA	Weight
166	23 + 5	628	***On*-site** LE: Post. Zone II. Stage 3. Plus Plan: Treatment LE ***Off*-site** LE: Post. Zone II. Stage 3. Plus Plan: Treatment LE	Type 1	36 + 4	2505
172	26 + 5	698	***On*-site** RE: Zone II. Stage 3. Pre-plus LE: Zone II. Stage 3. Pre-plus Plan: Treatment BE ***Off*-site** RE: Post. Zone II. Stage 3. Pre-plus LE: Post. Zone II. Stage 3. Plus Plan: Treatment BE	Type 1	36 + 2	2030
173	25 + 0	698	***On*-site** RE: Zone II. Stage 3. Plus LE: Zone II. Stage 3. Plus Plan: Treatment BE ***Off*-site** RE: Post. Zone II. Stage 3. Plus LE: Post. Zone II. Stage 3. Plus Plan: Treatment BE	Type 1	33 + 5	2080
12	28 + 3	1082	***On*-site** RE: Zone I by notch A-ROP. No plus Plan: Treatment RE ***Off*-site** RE: Zone I by notch A-ROP. No plus Plan: Treatment RE	Other Rapid ROP progression with hemorrhages	35 + 0	1915

Table 3. *Cont.*

ID	GA	BW	ROP Classification and Outcome	Indication	PMA	Weight
66	24 + 1	500	***On*-site** RE: Zone II. Stage 3. Pre-plus LE: Zone II. Stage 4A. Pre-plus Plan: Treatment BE ***Off*-site** RE: Zone II. Stage 3. Pre-plus LE: Zone II. Stage 3. Pre-plus Plan: Screening ≤ 1 week	Other worrisome structural ROP changes	42 + 6	3256
127	24 + 2	640	***On*-site** RE: Zone II. Stage 3. Pre-plus LE: Zone II. Stage 3. Pre-plus Plan: Screening ≤ 1 week ***Off*-site** RE: Post Zone II. Stage 3. Hybrid ROP Pre-plus LE: Zone II. Stage 3. Pre-plus Plan: Treatment BE	Other worrisome structural ROP changes	47 + 5	4100

Note: This table summarizes the patients, screened by the non-physician healthcare professional (NPHP), who received laser therapy treatment for ROP as the first treatment. Abbreviations: right eye (RE), left eye (LE), both eyes (BE), gestational age (GA), birth weight (BW), retinopathy of prematurity (ROP), and post-menstrual age (PMA).

The majority $n = 107$ (65%) had a lightly pigmented fundus, followed by 42 (25%) with a medium pigmented fundus, and lastly 16 (10%) had a dark fundus. Forty-five children (27%) were twins (twenty-two twin pairs, where one twin was excluded because screening was performed only by the on-site ophthalmologist).

3.2. Correlation between Image Quality, Satisfaction, and Fundus Pigmentation

In three (0.7%) screening sessions, the on-site ophthalmologist deemed the images unsatisfactory, while the NPHP had only flagged two of these sessions as unsatisfactory. In the first case, BIO was performed by the on-site ophthalmologist enabling visualization of the ridge, while the NPHP was similarly unsatisfied due to technical difficulties in imaging a darkly pigmented retina. In the second case, the on-site ophthalmologist was unsure whether there was a hemorrhage or an artifact on the images and performed BIO to rule out hemorrhages, while the NPHP was likewise not satisfied with the visualization of Zone II. In the last case, the on-site ophthalmologist supplemented the images with BIO but did not obtain new information; comparatively, the NPHP was satisfied with the image quality.

The off-site ophthalmologist was unsatisfied with two (0.5%) screening sessions. In one case, not all the images had been correctly uploaded to the imaging program; in another case, the ridge was not sufficiently visualized. The screening sessions deemed unsatisfactory by the on-site and off-site ophthalmologists did not overlap. The likelihood of deeming images unsatisfactory increased with greater retinal pigmentation for both the NPHP ($p = 0.0001$) and the on-site ophthalmologist ($p = 0.014$). However, this trend was not observed for the off-site ophthalmologist ($p = 0.26$).

3.3. Agreement on Screening Outcome between On-Site and Off-Site Ophthalmologists

The outcome of the screening session could be to treat ROP, screen again in ≤1 week, 1–2 weeks, 2 weeks, 2–3 weeks, or terminate the screening, based on the worst eye of each patient. We evaluated the level of agreement for the screening outcome between three on-site and one off-site ophthalmologists and found an 'almost-perfect' agreement between all ophthalmologists (k = 0.82, weighted kappa). The screening outcome deviated by one level in sixty-seven (16%) screening sessions, two levels in twenty (5%), and three levels in two (0.5%) screening sessions, see Table 4. No screening outcomes deviated by four or more levels. Although the frequency of disagreement regarding screening outcomes was slightly higher in darkly pigmented retinas, it was not significant. Overall, the frequency of agreement and disagreement did not vary significantly across the different pigmentation levels of light (79.2% and 20.8%), medium (79.3% and 20.7%), or dark (74% and 26%), respectively ($p = 0.69$).

Table 4. Level of agreement for screening outcome based on the most affected eye if unequal.

		Off-Site						
		Treat	**≤1 w**	**1–2 w**	**2 w**	**2–3 w**	**Terminate**	**Total**
***On*-site 1**	**Treat**	4	1	0	0	0	0	5
	≤1 w	0	33	5	0	0	0	38
	1–2 w	0	3	37	4	0	1	45
	2 w	0	0	11	33	0	4	48
	2–3 w	0	0	1	1	0	0	2
	Terminate	0	0	1	2	0	25	28
	Total	4	37	55	40	0	30	166
***On*-site 2**	**Treat**	0	0	0	0	0	0	0
	≤1 w	0	4	8	0	0	0	12
	1–2 w	0	0	27	5	0	0	32
	2 w	0	0	6	41	0	4	51
	2–3 w	0	0	1	0	0	3	4
	Terminate	0	0	0	2	0	49	51
	Total	0	4	42	48	0	56	150
***On*-site 3**	**Treat**	0	0	0	0	0	0	0
	≤1 w	1	12	5	0	0	0	18
	1–2 w	0	0	19	1	0	0	20
	2 w	0	0	5	16	0	1	22
	2–3 w	0	0	2	6	2	2	12
	Terminate	0	0	0	3	0	24	27
	Total	1	12	31	26	2	27	99
***On*-site all**	**Treat**	4	1	0	0	0	0	5
	≤1 w	1	49	18	0	0	0	68
	1–2 w	0	3	83	10	0	1	97
	2 w	0	0	22	90	0	9	121
	2–3 w	0	0	4	7	2	5	18
	Terminate	0	0	1	7	0	98	106
	Total	5	53	128	114	2	113	415

	Agreement	Expected agreement	Kappa, wgt (95% CI)	SE
On-site 1 × *off*-site	94.58%	69.79%	0.82 (0.73–0.88)	0.05
On-site 2 × *off*-site	94.00%	63.80%	0.83 (0.79–0.86)	0.06
On-site 3 × *off*-site	93.54%	67.69%	0.80 (0.77–0.84)	0.07
ALL × *off*-site	94.55%	68.40%	**0.82 (0.82–0.85)**	0.04

Note: Screening outcome tabulated between the *on*-site and *off*-site ophthalmologists' evaluation based on either eye with the most severe retinopathy of prematurity (ROP). The highlighted gray cells are decisions with full agreement. Abbreviations: week (w), weighted (wgt), confidence interval (CI), and standard error (SE).

3.4. Agreement on ROP Classification

Stage, zone, and plus disease did not differ significantly between the right and left eyes for each of the on- and off-site graders ($p > 0.05$). Data in this section are therefore presented for the right eye only.

Stage was categorized as Stage 0, Stage 1, Stage 2, Stage 3, A-ROP, and regression ROP. The level of agreement for ROP stage between the off-site and three on-site ophthalmologists was substantial (weighted kappa k = 0.69). ROP stage deviated by one level in twenty-eight (6%) screening sessions, two levels in twenty-three (5%), three levels in twenty-one (5%), four levels in two (0.5%), and by five levels in the last fifteen (3%) screening sessions, see Table 5.

Table 5. Level of agreement of ROP stage—Right eye.

				***Off*-Site**				
		Stage 0	**Stage 1**	**Stage 2**	**Stage 3**	**A-ROP**	**Reg ROP**	**Total**
***On*-site 1**	**Stage 0**	69	1	3	1	0	1	75
	Stage 1	0	1	0	0	0	0	1
	Stage 2	5	2	32	5	0	0	44
	Stage 3	1	0	5	21	0	2	29
	A-ROP	0	0	0	0	1	0	1
	Reg ROP	0	1	5	0	0	9	15
	Total	75	5	45	27	1	12	165
***On*-site 2**	**Stage 0**	100	0	2	0	0	3	105
	Stage 1	2	1	0	0	0	0	3
	Stage 2	8	1	19	0	0	1	29
	Stage 3	0	0	3	0	0	0	3
	A-ROP	0	0	0	0	0	0	0
	Reg ROP	3	0	5	0	0	2	10
	Total	113	2	29	0	0	6	150
***On*-site 3**	**Stage 0**	43	0	0	0	0	0	43
	Stage 1	0	2	0	0	0	0	2
	Stage 2	1	0	20	2	0	1	24
	Stage 3	0	0	4	9	0	0	13
	A-ROP	0	0	0	0	0	0	0
	Reg ROP	7	1	5	0	0	4	17
	Total	51	3	29	11	0	5	99
***On*-site all**	**Stage 0**	212	1	5	1	0	4	223
	Stage 1	2	4	0	0	0	0	6
	Stage 2	14	3	71	7	0	2	97
	Stage 3	1	0	12	30	0	2	45
	A-ROP	0	0	0	0	1	0	1
	Reg ROP	10	2	15	0	0	15	42
	Total	239	10	103	38	1	23	414

	Agreement	Expected agreement	Kappa, wgt (95% CI)	SE
On-site 1 × *off*-site	92.36%	66.23%	0.77 (0.77–0.83)	0.06
On-site 2 × *off*-site	89.67%	74.94%	0.59 (0.52–0.61)	0.07
On-site 3 × *off*-site	87.12%	60.56%	0.67 (0.65–0.74)	0.07
ALL × *off*-site	90.24%	68.45%	**0.69 (0.64–0.79)**	0.04

Note: Retinopathy of prematurity (ROP) stage tabulated between the on-site and off-site ophthalmologists for the right eyes. Stage evaluations with full agreement are marked in grey. Abbreviations: aggressive ROP (A-ROP), regressed ROP (reg ROP), weighted (wgt), confidence interval (CI), and standard error (SE).

Zone was categorized as Zone I by notch, Zone I, posterior Zone II, Zone II, and Zone III. The weighted kappa between the one off-site and three on-site ophthalmologists was k = 0.37, equivalent to a fair agreement. The frequency of deviations by one level was $n = 92$ (22%) and by two levels was $n = 1$ (0.2%), see Table 6.

Table 6. Level of agreement of ROP Zone—Right eye.

		Off-Site					
		Zone I Notch	**Zone I**	**Post Zone II**	**Zone II**	**Zone III**	**Total**
***On*-site 1**	**Zone I notch**	1	0	0	0	0	1
	Zone I	1	2	2	0	0	5
	Post Zone II	0	1	10	3	0	14
	Zone II	0	1	41	101	0	143
	Zone III	0	0	0	2	0	2
	Total	2	4	53	106	0	165
***On*-site 2**	**Zone I notch**	1	0	0	0	0	1
	Zone I	0	0	2	0	0	2
	Post Zone II	0	0	6	9	0	15
	Zone II	0	0	3	126	0	129
	Zone III	0	0	0	3	0	3
	Total	1	0	11	138	0	150
***On*-site 3**	**Zone I notch**	0	0	0	0	0	0
	Zone I	0	0	2	0	0	2
	Post Zone II	0	0	1	5	0	6
	Zone II	0	0	5	73	0	78
	Zone III	0	0	0	13	0	13
	Total	0	0	8	91	0	99
***On*-site all**	**Zone I notch**	2	0	0	0	0	2
	Zone I	1	2	6	0	0	9
	Post Zone II	0	1	17	17	0	35
	Zone II	0	1	49	300	0	350
	Zone III	0	0	0	18	0	18
	Total	3	4	72	335	0	414

	Agreement	Expected agreement	Kappa, wgt (95% CI)	SE
On-site 1 × *off*-site	92.12%	87.69%	0.36 (0.26–0.46)	0.05
On-site 2 × *off*-site	97.17%	93.99%	0.53 (0.41–0.59)	0.06
On-site 3 × *off*-site	91.58%	90.00%	0.16 (0.10–0.36)	0.05
ALL × *off*-site	94.32%	91.06%	**0.37 (0.37–0.40)**	0.04

Note: Retinopathy of prematurity (ROP) zone tabulated between the *on*-site and *off*-site ophthalmologists for the right eyes. Abbreviations: weighted (wgt), confidence interval (CI), and standard error (SE).

Plus disease was categorized as no plus, pre-plus, and plus. The weighted kappa regarding the presence of plus disease for the right eye was k = 0.69, corresponding to a substantial level of agreement. Deviations by one level were $n = 24$ (6%) on the right eyes, and $n = 25$ (6%) on the left eyes, when comparing all three ophthalmologists, see Table 7. No deviations by two levels occurred (plus versus no plus).

Table 7. Level of agreement of the presence of plus disease—Right eye.

		Off-Site			
		No Plus	**Pre-Plus**	**Plus**	**Total**
***On*-site 1**	**No plus**	134	11	0	145
	Pre-plus	3	16	0	19
	Plus	0	0	1	1
	Total	137	27	1	165
***On*-site 2**	**No plus**	144	3	0	147
	Pre-plus	1	2	0	3
	Plus	0	0	0	0
	Total	145	5	0	150
***On*-site 3**	**No plus**	82	2	0	84
	Pre-plus	4	11	0	15
	Plus	0	0	0	0
	Total	86	13	0	99
***On*-site all**	**No plus**	360	16	0	376
	Pre-plus	8	29	0	37
	Plus	0	0	1	1
	Total	368	45	1	414
	Agreement	Expected agreement	Kappa, wgt (95% CI)		SE
On-site 1 × *off*-site	95.76%	86.91%	0.68 (0.61–0.73)		0.07
On-site 2 × *off*-site	97.33%	94.80%	0.49 (0.06–0.92)		0.08
On-site 3 × *off*-site	93.94%	75.70%	0.75 (0.56–0.94)		0.10
ALL × *off*-site	94.20%	81.70%	**0.69 (0.59–0.77)**		0.05

Note: Presence of plus disease evaluation tabulated between the *on*-site and *off*-site ophthalmologists for the right eyes. Abbreviations: weighted (wgt), confidence interval (CI), and standard error (SE).

4. Discussion

4.1. Main Findings

In this paper, we investigated the feasibility of an NPHP performing ROP screening on prematurely born babies using wide-angle fundus photographs obtained by the ICON GO® camera. Images were evaluated independently by three *on*-site and one *off*-site ophthalmologist. The *on*-site ophthalmologist was present outside the screening room to ensure the safety of the study in cases where screening by the NPHP was deemed insufficient to reach a decision on the screening session outcome. Re-screening by the *on*-site ophthalmologist was performed in three out of four hundred and fifteen screening sessions and in two out of three, the re-examination was beneficial for reaching a decision. Photographs were re-evaluated by an *off*-site ophthalmologist who also had the final decision for the treatment of Type 1 ROP. There was an 'almost-perfect' level of agreement between the *on*-site and *off*-site ophthalmologists regarding the screening outcome, assessed by Cohen's kappa, followed by ROP stage and presence of plus disease, and lastly by ROP Zone in a descending order.

4.2. Defining Good Image Quality

High-quality images are important in order to classify ROP and decide the screening outcome. In our study, the certified NPHP was focused on image quality, including brightness, focus, and visualization of the retinal periphery. The degree of pigmentation of the ocular background played a significant role in the ease of obtaining images of sufficient quality as observed elsewhere [20]. The ophthalmologists had the possibility to improve the image brightness and contrast in the viewing software which was unavailable to the NPHP during the screening session. This indicates that slightly lower quality images may be still useful to make an adequate assessment, which supports the low rate of re-examinations observed in our study [12]. It is crucial to establish a standardized training program for NPHPs who operate widefield cameras during these screenings. The e-ROP study developed a thorough training program that included guidelines for imaging, selecting, and exporting retinal images [27]. This program can be adapted as a model for ROP telescreening, helping to ensure consistent and accurate results.

4.3. Potential Inclusion Bias

Our analysis indicated that the excluded patients were older than the included patients. These findings support the unequal distribution of ROP zone between the groups, with a higher frequency of Zone III involvement in the excluded screening sessions. These results were enhanced by the superior ability of examining Zone III with BIO compared to the camera. In summary, patients at high risk of acute ROP were primarily examined by the NPHP and the study results might overrepresent the most severe cases. Thus, considering the aim of the project, evaluating the feasibility of ROP telescreening performed with the ICON GO®, we do not believe that potential inclusion bias has a negative impact on the clinical implications of our findings.

4.4. Discrepancies in ROP Classification between Ophthalmologists

This is the first Danish study to analyze the feasibility and setup of a telescreening program in detecting ROP performed by an NPHP. Studies have been conducted elsewhere with non-physicians as the technicians [11–13,15,28,29]. These studies have shown promising results with some degree of variability in ROP classification, but a good level of agreement regarding ROP requiring treatment. The study by Campbell et al. presented the total percentage of image-based discrepancies between two experts for zone, stage, and plus disease, 8%, 40%, and 18%, respectively [15]. In comparison, our study showed discrepancies of 22.5% for zone, 19.5% for stage, and 5.7% for plus disease. The inconsistency between the studies can be explained by the fact that more categories were included in our study. For instance, the zone was categorized in I, II, and III, whereas we additionally had Zone I by notch and posterior Zone II. The agreement on defining the ROP zone was notably inconsistent in our study. Zone I is defined as a circular area centered on the optic nerve, with a radius equal to twice the distance from the macula to the optic disc center [3]. This definition does not account for the ocular growth during the neonatal period. A study aimed at predicting the Zone I area found that changes in axial length had the most significant impact [30]. This finding may help explain the discrepancies in ROP zone evaluations. Adopting a standardized template for defining Zone I based on the PMA of the child could potentially improve consistency in future research.

A previous Danish study investigated the inter-rater agreement regarding particularly plus disease. The available fundus photographs captured prior to ROP treatment were evaluated retrospectively by four experts. The level of agreement was inadequate for plus disease; however, a good agreement regarding treatment was presented, comparable to our study [31]. The variability in grading plus disease is concerning as it can determine whether a child receives treatment. This may lead experts to over-diagnose plus disease to meet the treatment criteria for Type 1. Conversely, if the camera applies pressure to the eye during imaging, the retinal vessels might misleadingly appear with less severe plus disease [19].

The level of agreement regarding ROP outcome analyzed with kappa statistics in this study was 'almost-perfect'. During our study, six patients fulfilled our criteria for receiving treatment, of whom three were due to Type 1 ROP and one due to A-ROP. In these cases, there was complete agreement regarding the indication for treatment. Lastly, two had late structural ROP complications, and disagreements regarding treatment occurred. Late structural changes due to ROP seen in children today are not described as part of the recommendations from the ETROP study conducted in 2004 and therefore disagreements among the graders were not surprising [22]. Treatment for ROP, outside the current recommendations, have been reported and are often related to Type 1 in the fellow eye, logistical considerations, Stage 3 with pre-plus, and concerning late structural changes due to ROP [32,33]. Further, these patients often have a PMA > 40 weeks, which also was the case in our study. It is nonetheless reassuring that our telescreening setup showed a 100% feasibility within the current treatment recommendations and additionally managed to represent these cases.

4.5. Strengths and Limitations

We evaluated the feasibility of ROP screening by an NPHP but did not compare to BIO performed on the same patients. We decided against performing both fundus photography and BIO due to the vulnerable condition of the children as this would significantly increase the duration of the examination. Some challenges must be addressed in using widefield cameras in screening for ROP. Firstly, it may prolong the examination time when the NPHP is striving for the best frames to be evaluated by the ophthalmologist compared to BIO performed by an experienced ophthalmologist. Additionally, the patient's family must wait for the ophthalmologist to review the images and cannot be informed about the screening outcome immediately after the screening session. Lastly, a thorough education of healthcare professionals in ROP screening with a widefield camera is essential to ensure patient safety. However, these challenges are deemed manageable, and lessons learned from other telescreening setups could be applied. So far, wide-angled cameras have been evaluated as a reliable supplement for BIO, the gold-standard within ROP screening, but has not yet replaced it [9,28]. With the exponential development of technology, a potential benefit of including artificial intelligence in telescreening for ROP has already been investigated and would expectedly support decision-making in ROP in the nearest future [34]. Telescreening in ROP would be a benefit due to optimized resources within staff, evaluation of ROP in a stressless environment, avoiding unnecessary transfer of preterm babies and their families between hospitals for evaluation, and the possibility of tracking regression and progression in ROP.

Despite a high number of included screening sessions in this study, the number of patients receiving ROP treatment was low. The strength of this study is that all ROP treatments were performed in the same center in Denmark; accordingly, all patients fulfilling our treatment criteria for Type 1 ROP were included.

5. Conclusions

Telescreening with the ICON GO® camera performed by an NPHP showed an 'almost-perfect' agreement regarding screening outcome and the need for re-examinations was negligible. A standardized education and certification for imaging ROP should be setup for healthcare professionals to ensure patient safety. This setup can open up possibilities for implementing telemedicine on a national level in Denmark.

Author Contributions: Conceptualization, C.S. and H.A.A.-A.; methodology, H.A.A.-A., L.K., R.B. and M.D.d.l.C.; software, H.A.A.-A.; validation, R.B. and M.K.; formal analysis, H.A.A.-A.; investigation, H.A.A.-A., R.B., M.K., C.F., A.-C.L., A.G.B. and K.K.; resources, M.B., C.S., R.B. and M.D.d.l.C.; data curation, H.A.A.-A.; writing—original draft preparation, H.A.A.-A.; writing—review and editing, H.A.A.-A., R.B., M.K., C.F., A.-C.L., A.G.B., C.S., K.K., M.B., M.D.d.l.C. and L.K.; visualization, H.A.A.-A.; supervision, H.A.A.-A., R.B., L.K. and M.D.d.l.C.; project administration, H.A.A.-A., L.K. and M.D.d.l.C.; funding acquisition, H.A.A.-A. All authors have read and agreed to the published version of the manuscript.

Funding: This research was funded by Synoptik-Fonden, Fight for sight, Denmark (Værn om Synet), The Danish Eye Research Foundation (Øjenfonden), Fabrikant Ejnar Willumsens Mindelegat (Nr. 500028) and Aase og Ejnar Danielsens Fond (Nr. 23-10-0403), Mette Warburgs foundation, and Dagmar Marshalls Fond.

Institutional Review Board Statement: The study was conducted in accordance with the Declaration of Helsinki and approved by the Institutional Review Board at the department of Ophthalmology—Rigshospitalet and Danish Data Protection Agency (protocol code P-2020-1206, 18th of December 2020). The Danish National Medical Research Ethics Committee (VMK) waived the need for ethical board approval (decision number VMK-protokol_200921_V1, 3rd of February 2022).

Informed Consent Statement: Patient consent was waived due to a decision from The Danish National Medical Research Ethics Committee. ROP screening with widefield camera is a routine part of standard care for all preterm infants meeting national screening criteria. There was no additional risk to patients beyond their usual clinical care.

Data Availability Statement: The fundus photographs generated and analyzed during the current study are not publicly available due to privacy concerns. As the images are identifiable and may reveal the identity of individual patients, they cannot be shared to protect patient confidentiality in accordance with ethical standards. The raw data supporting the conclusions of this article can be made available by the corresponding author on request.

Conflicts of Interest: The authors declare no conflicts of interest. The funders had no role in the design of the study; in the collection, analyses, or interpretation of data; in the writing of the manuscript; or in the decision to publish the results.

eferences

International Committee for the Classification of Retinopathy of Prematurity (ICROP). An international classification of retinopathy of prematurity. Prepared by an international committee. *Br. J. Ophthalmol.* **1984**, *68*, 690–697. [CrossRef] [PubMed]

International Committee for the Classification of Retinopathy of Prematurity (ICROP). The international classification of retinopathy of prematurity revisited: An international committee for the classification of retinopathy of prematurity. *Arch. Ophthalmol.* **2005**, *123*, 991–999. [CrossRef] [PubMed]

International Committee for the Classification of Retinopathy of Prematurity (ICROP). International Classification of Retinopathy of Prematurity, Third Edition. *Ophthalmology* **2021**, *128*, e51–e68. [CrossRef]

Smith, L.E.H. Pathogenesis of retinopathy of prematurity. *Semin. Neonatol.* **2003**, *8*, 469–473. [CrossRef]

Fledelius, H.C.; La Cour, M. Behandlingskrævende præmaturitetsretinopati i Danmark (Danish). *J. Dan. Med. Assoc.* **2004**, *166*, 4360–4362. Available online: https://ugeskriftet.dk/nyhed/behandlingskraevende-praematuritetsretinopati-i-danmark (accessed on 2 September 2024).

Li, J.-P.O.; Liu, H.; Ting, D.S.J.; Jeon, S.; Chan, R.V.P.; Kim, J.E.; Sim, D.A.; Thomas, P.B.M.; Lin, H.; Chen, Y.; et al. Digital technology, tele-medicine and artificial intelligence in ophthalmology: A global perspective. *Prog. Retin. Eye Res.* **2021**, *82*, 100900. [CrossRef]

Jackson, K.M.; Scott, K.E.; Zivin, J.G.; Bateman, D.A.; Flynn, J.T.; Keenan, J.D.; Chiang, M.F. Cost-Utility Analysis of Telemedicine and Ophthalmoscopy for Retinopathy of Prematurity Management. *Arch. Ophthalmol.* **2008**, *126*, 493–499. [CrossRef]

Trese, M.T. What is the real gold standard for ROP screening? *Retina* **2008**, *28*, S1–S2. [CrossRef]

Dhaliwal, C.; Wright, E.; Graham, C.; McIntosh, N.; Fleck, B.W. Wide-field digital retinal imaging versus binocular indirect ophthalmoscopy for retinopathy of prematurity screening: A two-observer prospective, randomised comparison. *Br. J. Ophthalmol.* **2009**, *93*, 355–359. [CrossRef]

). Brady, C.J.; D'amico, S.; Campbell, J.P. Telemedicine for Retinopathy of Prematurity. *Telemed. e-Health* **2020**, *26*, 556–564. [CrossRef]

l. Quinn, G.E.; Ying, G.-S.; Daniel, E.; Hildebrand, P.L.; Ells, A.; Baumritter, A.; Kemper, A.R.; Schron, E.B.; Wade, K.; e-ROP Cooperative Group. Validity of a Telemedicine System for the Evaluation of Acute-Phase Retinopathy of Prematurity. *JAMA Ophthalmol.* **2014**, *132*, 1178–1184. [CrossRef] [PubMed]

2. Morrison, D.; Bothun, E.D.; Ying, G.-S.; Daniel, E.; Baumritter, A.; Quinn, G. Impact of number and quality of retinal images in a telemedicine screening program for ROP: Results from the e-ROP study. *J. Am. Assoc. Pediatr. Ophthalmol. Strabismus* **2016**, *20*, 481–485. [CrossRef]

3. Simkin, S.K.; Misra, S.L.; Han, J.V.; McGhee, C.N.J.; Dai, S. Auckland regional telemedicine retinopathy of prematurity screening network: A 10-year review. *Clin. Exp. Ophthalmol.* **2019**, *47*, 1122–1130. [CrossRef] [PubMed]

4. Ho, T.; Lee, T.C.; Choe, J.Y.; Nallasamy, S. Evaluation of real-time video from the digital indirect ophthalmoscope for telemedicine consultations in retinopathy of prematurity. *J. Telemed. Telecare* **2020**, *28*, 502–507. [CrossRef]

5. Campbell, J.P.; Ryan, M.C.; Lore, E.; Tian, P.; Ostmo, S.; Jonas, K.; Chan, R.P.; Chiang, M.F. Diagnostic Discrepancies in Retinopathy of Prematurity Classification. *Ophthalmology* **2016**, *123*, 1795–1801. [CrossRef]

5. Greenwald, M.F.; Danford, I.D.; Shahrawat, M.; Ostmo, S.; Brown, J.; Kalpathy-Cramer, J.; Bradshaw, K.; Schelonka, R.; Cohen, H.S.; Chan, R.V.P.; et al. Evaluation of artificial intelligence-based telemedicine screening for retinopathy of prematurity. *J. AAPOS* **2020**, *24*, 160–162. [CrossRef]

17. Le Nguyen, T.A.; Raileanu, V.; Smith, B.; Griffin, A.; Shah, S. Excellent accuracy of trained neonatal nurses in the detection o referral-warranted retinopathy of prematurity within an established telemedicine screening programme. *J. Paediatr. Child Healt* **2024**, *60*, 369–374. [CrossRef]
18. Athikarisamy, S.E.; Lam, G.C.; Ross, S.; Rao, S.C.; Chiffings, D.; Simmer, K.; Bulsara, M.K.; Patole, S. Comparison of wide fiel imaging by nurses with indirect ophthalmoscopy by ophthalmologists for retinopathy of prematurity: A diagnostic accurac study. *BMJ Open* **2020**, *10*, e036483. [CrossRef]
19. Tan, Z.; Isaacs, M.; Zhu, Z.; Simkin, S.; He, M.; Dai, S. Retinopathy of prematurity screening: A narrative review of curren programs, teleophthalmology, and diagnostic support systems. *Saudi J. Ophthalmol.* **2022**, *36*, 283–295. [CrossRef]
20. Fan, K.C.; Read, S.P.; Patel, N.A.; Vanner, E.A.; Al-Khersan, H.; Laura, D.M.; Pakravan, P.; Negron, C.I.; Berrocal, A.M. Fundu Pigmentation in the Diagnosis and Treatment of Retinopathy of Prematurity. *Ophthalmology* **2021**, *128*, 1242–1244. [CrossRef]
21. Chan, R.V.P.; Chiang, M.F.; Jonas, K. Retinopathy of Prematurity: Case-Based Training. Available online: https://www.aao.org education/interactive-tool/retinopathy-of-prematurity-case-based-training (accessed on 2 September 2024).
22. Good, W.V. Final results of the early treatment for retinopathy of prematurity (ETROP) randomized trial. *Trans. Am. Ophthalmo Soc.* **2004**, *102*, 233–248. [PubMed] [PubMed Central]
23. Fierson, W.M. Screening examination of premature infants for retinopathy of prematurity. *Pediatrics* **2018**, *142*, e2018306 [CrossRef] [PubMed]
24. Sanghi, G.; Dogra, M.R.; Dogra, M.; Katoch, D.; Gupta, A. A hybrid form of retinopathy of prematurity. *Br. J. Ophthalmol.* **2012**, *9* 519–522. [CrossRef]
25. Landis, J.R.; Koch, G.G. The Measurement of Observer Agreement for Categorical Data. *Biometrics* **1977**, *33*, 159–174. [CrossRef
26. Kirkwood, B.R.; Sterne, J.A.C. *Essential Medical Statistics*, 2nd ed.; Blackwell Publishing Ltd.: Oxford, UK, 2003.
27. e-ROP Cooperative Group. Training retinal imagers for retinopathy of prematurity (ROP) screening. *Physiol. Behav.* **2017**, *17* 139–148. [CrossRef]
28. Maka, E.; Kovács, G.; Imre, L.; Gilbert, C.; Szabó, M.; Németh, J.; Nagy, Z.Z.; Somogyvári, Z. The validity of telemedicine-base screening for retinopathy of prematurity in the Premature Eye Rescue Program in Hungary. *J. Telemed. Telecare* **2021**, *27*, 367–37 [CrossRef]
29. Pasricha, M.V.; Ludwig, C.A.; Moshfeghi, D.M. Stanford University Network for Diagnosis of Retinopathy of Prematurit (SUNDROP): Truly Mobile Teleophthalmology. *Ophthalmic Surg Lasers Imaging Retin.* **2021**, *52*, 11–12. [CrossRef]
30. Wang, S.K.; Korot, E.; Zaidi, M.; Ji, M.H.; Al-Moujahed, A.; Callaway, N.F.; Kumm, J.; Moshfeghi, D.M. Modeling absolute zon size in retinopathy of prematurity in relation to axial length. *Sci. Rep.* **2022**, *12*, 4717. [CrossRef]
31. Slidsborg, C.; Forman, J.L.; Fielder, A.R.; Crafoord, S.; Baggesen, K.; Bangsgaard, R.; Fledelius, H.C.; Greisen, G.; la Cour, M Experts do not agree when to treat retinopathy of prematurity based on plus disease. *Br. J. Ophthalmol.* **2012**, *96*, 549–55 [CrossRef]
32. Lemaître, D.; Barjol, A.; Abdelmassih, Y.; Farnoux, C.; Martin, G.C.; Metge, F.; Chapron, T.; Caputo, G. Treatment outside th recommended guidelines for retinopathy of prematurity (Rop): Prevalence, characteristics, and issues. *J. Clin. Med.* **2022**, *11*, 3 [CrossRef]
33. Liu, T.; Tomlinson, L.A.; Ying, G.S.; Yang, M.B.; Binenbaum, G. Treatment of non–type 1 retinopathy of prematurity in th Postnatal Growth and Retinopathy of Prematurity (G-ROP) study. *J. AAPOS* **2019**, *23*, 332.e1–332.e6. [CrossRef] [PubMed]
34. Coyner, A.S.; Murickan, T.; Oh, M.A.; Young, B.K.; Ostmo, S.R.; Singh, P.; Chan, R.V.P.; Moshfeghi, D.M.; Shah, P.K.; Venkatapath N.; et al. Multinational External Validation of Autonomous Retinopathy of Prematurity Screening. *JAMA Ophthalmol.* **2024**, *14* 327–335. [CrossRef] [PubMed]

Journal of
*Personalized
Medicine*

MDPI

view

)cular Ultrasound in the Diagnosis of Optic Neuropathies: . Review of the Literature

essia Coppola, Giulia Abbinante, Ilaria De Pascale, Vincenzo Gagliardi, Giulio Salerno, Alfonso Pellegrino d Livio Vitiello *

Eye Unit, "Luigi Curto" Hospital, Azienda Sanitaria Locale Salerno, 84035 Polla, Italy;
ccc.coppolaa@aslsalerno.it (A.C.); ccc.abbinanteg@aslsalerno.it (G.A.); i.depascale@aslsalerno.it (I.D.P.);
v.gagliardi@aslsalerno.it (V.G.); gmed.salernog@aslsalerno.it (G.S.); al.pellegrino@aslsalerno.it (A.P.)
* Correspondence: livio.vitiello@gmail.com

Abstract: Background: Optic neuropathies represent one of the most frequent causes of vision loss, and they can manifest alone or in conjunction with neurological or systemic symptoms and signs. In recent years, the diagnostic techniques used to detect optic neuropathies have significantly improved, facilitating diagnosis and improving treatment. Among these, ocular ultrasound has assumed a fundamental role, although with conflicting results in the published scientific literature. For this reason, the aim of this review is to analyze the role of ocular ultrasound in the precise and targeted diagnosis of optic neuropathies to better understand the presumed potential of this precious diagnostic tool in the management of these ocular and neurological disorders. Methods: We carried out a search on PubMed and Scopus utilizing terms related to optic neuropathies and ocular ultrasound, including only relevant English full-length research articles, case reports, or case series. Results: Most of the papers published in the scientific literature use only the B-scan ultrasound technique without considering the more precise and objective standardized A-scan technique that allows for performing more accurate diagnostic tests, such as the "30-degree test" and the "optic nerve exercise test". Conclusions: Future clinical trials and research on optic neuropathies should also consider the use of the standardized A-scan technique in order to compare clinical findings not only with B-scan ultrasonography but also with other noninvasive procedures that could be helpful in reaching the correct diagnosis.

Keywords: glaucoma; ocular ultrasound; optic nerve; optic neuritis; optic neuropathies

1. Introduction

An isolated occurrence of vision loss associated with a more general neurological condition can be caused by disorders of the optic nerve, also known as optic neuropathies. There are many different neurological diseases for which optic neuropathy is frequently the presenting sign, with varied different etiologies [1].

Optic neuropathy is the term used to describe the malfunction and/or degeneration of the optic nerve's axons, which leads to optic nerve atrophy. Axonal injury and death of retinal ganglion cells are typical features of several optic neuropathies [2] (Table 1).

The two main degenerative causes of damage to the optic nerve are glaucoma and optic neuritis [2].

The site of the damage causing the visual loss is the only thing determined by the diagnosis of the optic neuropathy [3,4]. An optic neuropathy cannot be regarded as a disease unto itself; rather, physicians must first categorize the condition based on the assumed mechanism of the optic neuropathy before trying to use ancillary tests to determine the precise etiology of this pathological condition [5,6]. Understanding the impairments that commonly indicate optic neuropathy and the traits of the various causes aids clinicians in reducing a broad differential diagnosis and carrying out a successful diagnostic evaluation [7].

Table 1. Differential diagnosis of optic neuropathy.

Glaucoma
Inflammatory
- Idiopathic inflammatory optic neuritis (often associated with multiple sclerosis)
- Neuromyelitis optica
- Systemic inflammatory and autoimmune diseases
- Infectious diseases
Vascular
- Anterior or posterior
- Arteritic or non-arteritic
- Post-radiation therapy
Compressive or infiltrative
- Neoplastic
- Non-neoplastic
Paraneoplastic
Toxic
Nutritional
Hereditary
Traumatic

Ultrasonographic assessment of the optic nerve sheath diameter (ONSD) has been a popular tool for optic nerve examination in recent years [8–10]. In addition, ultrasonography is a quick, affordable, safe, non-invasive diagnostic technique that may be quite helpful for bedside evaluations of critically ill patients. However, a well-trained and skilled operator is needed to perform a reliable and well-executed ocular ultrasonography for optic nerve assessment, and several precautions should be taken in the exam execution as well as in the employed probe and technique to obtain trustworthy results [11–14].

For this reason, the aim of this review is primarily to illustrate the technique of performing ocular ultrasound for the evaluation of the optic nerve and secondarily to analyze the published scientific literature to highlight the potential role of ocular ultrasound in the evaluation of the optic nerve in cases of different optic neuropathies.

2. Materials and Methods

We utilized two medical databases, PubMed and Scopus, to perform our search. A preliminary general Google search was also performed in order to have a wider viewpoint. Terms like "ocular ultrasonography", "point-of-care ultrasound", "POCUS", "optic neuropathies", "glaucoma", and "optic neuritis" were entered in. The search sentences that were included in the text were either chosen straight from relevant bibliographies or with consideration for the body of current literature. Manual searches of the bibliographies were also carried out in order to find more inclusions. Only English full-length research articles, case reports, or case series pertaining to the ultrasonography assessment of the optic nerve in cases of optic neuropathies were included in this review.

3. Ultrasound Technique

Typically, a high-frequency and high-resolution (5–14 MHz) linear array probe is used for B-scan ultrasonography examinations. Generally, the patients are assessed while lying supine, with the head raised approximately 30–40 degrees.

Most clinicians gently apply a standard ultrasonic gel to the closed eyelid and orient the probe at the right angle to observe the optic nerve insertion.

Nevertheless, as the patient's gaze direction is not visible, this might result in mistakes in the evaluation and measurement of the ONSD and optic nerve. Considering this, skilled ophthalmologists typically perform this diagnostic exam with open lids and with the use of methylcellulose and anesthetic drops, increasing examination accuracy [15,16].

The optic disc is utilized as a reference point for measuring the ONSD from inner edge to inner edge at a distance of 3 mm behind the globe after adjusting the B-scan probe to better view the optic nerve insertion.

Apart from the B-scan examination, "standardized echography" is another well-known ultrasound method in the field of ophthalmology. It is often used with the ultrasonic probe in direct contact with the surface of the eye, combining the A, B, and Doppler methods [15]. This diagnostic method's uniqueness is directly related to the A-scan instrumentation's unique design and standardization. In fact, when analyzing the same structure, standardization enables each examiner to acquire the same echograms, resulting in similar and reproducible findings [15]. Moreover, a patient's age or overall health do not restrict the use of the standardized ultrasonography. However, sedation may be necessary for babies aged six months to three years in order to facilitate a comprehensive and exhaustive examination, while it is performed using only anesthetic drops in adults [15]. Standardized echography can measure the thickness of the optic nerve with an accuracy of +0.3 mm in the retrobulbar space and +0.5 mm in the posterior orbit [15]. Additionally, this ultrasonography method may identify pathological conditions, including meningioma and glioma, as well as neural swelling, increased thickness of the optic nerve sheaths, increased subarachnoid fluid, atrophy, and other disorders [15,17].

Regretfully, B-scan ultrasonography should not be considered an especially objective method of assessing the optic nerve. In fact, when evaluating small anatomical structures, such as the optic nerve, this ultrasound technique, which has been previously evaluated in the literature [18,19], has a number of drawbacks since the B-mode does not have a uniformity of the gain setting [20,21], also known as the "blooming effect" [15,22]. Consequently, this pitfall may be resolved by the standardized A-scan methodology, a blooming effect-free approach that employs an 8 MHz non-focused probe with a customized S-shaped amplification and enables more precise measurements, particularly in the case of the optic nerve assessment [15–23].

This method can also avoid the problem of calipers being positioned incorrectly and yield more accurate and exact findings by clearly showing strong reflecting spikes from the interface between arachnoid and subarachnoid fluid [15].

In addition, the standardized A-scan examination may be used to perform the "30-degree test" [11]. This test allows for clinicians to differentiate between an increase in ONSD caused by raised intracranial pressure related to increased subarachnoid fluid and an increase in ONSD caused by other disorders, such as optic neuritis or optic nerve meningioma. This maneuver is carried out with the patient looking straight ahead and then to the lateral side in healthy and cooperative patients. If this test demonstrates a decrease in the maximal diameter of at least 5%, it will demonstrate intracranial hypertension caused by increased subarachnoidal fluid, which causes ONSD distension; on the other hand, a solid lesion of the optic nerve or its inflammatory process will not lead to this reduction [11,15] (Figure 1).

Finally, the "optic nerve exercise test" can be used to rule out optic nerve compartment syndrome. In this case, the patient will be asked to look for 15 to 20 s at the very right and left lateral sides in turn throughout this test. This three-minute test is followed by a two-minute eye closure to allow for the subarachnoid fluid—which was driven out of the orbit during the exercise—to return to the baseline position. In healthy people, the orbital subarachnoid fluid frequently returns to its baseline level, unlike what happens in the presence of optic nerve compartment syndrome [14].

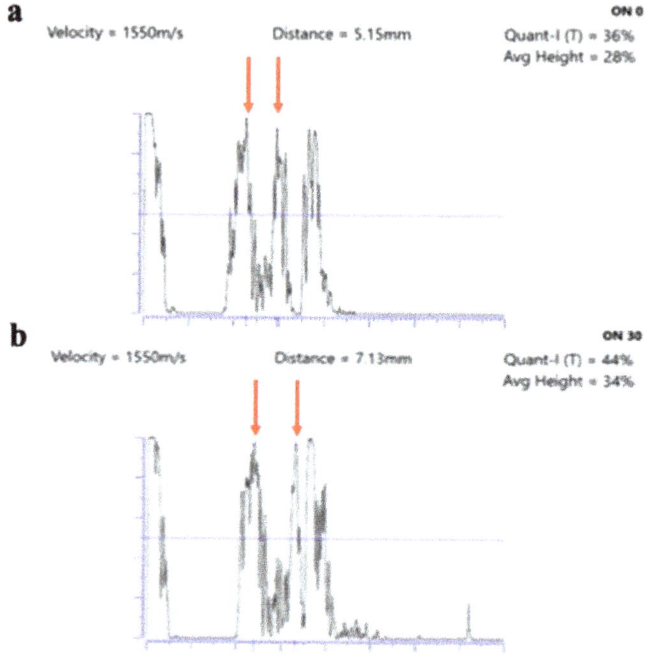

Figure 1. Standardized A-scan ultrasonography of a patient in the primary gaze position (**a**) with an enlargement of the optic nerve (5.15 mm). After the "30-degree test", (**b**) it is possible to observe the non-reduction in the distance between the hyperreflective peaks (red arrows—7.13 mm), thus demonstrating an increase in the thickness of the optic nerve not related to an increase in intracranial pressure.

4. Ocular Ultrasound in Glaucoma

Considering the previously described ultrasound technique [15], it can be used in the same way for the evaluation of the optic nerve in all the optic neuropathies. In particular, for the B-scan, the probe is placed in the temporal portion of the open eye in the primary gaze direction and is tilted until the optic nerve insertion is visualized; on the other hand, when the standardized A-scan technique is performed, the probe is always placed temporally, but this time, the peaks corresponding to the medial rectus muscle are first visualized using it as a reference point. Subsequently, the probe is tilted to identify the peaks corresponding to the optic nerve so that its measurement can be carried out [15]. However, as previously stated, the standardized A-scan technique requires the operator to be skilled in this type of diagnostic evaluation [16–23].

One of the main and most widespread diseases of the optic nerve is certainly glaucoma. Kerlen, in the 1980s, already stated how the optic nerve of glaucomatous patients could be evaluated through excavation of the disc with B-scan ultrasonography, even with media opacities [24]. Conversely, the use of ocular ultrasound in glaucomatous patients to evaluate any other alterations affecting the optic nerve is quite controversial, considering that there are also few published papers on this challenging topic [25–28].

Abegão Pinto and colleagues [25] were the first to investigate with B-scan ultrasound how ONSD differs between glaucomatous patients and healthy people. They enrolled 46 patients with normal-tension glaucoma (NTG) (patients with optic disc damage and visual field loss), 61 patients with primary open-angle glaucoma (POAG) (patients with untreated intraocular pressure of 21 mmHg or above), and 42 healthy control subjects. They found that ONSD did not significantly differ between healthy, NTG, and POAG patients, with no correlation between visual field damage and ONSD in either of the glaucoma groups. On the other hand, ONSD was found to be correlated with intraocular pressure only in NTG patients. For this reason, the authors hypothesized that the translaminar pressure gradient may play a special role in this particular form of glaucoma [25].

Willekens et al. [26] tried to determine the influence of retrobulbar hemodynamics on ONSD values in glaucomatous patients evaluated by ultrasound color Doppler imaging. In particular, they assessed 88 POAG patients, 58 NTG patients, and 51 healthy controls, and they did not find any significant differences in ONSD between the three study groups, while ONSD was found to be negatively correlated with retrobulbar blood flow velocities in glaucomatous patients but not in healthy controls.

In 2018, Liu et al. [27] studied the optic nerve with ultrasound in 40 NTG patients and 42 POAG patients, comparing them with 46 healthy controls, analyzing the effect that low cerebrospinal fluid pressure in the subarachnoid space of the retrobulbar optic nerve (ONSASA) has on the trans-lamina cribrosa pressure difference in NTG. The results showed that ONSASA was significantly smaller in the NTG group compared to the POAG or control groups, confirming the importance that cerebrospinal fluid pressure has on the trans-lamina cribrosa pressure difference in the NTG etiopathogenesis.

Finally, Omatiga and co-authors [28] evaluated 60 glaucomatous adults and 60 healthy age- and sex-matched individuals to sonographically assess potential changes in the ONSD between the two groups, finding the ONSD of the glaucomatous eyes to be substantially thinner compared to the matching control eyes.

In conclusion, considering the conflicting results and the presence of few clinical studies, further studies are needed to better understand the potential role of the ultrasound ONSD and ocular ultrasonography in the diagnosis and management of glaucoma.

5. Ocular Ultrasound in Acute Optic Neuritis

The usefulness of ocular ultrasound in evaluating the optic nerve in cases of inflammatory processes, such as optic neuritis, has been known since the 1980s [15,24,29]. In fact, with B-scan ultrasonography, it is also possible to appreciate the presence of papilledema at the optic nerve insertion, with an elevation of the optic disc (Figure 2).

Several published papers already analyzed the role of ocular ultrasonography in the diagnosis and management of acute optic neuritis.

In the 1990s, a great emphasis was placed on the analysis of the optic nerve with the standardized A-scan method, and Dees et al. [30] performed a pilot study of 27 patients by performing B-scan and standardized A-scan ultrasound on patients presenting with optic neuritis. The 30-degree test was considered to be positive if the swelling decreased by at least 10% on abduction. They classified three groups of patients according to their ultrasound characteristics: normal nerves, swollen nerves with a positive 30-degree test, and swollen nerves with a negative 30-degree test. The results showed a substantial increase in optic nerve diameter in 74% of cases and a positive correlation between nerve swelling and the severity of initial visual loss.

During the same years, Elvin et al. [31] emphasized the importance of Doppler ultrasonography in optic neuritis to determine nerve morphology, nerve swelling, and resistance to flow in the central retinal artery, correlating them with magnetic resonance imaging and visual evoked potentials. The ultrasound examinations were performed on a dynamic scanner with a 7.5 MHz linear transducer within a mean of 27 days of the onset of symptoms. A statistically significant difference was found in the optic nerve diameter and in the resistance to flow in the central retinal artery between the affected and unaffected eyes, confirming the possibility of using Doppler as an indicator of optic nerve inflammation activity.

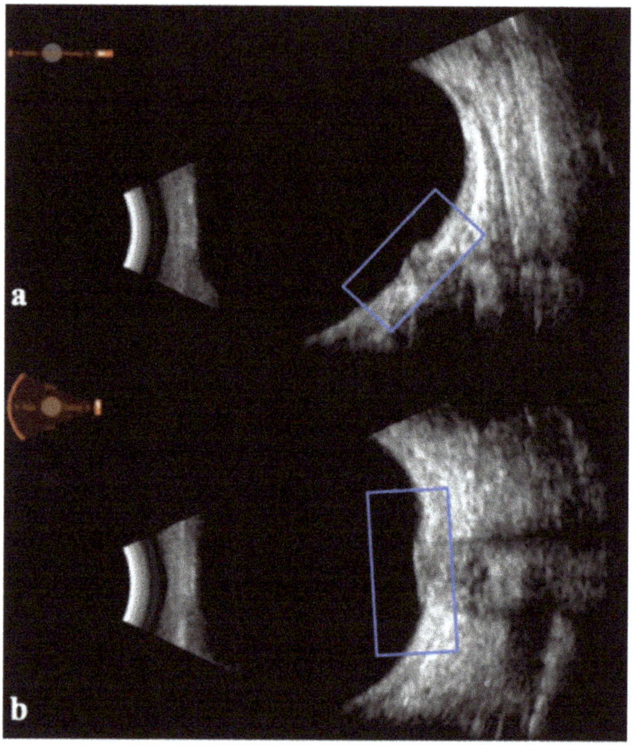

Figure 2. B-scan ultrasonography of the optic nerve insertion in the sagittal (**a**) and transversal (**b**) planes in a patient with papilledema. It is possible to observe the prominence of the optic disc (blue box).

The possibility of increasing the quality of diagnosis with Doppler ultrasound of the optic nerve was also taken up some years later by Karaali et al. [32] and Karami et al. [33].

The first ones evaluated orbital blood flow velocities with Doppler sonography in 20 patients with acute unilateral optic neuritis, and they found that peak systolic and end diastolic velocities in the ophthalmic artery were significantly increased in the affected orbits.

On the other hand, Karami et al. [33] subverted the conception of Doppler ultrasound for studying the optic nerve because, contrary to the previous studies [31,32], they showed that there were no significant differences in orbital blood flow parameters between the eye with optic neuritis and the healthy contralateral eye of the 23 enrolled patients.

Lochner and colleagues [34–36] also utilized B-scan ultrasonography to evaluate the possibility to measure optic nerve diameter and ONSD in patients affected by unilateral optic neuritis, comparing them with healthy controls. They found a statistically significant difference between the two groups in all their clinical research, with a significant thickening of the ONSD in the patients affected by optic neuritis.

In addition, several case reports and case series analyzed the role of ocular ultrasound in detecting optic neuritis in the emergency department [37–39].

Wayman and Carmody [37] assessed a 37-year-old diabetic patient complaining of visual loss in the left eye, initially without pain and then with a feeling of pressure on the eye. He underwent a B-scan ultrasonography, which revealed an ONSD dilatation of 6.21 mm and an elevation of the optic disc, both consistent with papilledema or an optic disc swelling. The diagnosis of optic neuritis was then confirmed following an ophthalmological and neurological consultation, also performing a brain magnetic resonance imaging.

Similarly, in two other case series [38,39], the authors were able to make a diagnosis of optic neuritis thanks to the patient's symptoms and clinical signs and by carrying out an ocular ultrasound with the B-scan method, which revealed a notable thickening of the affected ONSD compared to the healthy contralateral eye.

6. Ocular Ultrasound in Optic Neuritis Related to Demyelinating Disorders

Optic neuritis, particularly retrobulbar optic neuritis, can also represent the initial symptom of a central nervous system disease: in particular, demyelinating disorders such as multiple sclerosis [40].

The role of optic nerve ultrasound examination in evaluating retrobulbar optic neuritis was studied in 2005 by Titlić et al. [41] and in 2010 by Stefanović et al. [42].

Titlić et al. [41] prospectively evaluated 20 patients with multiple sclerosis and compared the results with those obtained by magnetic resonance imaging. They found that the diameter of the optic nerve with retrobulbar neuritis showed statistically significant differences from the healthy one and correlated significantly with the number of multiple sclerosis brain lesions.

Stefanović et al. [42], instead, used the B-scan method in 23 patients presenting with retrobulbar optic neuritis and papillitis. Similar to the study performed by Dees et al. [30], they also performed the 30-degree test during the optic nerve assessment. The results showed that the retrobulbar region of the optic nerve was thicker in 94% of the patients with retrobulbar neuritis and in all the patients with papillitis, also finding a correlation between the reduction in visual acuity and the thickening of the retrobulbar region of the optic nerve.

Raeesmohammadi and colleagues [43] sonographically evaluated 60 patients affected by multiple sclerosis who had not recently received an optic neuritis diagnosis, comparing them with 60 healthy sex- and age-matched volunteers. They found that, when optic nerve diameter and ONSD were evaluated by ocular ultrasound, the patients affected by multiple sclerosis who were not currently experiencing an optic neuritis had considerably lower levels than their healthy controls, indicating a gradual subclinical axonal loss.

Similar results were also detected by De Masi et al. [44] and Schroeder et al. [45] who found optic nerve diameter and ONSD evaluated with ocular ultrasound were smaller in patients affected by multiple sclerosis compared to healthy controls, suggesting a chronic depletion of axons in this demyelinating disorder.

Conversely, Elkholy et al. [46] assessed 25 patients with a first attack of an acute demyelinating optic neuritis compared to 25 healthy subjects using ocular ultrasound, showing a significant thickening of ONSD compared to the controls. Furthermore, they also found the ONSD thickness and visual acuity to be significantly inversely correlated.

An increased ultrasound ONSD in the case of patients with optic neuritis related to multiple sclerosis was also found by Saigh et al. [47] and Kwon et al. [48], while Koraysha and colleagues [49] found no significant differences of optic nerve diameter and ONSD between the patients' group and control group.

In addition, Krogias et al. [50] evaluated 34 optic nerves from 17 patients affected by chronic inflammatory demyelinating polyradiculoneuropathy compared to 30 optic nerves from 15 healthy subjects. Optic nerve diameter and ONSD were sonographically measured, with no significant differences between the two study groups.

Finally, Candeliere Merlicco and co-authors [51] aimed to evaluate the utility of transorbital ultrasonography in the quantification of optic nerve atrophy in multiple sclerosis patients and to determine whether optic nerve atrophy correlates with the disease duration and disability. They enrolled 59 patients diagnosed with relapsing–remitting multiple sclerosis and 36 healthy controls. The ultrasound ONSD was found to be smaller in the patients with multiple sclerosis and to be correlated with the Expanded Disability Status Scale and with the duration of the disease without being interfered by the previous history of optic neuritis.

In conclusion, in cases of demyelinating diseases, the results present in the literature are conflicting, as the thickness of the ONSD measured with ocular ultrasound is variable based on the state of the disease and the presence of acute inflammation of the optic nerve. In fact, in the presence of an acute inflammatory process, the ONSD is increased in thickness, while in the presence of a demyelinating disorder alone, the ONSD is reduced in size compared to healthy controls.

The main findings published in the scientific literature related to optic neuritis are summarized in Table 2.

Table 2. Summary of the studies analyzing the role of ocular ultrasound in optic neuritis.

Authors (Year)	Ref.	N. Patients	Ultrasound Technique	Outcomes
Dees et al. (1995)	[30]	27 patients with idiopathic optic neuritis	B-scan and standardized A-scan techniques	Substantial increase in optic nerve diameter in 74% of cases and a positive correlation between nerve swelling and the severity of initial visual loss.
Elvin et al. (1998)	[31]	18 patients with a clinical diagnosis of optic neuritis	Doppler ultrasonography	A statistically significant difference was found in the optic nerve diameter and in the resistance to flow in the central retinal artery between the affected and unaffected eyes, confirming the possibility of using Doppler as an indicator of optic nerve inflammation activity.
Karaali et al. (2003)	[32]	20 patients with acute unilateral optic neuritis	Doppler ultrasonography	Peak systolic and end diastolic velocities in the ophthalmic artery were significantly increased in the affected eyes.
Karami et al. (2012)	[33]	23 patients with acute unilateral optic neuritis	Doppler ultrasonography	No significant differences were found in orbital blood flow parameters between the eye with optic neuritis and the healthy contralateral eye.
Lochner et al. (2017)	[34]	23 patients with unilateral optic neuritis and 19 sex- and age-matched healthy controls	B-scan ultrasonography	Optic nerve sheath diameter and optic nerve diameter are increased in the affected eye.
Lochner et al. (2014)	[35]	21 patients with unilateral optic neuritis and 21 sex- and age-matched healthy controls	B-scan ultrasonography	The median optic nerve sheath diameter and optic nerve diameter were thicker on the affected side compared with the nonaffected side and controls.
Lochner et al. (2017)	[36]	45 patients with newly diagnosed optic neuritis	B-scan ultrasonography	The median optic nerve sheath diameter was thicker on the affected side compared with the nonaffected side.
Wayman and Carmody (2014)	[37]	37-year-old diabetic patient complaining of visual loss in the left eye	B-scan ultrasonography	Optic nerve sheath diameter was found to be 6.21 mm with an elevation of the optic disc. The diagnosis of optic neuritis was then confirmed following an ophthalmological and neurological consultation, also performing a brain magnetic resonance imaging.
Badron and Ong (2019)	[38]	15-year-old girl with optic neuritis	B-scan ultrasonography	Transorbital ultrasound revealed an irregularly enlarged optic nerve sheath with increased optic nerve sheath diameter (5.1 mm) and an elevated optic disc height (0.5 mm). The ultrasound findings correlated well with her magnetic resonance imaging of her orbit.
Yee et al. (2019)	[39]	A 35-year-old man, a 48-year-old man, a 34-year-old female, and a 28-year-old female with optic neuritis	B-scan ultrasonography	Optic nerve sheath diameters of the affected eyes were all found to be more than 5.5 mm.
Titlić et al. (2005)	[41]	20 patients with multiple sclerosis and retrobulbar neuritis	B-scan ultrasonography	The diameter of the optic nerve with retrobulbar neuritis showed statistically significant differences from the healthy one and correlated significantly with the number of multiple sclerosis brain lesions.
Stefanović et al. (2010)	[42]	23 patients presenting with retrobulbar optic neuritis and papillitis	B-scan and standardized A-scan techniques	The retrobulbar region of the optic nerve was found to be thicker in 94% of the patients with retrobulbar neuritis and in all the patients with papillitis, also finding a correlation between the reduction in visual acuity and the thickening of the retrobulbar region of the optic nerve.
Raeesmohammadi et al. (2020)	[43]	60 patients affected by multiple sclerosis who had not recently received an optic neuritis diagnosis, and 60 healthy sex- and age-matched volunteers.	B-scan ultrasonography	Patients affected by multiple sclerosis who were not currently experiencing an optic neuritis had considerably lower levels of optic nerve sheath diameter and optic nerve diameter than their healthy controls, indicating a gradual subclinical axonal loss.
De Masi et al. (2016)	[44]	60 unselected relapse-free multiple sclerosis patients and 35 matched healthy controls	B-scan ultrasonography	Optic nerve diameter and optic nerve sheath diameter evaluated with ocular ultrasound were found to be smaller in patients affected by multiple sclerosis compared to healthy controls, suggesting a chronic depletion of axons.

Table 2. *Cont.*

Authors (Year)	Ref.	N. Patients	Ultrasound Technique	Outcomes
Schroeder et al. (2020)	[45]	78 patients with a history of demyelinating disorders	B-scan ultrasonography	Optic nerve diameter and optic nerve sheath diameter evaluated with ocular ultrasound were found to be smaller in patients affected by multiple sclerosis compared to healthy controls, suggesting a chronic depletion of axons.
Elkholy et al. (2020)	[46]	25 patients with a first attack of an acute demyelinating optic neuritis compared to 25 healthy subjects	B-scan ultrasonography	A significant thickening of optic nerve sheath diameter was found compared to controls. Furthermore, optic nerve sheath diameter thickness and visual acuity were found to be significantly inversely correlated.
Saigh et al. (2019)	[47]	59-year-old female patient with progressive unilateral visual loss while she was receiving outpatient treatment for relapsing–remitting multiple sclerosis	B-scan ultrasonography	Transorbital ultrasound revealed a disparity between the optic nerve sheath diameters of the affected and nonaffected eyes and striking optic nerve edema in the affected eye, thus diagnosing an acute optic neuritis.
Kwon et al. (2019)	[48]	17 patients with first-attack unilateral acute optic neuritis	B-scan ultrasonography	Ocular ultrasonography revealed thickening of the optic nerve diameter and optic nerve sheath diameter on the affected side compared with the unaffected side.
Koraysha et al. (2019)	[49]	23 patients affected by relapsing–remitting multiple sclerosis with a history of optic neuritis, 26 patients affected by relapsing–remitting multiple sclerosis without a history of optic neuritis, and 50 age- and sex-matched healthy controls	B-scan ultrasonography	No significant differences of optic nerve diameter and optic nerve sheath diameter were found between the patients' group and control group.
Krogias et al. (2016)	[50]	17 patients affected by chronic inflammatory demyelinating polyradiculoneuropathy compared to 15 healthy subjects	B-scan ultrasonography	Optic nerve diameter and optic nerve sheath diameter showed no significant differences between the two study groups.
Candeliere Merlicco et al. (2018)	[51]	59 patients diagnosed with relapsing–remitting multiple sclerosis and 36 healthy controls	B-scan ultrasonography	The ultrasound optic nerve sheath diameter was found to be smaller in patients with multiple sclerosis and to be correlated with the Expanded Disability Status Scale and with the duration of the disease without being interfered by the previous history of optic neuritis.

7. Ocular Ultrasound in Other Optic Neuropathies

In 1997, Gerling et al. [52] used ultrasound to study optic nerve diameter in idiopathic optic neuritis and anterior ischemic optic neuropathy. They evaluated 25 patients, 16 with idiopathic optic neuritis and 9 with anterior ischemic optic neuropathy, with a B-scan ultrasound (10 MHz); the probe was placed on the closed upper eyelid while the patient looked temporally. The optic nerve diameter in the patients with optic neuritis with and without disc swelling was significantly larger than that in the contralateral healthy eye. This difference was not confirmed in the patients with anterior ischemic optic neuropathy, and this can be explained by the fact that, in the patients with idiopathic optic neuritis with and without disc swelling, the enlargement of the optic disc is probably caused by an inflammatory edema, which is not present in the case of a vascular optic neuropathy.

Similarly, Dehghani and colleagues [53] evaluated the usefulness of B-scan ultrasonography in distinguishing optic neuritis from non-arteritic anterior ischemic optic neuropathy by measuring the diameter of the optic nerve. They compared 10 consecutive patients with optic neuritis, 10 patients with non-arteritic anterior ischemic optic neuropathy, 10 young controls, and 10 elderly controls. The diameter of the optic nerve was measured using B-scan ultrasonography (13 MHz) by a single radiologist who was not aware of the diagnosis or the side of the lesion. In the optic neuritis patients, the mean diameter of the affected nerve was significantly larger than that of the unaffected nerve and also larger than that of the healthy controls. On the other hand, in the non-arteritic anterior ischemic optic neuropathy patients, there was no significant difference between the mean diameter of the affected nerves and the control group. Moreover, the diameter of the affected nerve was significantly larger in the optic neuritis patients than in the non-arteritic anterior ischemic optic neuropathy patients. For this reason, the authors concluded that B-scan ultrasonography is helpful in the early stages of optic neuropathy to distinguish optic neuritis from non-arteritic anterior ischemic optic neuropathy in those cases for which the diagnosis is still uncertain after clinical evaluation.

Finally, Ji et al. [54] evaluated the ONSD in eyes with dysthyroid optic neuropathy (DON) and its relationship with clinical characteristics and disease severity. A total of 47 healthy eyes, 36 thyroid-associated ophthalmopathy (TAO) eyes without DON, and 33 eyes with DON were studied. All subjects underwent transbulbar B-scan ultrasonography performed by a single investigator using a 10 MHz probe. The authors demonstrated that ONSDs measured at 3 mm and 6 mm of DON eyes were significantly higher than those in non-DON eyes and healthy eyes, showing that ONSD can be potentially used to distinguish DON eyes from non-DON eyes, although the ultrasound ONSD characteristics of chronic DON eyes need to be further examined.

8. Discussion

Nowadays, optic neuropathy represents a very dangerous pathological disorder for vision as well as often being the presenting sign of more complex systemic diseases [1,2]. For this reason, a quick and timely diagnosis of this pathological condition could be crucial in order to best manage and treat this clinical entity, thus limiting complications.

This gap may be filled by using ultrasound measurement of ONSD, which has been demonstrated to be a safe, noninvasive bedside diagnostic method that allows for the early start of therapy and the real-time assessment of optic neuropathies. In this therapeutic context, it appears to have unrealized potential even though it is not a revolutionary method [15].

Currently, the biggest pitfall is the substantial variation in ultrasound ONSD reported in the clinical research, as evidenced by conflicting cut-off value results and morphological findings from the published scientific literature pertaining to various optic neuropathies, particularly optic neuritis and glaucoma. Since the B-scan is the diagnostic tool that clinicians use most frequently to assess optic nerves, it is possible that the primary cause of this problem is the lack of uniformity in this ultrasound method. In fact, as previously mentioned in this review, B-scan ultrasonography—which is known to be affected by the "blooming effect" that is connected to the lack of a uniform gain setting—was used in all of the included articles [25–54] with the exception of the papers by Dees et al. [30] and Stefanović et al. [42]. Indeed, these papers appear to be the most methodically correct studies because A-scan analysis and the 30-degree test were performed to avoid bias, as previously suggested by Ossoinig [15], even though they are almost 30-year-old and 14-year-old studies, respectively, and they did not analyze a large number of patients.

Considering the "blooming effect", bias may also have an impact on the calipers' position when performing ONSD measurements, changing the objectivity and dependability of the results. Furthermore, the B-scan examination was carried out with the patient's eyelids closed in all of these publications [25–54], which might have resulted in mistakes in the evaluation and measurement of ONSD since the patient's gaze direction was not clearly visible.

For all the above-mentioned B-scan ultrasonography drawbacks, it is recommended to combine the B-scan technique with the standardized A-scan technique [11–23] to provide data that are as exact, unbiased, consistent, and accurate as feasible. In this way, it is possible to undertake a thorough ultrasound examination with far less bias and no loss of important clinical information, leading to more accurate clinical findings.

Currently, regardless of the potential usefulness of ocular ultrasound in the evaluation of the optic nerve, its use is still limited in the management of optic neuropathies, considering the conflicting scientific results and that they can also be identified clinically. However, the role of ocular ultrasound can be decisive in distinguishing a thickening of the optic nerve linked to an inflammatory process or to an increase in subarachnoid fluid, thanks to the use of the "30-degree test" previously described [15].

The main limitations of this review are its non-systematic and basically narrative nature and having used only two scientific databases (PubMed and Scopus) for its drafting.

9. Conclusions

In conclusion, in order to compare clinical findings not just with B-scan ultrasonography but also with other noninvasive procedures that could be helpful in reaching the correct diagnosis in cases of optic neuropathies, future clinical trials and research carried out on this pathological condition should also utilize the standardized A-scan technique. Furthermore, rather than relying on only ultrasound ONSD, it is crucial to highlight that the assessment of optic neuropathies should be carried out in tandem with accessible data from clinical examinations and other diagnostic techniques, correlating them with each other.

Author Contributions: A.C., G.A., I.D.P., V.G. and G.S. analyzed the literature and wrote the original draft. A.P. and L.V. conceived the article and reviewed the manuscript. All authors have read and agreed to the published version of the manuscript.

Funding: This research received no external funding.

Institutional Review Board Statement: Not applicable.

Informed Consent Statement: Not applicable.

Data Availability Statement: No new data were created or analyzed in this study. Data sharing is not applicable to this article.

Conflicts of Interest: The authors declare no conflicts of interest.

References

Biousse, V.; Newman, N.J. Diagnosis and clinical features of common optic neuropathies. *Lancet Neurol.* **2016**, *15*, 1355–1367. [CrossRef] [PubMed]

You, Y.; Gupta, V.K.; Li, J.C.; Klistorner, A.; Graham, S.L. Optic neuropathies: Characteristic features and mechanisms of retinal ganglion cell loss. *Rev. Neurosci.* **2013**, *24*, 301–321. [CrossRef] [PubMed]

Sandbach, J.M.; Newman, N.J. Retinal masqueraders of optic nerve disease. *Ophthalmol. Clin. N. Am.* **2001**, *14*, 41–59.

Weerasinghe, D.; Lueck, C. Mimics and chameleons of optic neuritis. *Pract. Neurol.* **2016**, *16*, 96–110. [CrossRef]

Shapey, J.; Sabin, H.I.; Danesh-Meyer, H.V.; Kaye, A.H. Diagnosis and management of optic nerve sheath meningiomas. *J. Clin. Neurosci.* **2013**, *20*, 1045–1056. [CrossRef]

Gaier, E.D.; Boudreault, K.; Rizzo, J.F., 3rd; Falardeau, J.; Cestari, D.M. Atypical Optic Neuritis. *Curr. Neurol. Neurosci. Rep.* **2015**, *15*, 76. [CrossRef]

Rizzo, J.F., 3rd; Lessell, S. Optic neuritis and ischemic optic neuropathy. Overlapping clinical profiles. *Arch. Ophthalmol.* **1991**, *109*, 1668–1672. [CrossRef]

Lochner, P.; Leone, M.A.; Coppo, L.; Nardone, R.; Zedde, M.L.; Cantello, R.; Brigo, F. B-mode transorbital ultrasononography for the diagnosis of acute optic neuritis. A systematic review. *Clin. Neurophysiol.* **2016**, *127*, 803–809. [CrossRef] [PubMed]

Rosa, N.; De Bernardo, M.; Di Stasi, M.; Cione, F.; Capaldo, I. A-Scan Ultrasonographic Evaluation of Patients with Idiopathic Intracranial Hypertension: Comparison of Optic Nerves. *J. Clin. Med.* **2022**, *11*, 6153. [CrossRef]

10. Rosa, N.; De Bernardo, M.; Abbinante, G.; Vecchio, G.; Cione, F.; Capasso, L. Optic Nerve Drusen Evaluation: A Comparison between Ultrasound and OCT. *J. Clin. Med.* **2022**, *11*, 3715. [CrossRef]

11. De Bernardo, M.; Vitiello, L.; Rosa, N. A-scan ultrasonography and optic nerve sheath diameter assessment during acute elevations in intra-abdominal pressure. *Surgery* **2020**, *167*, 1023–1024. [CrossRef] [PubMed]

12. De Bernardo, M.; Vitiello, L.; Rosa, N. Optic nerve sheath diameter ultrasonography in differentiation of ischemic and hemorrhagic strokes. *Am. J. Emerg. Med.* **2019**, *37*, 1384–1385. [CrossRef] [PubMed]

13. De Bernardo, M.; Vitiello, L.; Capone, M.; Rosa, N. A-scan ultrasonography and optic nerve sheath diameter evaluation in children with acute liver failure. *Liver Int.* **2020**, *40*, 1504. [CrossRef]

14. De Bernardo, M.; Vitiello, L.; Rosa, N. Ocular ultrasonography to detect intracranial pressure in aneurysmal subarachnoid hemorrhage. *Ann. Clin. Transl. Neurol.* **2020**, *7*, 1459–1460. [CrossRef]

15. Ossoinig, K.C. Standardized echography of the optic nerve. In *Documenta Ophthalmologica Proceedings Series*; Ophthalmic Echography 13; Till, P., Ed.; Springer: Dordrecht, The Netherlands, 1990; Volume 55, pp. 3–99.

16. De Bernardo, M.; Vitiello, L.; De Pascale, I.; Capasso, L.; Cornetta, P.; Rosa, N. Optic Nerve Ultrasound Evaluation in Idiopathic Intracranial Hypertension. *Front. Med.* **2022**, *9*, 845554. [CrossRef] [PubMed]

17. De Bernardo, M.; Vitiello, L.; Rosa, N. Ultrasound optic nerve sheath diameter measurement in optic neuritis. *Am. J. Emerg. Med.* **2019**, *37*, 1595–1596. [CrossRef]

18. De Bernardo, M.; Vitiello, L.; Rosa, N. Ultrasound optic nerve sheath diameter evaluation in patients undergoing robot-assisted laparoscopic pelvic surgery. *J. Robot. Surg.* **2019**, *13*, 709–710. [CrossRef]

19. Abbinante, G.; Vitiello, L.; Coppola, A.; Salerno, G.; Gagliardi, V.; Pellegrino, A. Optic Nerve Ultrasound Evaluation in Childrer A Review. *Diagnostics* **2023**, *13*, 535. [CrossRef]
20. Vitiello, L.; De Bernardo, M.; Capasso, L.; Cornetta, P.; Rosa, N. Optic Nerve Ultrasound Evaluation in Animals and Norma Subjects. *Front. Med.* **2022**, *8*, 797018. [CrossRef]
21. De Bernardo, M.; Vitiello, L.; Rosa, N. Optic nerve ultrasound measurement in multiple sclerosis. *Acta Neurol. Scand.* **2019**, *139* 399–400. [CrossRef]
22. De Bernardo, M.; Vitiello, L.; De Luca, M.; La Marca, A.; Rosa, N. Optic Nerve Changes Detected with Ocular Ultrasonography during Different Surgical Procedures: A Narrative Review. *J. Clin. Med.* **2022**, *11*, 5467. [CrossRef] [PubMed]
23. Vitiello, L.; Salerno, G.; De Bernardo, M.; D'Aniello, O.; Capasso, L.; Marotta, G.; Rosa, N. Ultrasound Detection of Intracrania Hypertension in Brain Injuries. *Front. Med.* **2022**, *9*, 870808. [CrossRef]
24. Kerlen, C.H. B-scan ultrasonography in optic nerve lesions. *Doc. Ophthalmol.* **1982**, *52*, 317–325. [CrossRef]
25. Abegão Pinto, L.; Vandewalle, E.; Pronk, A.; Stalmans, I. Intraocular pressure correlates with optic nerve sheath diameter in patients with normal tension glaucoma. *Graefes Arch. Clin. Exp. Ophthalmol.* **2012**, *250*, 1075–1080. [CrossRef] [PubMed]
26. Willekens, K.; Abegão Pinto, L.; Vandewalle, E.; Marques-Neves, C.; Stalmans, I. Higher optic nerve sheath diameters are associated with lower ocular blood flow velocities in glaucoma patients. *Graefes Arch. Clin. Exp. Ophthalmol.* **2014**, *252*, 477–483 [CrossRef]
27. Liu, H.; Yang, D.; Ma, T.; Shi, W.; Zhu, Q.; Kang, J.; Wang, N. Measurement and Associations of the Optic Nerve Subarachnoic Space in Normal Tension and Primary Open-Angle Glaucoma. *Am. J. Ophthalmol.* **2018**, *186*, 128–137. [CrossRef] [PubMed]
28. Omatiga, A.G.; Onakpoya, O.H.; Idowu, B.M.; Asaleye, C.M.; Adegbehingbe, B.O.; Aderibigbe, A.S. B-mode sonographic evaluation of optic nerve sheath diameter and lens thickness in Nigerian adults with glaucoma. *Afr. Health Sci.* **2018**, *18*, 343–351 [CrossRef] [PubMed]
29. Coleman, D.J.; Carroll, F.D. Evaluation of optic neuropathy with B-scan ultrasonography. *Am. J. Ophthalmol.* **1972**, *74*, 915–920 [CrossRef]
30. Dees, C.; Buimer, R.; Dick, A.D.; Atta, H.R. Ultrasonographic investigation of optic neuritis. *Eye* **1995**, *9 Pt 4*, 488–494. [CrossRef]
31. Elvin, A.; Andersson, T.; Söderström, M. Optic neuritis. Doppler ultrasonography compared with MR and correlated with visual evoked potential assessments. *Acta Radiol.* **1998**, *39*, 243–248.
32. Karaali, K.; Senol, U.; Aydin, H.; Cevikol, C.; Apaydin, A.; Lüleci, E. Optic neuritis: Evaluation with orbital Doppler sonography *Radiology* **2003**, *226*, 355–358. [CrossRef]
33. Karami, M.; Janghorbani, M.; Dehghani, A. Orbital Doppler evaluation of blood flow velocities in optic neuritis. *Korean J. Ophthalmol.* **2012**, *26*, 116–122. [CrossRef]
34. Lochner, P.; Cantello, R.; Fassbender, K.; Lesmeister, M.; Nardone, R.; Siniscalchi, A.; Clemente, N.; Naldi, A.; Coppo, L.; Brigo, F. et al. Longitudinal Assessment of Transorbital Sonography, Visual Acuity, and Biomarkers for Inflammation and Axonal Injury in Optic Neuritis. *Dis. Markers* **2017**, *2017*, 5434310. [CrossRef]
35. Lochner, P.; Cantello, R.; Brigo, F.; Coppo, L.; Nardone, R.; Tezzon, F.; Raymkulova, O.; Strigaro, G.; Comi, C.; Leone, M.A. Transorbital sonography in acute optic neuritis: A case-control study. *AJNR Am. J. Neuroradiol.* **2014**, *35*, 2371–2375. [CrossRef] [PubMed]
36. Lochner, P.; Leone, M.A.; Fassbender, K.; Cantello, R.; Coppo, L.; Nardone, R.; Zorzi, G.; Lesmeister, M.; Comi, C.; Brigo, F. Transorbital Sonography and Visual Outcome for the Diagnosis and Monitoring of Optic Neuritis. *J. Neuroimaging* **2017**, *27*, 92–96 [CrossRef]
37. Wayman, D.; Carmody, K.A. Optic neuritis diagnosed by bedside emergency physician-performed ultrasound: A case report. *J. Emerg. Med.* **2014**, *47*, 301–305. [CrossRef] [PubMed]
38. Badron, J.; Ong, G.Y. Bedside Transorbital Ultrasound in the Clinical Evaluation of Pediatric Optic Neuritis in the Emergency Department. *J. Emerg. Med.* **2019**, *56*, 417–420. [CrossRef] [PubMed]
39. Yee, N.P.; Kashani, S.; Mailhot, T.; Omer, T. More than meets the eye: Point-of-care ultrasound diagnosis of acute optic neuritis in the emergency department. *Am. J. Emerg. Med.* **2019**, *37*, 177.e1–177.e4. [CrossRef]
40. Rovira, À.; Vidal-Jordana, A.; Auger, C.; Sastre-Garriga, J. Optic Nerve Imaging in Multiple Sclerosis and Related Disorders *Neuroimaging Clin. N. Am.* **2024**, *34*, 399–420. [CrossRef]
41. Titlić, M.; Erceg, I.; Kovacević, T.; Gabrić, N.; Karaman, K.; Zuljan, I.; Orsolić, K.; Kalajzić, J. The correlation of changes of the optic nerve diameter in the acute retrobulbar neuritis with the brain changes in multiple sclerosis. *Coll. Antropol.* **2005**, *29*, 633–636.
42. Stefanović, I.B.; Jovanović, M.; Krnjaja, B.D.; Veselinović, D.; Jovanović, P. Influence of retrobulbar neuritis and papillitis on echographically measured optic nerve diameter. *Vojnosanit. Pregl.* **2010**, *67*, 32–35. [CrossRef]
43. Raeesmohammadi, L.; Esmaeili, S.; Abbasi, M.H.; Mehrpour, M.; Mirzaasgari, Z.; Baradaran, H.R.; Deilami, P.; Motamed, M.R. Transbulbar B-mode sonography in multiple sclerosis without optic neuritis; clinical relevance. *Brain Res.* **2020**, *1734*, 146723 [CrossRef] [PubMed]
44. De Masi, R.; Orlando, S.; Conte, A.; Pasca, S.; Scarpello, R.; Spagnolo, P.; Muscella, A.; De Donno, A. Transbulbar B-Mode Sonography in Multiple Sclerosis: Clinical and Biological Relevance. *Ultrasound Med. Biol.* **2016**, *42*, 3037–3042. [CrossRef] [PubMed]

Schroeder, C.; Katsanos, A.H.; Ayzenberg, I.; Schwake, C.; Gahlen, A.; Tsivgoulis, G.; Voumvourakis, K.; Gold, R.; Krogias, C. Atrophy of optic nerve detected by transorbital sonography in patients with demyelinating diseases of the central nervous system. *Eur. J. Neurol.* **2020**, *27*, 626–632. [CrossRef]
Elkholy, S.H.; El-Jaafary, S.I.; Kotb, M.S.; El Gohary, A.M.; Elbhy, B.A. Trans-orbital sonography versus visual evoked potentials in acute demyelinating optic neuritis. *Mult. Scler. Relat. Disord.* **2020**, *40*, 101934. [CrossRef]
Saigh, M.P.; Plauché, H.M.; Butts, C.; Karam, A.K.; Suau, S.J.; Moreno-Walton, L. Acute Optic Neuritis Diagnosed by Bedside Ultrasound in an Emergency Department. *J. Emerg. Med.* **2019**, *57*, 207–211. [CrossRef] [PubMed]
Kwon, Y.J.; Kim, Y.H.; Baek, S.H.; Son, M.H.; Lee, J.H.; Kim, B.J. Transorbital ultrasonography in acute optic neuritis: Can it be a supportive diagnostic tool? *Mult. Scler. Relat. Disord.* **2019**, *31*, 54–58. [CrossRef]
Koraysha, N.A.; Kishk, N.; Hassan, A.; Samy El Gendy, N.M.; Shehata, H.S.; Al-Azayem, S.A.; Kamal, Y.S. Evaluating optic nerve diameter as a possible biomarker for disability in patients with multiple sclerosis. *Neuropsychiatr. Dis. Treat.* **2019**, *15*, 2571–2578. [CrossRef]
Krogias, C.; Ayzenberg, I.; Schroeder, C.; Grüter, T.; Gold, R.; Yoon, M.S. Transorbital sonography in CIDP patients: No evidence for optic nerve hypertrophy. *J. Neurol. Sci.* **2016**, *362*, 206–208. [CrossRef]
Candeliere Merlicco, A.; Gabaldón Torres, L.; Villaverde González, R.; Fernández Romero, I.; Aparicio Castro, E.; Lastres Arias, M.C. Transorbital ultrasonography for measuring optic nerve atrophy in multiple sclerosis. *Acta Neurol. Scand.* **2018**, *138*, 388–393. [CrossRef]
Gerling, J.; Janknecht, P.; Hansen, L.L.; Kommerell, G. Diameter of the optic nerve in idiopathic optic neuritis and in anterior ischemic optic neuropathy. *Int. Ophthalmol.* **1997**, *21*, 131–135. [CrossRef] [PubMed]
Dehghani, A.; Giti, M.; Akhlaghi, M.R.; Karami, M.; Salehi, F. Ultrasonography in distinguishing optic neuritis from nonarteritic anterior ischemic optic neuropathy. *Adv. Biomed. Res.* **2012**, *1*, 3. [CrossRef] [PubMed]
Ji, X.; Xiao, W.; Ye, H.; Chen, R.; Wu, J.; Mao, Y.; Yang, H. Ultrasonographic measurement of the optic nerve sheath diameter in dysthyroid optic neuropathy. *Eye* **2021**, *35*, 568–574. [CrossRef] [PubMed]

Journal of
Personalized
Medicine

Article

Subclinical Ocular Motility Dysfunction and Extraocular Muscle Changes in Inactive Graves' Orbitopathy

Filippo Lixi [1,†], Alberto Cuccu [1,†], Giuseppe Giannaccare [1,*], Matteo Onnis [1], Mihaela Madalina Timofte Zorila [2,3], Stefano Mariotti [4], Rosanna Vacca [4], Paola Elisa Meloni [4], Michela Pisu [4], Chiara Mura [4] and Francesco Boi [4]

1 Eye Clinic, Department of Surgical Sciences, University of Cagliari, 09124 Cagliari, Italy; f.lixi1@studenti.unica.it (F.L.); a.cuccu@aoucagliari.it (A.C.); m.onnis15@studenti.unica.it (M.O.)
2 Department of Ophthalmology, Cai Ferate Clinical Hospital, 1 Garabet Ibraileanu Street, 700506 Iasi, Romania; mihaela-madalina.timofte-zorila@d.umfiasi.ro
3 Faculty of Medicine, "Grigore T. Popa" University of Medicine and Pharmacy, 16 Universitatii Street, 700115 Iasi, Romania
4 Endocrinology Unit, Department of Medical Sciences and Public Health, University of Cagliari, 09124 Cagliari, Italy; mariotti@medicina.unica.it (S.M.); rosanna.vacca23@gmail.com (R.V.); dottoressapisu@gmail.com (M.P.); chiara.mura@unica.it (C.M.); francesco.boi@unica.it (F.B.)
* Correspondence: giuseppe.giannaccare@unica.it
† These authors share co-first authorship.

Abstract: This study aimed to investigate the presence of structural and functional changes in extraocular muscles (EMs) among patients with inactive Graves' orbitopathy (GO) classified according to the Clinical Activity Score (CAS). Sixty-seven patients with Graves' disease (GD) and inactive GO were included. The data collected included clinical parameters, thyroid function, autoantibody levels, EOM morphology via orbital ultrasound (US), and ocular motility. Patients were stratified into Red Filter Test (RFT)-positive or RFT-negative groups based on the presence or absence of latent diplopia during the RFT examination. Thirty-three patients (49.25%) exhibited latent diplopia on the RFT, despite not reporting double vision during standard ocular motility tests. Significant differences were observed between the two groups in terms of age, disease duration, intraocular pressure (IOP) elevation in up-gaze, and medial rectus muscle thickness ($p < 0.05$). No significant differences were found in thyroid status, TRAb and ATA levels, CASs, exophthalmos, or lateral rectus thickness between the two groups. This study revealed that in inactive GO, subclinical EM dysfunction and morphological changes may be present, which might not be apparent through routine ocular examinations. The RFT is effective in detecting latent diplopia, highlighting its utility in identifying subtle ocular motility issues and subclinical muscle involvement. Comprehensive evaluations combining functional tests like the RFT and imaging are essential for early detection of GO-related abnormalities, enabling tailored and prompt management and improving patient outcomes.

Keywords: thyroid eye disease; Graves' orbitopathy; Red Filter Test; CAS

1. Introduction

Graves' Disease (GD) is an autoimmune disorder, known as the leading cause of hyperthyroidism, responsible for 50–80% of cases globally [1–3]. The disease is typically triggered by thyrotropin receptor autoantibodies (TRAb), which bind to and activate the thyroid-stimulating hormone receptor (TSHR), causing an overproduction of thyroid hormones [4].

Graves' orbitopathy (GO) is the most frequent extra-thyroidal manifestation of GD, affecting about 50% of those with Graves' hyperthyroidism. It is noteworthy that individuals with Hashimoto's thyroiditis or even those without evident thyroid disease can also develop GO [5,6].

As an immune-mediated disease, GO is triggered by auto-reactive T lymphocytes recognizing one or more antigens shared by the thyroid and orbital tissues, primarily the TSHR [7]. This inflammatory process causes the expansion of orbital fibro-adipose tissue, the infiltration and enlargement of extraocular muscles (EMs), leading to clinical manifestations such as exophthalmos, diplopia, ocular soft tissue changes, and possible optic nerve compression [8,9].

The Clinical Activity Score (CAS), proposed by Mourits and colleagues, is based on a set of criteria, with each criterion being scored as present or absent, and aims to distinguish patients with active GO from those with inactive disease [10].

However, it is well known that GD patients with inactive GO may present morphologic alterations of EMs and/or fibro-adipose tissue changes detectable with different imagine techniques [11]. Moreover, the dysfunction of EMs can cause eye movement-related impairment, significantly altering the quality of patients' life and presenting as a treatment challenge [12].

This study aimed to investigate the presence of alteration in EMs' function, evaluated by means of the Red Filter test (RFT) among patients with inactive Graves' orbitopathy (GO) without frank diplopia.

2. Materials and Methods

This was a retrospective study conducted at the University Hospital of Cagliari, Italy. The study received approval by the Institutional Review Board (IRB) of the University of Cagliari (PG/2015/3455; 26 February 2015). All subjects provided written informed consent and the study was performed in accordance with the Declaration of Helsinki.

2.1. *Patients' Selection and Data Collection*

A total of 67 consecutive patients with GD and inactive GO according to CAS were examined. Patients were enrolled consecutively between January 2011 and December 2014 at a single center (University Hospital of Cagliari, Cagliari, Italy). The following data were collected from each patient's medical file: age, sex, disease duration, CAS class, free thyroxine (FT4), free triiodothy-ronine (FT3) and thyroid-stimulating hormone (TSH), thyrotropin receptor antibody (TRAb) [TRAb levels were considered as a low titer (1–2 IU/L), moderate titer (2–10 IU/L) and high titer (>10 IU/L)], Anti-Thyroid Antibody (ATA) levels [ATA levels were considered positive if anti-thyroglobulin (TG) antibodies were equal to or higher than 4.5 IU/mL, or if anti-thyroid peroxidase (TPO) antibodies were equal to or higher than 60 IU/mL], intraocular pressure (IOP) measurement in primary and up-gaze for both eyes, best-corrected visual acuity (BCVA), slit lamp examination, eye motility, RFT and exophthalmometry. Patients were categorized into 2 groups based on positive (RFT-positive) or negative diplopia (RFT-negative) on RFT.

2.2. *Ophthalmic Assessment*

Ocular motility tests were performed by the same experienced ophthalmologist (A.C.) to evaluate latent or manifest deficits. Manifest diplopia was assessed by asking the patients to follow a small tool moved from the center of the visual field towards its periphery in the four main directions. The presence of latent diplopia was investigated using the RFT: a red glass was placed in front of the patient's right eye, and the patient was asked to focus on a single white light source directly in front of them, maintaining a primary gaze. The patient was then instructed to look at the light source from various positions of gaze, including the primary position and the eight cardinal positions. If there was a muscle dysfunction, the patient reported diplopia (perception of two lights: white and red). The direction of gaze that resulted in diplopia or showed the greatest separation of the images could suggest which structures were involved. IOP was measured first in primary gaze and then in up-gaze. The measurement of eye proptosis was assessed with Hertel's exophtalmometer. The normal range of values was considered 12–21 mm. Values above the upper limit or the difference between the two eyes $\geq$ 3 mm were considered positive.

2.3. Imaging Evaluation

Orbital US was performed by the same experienced echographer (A.C.) using a B-mode MYLAB 70XV Echo-scan (ESAOTE, Genova, Italy) with a 10 MHz transducer. The medial and lateral rectus muscles were examined in both eyes, while the vertical recti were measured only occasionally. During the examination, the patients were asked to look straight ahead, maintaining a primary gaze position. The probe was placed on the closed eyelid, on the opposite side of the muscle that was examined. Suitable sections were frozen on the screen when the trans-bulbar muscle stripe appeared as distinctly as possible. The thickest section of the muscle was then measured at the point of greatest enlargement, perpendicular to the muscle axis, using calipers. Muscles were considered normal if the thickness was < 4 mm, thickened if the thickness was between 4 and 6 mm, and very thickened if the thickness was > 6 mm.

2.4. Statistical Analysis

Statistical analysis was performed using the Statistical Package for Social Science software (IMB SPSS Statistics, version 25 for Windows). Means ± standard deviations (SDs)/median for continuous variables were estimated or percent distributions were presented. The distribution of variables was assessed with Shapiro–Wilk tests. Visual acuity was converted in logMAR for statistical analysis. Fisher's test and Chi-squared test were used to compare categorical variables. Parametric (*t*-test) and non-parametric (Mann–Whitney U test) tests were used to compare normally and non-normally distributed variables, respectively, between groups. A p value of <0.05 was considered statistically significant.

3. Results

3.1. Demographic, Laboratories and Clinical Characteristics of Study Population

All patients were Caucasians. A total of 134 eyes of 67 patients were included in this study. The medical records of 46 females and 21 males with a mean age 46.0 ± 12.1 (range 18–72 years) were evaluated. Thirty-six (53.73%) patients were hyperthyroid, twenty-eight (41.79%) were euthyroid, and three (4.47%) were hypothyroid. The mean duration of thyroid disease was 29.00 ± 41.21 months. TSH mean value was 1.57 mU/L (median 0.50 mU/L), FT4 mean value was 2.45 ng/dL (median 1.40 ng/dL), and FT3 mean value was 4.47 pg/mL (median 3.36 pg/mL). TRAb values were positive in 51 (76.11%) patients, with a low titer in 22 subjects (32.83%), moderate titer in 16 (23.88%) and high titer in 13 (19.40%). Sixteen (23.88%) patients were negative for TRAb. ATAs were positive in 48 (71.64%) and negative in 19 (28.36%) patients. All patients presented CAS ≤ 2. Thirty-six (53.73%) patients were CAS 0, twenty-six (38.80%) were CAS 1 and five (7.46%) were CAS 2. Eight (11.94%) patients presented mild exophthalmos (1–2 mm proptosis above the upper limit or 3–4 mm of difference compared to the fellow eye). No patients complained of diplopia upon evaluation of ocular motility. BCVA was logMAR 0.02 ± 0.09. Mean IOP in primary gaze was 14.46 ± 2.76 mmHg. Mean IOP in up-gaze was 16.64 ± 4.07. In the US exam, considering both orbits, medial rectus resulted normal in 69 (51.49%), thickened in 57 (42.54%) and very thickened in 8 eyes (5.97%). Lateral rectus was normal in 109 (81.34%), thickened in 22 (16.42%) and very thickened in 3 eyes (2.24%). During the ocular motility examination, no patients reported manifest diplopia. Conversely, in the RFT, 33 (49.25%) patients exhibited latent diplopia in the vertical gaze position.

Demographic, laboratory and clinical characteristics are displayed in Table 1.

Table 1. Demographic, laboratory and clinical data of patients.

	All Patients (n = 67) *n (%)*
Gender	
Male	21 (31.3%)
Female	46 (68.7%)
Mean age (SD)	46 (12.1)
Thyroid status	
Hyperthyroid	36 (53.7%)
Euthyroid	28 (41.8%)
Hypothyroid	3 (4.4%)
Mean duration of disease (months)	29.0 (41.21)
Mean thyroid hormones (SD)	
TSH (mU/L)	1.57 (3.02)
FT4 (ng/dL)	2.45 (3.90)
FT3 (pg/mL)	4.47 (4.47)
TRAb title	
Negative	16 (22.8%)
Low(1–2 IU/L)	22 (32.8%)
Moderate (2–10 IU/L)	16 (22.8%)
High (>10 IU/L)	13 (19.4%)
ATA levels	
Positive (Anti-TG ≥ 4.5 IU/mLorAnti-TPO ≥ 60 IU/mL)	48 (71.6%)
Negative (Anti-TG < 4.5 IU/mLorAnti-TPO < 60 IU/mL)	19 (28.4%)
CAS	
CAS 0	36 (53.7%)
CAS 1	26 (38.8%)
CAS 2	5 (7.4%)
Exophthalmos (>21 mm or difference between the two eyes ≥ 3 mm)	8 (11.9%)
BCVA (logMAR) (SD)	0.02 (0.09)
Mean IOP (mmHg) (SD)	
Primary gaze	14.46 (2.76)
Up-gaze	16.64 (4.07)
US Medial Rectus	
Normal (<4 mm)	69 (51.5%)
Thickened (4–6 mm)	57 (42.5%)
Very Thickened (>6 mm)	8(6.0%)
US Lateral Rectus	
Normal (<4 mm)	109 (81.3%)
Thickened (4–6 mm)	22 (16.4%)
Very Thickened (>6 mm)	3 (2.2%)

TSH = thyroid-stimulating hormone; FT4 = free thyroxine; FT3 = free triiodothy-ronine; TRAb = thyrotropin receptor antibody; Anti-TG = Anti-thyroglobulin; Anti-TPO = Anti-thyroid peroxidase; CAS = Clinical Activity Score; BCVA = Best-corrected visual acuity; IOP = Intraocular pressure; US = Ultrasound.

3.2. Analysis of RFT-Positive vs. RFT-Negative Patients

Study subjects were divided into two groups according to positive (RFT-positive, n = 33) or negative diplopia on RFT (RFT-negative, n = 34). The characteristics of two groups are displayed in Table 2.

Table 2. Demographic, laboratory and clinical characteristics of two groups.

	RFT-Positive (n = 33) *n (%)*	*RFT-Negative (n = 34)* *n (%)*	*p-Value*
Gender			1 *
Male	10 (30.3%)	11 (32.4%)	
Female	23 (69.7%)	23 (67.6%)	
Mean age (SD)	49.1 (12.3)	43.0 (11.3)	0.03 †
Thyroid status			0.75 χ
Hyperthyroid	17 (51.5%)	19 (55.9%)	
Euthyroid	15 (45.5%)	13 (38.2%)	
Hypothyroid	1 (3.0%)	2 (5.9%)	
Mean duration of disease (months) (SD)	34.1 (37.6)	24.1 (44.5)	0.04 ‡
Mean thyroid hormones (SD)			
TSH (mU/L)	1.03 (1.27)	2.10 (4.08)	0.71 ‡
FT4 (ng/dL)	2.38 (3.17)	2.52 (4.54)	0.23 ‡
FT3 (pg/mL)	5.13 (5.85)	3.83 (2.45)	0.23 ‡
TRAb title			0.55 χ
Negative	6 (18.2%)	10 (29.4%)	
Low (1–2 IU/L)	10 (30.3%)	12 (35.3%)	
Moderate (2–10 IU/L)	9 (27.3%)	7 (20.6%)	
High (>10 IU/L)	8 (24.2%)	5 (14.7%)	
ATA levels			1 *
Positive (Anti-TG ≥ 4.5 IU/mLorAnti-TPO ≥ 60 IU/mL)	24 (72.7%)	24 (70.6%)	
Negative (Anti-TG < 4.5 IU/mLorAnti-TPO < 60 IU/mL)	9 (27.3%)	10 (29.4%)	
CAS			0.30 χ
CAS 0	18 (54.6%)	18 (53.0%)	
CAS 1	11 (33.3%)	15 (44.1%)	
CAS 2	4 (12.1%)	1 (2.9%)	
Exophthalmos (>21 mm or difference between the two eyes ≥ 3 mm)	3 (9.1%)	5 (14.7%)	0.71 *
BCVA (logMAR)(SD)	0.01 (0.01)	0.03 (0.01)	0.27 ‡
Mean IOP (mmHg) (SD)			
Primary gaze	14.20 (2.80)	14.71 (2.72)	0.46 ‡
Up-gaze	18.15 (4.56)	15.18 (2.87)	0.00005 ‡
US Medial Rectus			0.003 χ
Normal (<4 mm)	27 (40.9%)	42 (61.8%)	
Thickened (4–6 mm)	31 (47.0%)	26 (38.2%)	
Very Thickened (>6 mm)	8 (12.1%)	0 (0.0%)	
US Lateral Rectus			0.10 χ
Normal (<4 mm)	50 (75.8%)	59 (86.8%)	
Thickened (4–6 mm)	13 (19.7%)	9 (13.2%)	
Very Thickened (>6 mm)	3 (4.5%)	0 (0.0%)	

* = Fisher's exact test; † = *t*-test; ‡ = Mann–Whitney U test; χ = Chi-squared test. TSH = thyroid-stimulating hormone; FT4 = free thyroxine; FT3 = free triiodothy-ronine; TRAb = thyrotropin receptor antibody; Anti-TG = Anti-thyroglobulin; Anti-TPO = Anti-thyroid peroxidase; CAS = Clinical Activity Score; BCVA = Best-corrected visual acuity; IOP = Intraocular pressure; US = Ultrasound.

The gender distribution was similar across both groups ($p = 1$). The RFT-positive group had a significantly higher mean age (49.1 ± 12.3 years vs. 43.0 ± 11.3 years, $p = 0.03$) and a longer mean disease duration (34.1 ± 37.6 months vs. 24.1 ± 44.5 months, $p = 0.04$). Thyroid status, thyroid hormone levels (TSH, FT4, FT3), TRAb levels, ATA, CASs, exophthalmos presence and BCVA showed no significant differences between the groups. The mean IOP exhibited a significant increase from 14.20 ± 2.80 mmHg in primary gaze to 18.15 ± 4.56 mmHg in up-gaze ($p < 0.001$, Mann–Whitney U test), corresponding to a 27.8% elevation in the RFT-positive group. Concerning the RFT-negative group, the mean IOP exhibited an increase from

14.71 ± 2.72 mmHg in primary gaze to 15.18 ± 2.87 mmHg in up-gaze ($p = 0.35$, Mann–Whitney U test), corresponding to a 3.2% elevation in the RFT-negative group. In up-gaze, the mean IOP was significantly higher in the RFT-positive group compared to the RFT-negative group ($p = 0.00005$). Ultrasound measurements revealed that the medial rectus muscle was more frequently thickened in the RFT-positive group (59.1% vs. 38.2%, $p = 0.003$), while the lateral rectus muscle thickness did not differ significantly between the groups (24.2% vs. 13.2, $p = 0.10$).

4. Discussion

External eye muscles play a critical role in the pathophysiology of GO, being involved in both active and inactive phases of the disease. In these conditions, the muscles may become edematous and infiltrated or undergo fibrosis, which can alter eye motility [12,13].

Double vision or diplopia is a common and debilitating symptom of GO [14]. The European Group on Grave's Orbitopathy (EU-GOGO) reported that 49% of patients with GO presented some degree of eye movement dysfunction [15]. Additionally, patients with diplopia pose a major burden for public health systems due to potential occupational impairments, especially when double vision occurs in the primary and reading position [16].

Diplopia may be latent or manifest. The former occurs when the eyes tend to deviate from their normal position, but this misalignment is typically kept in check by the brain's fusion mechanism. In latent diplopia, double vision does not usually occur because the brain compensates and corrects the misalignment. However, under certain conditions, the brain's ability to maintain proper alignment can weaken, potentially leading to eye strain or double vision. Conversely, manifest diplopia is a condition where there is a constant and noticeable misalignment of the eyes, leading to persistent double vision which the brain cannot correct [17].

Several classifications have been developed and used to evaluate GO. VISA and EUGOGO both subjectively assess the presence of diplopia, noting whether it is vertical or horizontal, constant or intermittent, and if it worsens in the morning [18]. None of these scores can detect latent diplopia or measure the level of involvement of all EMs throughout the eye disease. This gap in the ocular evaluations highlights the need for some methods to be implemented in current practice to comprehensively assess diplopia. Accordingly, while the Hess Lancaster test is considered the gold standard for evaluating diplopia, it requires specialized equipment and trained technicians. In contrast, the RFT is a straightforward, cost-effective, and reliable method that can be easily performed in a clinical setting without specialized instruments [19]. Therefore, RFT can offer a valid alternative to rapidly and non-invasively evaluating diplopia in these patients.

In the studied populations, 33 (49.25%) patients with inactive GO exhibited positive diplopia on RFT in vertical gaze, which they had previously not complained of during the ocular motility examination. This could be due to the ability of RFT to evaluate the total deviation (both manifest and latent) by disrupting fusional mechanisms through stark color differences between the eyes [20]. This finding highlights that even in the absence of active disease, subclinical changes in EM function can still be present. Therefore, while CAS is an effective score for categorizing disease activity, it may not fully capture subtle changes in muscle morphology or function.

In terms of structural alterations, a significant difference in IOP between primary and up-gaze positions is well-established in patients with GO as an indicator of inferior rectus muscle thickening. Specifically, in the up-gaze position, the pulling of inferior rectus muscle in patients with GO causes the superior rectus muscle to use greater force to elevate the eyeball. This additional force acts on the eyeball wall and the compression of the superior and inferior rectus muscle significantly elevates the IOP [21]. Despite the lack of a thickness measurement of the vertical recti in our cohort due to different limitations of US in evaluating superior and inferior rectus [22], the significant IOP increment in the RF-positive group may reflect increased resistance from a stiffened inferior rectus muscle.

Ultrasounds represent a cheap, rapid and effective tool for assessing eye muscle involvement in patients with GO, especially compared with more invasive exams like computed tomography (CT) and magnetic resonance imaging (MRI) [23].

B-scan images showed that the horizontal recti had different thickening rates between the two groups, with more thickening of the medial rectus in the RFT-positive group. This finding is consistent with the literature, which indicates that the medial rectus is primarily involved in GO, after the inferior rectus [24]. No significant difference was observed in the lateral rectus thickness between the two groups, likely because the latter is the least affected muscle in GO, followed by the oblique muscles. [25]. Despite these results, the RFT was positive in vertical gaze, likely because the maximum vertical disparity that can be fused is only about 3–5 Δ, significantly less than the horizontal fusion amplitude of 15–20 Δ [26].

The factors of disease duration and age of patients exhibited a significant difference between the two groups. These could lead to an increased cumulative exposure to autoimmune inflammation and subsequently more significant tissue damage and fibrosis over time, which could be reflected in imaging and functional test alterations. Additionally, age-related changes in the ocular muscles and overall tissue elasticity reduction could contribute to the observed differences between the groups [27].

Patients with GO may have hyperthyroidism, hypothyroidism, or euthyroidism [5]. The distribution of thyroid status did not significantly differ between the RFT-positive and RFT-negative groups, suggesting that latent diplopia is not directly influenced by the current thyroid status. Similarly, sex and patients with some degree of exophthalmos did also not differ between the two groups.

The role of TRAb and ATA in the pathogenesis of GD and GO has been extensively investigated [28]. However, the lack of a significant difference between the groups suggests that these antibodies alone do not determine the presence of diplopia, as already shown in previous reports [29,30].

These findings suggest that even in inactive GO, there can be subtle yet clinically relevant changes in EOM function and morphology. The early detection of these changes could significantly influence the progression and prognosis of the disease by facilitating a dedicated management plan to mitigate disease advancement. This plan might involve more rigorous follow-up schedules to monitor the patient closely and implement timely interventions. Preventive measures, such as protecting the eyes from sun and wind exposure and encouraging patients to quit smoking, can help reduce risk factors associated with disease exacerbation [31]. Ensuring optimal thyroid hormone levels by tailoring anti-thyroid therapy to achieve euthyroidism and avoiding hormonal fluctuations is also crucial in stabilizing the condition. Furthermore, considering selenium's potential benefits in slowing disease progression, initiating therapy with 200 mcg/day could be a viable option for such patients [32]. Through these strategies, early intervention may improve disease progression and patient outcomes.

Nonetheless, the study had several limitations. Firstly, the retrospective design of the study inherently limits the generalizability of our findings. Secondly, the research was conducted at a single center with a cohort composed entirely of Caucasian patients, which may restrict the generalizability of the results to other populations or settings. Thirdly, the relatively small sample size of 67 patients could affect the robustness and statistical power of the study [the statistical power of the study, calculating by using G*Power software (version 3.1.9.6) [33], given a total sample size of 67 (with groups of 33 and 34 participants) a significance level of 0.05, and an effect size of 0.5, is approximately 0.65]. Additionally, the reliance on the RFT for assessing latent diplopia may not account for all potential functional deficits, suggesting the need for additional functional assessments in future research.

5. Conclusions

The present study identifies subclinical EM dysfunction and changes in inactive GO patients. Clinicians should consider comprehensive ocular evaluations, including imaging studies and functional tests like the RFT, which can be integrated into the standard VISA or EUGOGO evaluation to facilitate a better assessment of the extent of EOM involvement in GO. The early detection of latent diplopia and muscular abnormalities, as well as appropriate therapeutic options, might influence the progression and prognosis of more severe manifestations of late fibrotic alterations, thereby improving patient outcomes. Future research should focus on larger, multi-center studies with advanced imaging and functional assessments to gain a deeper understanding of EM dysfunction in inactive GO, and refine treatment approaches.

Author Contributions: Conceptualization, F.L., A.C., G.G. and F.B.; Data curation, F.L., M.O., M.M.T.Z. and R.V.; Formal analysis, F.L. and M.O.; Investigation, S.M., R.V., P.E.M., M.P. and F.B.; Methodology, F.L., A.C., G.G., M.O., P.E.M. and M.P.; Project administration, A.C., G.G. and F.B.; Software, F.L.; Supervision, G.G. and F.B.; Visualization, G.G. and S.M.; Writing—original draft, F.L., A.C. and M.M.T.Z.; Writing—review and editing, F.L., A.C., G.G. and C.M. All authors have read and agreed to the published version of the manuscript.

Funding: This research received no external funding.

Institutional Review Board Statement: The study was conducted in accordance with the Declaration of Helsinki and approved by the Institutional Review Board of Comitato Etico AOU Cagliari (PG/2015/3455; 26 February 2015).

Informed Consent Statement: Informed consent was obtained from all subjects involved in the study.

Data Availability Statement: The data presented in this study are available on request from the corresponding author.

Conflicts of Interest: The authors declare no conflicts of interest.

eferences

Brent, G.A. Clinical practice. Graves' disease. *N. Engl. J. Med.* **2008**, *358*, 2594–2605. [CrossRef] [PubMed]

Cooper, D.S. Hyperthyroidism. *Lancet* **2003**, *362*, 459–468. [CrossRef] [PubMed]

Weetman, A.P. Graves' Disease. *N. Engl. J. Med.* **2000**, *343*, 1236–1248. [CrossRef] [PubMed]

Eckstein, A.K.; Johnson, K.T.M.; Thanos, M.; Esser, J.; Ludgate, M. Current insights into the pathogenesis of Graves' orbitopathy. *Horm. Metab. Res.* **2009**, *41*, 456–464. [CrossRef] [PubMed]

Bartalena, L.; Tanda, M.L. Current concepts regarding Graves' orbitopathy. *J. Intern. Med.* **2022**, *292*, 692–716. [CrossRef] [PubMed] [PubMed Central]

Bartalena, L.; Tanda, M.L. Clinical practice. Graves' ophthalmopathy. *N. Engl. J. Med.* **2009**, *360*, 994–1001. [CrossRef] [PubMed]

Scarabosio, A.; Surico, P.L.; Singh, R.B.; Tereshenko, V.; Musa, M.; D'Esposito, F.; Russo, A.; Longo, A.; Gagliano, C.; Agosti, E.; et al. Thyroid Eye Disease: Advancements in Orbital and Ocular Pathology Management. *J. Pers. Med.* **2024**, *14*, 776. [CrossRef] [PubMed] [PubMed Central]

Bahn, R.S. Graves' Ophthalmopathy. *N. Engl. J. Med.* **2010**, *362*, 726–738. [CrossRef] [PubMed]

Smith, T.J. Pathogenesis of Graves' orbitopathy: A 2010 update. *J. Endocrinol. Investig.* **2010**, *33*, 414–421. [CrossRef]

Mourits, M.P.; Koornneef, L.; Wiersinga, W.M.; Prummel, M.F.; Berghout, A.; van der Gaag, R. Clinical criteria for the assessment of disease activity in Graves' ophthalmopathy: A novel approach. *Br. J. Ophthalmol.* **1989**, *73*, 639–644. [CrossRef]

Lennerstrand, G.; Tian, S.; Isberg, B.; Landau Högbeck, I.; Bolzani, R.; Tallstedt, L.; Schworm, H. Magnetic resonance imaging and ultrasound measurements of extraocular muscles in thyroid-associated ophthalmopathy at different stages of the disease. *Acta Ophthalmol. Scand.* **2007**, *85*, 192–201. [CrossRef] [PubMed]

Nagy, E.V.; Toth, J.; Kaldi, I.; Damjanovich, J.; Mezosi, E.; Lenkey, A.; Toth, L.; Szabo, J.; Karanyi, Z.; Leovey, A. Graves' ophthalmopathy: Eye muscle involvement in patients with diplopia. *Eur. J. Endocrinol.* **2000**, *142*, 591–597. [CrossRef] [PubMed]

Jankauskiene, J.; Imbrasiene, D. Investigations of ocular changes, extraocular muscle thickness, and eye movements in Graves' ophthalmopathy. *Medicina* **2006**, *42*, 900–903. [PubMed]

Johnson, B.T.; Jameyfield, E.; Aakalu, V.K. Optic neuropathy and diplopia from thyroid eye disease: Update on pathophysiology and treatment. *Curr. Opin. Neurol.* **2021**, *34*, 116–121. [CrossRef] [PubMed] [PubMed Central]

Prummel, M.F.; Bakker, A.; Wiersinga, W.M.; Baldeschi, L.; Mourits, M.P.; Kendall-Taylor, P.; Perros, P.; Neoh, C.; Dickinson, A.J.; Lazarus, J.H.; et al. Multi-center study on the characteristics and treatment strategies of patients with Graves' orbitopathy: The first European Group on Graves' Orbitopathy experience. *Eur. J. Endocrinol.* **2003**, *148*, 491–495. [CrossRef] [PubMed]

Ponto, K.A.; Merkesdal, S.; Hommel, G.; Pitz, S.; Pfeiffer, N.; Kahaly, G.J. Public health relevance of Graves' orbitopathy. *J. Clin. Endocrinol. Metab.* **2013**, *98*, 145–152. [CrossRef] [PubMed]

Gräf, M.; Lorenz, B. How to deal with diplopia. *Rev. Neurol.* **2012**, *168*, 720–728. [CrossRef] [PubMed]

18. Barrio-Barrio, J.; Sabater, A.L.; Bonet-Farriol, E.; Velázquez-Villoria, Á.; Galofré, J.C. Graves' Ophthalmopathy: VISA versus EUGOGO Classification, Assessment, and Management. *J. Ophthalmol.* **2015**, *2015*, 249125. [CrossRef] [PubMed] [PubMed Central]
19. Yoo, H.S.; Park, E.; Rhiu, S.; Chang, H.J.; Kim, K.; Yoo, J.; Heo, J.H.; Nam, H.S. A computerized red glass test for quantifyin diplopia. *BMC Ophthalmol.* **2017**, *17*, 71. [CrossRef] [PubMed] [PubMed Central]
20. Bitner, D.P.; Adesina, O.O.; Ding, K.; Farris, B.K.; Michael Siatkowski, R. Comparison of Objective and Subjective Techniques c Strabismus Measurement in Adults With Normal Retinal Correspondence. *J. Pediatr. Ophthalmol. Strabismus.* **2017**, *54*, 216–22 [CrossRef] [PubMed]
21. Li, X.; Bai, X.; Liu, Z.; Cheng, M.; Li, J.; Tan, N.; Yuan, H. The Effect of Inferior Rectus Muscle Thickening on Intraocular Pressur in Thyroid-Associated Ophthalmopathy. *J. Ophthalmol.* **2021**, *2021*, 9736247. [CrossRef] [PubMed] [PubMed Central]
22. Karhanova, M.; Kovar, R.; Frysak, Z.; Sin, M.; Zapletalova, J.; Rehak, J.; Herman, M. Correlation between magnetic resonanc imaging and ultrasound measurements of eye muscle thickness in thyroid-associated orbitopathy. *Biomed. Pap. Med. Fac. Uni Palacky. Olomouc Czech Repub.* **2015**, *159*, 307–312. [CrossRef] [PubMed]
23. Fledelius, H.C.; Zimmermann-Belsing, T.; Feldt-Rasmussen, U. Ultrasonically measured horizontal eye muscle thickness i thyroid associated orbitopathy: Cross-sectional and longitudinal aspects in a Danish series. *Acta Ophthalmol. Scand.* **2003**, *8* 143–150. [CrossRef] [PubMed]
24. Szelog, J.; Swanson, H.; Sniegowski, M.C.; Lyon, D.B. Thyroid Eye Disease. *Mo. Med.* **2022**, *119*, 343–350. [PubMed] [PubMed Central]
25. Yang, J.; Chen, J.; Shi, B.; You, Y.; Pi, X.; Zhao, G.; Jiang, F. Effects of various extraocular muscle enlargement patterns on muscl diameter index in graves ophthalmopathy patients: A retrospective cohort study. *Sci. Rep.* **2023**, *13*, 16939. [CrossRef] [PubMed] [PubMed Central]
26. Bharadwaj, S.R.; Hoenig, M.P.; Sivaramakrishnan, V.C.; Karthikeyan, B.; Simonian, D.; Mau, K.; Rastani, S.; Schor, C.M. Variatio of binocular-vertical fusion amplitude with convergence. *Investig. Ophthalmol. Vis. Sci.* **2007**, *48*, 1592–1600. [CrossRef] [PubMed] [PubMed Central]
27. Perros, P.; Crombie, A.L.; Matthews, J.N.; Kendall-Taylor, P. Age and gender influence the severity of thyroid-associate ophthalmopathy: A study of 101 patients attending a combined thyroid-eye clinic. *Clin. Endocrinol.* **1993**, *38*, 367–372. [CrossRef] [PubMed]
28. Hesarghatta Shyamasunder, A.; Abraham, P. Measuring TSH receptor antibody to influence treatment choices in Graves' diseas *Clin. Endocrinol.* **2017**, *86*, 652–657. [CrossRef] [PubMed]
29. Nicolì, F.; Lanzolla, G.; Mantuano, M.; Ionni, I.; Mazzi, B.; Leo, M.; Sframeli, A.; Posarelli, C.; Maglionico, M.N.; Figus, M et al. Correlation between serum anti-TSH receptor autoantibodies (TRAbs) and the clinical feature of Graves' orbitopathy. *J. Endocrinol. Investig.* **2021**, *44*, 581–585. [CrossRef] [PubMed]
30. Tabasum, A.; Khan, I.; Taylor, P.; Das, G.; Okosieme, O.E. Thyroid antibody-negative euthyroid Graves' ophthalmopathy *Endocrinol. Diabetes Metab. Case Rep.* **2016**, *2016*, 160008. [CrossRef] [PubMed] [PubMed Central]
31. Bartalena, L.; Kahaly, G.J.; Baldeschi, L.; Dayan, C.M.; Eckstein, A.; Marcocci, C.; Marinò, M.; Vaidya, B.; Wiersinga, W.M EUGOGO. The 2021 European Group on Graves' orbitopathy (EUGOGO) clinical practice guidelines for the medical managemen of Graves' orbitopathy. *Eur. J. Endocrinol.* **2021**, *185*, G43–G67. [CrossRef] [PubMed]
32. Lanzolla, G.; Marinò, M.; Marcocci, C. Selenium in the Treatment of Graves' Hyperthyroidism and Eye Disease. *Front. Endocrino* **2021**, *11*, 608428. [CrossRef] [PubMed] [PubMed Central]
33. Kang, H. Sample size determination and power analysis using the G*Power software. *J. Educ. Eval. Health Prof.* **2021**, *18*, 1 [CrossRef] [PubMed] [PubMed Central]

Journal of
*Personalized
Medicine*

MDPI

rticle

ntraocular Pressure Measurements in Standing, Sitting, Prone, nd Supine Positions

laddalena De Bernardo, Ferdinando Cione *, Ilaria De Pascale, Sergio Pagliarulo and Nicola Rosa

Eye Unit, Department of Medicine Surgery and Dentistry, "Scuola Medica Salernitana", University of Salerno, 84081 Salerno, Italy; mdebernardo@unisa.it (M.D.B.)
* Correspondence: fcione@unisa.it

Abstract: In this study, intraocular pressure (IOP) was measured in sitting, supine, prone, and standing (ST) positions and again five minutes after standing (ST-5) utilizing a Tono-Pen AVIA in 124 eyes of 62 healthy subjects with ages ranging from 21 to 59 years (mean 30 ± 10 years). In each subject, the average IOP of both eyes was used for the statistical evaluation. The mean IOP difference between the ST and sitting positions was −0.13 ± 1.63 mmHg (p = 0.548); between ST-5 and sitting, it was 0.53 ± 1.24 mmHg (p = 0.001); between supine and sitting, it was 1.30 ± 1.48 mmHg (p < 0.001); between ST and supine, it was −1.43 ± 1.74 mmHg (p < 0.001); between ST-5 and supine, it was −0.77 ± 1.59 mmHg (p < 0.001); between prone and supine, it was 2.24 ± 1.92 mmHg (p < 0.001); between ST and ST-5, it was −0.67 ± 1.84 mmHg (range: −7.5 to 5 mmHg) (p = 0.007); between prone and ST, it was 3.46 ± 2.01 mmHg (p < 0.001); between ST-5 and prone, it was −2.46 ± 1.67 mmHg (p < 0.001); and between sitting and prone, it was −3.22 ± 1.56 mmHg (p < 0.001). The results show a significant IOP increase in the ST-5 position, suggesting that such measurements need to be performed in an attempt to explain the progression of glaucoma in apparently normal-tension patients.

Keywords: intraocular pressure; hand-held tonometer; standing position; supine position; sitting position; normal-tension glaucoma

1. Introduction

The increase in intraocular pressure (IOP) is a well-established risk factor for glaucoma development and progression [1–3]. Given improvements in understanding glaucoma pathophysiology, IOP remains the only variable that therapy can improve [4]. For this reason, IOP measurement is part of routine ophthalmic examinations. Unfortunately, these examinations represent only a snapshot of the real IOP due to its circadian fluctuations that may influence glaucoma progression [5–7].

Among the variables that can influence this fluctuation, the position of the body can play a major role in nocturnal IOP elevation; in fact, several studies have demonstrated that the IOP may rise significantly when the patient assumes a supine position compared to a sitting position [8–10]. In some cases, this could explain why glaucomatous damage continues to progress despite the detection of a low IOP during routine ophthalmic examinations, suggesting that some high-risk patients should sleep with their head elevated [11]. It should be taken in account that many people can spend hours in a standing position during the day, and for this reason, it could be helpful to know if pressure changes occur in this situation. In a PubMed literature search, it was possible to find just four papers that reported some information about this topic [12–15]. Among these, in one paper, IOP measurements taken in a standing position were compared with those taken an unusual position, suspending the patients by the ankles from a gravity inversion device [12], while another study was performed on a very limited number of patients [13], and two others used rebound tonometers (Icare Pro–ICP) [14,15].

The rebound principle upon which Icare is based is different from the applanation principle of Goldmann applanation tonometry (GAT), which is still considered the gold standard in IOP measurement. Also, Tono-Pen AVIA (TPA) uses the same physical principle to measure the IOP, but it has two advantages:

(1) The applanated area is much smaller, because the transducer tip has a diameter of 1.0 mm.
(2) TPA is portable and it does not need to be installed on a slit-lamp, and therefore it can be used to measure IOP in different IOP positions [16].

A previous paper published by De Bernardo et al. evaluated TPA and rebound tonometers in different body positions, but they carried out their study on a small number patients and not all body positions were analyzed [16]. On these bases, in continuity with previously published evidence, the aim of this study was to evaluate IOP measurements performed with an applanation-based tonometer by checking if similar changes were observed in a larger population after 5 min or more in a standing position and in a prone position.

2. Materials and Methods

One hundred and twenty-four eyes of 62 healthy subjects (16 males) with an age ranging from 21 to 59 years old (mean 30 ± 10 years) and a refractive error ranging from −6.50 to +1.25 D (mean −2.07 ± 2.13 D) were included in this prospective observational study.

The study was conducted in adherence to the tenets of the World Medical Association's Declaration of Helsinki. The purpose of the study was explained to all participants, who provided written informed consent. The study was approved by the Institutional Review Board of the University of Salerno (Cometico Campania Sud, Naples., Italy, Protocol No. 16544). Each subject underwent a general physical checkup to rule out any systemic disease.

The participants underwent a comprehensive ophthalmic examination that included the following:

- Best corrected visual acuity;
- Refractive error, performed with an objective method and perfected with a subjective method;
- Fundus examination;
- Axial eye length (AL), evaluated with an IOLMaster (Zeiss, Jena, Germany, version 5.4.4.00006);
- Central corneal thickness (CCT) measured with a Pentacam HR (Oculus, Wetzlar, Germany, version 1.19r11). IOP measurements were taken with TPA (Reichert Inc., Depew, NY, USA).

IOP was measured between ten and twelve a.m. by a single observer. TPA used the same physical principle as GAT to measure IOP, but the applanated area is much smaller. Before each measurement, the eyes were anesthetized with oxibuprocaine eye drops and the TPA probe tip was covered with a new latex tip cover. When ten valid readings were obtained by slightly touching the central cornea, the mean IOP readings were automatically averaged by the instrument. The measurement was shown on the liquid crystal display, situated on the device side, together with the "statistical confidence indicator", indicating that the standard deviation of the valid measurements was 5% or less of the number shown: the higher the value, the more reliable the measurements [16]. Only values higher than 90 were accepted.

The measurements were obtained in a sitting position, a supine position after five minutes of lying down, a prone position, a standing (ST) position, and after five minutes in a standing position (ST-5) in a random sequence [14]. The measurements in a prone position were taken with the patient's head protruding beyond the bed, with the chin resting on the bed and the eyes looking downwards. Unfortunately, not all patients were able to position their body to perform correct IOP measurements in a prone position: for this reason, prone measurements were taken in 23 patients. In addition, in 4 patients, the IOP measurements in an ST position were not performed. In each patient, the average of both eyes' IOP was analyzed using the paired Student's *t*-test. Single pairwise comparisons through T-tests were preferred to repeated-measures ANOVA tests because of the different sample sizes available. Correlations analyses were performed with Pearson's test (r: correlation coefficient according to Pearson). All statistical analyses were performed with Microsoft Excel software, and they were double-checked with SPSS software (Version 26.0 IBM Inc., Chicago, IL, USA). Data were expressed as means ± standard deviations and p values < 0.050 was considered significant. The preliminary required sample size was computed with G*Power software (Version 3.1.9.7) by using the T test family option, two-tailed. Given an effect size dz of 0.786, determined with G*Power software, it was estimated that a sample size of 20 subjects would be necessary, with a significance level of 0.05 and a test power of 0.90.

3. Results

IOP measurements in the different positions (Table 1) and the statistical differences summarized in Figures 1–9 and Table 2 clearly show that:

- In the ST-5 and supine positions, the IOP is higher than in the sitting position ($p < 0.001$) in both cases (Figures 1 and 2, correspondingly);
- In the prone position, the IOP is higher than in the supine position ($p < 0.001$, Figure 3);
- In the supine position, the IOP is higher than in the ST position ($p < 0.001$, Figure 4), and this difference decreases with increasing time (ST-5 min, Figure 5);
- In the ST-5 min position, the IOP is higher than in the ST position ($p = 0.007$, Figure 6).

Table 1. Intraocular pressure measurements (in mmHg) in the different positions with a Tono-Pen Avia tonometer.

	Sitting	Supine	ST *	ST-5	Prone **
Mean	14.63	15.93	14.38	15.16	18.15
SD	2.82	3.27	2.96	3.18	3.19
Min	9.50	10.00	9.50	10.00	13.00
Max	22.50	25.50	24.00	24.00	23.00

ST: measurements obtained immediately after assuming a standing position; ST-5: measurements obtained after five minutes in a standing position; SD: standard deviation. * ST data are avilable only for 58 patients; ** prone position data are available only for 23 patients.

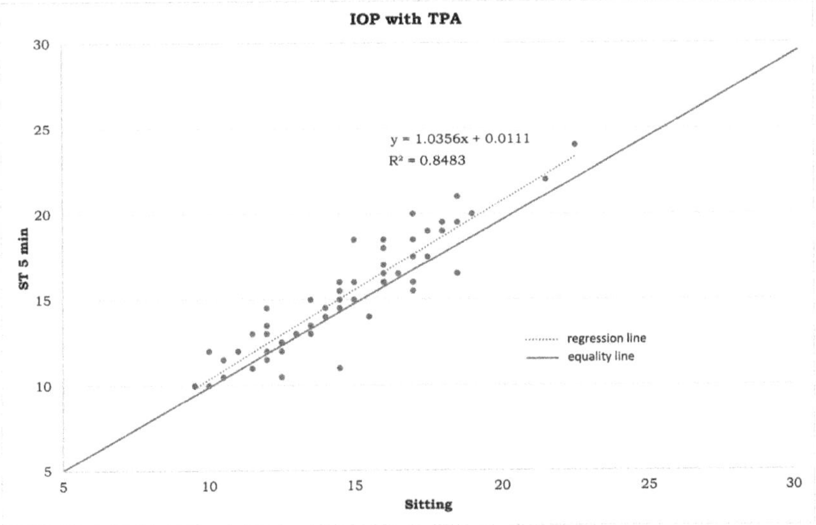

Figure 1. Plot between the IOP measurements in a sitting position on the horizontal axis and IOP measurements in the ST-5 min position on the vertical axis (in mmHg). IOP: intraocular pressure. TPA: Tono-Pen AVIA. ST-5 min: measurements obtained after five minutes in a standing position.

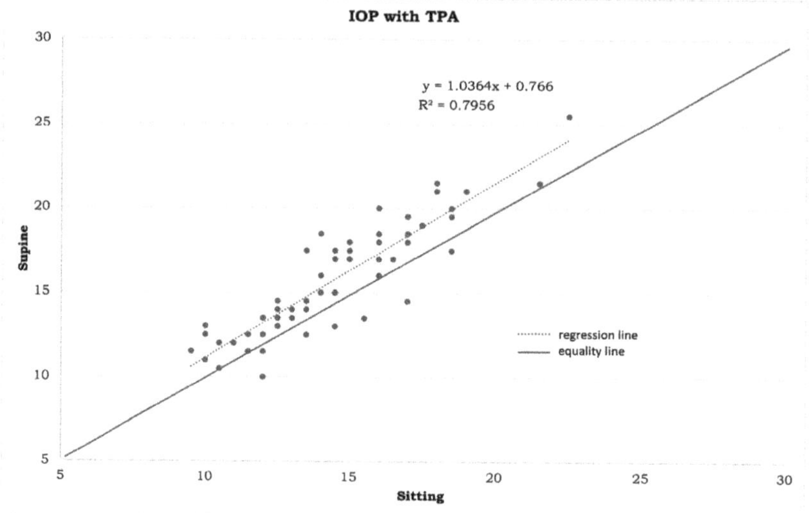

Figure 2. Plot between the IOP measurements in a sitting position on the horizontal axis and IOP measurements in a supine position on the vertical axis (in mmHg). IOP: intraocular pressure. TPA: Tono-Pen AVIA.

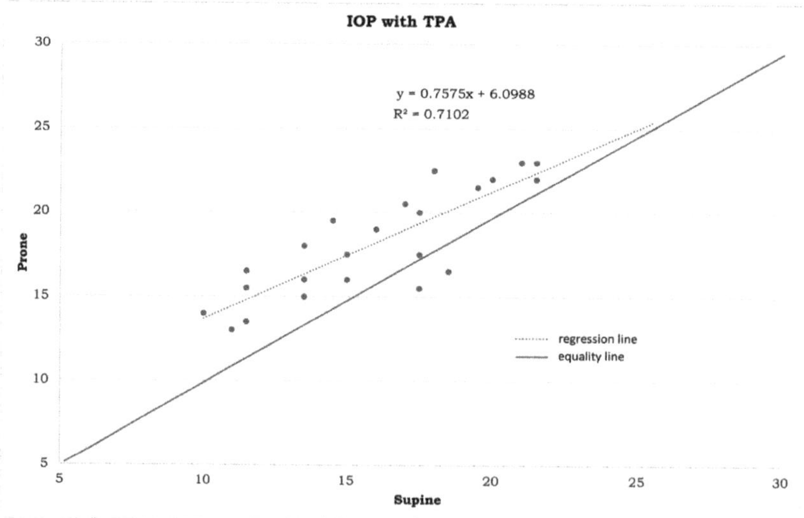

Figure 3. Plot between the IOP measurements in a supine position on the horizontal axis and IOP measurements in a prone position on the vertical axis (in mmHg). IOP: intraocular pressure. TPA: Tono-Pen AVIA.

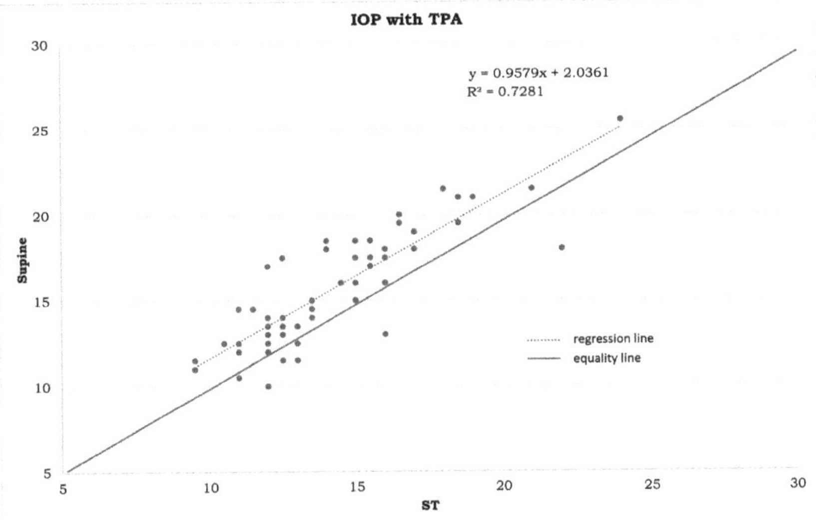

Figure 4. Plot between the IOP measurements in an ST position on the horizontal axis and IOP measurements in a supine position on the vertical axis (in mmHg). IOP: intraocular pressure. TPA: Tono-Pen AVIA. ST: measurements obtained immediately after assuming a standing position.

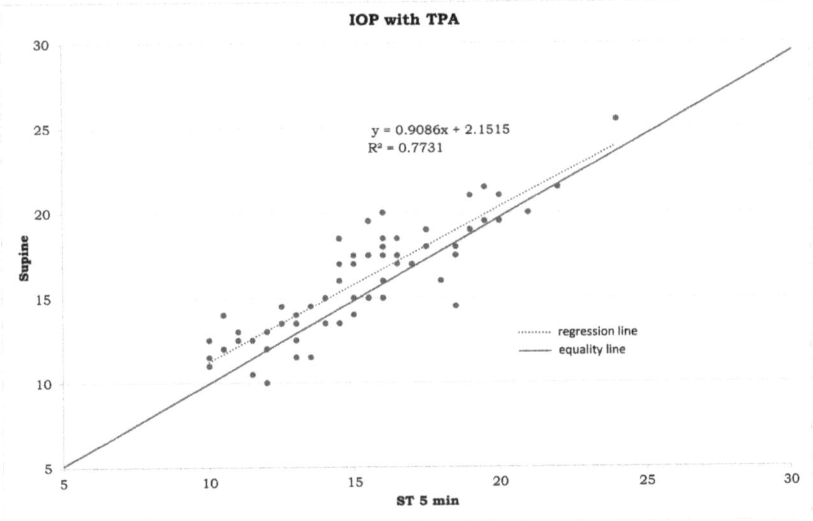

Figure 5. Plot between the IOP measurements in the ST-5 min position on the horizontal axis and IOP measurements in a supine position on the vertical axis (in mmHg). IOP: intraocular pressure. TPA: Tono-Pen AVIA. ST-5 min: measurements obtained after five minutes in a standing position.

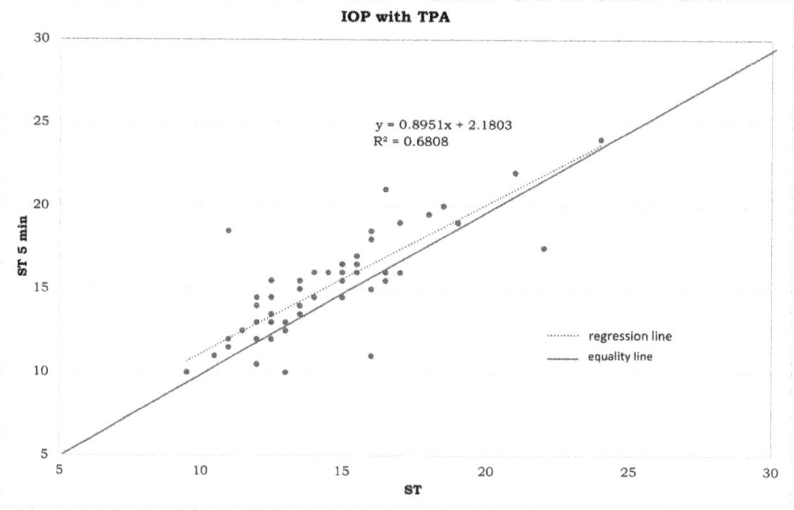

Figure 6. Plot between the IOP measurements in a ST position on the horizontal axis and IOP measurements in the ST-5 min position on the vertical axis (in mmHg). IOP: intraocular pressure. TPA: Tono-Pen AVIA. ST-5 min: measurements obtained after five minutes in a standing position. ST: measurements obtained immediately after assuming a standing position.

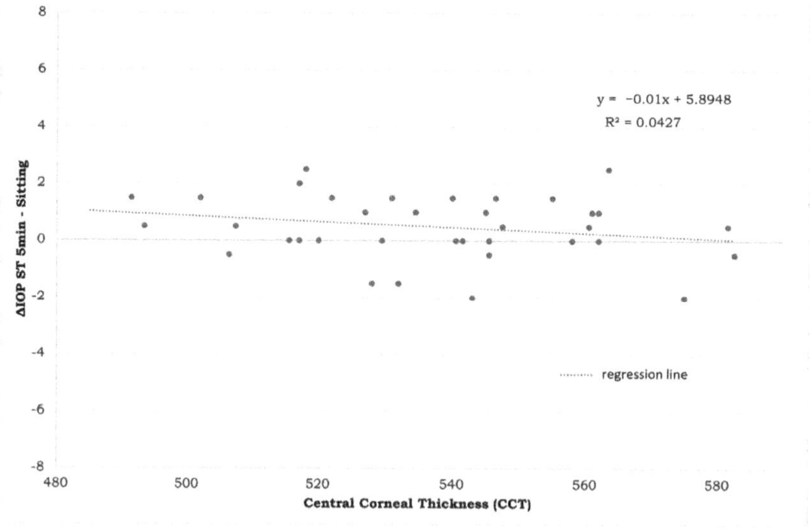

Figure 7. Plot between the CCT mean of both eyes of each subject on the horizontal axis (in micron) and difference in IOP measurements between the ST-5 and sitting positions on the vertical axis (in mmHg). CCT: central corneal thickness. IOP: intraocular pressure. ST-5 min: measurements obtained after five minutes in a standing position.

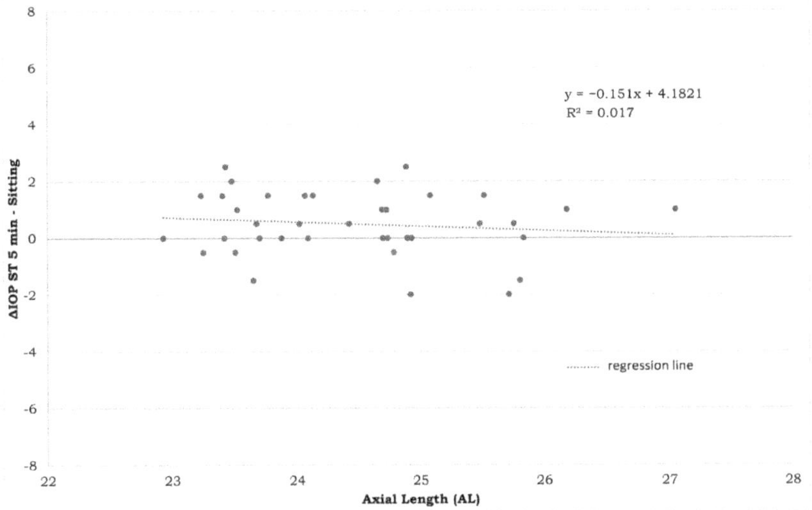

Figure 8. Plot between the AL mean of both eyes of each subject on the horizontal axis (in mm) and difference in IOP measurements between the ST-5 and sitting positions on the vertical axis (in mmHg). IOP: intraocular pressure. ST-5 min: measurements obtained after five minutes in a standing position.

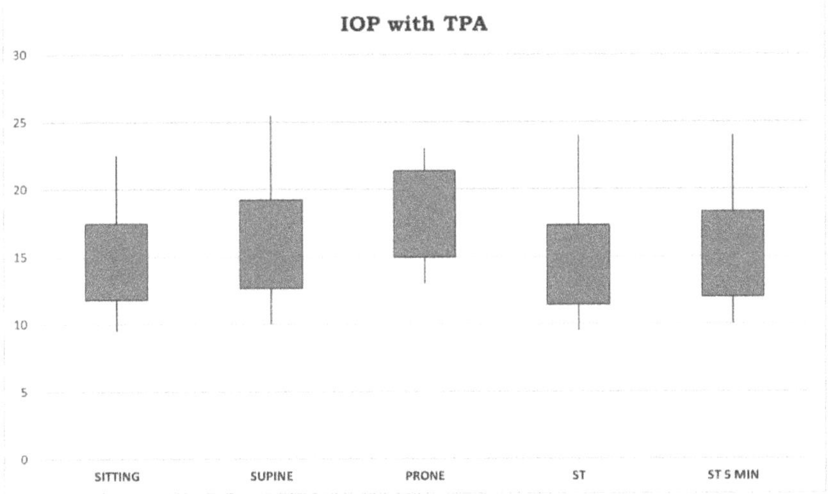

Figure 9. Standard deviations and minimum/maximum values for IOP measurements in the sitting, supine, prone, ST and ST-5 min positions (in mmHg). IOP: intraocular pressure. TPA: Tono-Pen AVIA. ST 5 MIN: measurements obtained after five minutes in a standing position. ST: measurements obtained immediately after assuming a standing position.

Table 2. Intraocular pressure difference (in mmHg) measured with a Tono-Pen AVIA tonometer between different positions, with statistical differences.

	Difference ST/Sitting	Difference ST-5/Sitting	Difference Supine/Sitting	Difference ST/Supine	Difference ST-5/Supine
Mean	−0.13	0.53	1.30	−1.43	−0.77
SD	1.63	1.24	1.48	1.74	1.59
95%CI	−0.56/0.30	0.22/0.85	−0.19/1.68	−1.89/−0.97	−1.16/−0.36
p	0.548	0.001	<0.001	<0.001	<0.001
	Difference Prone/Supine	**Difference ST/ST-5**	**Difference Prone/ST**	**Difference ST-5/Prone**	**Difference Sitting/Prone**
Mean	2.24	−0.67	3.46	−2.46	−3.22
SD	1.92	1.84	2.01	1.67	1.56
95%CI	1.41/3.06	−1.16/−0.19	2.59/4.33	−3.18/−1.73	−3.89/−2.54
p	<0.001	0.007	<0.001	<0.001	<0.001

ST: measurements obtained immediately after assuming a standing position; ST-5 min: measurements obtained after five minutes in a standing position; SD: standard deviation; 95%CI: 95% confidence interval around the mean; *p*: level of significance of paired *t*-test.

The CCT measured with the Pentacam HR was 535 ± 32 μm (range: 452 to 598 μm).

The AL obtained from the IOLMaster was 24.47 ± 1.28 mm (range: 21.70 to 27.16 mm).

IOP differences in the sitting and ST-5 min positions presented no correlation with CCT (Figure 7) and AL (Figure 8).

Means and standard deviations for IOP measurements in the sitting, supine, prone, ST, and ST-5 min positions (in mmHg) are shown in Figure 9.

Figures and Tables

Table 1 synthesizes the IOP values obtained with the TPA in all positions, while Table 2 shows the mean differences between IOPs measured in all positions, with the level of significance. We should reiterate that comparisons with ST data were performed based on 58 patients; meanwhile, analysis with prone position data were carried out on 23 patients.

Figures 1–6 represent the correlation analysis between IOP values in different body positions. A strong positive correlation was found

- between sitting and ST-5 IOP (r = 0.921);
- between sitting and supine IOP (r = 0.891);
- between supine and prone IOP (r = 0.843);
- between ST and supine IOP (r = 0.853);
- between ST-5 and supine IOP (r = 0.879);
- between ST and ST-5 IOP (r = 0.825).

For brevity, only the most clinically relevant correlations were reported.

The correlations between biometric parameters and IOP changes are shown in Figures 7 and 8. A low correlation rate was found between both AL and CCT and ΔIOP ST-5/sitting (r: −0.330 and r: −0.439, respectively), meaning that biometric parameters are less involved in IOP changes across different body positions. For brevity, only the most clinically relevant correlations were reported. Figure 9 reports graphically descriptive statistic data of IOP values in different body positions.

A cluster analysis based on patients' age was carried out in order to verify personalized responses. Due to the low number of prone measurements, these data were not considered in cluster analysis to avoid a too low sample size. The median age of subjects (25 years) was considered as the cut-off value for age range analysis. Overall, 35 subjects (31 in standing position) were evaluated in subgroup A (patients' age ≤ 25 years), while 27 subjects were evaluated in subgroup B (patients' age > 25 year). The results are reported in Table 3.

Table 3. Intraocular pressure difference (in mmHg) measured with a Tono-Pen AVIA tonometer between different positions divided by patients' age, with statistical differences.

A	Difference ST-5/Sitting	Difference ST-5/Supine	Difference ST/ST-5	Difference Supine/Sitting	Difference ST/Sitting	Difference ST/Supine
Mean	0.26	−0.93	−0.79	1.19	−0.55	−1.73
SD	1.26	1.61	2.02	1.60	1.65	1.58
95%CI	−0.17/0.69	−1.48/−0.38	−1.53/−0.05	0.63/1.74	−1.15/0.06	−2.31/−1.15
p	0.237	0.002	0.037	<0.001	0.074	<0.001
B	**Difference ST-5/Sitting**	**Difference ST-5/Supine**	**Difference ST/ST-5**	**Difference Supine/Sitting**	**Difference ST/Sitting**	**Difference ST/Supine**
Mean	0.89	−0.56	−0.54	1.44	0.35	−1.09
SD	1.13	1.56	1.63	1.32	1.49	1.87
95%CI	0.44/134	−1.17/0.06	−1.18/0.11	0.92/1.97	−0.23/0.94	−1.83/−0.35
p	<0.001	0.075	0.100	<0.001	0.232	0.005

A: patients' age ≤ 25 years; B: patients' age > 25 years; ST: measurements obtained immediately after assuming a standing position; ST-5 min: measurements obtained after five minutes in a standing position; SD: standard deviation; 95%CI: 95% confidence interval around the mean; *p*: level of significance of paired *t*-test; in bold: similar level of significance compared to the general population (Table 2).

The same trend was noted both in the general population and in the age-divided subgroups for supine/sitting and ST/supine. The difference in ST/sitting was not statistically significant in all groups, and instead a lower difference for ST-5/sitting was found in younger patients and a lower difference for ST-5/supine and ST/ST-5 was found in older patients.

4. Discussion

Goldmann applanation tonometry (GAT) is considered to be the gold standard in IOP measurements, but unfortunately it has several limitations, including that it needs to be mounted on a slit lamp, and for this reason, it is almost impossible to use in patients in a supine or a standing position; for this reason, this study was conducted with TPA, which has been reported to give reliable measurements compared to GAT in a sitting position [17].

In a PubMed literature search, it was possible to find several papers where the IOP was measured in sitting and supine position with different devices, some with the Tonopen [18–22], some others with the Icare [23], others with both tonometers [24–26], and only one with TPA [24]. However, just four papers investigated the IOP in a standing position, and they made different comparisons [12,13], or the authors used an ICP [14,15].

LeMarr et al. [12], in a group of 26 young subjects, evaluated the IOP changes between a standing and a head-down position. They found an increase in IOP in the head-down position, which a very unusual position; moreover, no comparison was made with a sitting or supine position.

Singleton et al. [13] evaluated the changes in IOP with postural changes (supine, sitting, and standing) in just 11 normal subjects, comparing them to the changes that occur in several groups of patients with different kinds of autonomic dysfunction. In this very small group of normal subjects, they found that the changes in IOP with postural changes were not statistically significant.

Meanwhile, some studies have measured the IOP disparity between sitting and supine postures. Lee et al. [17] examined 19 healthy young Korean participants, comparing the IOP in a sitting and supine position with a Tonopen XL: they observed an increase of approximately 3 mmHg when moving from a sitting to a supine position.

In another study, Lee et al. [23] measured the IOP in 40 eyes of 20 healthy Korean subjects using an Icare tonometer and found a statistically significant mean increase in IOP ($p < 0.001$) of about 2 mmHg when shifting from a sitting to a supine position.

Moster et al. [20] measured the IOP in both a sitting and a supine position in 45 glaucoma patients and 46 healthy subjects with a Tonopen. In each group, the authors found a statistically significant mean IOP increase from a sitting to a supine position, being higher in glaucomatous patients (2.3 mmHg) than in healthy subjects (1.2 mmHg).

Barkana et al. tested the IOP with a Tonopen XL in 19 healthy subjects [21], first sitting then lying for 15 ± 5 min and 45 ± 5 min in a supine position; the same authors in another study measured the IOP with a Tonopen XL in twenty-one eyes of 21 healthy subjects [24], first in a sitting position and then after 10 min in a supine position. In both studies, the authors found an increase in IOP from a sitting to a supine position; furthermore, in the first study, the IOP after 45 min in a supine position was less than that measured after 15 min, without statistically significant differences.

Schweier et al. [25], in 36 eyes of 36 healthy individuals, measured IOP with ICP, TPA, and GAT in a sitting position and 10 min after reclining. They found the IOP to be lower in the sitting position compared to the reclining position with both hand-held tonometers, and the mean difference was greater with TPA (1.8 mmHg) than with ICP (0.8 mmHg) [25].

Sobczak et al. [26], in 71 healthy subjects, found no statistically significant differences between IOP measurements in sitting and supine positions using an ICP tonometer.

Our results regarding the IOP changes in a standing position cannot be compared with the previously published papers by LeMarr [12] and Singleton [13], due to the lack of measurements in the sitting position in the first case and the limited number of patients in the second case.

The results of the present study agree with those published by De Bernardo et al. [14], indicating that utilizing the ICP revealed a non-significant increase in the ST position compared to the sitting position, followed by a statistically significant increase in the ST-5 min position compared to the ST position. Mayali et al. [15], on the other hand, using rebound tonometry (ICP), found no IOP differences in the standing position versus other body positions.

Compared with other papers that considered only measurements in sitting and supine positions, the present study, performed with TPA, confirms these findings. However, our finding of a significant increase in the IOP in a prolonged standing position could be an interesting new finding, even if it is less than the increase in a supine position.

The IOP increase in the supine position may have different explanations; in particular, some researchers have indicated that this is due to an increase, in the supine position, in the episcleral venous pressure [27]. Other authors suggest that this could be due to choroidal vascular engorgement caused by the redistribution of bodily fluids in the supine position [28].

The results displayed in Figures 7 and 8 clearly show that the IOP measured in the different postures is not related to the CCT or to the AL. The reason for the increase in prolonged standing position is not as obvious. One hypothesis could be that, even if the exact mechanism of the IOP regulation is unknown, it may be under systemic vascular control, through the autonomous nervous system, which contributes to maintaining relatively constant blood flow to the tissue despite perfusion pressure fluctuations. Local myogenic, metabolic, and circulating humoral factors are involved in the autoregulation process [13,29]. However, future studies correlating the postural changes in IOP with eventual changes in blood pressure, heart rate, ocular perfusion pressure, and peripheral vasoconstriction could be useful to better understand the reason for these IOP modifications.

Although the sample in our study is not representative for all age groups, previous studies suggest that the IOP change associated with different body positions is not age-related [15]; a cluster analysis based on patients' age was carried out in order to verify if the same trend in IOP changes persists in different age ranges. As reported in Table 3, younger subjects showed a lower difference between the ST-5 and sitting positions than the general population; on the other hand, differences between ST-5 and both the supine and ST positions were lower in older patients. A more valid vascular flow redistribution could explain the lower difference between the first (sitting position) and the last (ST-5 position) IOP measurements in younger patients. On the other hand, a more stable choroidal vascular engorgement could explain the lower differences between ST-5 and both the ST and supine positions in older subjects. These findings could help in a personalized analysis of IOP changes in normal subjects and glaucomatous patients, according to their age range. Unfortunately, due to only male subjects being examined in this study, a gender-based analysis of IOP changes in different positions was inexecutable.

One criticism that could be applied to this study is that the TPA was used instead of the GAT, which, introduced in 1957 by Hans Goldmann, represents the gold standard in measuring IOP [30]. Unfortunately, it is well known that the measured IOP value is influenced by several corneal parameters, such as biomechanical properties, CCT [31–35], corneal irregularities [36], and corneal refractive surgery [37,38]. Albis-Donado et al. evaluated different external factors that can influence GAT reliability: CCT is crucial, but the authors also emphasized the role of altitude [32]. In fact, they found a higher risk of underestimating IOP not only with thinner corneas, but also with a higher altitude. These outcomes are valid for GAT; on the other hand, dynamic contour tonometry (DCT) seems to be less affected by external factors [32]. Chen et al. demonstrated that CCT influences IOP measured not only with GAT, but also with rebound tonometry and with non-contact tonometry (NCT) [34]; they observed that NCT was mostly influenced by CCT, while GAT was less dependent on CCT.

Regarding corneal abnormalities, Knauf et al. reported that IOP measurement is challenging at various stages of keratoconus (KC), depending on the corneal thickness and biomechanical properties [35]. These features are altered in KC eyes. For similar reasons, IOP is difficult after corneal refractive surgery: changes in corneal thickness and corneal curvature affect IOP measurement reliability with different instruments, and topical steroids used postoperatively may mask the incidence and severity of steroid-induced ocular hypertension in the short term [38].

Since the purpose of this study was to compare IOP measurements in different positions, and GAT cannot be used when a patient is unable to sit at a slit lamp (small children, bed-ridden persons) or in situations such as taking measurements in a standing or supine position, TPA was chosen, among the hand-held IOP measuring devices, because it is one of the most widely used, and so far has not been tested for such a purpose.

5. Conclusions

In conclusion, the results of this study confirm the importance of measuring IOP in a supine position, but more importantly suggest that such measurements should also be performed after five minutes in a standing position, as in some jobs (e.g., waiters, policemen, chefs. . .) people can spend a significant amount of time standing, and this information could be helpful in understanding some cases of optic nerve damage or glaucoma progression, despite an apparently normal IOP.

Author Contributions: Conceptualization, I.D.P. and N.R.; methodology, F.C.; software, M.D.B. and N.R.; validation, S.P., M.D.B. and N.R.; formal analysis, F.C.; investigation, M.D.B.; resources, M.D.B. and I.D.P.; data curation, M.D.B.; writing—original draft preparation, S.P.; writing—review and editing, S.P.; visualization, N.R.; supervision, M.D.B.; project administration, N.R. All authors have read and agreed to the published version of the manuscript.

Funding: This research received no external funding.

Institutional Review Board Statement: This study was conducted in accordance with the Declaration of Helsinki and approved by the Institutional Review Board of Cometico Campania Sud, Italy (protocol code n° 16544).

Informed Consent Statement: Informed consent was obtained from all subjects involved in this study.

Data Availability Statement: The datasets generated and analyzed during the current study are available from the corresponding author upon reasonable request.

Conflicts of Interest: The authors declare no conflict of interest.

References

1. Heijl, A.; Leske, M.C.; Bengtsson, B.; Hyman, L.; Bengtsson, B.; Hussein, M.; Early Manifest Glaucoma Trial Group. Reduction c intraocular pressure and glaucoma progression: Results from the Early Manifest Glaucoma Trial. *Arch. Ophthalmol.* **2002**, 8 1268–1279. [CrossRef] [PubMed]
2. Kass, M.A.; Heuer, D.K.; Higginbotham, E.J.; Johnson, C.A.; Keltner, J.L.; Miller, J.P.; Parrish, R.K.; Wilson, M.R.; Gordon, M.O Ocular Hypertension Treatment Study Group. The Ocular Hypertension Treatment Study: A randomized trial determines tha topical ocular hypotensive medication delays or prevents the onset of primary open-angle glaucoma. *Arch. Ophthalmol.* **2002**, 12 701–713. [CrossRef] [PubMed]
3. Leske, M.C.; Heijl, A.; Hussein, M.; Bengtsson, B.; Hyman, L.; Komaroff, E.; Early Manifest Glaucoma Trial Group. Factor for glaucoma progression and the effect of treatment: The Early Manifest Glaucoma Trial. *Arch. Ophthalmol.* **2003**, *121*, 48–5 [CrossRef] [PubMed]
4. Weinreb, R.N.; Aung, T.; Medeiros, F.A. The Pathophysiology and Treatment of Glaucoma: A Review. *JAMA* **2014**, *311*, 1901–191 [CrossRef] [PubMed]
5. Asrani, S.; Zeimer, R.; Wilensky, J.; Gieser, D.; Vitale, S.; Lindenmuth, K. Large diurnal fluctuations in intraocular pressure are a independent risk factor in patients with glaucoma. *J. Glaucoma* **2000**, *9*, 134–142. [CrossRef] [PubMed]
6. Caprioli, J. Intraocular pressure fluctuation: An independent risk factor for glaucoma? *Arch. Ophthalmol.* **2007**, *125*, 1124–112 [CrossRef] [PubMed]
7. Caprioli, J.; Coleman, A.L. Intraocular pressure fluctuation: A risk factor for visual field progression at low intraocular pressure in the Advanced Glaucoma Intervention Study. *Ophthalmology* **2008**, *115*, 1123–1129. [CrossRef] [PubMed]
8. Tarkkanen, A.; Leikola, J. Postural variations of the intraocular pressure as measured with the Mackay-Marg tonometer. *Act Ophthalmol.* **1967**, *45*, 569–575. [CrossRef] [PubMed]
9. Jain, M.R.; Marmion, V.J. Rapid pneumatic and Mackey-Marg applanation tonometry to evaluate the postural effect on intraocula pressure. *Br. J. Ophthalmol.* **1976**, *60*, 687–693. [CrossRef]
10. Krieglstein, G.; Langham, M.E. Influence of body position on the intraocular pressure of normal and glaucomatous eye *Ophthalmologica* **1975**, *171*, 132–145. [CrossRef]
11. Buys, Y.M.; Alasbali, T.; Jin, Y.P.; Smith, M.; Gouws, P.; Geffen, N.; Flanagan, J.G.; Shapiro, C.M.; Trope, G.E. Effect of sleeping in head-up position on intraocular pressure in patients with glaucoma. *Ophthalmology* **2010**, *117*, 1348–1351. [CrossRef] [PubMed
12. LeMarr, J.D.; Golding, L.A.; Adler, J.G. Intraocular pressure response to inversion. *Am. J. Optom. Physiol. Opt.* **1984**, *61*, 679–68 [CrossRef] [PubMed]
13. Singleton, C.D.; Robertson, D.; Byrne, D.W.; Joos, K.M. Effect of posture on blood and intraocular pressures in multiple systen atrophy, pure autonomic failure, and baroreflex failure. *Circulation* **2003**, *108*, 2349–2354. [CrossRef] [PubMed]
14. De Bernardo, M.; Borrelli, M.; Cembalo, G.; Rosa, N. Intraocular Pressure Measurements in Standing Position with a Rebounc Tonometer. *Medicina* **2019**, *55*, 701. [CrossRef] [PubMed]
15. Mayalı, H.; Tekin, B.; Kayıkçıoğlu, Ö.R.; Kurt, E.; İlker, S.S. Evaluation of the Effect of Body Position on Intraocular Pressur Measured with Rebound Tonometer. *Turk J. Ophthalmol.* **2019**, *49*, 6–9. [CrossRef] [PubMed]
16. De Bernardo, M.; Abbinante, G.; Borrelli, M.; Di Stasi, M.; Cione, F.; Rosa, N. Intraocular Pressure Measurements in Standing Sitting, and Supine Position: Comparison between Tono-Pen Avia and Icare Pro Tonometers. *J. Clin. Med.* **2022**, *11*, 623 [CrossRef] [PubMed]
17. Berk, T.A.; Yang, P.T.; Chan, C.C. Prospective comparative analysis of 4 different intraocular pressure measurement technique and their effects on pressure readings. *J. Glaucoma* **2017**, *26*, 194–195. [CrossRef] [PubMed]
18. Lee, J.Y.; Yoo, C.; Jung, J.H.; Hwang, Y.H.; Kim, Y.Y. The effect of lateral decubitus position on intraocular pressure in health young subjects. *Acta Ophthalmol* **2012**, *90*, e68–e72. [CrossRef] [PubMed]
19. Fogagnolo, P.; Orzalesi, N.; Ferreras, A.; Rossetti, L. The circadian curve of intraocular pressure: Can we estimate its characteristic during office hours? *Investig. Ophthalmol. Vis. Sci.* **2009**, *50*, 2209–2215. [CrossRef]
20. Moster, S.J.; Fakhraie, G.; Venketesh, R.; Moster, M.L.; Zhao, Y.; Moster, M.R. Relationship of central corneal thickness to postura IOP changes in patients with and without glaucoma in southern India. *Int. Ophthalmol.* **2012**, *32*, 307–311. [CrossRef]
21. Barkana, Y. Postural change in intraocular pressure: A comparison of measurement with a Goldmann tonometer, Tonopen XL Pneumatonometer, and HA-2. *J. Glaucoma* **2014**, *23*, e23–e28. [CrossRef] [PubMed]
22. Huang, R.; Ge, J.; Chen, G.; Gao, X.; Laties, A.M.; Zhang, X. Four measures of intraocular pressure fluctuation: Which correlate most optimally with actual office-hour readings? *J. Glaucoma* **2015**, *24*, 550–555. [CrossRef] [PubMed]
23. Lee, T.E.; Yoo, C.; Kim, Y.Y. Effects of different sleeping postures on intraocular pressure and ocular perfusion pressure in health young subjects. *Ophthalmology* **2013**, *120*, 1565–1570. [CrossRef] [PubMed]
24. Barkana, Y.; Gutfreund, S. Measurement of the difference in intraocular pressure between the sitting and lying body positions in healthy subjects: Direct comparison of the Icare Pro with the Goldmann applanation tonometer, Pneumatonometer and Tonoper XL. *Clin. Exp. Ophthalmol.* **2014**, *42*, 608–614. [CrossRef] [PubMed]
25. Schweier, C.; Hanson, J.V.; Funk, J.; Töteberg-Harms, M. Repeatability of intraocular pressure measurements with Icare PRO rebound, Tono-Pen AVIA, and Goldmann tonometers in sitting and reclining positions. *BMC Ophthalmol.* **2013**, *13*, 44. [CrossRef [PubMed]

Sobczak, M.; Asejczyk, M.; Geniusz, M. Does body position, age, and heart rate induce IOP's changes? *Eur. J. Ophthalmol.* **2022**, *32*, 1530–1537. [CrossRef] [PubMed]

Sultan, M.; Blondeau, P. Episcleral venous pressure in younger and older subjects in the sitting and supine positions. *J. Glaucoma* **2003**, *12*, 370–373. [CrossRef] [PubMed]

Malihi, M.; Sit, A.J. Effect of head and body position on intraocular pressure. *Ophthalmology* **2012**, *119*, 987–991. [CrossRef] [PubMed]

Cowley, A.W.; Franchini, K.G. Neurogenic control of blood vessels. In *Primer on the Autonomic Nervous System*; Robertson, D., Low, P.A., Polinsky, R.J., Eds.; Academic Press: New York, NY, USA, 1996; pp. 49–55.

Whitacre, M.M.; Stein, R. Sources of error with use of Goldmann-type tonometers. *Surv. Ophthalmol.* **1993**, *38*, 1–30. [CrossRef]

Rosa, N.; De Bernardo, M.; Pepe, A.; Vitiello, L.; Marotta, G.; Imparato, R.; Capasso, L. Corneal thickness evaluation in healthy eyes: Comparison between two different Scheimpflug devices. *PLoS ONE* **2020**, *15*, e0243370. [CrossRef]

Albis-Donado, O.; Ramirez-Neria, P.; Rios-Acosta, N.; Stalmans, I. The influence of altitude on the differences between Goldmann tonometry and Pascal dynamic contour tonometry: An ecological meta-analysis. *Indian J. Ophthalmol.* **2024**, *72* (Suppl. 3), S398–S403. [CrossRef] [PubMed]

De Bernardo, M.; Vitiello, L.; Abbinante, G.; De Pascale, I.; Capasso, L.; Marotta, G.; Rosa, N. Comparison between two devices in the detection of corneal thickness changes after cataract surgery. *Sci. Rep.* **2021**, *11*, 6709. [CrossRef] [PubMed]

Chen, M.; Zhang, L.; Xu, J.; Chen, X.; Gu, Y.; Ren, Y.; Wang, K. Comparability of three intraocular pressure measurement: iCare pro rebound, non-contact and Goldmann applanation tonometry in different IOP group. *BMC Ophthalmol.* **2019**, *19*, 225. [CrossRef] [PubMed]

De Bernardo, M.; Casaburi, C.; De Pascale, I.; Capasso, L.; Cione, F.; Rosa, N. Comparison between dynamic contour tonometry and Goldmann applanation tonometry correcting equations. *Sci. Rep.* **2022**, *12*, 20190. [CrossRef] [PubMed]

Knauf, D.; Seitz, B.; Schießl, G.; Zemova, E.; Flockerzi, E. Analysis of Various Modalities for Intraocular Pressure Measurement in Relation to Keratoconus Severity in 246 Eyes of the Homburg Keratoconus Center. *Cornea* **2023**, *42*, 829–836. [CrossRef] [PubMed]

De Bernardo, M.; Capasso, L.; Caliendo, L.; Vosa, Y.; Rosa, N. Intraocular pressure evaluation after myopic refractive surgery: A comparison of methods in 121 eyes. *Semin. Ophthalmol.* **2016**, *31*, 233–242. [CrossRef]

Ang, R.E.T.; Bargas, N.V.R.; Martinez, G.H.A.; Sosuan, G.M.N.; Nabor-Umali, M.I. Comparison of Three Tonometers in Measuring Intraocular Pressure in Eyes That Underwent Myopic Laser in situ Keratomileusis and Photorefractive Keratectomy. *Clin. Ophthalmol.* **2022**, *16*, 1623–1637. [CrossRef]

Journal of
Personalized
Medicine

MDPI

Review

Ocular Manifestations and Complications of Patent Foramen Ovale: A Narrative Review

Filippo Lixi [1], Luca Fazzini [2], Claudia Cannas [1], Roberta Montisci [2] and Giuseppe Giannaccare [1,*]

[1] Eye Clinic, Department of Surgical Sciences, University of Cagliari, 09124 Cagliari, Italy; f.lixi1@studenti.unica.it (F.L.); claudiacannas.94@gmail.com (C.C.)
[2] Clinical Cardiology Unit, Department of Medical Sciences and Public Health, University of Cagliari, 09124 Cagliari, Italy; luca.fazzini10@gmail.com (L.F.); rmontisci@unica.it (R.M.)
* Correspondence: giuseppe.giannaccare@unica.it

Abstract: Patent foramen ovale (PFO) is a prevalent congenital cardiac anomaly associated with a persistent opening between the atrial septum, allowing communication between the left and right atria. Despite often being asymptomatic, PFO can lead to various clinical presentations, including cryptogenic stroke and other embolic events. Transient visual disturbances, alterations in the visual field, migraine with aura, impaired eye movement and endogenous eye infections may prompt patients to seek ophthalmological consultation. Understanding these diverse clinical scenarios is crucial for early detection, appropriate management and mitigating the morbidity burden associated with PFO. This narrative review aims at examining the spectrum of clinical presentations of ocular pictures associated with PFO. The pathophysiology, diagnosis and treatment methods for PFO will be described, emphasizing the importance of a multidisciplinary approach involving ophthalmologists, cardiologists, neurologists and imaging specialists. In the future, prospective studies and clinical trials are warranted to provide further insights into the preventive role and optimal therapeutic strategies for managing PFO-related ocular complications, ultimately guiding clinical decision making and optimizing patient care.

Keywords: patent foramen ovale; eye; eye disorders; retinal artery occlusion; migraine with aura; impaired eye movement

1. Introduction

Patent foramen ovale (PFO) is a common congenital cardiac anomaly characterized by a persistent opening between the atrial septum, which allows for communication between the left and right atria [1]. After birth, changes in blood pressure lead to the closure of the foramen ovale in about 75% of newborns. As a result, its prevalence is estimated to be around 25–30% in the general population [2–4]. This defect creates a potential pathway for paradoxical embolism, allowing venous thrombi or other embolic material to bypass pulmonary circulation and enter systemic circulation, leading to deleterious clinical consequences [5].

Despite often being asymptomatic, PFO has been associated with various clinical presentations, ranging from cryptogenic stroke to different embolic events [5,6]. To highlight the impact of PFO, patients with cryptogenic stroke have a 2.9 times higher likelihood of having it compared to controls [7]. PFO may be implicated in approximately two-thirds of cryptogenic stroke cases and potentially up to 80% in younger patients [8]. In addition to the well-known and extensively studied complications documented in the literature, more potential clinical presentations have been linked to PFO. These presentations may encompass heterogeneous, less common, yet clinically relevant symptoms that may prompt patients to seek ophthalmic consultation. These symptoms could include transient visual disturbances, alterations in the visual field, migraine and other oculomotor signs that raise suspicion of possible PFO-related complications [9,10]. Several studies and case reports have described acute retinal ischemic events, including transient visual loss and retinal artery occlusions. Understanding the potential clinical manifestations of PFO is crucial for early detection and appropriate management, particularly considering the highly significant prevalence of this condition. Recognizing these manifestations early can facilitate prompt referral to cardiology, appropriate diagnostic work-up and consideration for available PFO closure treatment [11].

In this review, we will analyze the spectrum of clinical presentations associated with PFO, primarily focusing on manifestations that may drive patients to ophthalmological evaluation, also trying to highlight the importance of mitigating the morbidity burden associated with PFO, given its high prevalence in the general population.

2. Materials and Methods

We utilized the PubMed medical database for our search. The term "patent foramen ovale" was combined with the words "eye", "eye disorders", "eye diseases", "retina", "ophthalmology", "eye palsy", "migraine with aura". The text keywords were chosen using information from pertinent bibliographies and the latest literature. The earliest publishing date of the search was set for January 1990, and it ended in March 2024.

Only English-language articles and reviews were analyzed, even though no language limits were placed on the searches. Moreover, manual searches were conducted within initial findings to identify further bibliographic references.

A total of 801 full-text articles were identified on PubMed, 679 of which were excluded after the first screening. The remaining 122 articles were evaluated for eligibility. After a full-text evaluation, 73 papers were retained as relevant articles and were used in this review.

3. Results

3.1. Patent Foramen Ovale: Pathophysiology, Diagnosis and Screening

PFO is derived from embryological folding misplacement. Briefly, the septum primum originates from the upper part of the atrium. The septum secundum forms through a folding of the atrial walls, creating the ostium secundum, which serves as a passage for oxygenated blood to flow from right to left during fetal life. A PFO occurs when the septum primum and septum secundum remain unjoined near the anterior and superior edge of the oval fossa. PFO size in adults is heterogeneous, ranging from 1 mm to 15–19 mm [4]. Of note, larger size and specific morphologies have been shown to correlate with enhanced risk of cerebrovascular accidents [12,13].

Usually, the diagnosis of PFO is made incidentally during routine imaging studies or after the patient presents with a potential clinical manifestation, prompting further imaging evaluation. The diagnosis is pursued through multimodality ultrasound imaging, including transthoracic echocardiography (TTE), transesophageal echocardiography (TEE) and transcranial Doppler using aerated saline as a contrast agent. TTE is often the initial screening tool, providing valuable information about the cardiac structure and function. However, its sensitivity in detecting PFO may be limited due to technical factors and the position of the septum, probably leading to minimal shunting miss [14,15]. Conversely, TEE offers higher sensitivity and specificity that reaches 100% when a contrast agent is used [16,17], allowing for closer visualization of the interatrial septum and providing detailed images of the fossa ovalis properly describing the PFO size and morphology [17]. It is particularly useful in cases in which TTE results are inconclusive or when a higher level of detail is required. Additionally, TEE enables the assessment of associated cardiac anomalies and facilitates the guidance of percutaneous closure procedures. Complementing echocardiographic techniques, by monitoring cerebral blood flow, transcranial Doppler can detect microembolic signals arising from right-to-left shunting through the PFO, especially when contrast injection is performed before Valsalva maneuver [18]. Its sensitivity was shown to be heterogeneous compared to intracardiac imaging [19–22]. However, these imaging modalities together play a crucial role in the comprehensive evaluation and management of patients with suspected PFO.

Screening for a PFO should be selectively conducted among individuals who have recently experienced clinical events potentially suggestive of PFO presence and who stand to benefit from PFO treatment. TEE is indicated in patients with a higher likelihood of having a PFO, for example, when assessing young individuals with unexplained strokes or any other plausible symptom linked to PFO; for patients with a lower probability of PFO, contrast TTE or transcranial Doppler may serve as reasonable initial diagnostic methods.

3.2. PFO and Acute Retinal Ischemic Events

Transient monocular vision loss (TMVL)/amaurosis fugax (AF), central retinal artery occlusion (CRAO), branch retinal artery occlusion (BRAO) and cilioretinal artery occlusion (CLRAO) are acute retinal ischemic events manifesting as sudden, painless monocular visual losses with different degrees of severity. The occlusion of the retinal artery can be transient or permanent and may result in impaired blood flow in the ocular circulation, which is associated with a high cardiovascular morbidity and mortality risk [23].

TMVL/AF is a condition characterized by a transient episode of monocular blindness that typically lasts for seconds to minutes. It occurs due to a temporary interruption of blood flow at the level of the ophthalmic artery or central retinal artery and its branches. The most common cause of TMVL/AF in the elderly population is embolism, characterized by a small clot or debris traveling through the bloodstream and blocking a blood vessel. These emboli can originate from various sites, including the carotid arteries, heart or other blood vessels [24]. Although in younger people, TMVL/AF is often associated with temporary spasm at the level of ocular circulation, monocular TMVL/AF may be the consequence of cardiogenic emboli secondary to cardiac malformations. Accordingly, in a recent cohort study, 15% of patients with TMVL/AF were found to have a PFO [25].

CRAO is a disease in which the main artery supplying blood to the retina becomes occluded. It manifests as an acute loss of vision, typically resulting in visual acuity of 20/400 or poorer; its incidence is 1 in 100,000 individuals, with a mean age of presentation of 60 years (Figure 1A–C) [26].

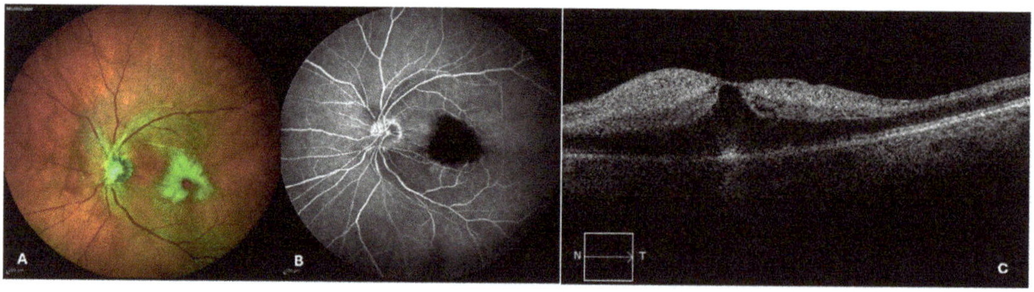

Figure 1. Retinal ischemic events related to PFO: (**A**) Multimodal imaging of a CRAO. On fundus photography, the retina at the posterior pole appears pale and opaque due to the ischemia; a distinctive cherry-red spot is visible at the fovea, which remains red due to the underlying choroidal circulation. The retinal arteries are thin and narrowed. (**B**) Fluorescein angiography reveals a hypofluorescent macular spot secondary to the ischemia of retinal layers. (**C**) The latter is confirmed by optical coherence tomography (OCT), which shows hyper-reflective and edematous inner retinal layers.

BRAO is a disorder in which one of the branches of the central retinal artery becomes blocked, leading to restricted blood flow to a portion of the retina; its incidence is closer to 5 per 100,000 persons per year [27]. The symptoms of BRAO can vary depending on the severity and location of the occlusion, but usually, the prognosis is better than in CRAO, resulting in a localized scotoma or in a sectoral visual field defect. Both of these ischemic disorders can be linked to PFO [28].

Another distinct clinical entity is the CLRAO. The cilioretinal artery arises from the short posterior ciliary vessels, and its prevalence ranges from 6.9% to 49.5%. It may play a role in providing additional blood supply to the macular region of the retina, thus preserving central vision, in cases where the main retinal vasculature is compromised, such as in CRAO [29]. CLRAO can be a consequence of a hemodynamic blockage of the artery caused by a rise in intraluminal pressure in retinal vasculature exceeding the level of perfusion pressure, or it can be secondary to embolism or thrombosis, or it can recognize an arteritic etiology. Symptoms of CLRAO may include sudden blurring, scotoma or distortion of central vision. Since CLRAO has been linked to PFO through an embolic mechanism, the presence of an underlying cardiac defect should be excluded in young people presenting this disorder [28,30,31].

The diagnosis of acute retinal ischemic events is clinical and based on different possible morphologic findings detectable on fundus examination, such as retinal afferent pupillary defect (RAPD), retinal whitening, macular cherry-red spot and intra-arterial emboli. Retinal fluorescein angiography, optical coherence tomography (OCT) and OCT angiography (OCTA) can confirm the diagnosis, showing delayed arterial filling, retinal ischemia and hyper-reflective inner retinal layers [31–33]. Therapeutical approaches, including anterior chamber paracentesis, drug-lowering intraocular pressure and ocular massage, are often useless [34].

Despite being rare among younger patients, retinal arterial obstructions are described to be linked to underlying cardiac abnormalities in 45% of individuals below the age of 45 [35]. Numerous reports have detailed the connection between PFO and retinal ischemic disorders [25,28,30–33,36–51] (Table 1). In a cohort of 18 patients diagnosed with either central or branch retinal artery occlusion, TEE was conducted to probe potential underlying cardiac or aortic disorders as sources of retinal emboli. The investigation unveiled that 17% of the patients exhibited a PFO [48]. Fekri and colleagues analyzed 23 cases of retinal ischemic events in the presence of PFO, revealing a comparable incidence of BRAO and CRAO. Most cases were under 50 years old (78.3%), and roughly 50% of patients underwent uncomplicated PFO closure. TEE exhibited higher sensitivity than TTE in diagnosing the underlying cardiac disease (71.4% versus 28.6%) [28]. Similar findings were reported by Wieder et al., demonstrating that TEE detected PFO in 85.7% of cases compared to 14.3% with TTE in the context of ischemic retinal disorders in patients with a mean age of 42.4 years [32].

Table 1. Summary of the studies showing retinal ischemic events in patients with PFO.

Author (Year)	Reference	Type of Study	Population	Outcomes
Sverdlichenko et al. (2024)	[25]	Prospective cohort study	20 cases under 45 years of age with TMVL (4 men and 16 women)	All patients included were referred for neuroimaging and cardiac investigations. Two of the thirteen patients who completed echocardiography had PFO (15%).
Fekri et al. (2024)	[28]	Case-study-based review	23 cases of CRAO (n = 10), BRAO (n = 10) and CILRAO (n = 3) with PFO	A total of 78.3% of the cases were under 50 years of age. A high RoPE score (≥7, suggestive of paradoxical embolism via PFO) was estimated for 71.4% of patients. TEE exhibited higher sensitivity than TTE in diagnosing the underlying cardiac disease (71.4% versus 28.6%). Approximately half of the patients underwent percutaneous closure of the PFO with no complications.
Jurgens et al. (2022)	[31]	Review and case report	1 case	A pregnant woman developed cilioretinal artery occlusion of thromboembolic origin associated with PFO. OCTA enabled risk-free imaging of retinal vessel perfusion during pregnancy.
Wieder et al. (2021)	[32]	Review and case report	1 case	A 43- year-old man presented with CRAO in the setting of PFO. TEE appeared more sensitive than TTE in diagnosing PFO (85.7% versus 14.3%).
Chatziralli et al. (2015)	[33]	Case report	1 case	A 35-year-old man presented with a left inferior BRAO. Cardiologic examination with TEE revealed a right-to-left shunt across PFO. The patient developed no other embolic event at the 9-month follow-up, having undergone an operation for PFO repair.

Table 1. *Cont.*

Author (Year)	Reference	Type of Study	Population	Outcomes
Inatomi et al. (2001)	[36]	Retrospective study	22 cases	A total of 22 patients with retinal artery occlusion (RAO) were analyzed. TEE findings were abnormal in 13 (59%) of the 22 patients. PFO was observed in 9% of patients.
Tayyab et al. (2023)	[37]	Case report	1 case	A teenage girl presented with CRAO in the right eye, which was accompanied by frontal headaches and vertigo. Investigations to rule out hematologic, vascular and cardiac causes were performed. TEE revealed PFO as the cause of this cryptogenic stroke.
Ho and Spaide (2007)	[38]	Case report	1 case	A healthy 15-year-old boy developed a CRAO with cilioretinal artery sparing after a fractured clavicle. Initially, no abnormalities were found after extensive systemic examinations. Subsequently, PFO was revealed by TEE, and the patient was scheduled for cardiac surgery.
Gabrielian et al. (2009)	[39]	Case report	1 case	A healthy 17-year-old male presented with sudden, painless loss of vision in his right eye while playing basketball. Fundus examination and fluorescein angiography confirmed a retinal artery occlusion. The hematological/infectious work-up, including TTE, was negative. However, TEE showed PFO. The patient underwent a successful percutaneous femoral catheterization to close the defect.
Nakagawa et al. (2004)	[40]	Case report	1 case	A 43-year-old woman presented a bilateral CRAO within one month. The patient was treated with urokinase and with an anticoagulant. The corrected VA recovered completely in the right eye and partially in the left eye. After extensive examination, TEE revealed a right-to-left shunt through PFO. The patient was treated with anticoagulants and has suffered no recurrence of CRAO.
Ascuitto et al. (2021)	[41]	Case report	1 case	A patient presented with painless, sudden visual loss in his left eye. He was diagnosed with CRAO, likely from a paradoxical embolus associated with an atrial septal aneurysm containing PFO. The patient underwent successful percutaneous closure of the PFO without complication.
Shoeibi et al. (2013)	[42]	Case report	1 case	A 29-year-old female patient presented a BRAO. The patient was treated with oral acetazolamide, topical timolol, ocular massage and anterior chamber paracentesis. The visual field defect partially recovered. After an extensive work-up, a small-sized PFO was detected by TEE. Low-dose aspirin therapy was initiated, and over the subsequent two years, no other embolic event occurred.
Wisotsky et al. (1993)	[43]	Case report	2 cases	A 28-year-old man and a 19-year-old woman presented BRAO. In each patient, PFO was demonstrated via transesophageal echocardiography after a transthoracic study disclosed no abnormalities.
Liu et al. (2017)	[44]	Case report	1 case	A 21-year-old man presented with an eight-day history of a blurry patch of vision in the right eye. A BRAO was diagnosed after fundus and OCT examinations. A TTE bubble contrast study showed a large right-to-left shunt at the atrial level. Percutaneous closure of the PFO was undertaken. Normal visual acuity after 12 months was recovered.
Grudzińska et al. (2021)	[45]	Case report	1 case	A 33-year-old Caucasian man presented a superior nasal loss of visual field and central scotoma in his left eye. A BRAO was diagnosed. The patient underwent standard TTE without any pathological findings. TEE revealed a marked leak through PFO, and cardiologists decided on foramen ovale closure.

Table 1. *Cont.*

Author (Year)	Reference	Type of Study	Population	Outcomes
Sheth et al. (2009)	[46]	Case report	1 case	An 18-year-old male claimed sudden-onset left visual loss. Ophthalmological examination revealed an afferent pupillary defect secondary to left hemiretinal artery occlusion. A subsequent cardiology review with TEE revealed PFO, which was closed surgically.
Sabanis et al. (2020)	[47]	Case report	1 case	A patient with no significant comorbidities experienced a paradoxical thromboembolic episode of CRAO. After a comprehensive examination, PFO was diagnosed after a bubble contrast TTE.
Kramer et al. (2001)	[48]	Retrospective observational case series	18 cases	A total of 18 patients who were diagnosed with retinal artery occlusion (7 CRAO, 11 BRAO) were analyzed. Cardiac or thoracic aortic pathologic conditions, which were a possible source of the retinal emboli, were detected by TEE in 13 of the 18 patients (72%). They included aortic arch atheroma (n = 7), mitral annulus calcification (n = 4), left atrial appendage thrombus (n = 2), valvular abnormalities (n = 5), left atrial smoke (n = 3) and PFO (n = 3). TEE showed higher sensitivity than TTE in detecting the cardiac emboli source.
Zhu et al. (2021)	[49]	Case report	1 case	A 46-year-old woman presented an amaurosis fugax lasting 20 min and a persistent visual alteration in her left eye. Fundus examination did not reveal significant abnormalities. Fundus fluorescein angiography showed a long arm–retina circulation time. Imaging examinations revealed bilateral internal carotid artery (ICA) hypoplasia and a variation in the circle of Willis. Furthermore, TEE showed the presence of a PFO and a cardiogenic embolic event. Aspirin 100 mg/day was given to the patient, and PFO occlusion surgery was recommended.
Si et al. (2023)	[50]	Review and case report	1 case	A 40-year-old woman reported a gradual decline in visual acuity, with visual field defects that had developed in two stages after HA injection as facial filler into the nasal root. Multiple retinal artery occlusions were diagnosed. PFO was detected by TEE. The patient was treated with intravenous dexamethasone and cobamamide, as well as extracorporeal counterpulsation therapy. Visual acuity improved from counting fingers at 30 cm to 20/133 within 3 days.
Pipolo et al. (2023)	[51]	Case report	1 case	A 28-year-old woman presented at the clinic 20 h after an acute visual field defect in the right eye. At that time, she was 18 weeks pregnant and had no report of complications in her previous pregnancy. After ophthalmological evaluation, BRAO was diagnosed. A transcranial Doppler with contrast indicated a right-to-left intracardiac shunt, confirmed by the presence of PFO at the TEE. Thrombophilic conditions were excluded. Enoxaparin 1 mg/kg was started and kept until the delivery. Then, a surgical closure of PFO was programmed.

While the exact pathogenesis of retinal arterial blockage in individuals with PFO remains incompletely understood, several mechanisms have been proposed. These include emboli formation within the atrial septum, transient arrhythmias leading to thrombus formation and paradoxical emboli originating from the peripheral venous system, which reach the head circulation occluding the ophthalmic artery and its branches [33,37].

Once diagnosed, considering PFO closure may be advisable to reduce the risk of additional ischemic vasculo-occlusive events [28,33,39,41,44–46].

Moreover, in addition to well-known risk factors like smoke and hypertension, an association with conditions such as internal carotid artery (ICA) hypoplasia, filler injections and pregnancy has also been described in patients with PFO developing retinal ischemic events [26,31,32,36,41,49–51].

ICA is one of the most important blood sources to the head, and its hypoplasia is rare. Many cases of abnormal development of ICA are asymptomatic, thanks to the compensatory action of collateral circulation. However, Zhu and co-authors reported a case of an apparently healthy woman who developed an AF due to the presence of a concomitant PFO in association with ICA hypoplasia that resulted in an embolism at the level of the retinal artery [49].

Facial filler with hyaluronic acid (HA) has previously been linked to visual loss. The retrograde flow mechanism is widely recognized as the primary explanation for sudden vision loss following HA injection for facial filler procedures. This phenomenon occurs when the injected filler material inadvertently enters a blood vessel, leading to its backward movement against the natural blood flow direction until it reaches the ocular circulation [52]. Nevertheless, in a recent report, a young woman presented multiple retinal artery ischemic events occurring in a peculiar pattern. Indeed, the patient's visual loss presented in two stages, rather than directly after injection, and was associated with dyspnea. Hence, the authors speculated that the HA entered systemic venous circulation, reached the right heart, passed directly into the left heart through a PFO and then caused retinal artery occlusion [50].

Various physiological adaptations, encompassing complex cardiovascular, coagulative, hormonal and immunological changes, occur during pregnancy and can trigger vascular occlusive events. The concomitant presence of PFO increases the risk of ocular thromboembolic events, as demonstrated by retinal vascular occlusion episodes described in two different reports. In these situations, OCTA, as a dye-free, non-invasive tool, represents a valuable option to diagnose and analyze the retinal perfusion status in pregnancy [31,51].

Therefore, PFO should be considered in cases of young patients who develop unexplained acute retinal ischemic events.

3.3. PFO and Migraine with Aura

Migraine is a neurological disorder characterized by recurrent, severe headaches, often accompanied by other symptoms, such as nausea, vomiting, sensitivity to light and visual disorder. Migraine attacks can cause significant pain and discomfort, sometimes lasting for hours to days, and can greatly disrupt daily life activities. Migraine with aura is a type of migraine characterized by specific neurological and visual symptoms, known as "aura", which usually occurs before the headache phase. The aura symptoms can vary widely among individuals but commonly include visual disturbances, such as flashing lights, blind spots or zigzag patterns which are usually bilateral. Other sensory disorders like tingling sensations in the face or hands, speech difficulties and confusion can be present. These symptoms develop gradually over a few minutes and last for about 20–60 min before the headache phase begins [53]. Multifactorial causative mechanisms, such as genetic, environmental and neurological factors, are recognized to be involved in migraine. Different triggers include stress, bright lights, certain foods, changes in sleep patterns, hormonal variations, sensory stimuli, weather changes and strong odors [53].

Migraine prevalence varies across different populations and regions, with a higher incidence among females [54]. The association between PFO and migraine has been widely described in the literature [10,55,56] (Table 2). Specifically, the relationship between PFO and migraine with aura was first described in a study carried out by Del Sette and colleagues. Among 80 migraineurs with aura, with an average age of 37.24 years, 36 individuals (45%) were found to have a cardiac right-to-left shunt [55]. Furthermore, migraine with aura appears to be more prevalent in individuals with PFO, and the latter is more common in migraineurs with aura than in the general population. Accordingly, a meta-analysis conducted by Schwedt et al. demonstrated a higher prevalence of PFO among migraine patients with aura (40.9–72.0%) compared to migraineurs without aura (16.2–33.7%). Moreover, the prevalence of migraine in individuals with PFO varied from 22.3% to 64.3% [10].

Table 2. Summary of the studies showing correlation between migraine and PFO.

Author (Year)	Reference	Type of Study	Population	Outcomes
Schwedt et al. (2008)	[10]	Systematic review	18 studies, 1517 patients	The aim of this study was to examine the prevalence of migraine in patients with PFO, the prevalence of PFO in migraineurs and the effect of PFO closure on migraine. The estimated strength of association between PFO and migraine, reflected by summary odds ratios (ORs), was 5.13 [95% confidence interval (CI) 4.67, 5.59], and between PFO and migraine with aura, the OR was 3.21 (95% CI 2.38, 4.17). The association between migraine and PFO was OR 2.54 (95% CI 2.01, 3.08). Six studies on PFO closure suggested improvement in migraine. The low-to-moderate grade of evidence from observational studies supports an apparent association between PFO and migraine. PFO closure seemed to affect migraine patterns favorably.
Del Sette et al. (2008)	[55]	Prospective study	87 patients	The objective of this study was to clarify the relationship between right-to-left shunt (RLS) and white matter lesions (WMLs) in patients with migraine with aura (MA). Among 80 migraineurs with aura, with an average age of 37.24 years, 36 individuals (45%) were found to have a cardiac right-to-left shunt. The comparison of T2-weighted MRI scans revealed no significant difference in the number of lesions or lesion loads between patients with and without RLS. In conclusion, RLS does not increase the likelihood of finding WMLs in migraineurs.
Liu et al. (2020)	[56]	Narrative review	99 articles	In this article, the potential pathophysiological mechanisms of migraine, the clinical symptoms of migraine with PFO and the clinical features of PFO with migraine were described. The incidence of PFO in migraine patients is higher than that in the general population, suggesting that PFO and migraine may be risk factors for each other, but more research is needed to confirm this speculation. An increasing number of studies have found that migraines with aura are more closely associated with PFO, and the presence of right-to-left shunt (RLS) increased the likelihood of aura attacks. The evidence supports a "dose–response" relationship between migraine and PFO, although more work needs to be conducted in terms of patient selection as well as the inclusion of an antiplatelet control group for PFO closure interventions to uncover possible beneficial results in clinical trials.
Wilmshurst (2018)	[57]	Randomized controlled trial	147 patients	The Migraine Intervention with STARFlex Technology (MIST) trial was a randomized double-blind trial in patients with severe intractable migraine with aura and moderate–large PFO that compared the implantation of STARFlex devices with the intention of closing their PFO versus a sham procedure. The results showed no significant difference in migraine outcomes between those receiving the STARFlex implant and those in the sham group.
Dowson et al. (2008)	[58]	Randomized controlled trial	432 patients	The aim of this study was to investigate whether closing patent foramen ovale (PFO) could effectively treat migraine with aura. Patients were randomly assigned to transcatheter PFO closure with the STARFlex implant or to a sham procedure. No significant difference was observed in the primary endpoint of migraine headache cessation between the implant and sham groups.
Mattle et al. (2016)	[59]	Randomized controlled trial	107 patients	The Percutaneous Closure of Patent Foramen Ovale In Migraine with Aura (PRIMA) study aimed to evaluate the efficacy of percutaneous patent foramen ovale (PFO) closure in reducing migraine symptoms in patients diagnosed with migraine with aura. Patients were divided in two groups and treated with a PFO closure or medical treatment. Despite the safety of the procedure, PFO closure did not reduce overall monthly migraine days.
Tobis et al. (2017)	[60]	Randomized controlled trial	230 patients	The Prospective, Randomized Investigation to Evaluate Incidence of Headache Reduction in Subjects With Migraine and PFO Using the AMPLATZER PFO Occluder to Medical Management (PREMIUM) study investigated migraine reduction in subjects with persistent migraines and PFO. It compared medical therapy alone to therapy combined with PFO closure using the Amplatzer device. The trial found no superior reduction in migraine attacks with PFO closure compared to sham control. However, it did show a significant decrease in headache days among subjects with or without aura following PFO closure.

Table 2. *Cont.*

Author (Year)	Reference	Type of Study	Population	Outcomes
Giardini et al. (2006)	[61]	Prospective study	38 patients	This study evaluated the long-term outcomes of transcatheter patent foramen ovale (PFO) closure on migraine headache with aura (MHA) and recurrent stroke risk. Among 38 patients followed for at least 3 years after the procedure, 92% reported complete resolution of MHA after an average of 4.9 years. Recurrent stroke occurred in 5.3% of cases within 5 years, predominantly within the first 15 months after the procedure. Overall, the MIDAS scores significantly decreased (from 38.6 ± 26.3 to 4.4 ± 5.1, $p < 0.0001$) following intervention.
Yan et al. (2024)	[62]	Retrospective study	78 patients	This study aimed to investigate the therapeutic efficacy of patent foramen ovale (PFO) closure in migraine patients with a massive right-to-left shunt (RLS). The study included 51 patients without white matter lesions (WMLs) (control group, CG) and 27 patients with white matter lesions (WMLs) (observation group, OG). PFO closure proved effective and safe in treating migraine patients with RLS. However, for those with WMLs, clinical attention should be directed toward the treatment of WMLs.
Elbadawi et al. (2018)	[63]	Meta-analysis	3 studies, 484 patients	The analysis included three key studies: the MIST, PRIMA and PREMIUM trials. The primary outcome demonstrated a significant reduction in monthly migraine attacks, favoring PFO closure over control groups ($p = 0.01$). Although complete resolution of migraine attacks showed a trend favoring PFO closure, the difference did not achieve statistical significance. In patients with predominant aura migraine attacks, PFO closure demonstrated a significant reduction in migraine attacks. No significant differences in responders' rate between PFO closure and control groups were found.
Shi et al. (2017)	[64]	Meta-analysis and systematic review	8 articles, 546 patients	The study investigated how the closure of patent foramen ovale (PFO) affected migraine in 546 patients, distinguishing between those with migraine with aura (MA) and migraine without aura (MwoA). Following PFO closure, migraine symptoms improved in 81% of MA patients and 63% of MwoA patients. The benefits of PFO closure were significantly greater for patients with MA compared to patients with MwoA ($p = 0.03$).
Zhang et al. (2022)	[65]	Meta-analysis	3 RCTs, 1 pooled study, 8 case series, 1165 patients	The aim of the study was to evaluate the impact of patent foramen ovale (PFO) closure on migraine. The findings revealed a statistically significant reduction in both monthly migraine attacks and migraine days, along with a substantial decrease in migraine frequency and severity in patients undergoing PFO closure, particularly those with migraines accompanied by aura (MA). The meta-analysis supports PFO closure as a potentially effective and safe therapeutic option for reducing the migraine burden, particularly in patients with MA.
Zhang et al. (2021)	[66]	Meta-analysis	3 RCTs, 4 observation studies, 887 patients	The meta-analysis findings indicate that PFO closure leads to a substantial reduction in both monthly migraine attacks and migraine days per month compared to control groups. This effect was particularly pronounced in patients with migraine accompanied by aura, where there was a notable increase in the rate of complete cessation of migraine attacks following the procedure. These results underscore the potential of PFO closure as an effective therapeutic option for managing migraine, especially in cases where traditional treatments have been insufficient.

The pathophysiology of migraine with aura in patients with PFO remains uncertain. Various vasoactive substances, including serotonin or 5-hydroxytryptamine, typically processed through the pulmonary circulation, may bypass this route via the PFO, potentially triggering migraines. Additionally, small emboli passing through the PFO into the arterial system could lead to microinfarctions or cortical spreading depression, precipitating migraine attacks. Furthermore, focal areas of reduced blood flow near the ischemic threshold in the occipital regions may lead to visual symptoms during the aura episode [56,57].

Although multiple studies have investigated the effect of closing PFO on migraine, the therapeutic effect of this surgical procedure is still controversial. The MIST trial found no significant difference between patients who underwent PFO closure and those who did not [58]. On the other hand, the PRIMA trial did not demonstrate a reduction in its primary endpoint based on decreasing migraine days [59], while the PREMIUM trial showed a statistically significant decrease in headache days but failed to achieve a reduction in its primary outcome, defined as a responder rate with a 50% decrease in migraine attacks [60]. Conversely, other reports showed a significant decrease in the frequency of migraine attacks following PFO closure in patients with migraine with aura [61–66]. Specifically, an overall reduction in the frequency of migraine attacks per day and a decrease in the number of headache days were observed over one month [65,66]. Moreover, in patients whose migraine episodes were with aura, there was a decrease in migraine attacks following PFO closure compared to control groups [63].

Considering that visual symptoms usually precede the headache, ophthalmologists play an important role in diagnosing migraine with aura and differentiating it from other ophthalmic conditions that may present with similar symptoms, such as retinal ischemia or retinal detachment. Additionally, ophthalmologists may collaborate with neurologists in the management of migraine with aura, providing guidance on lifestyle modifications and strategies to manage migraine triggers (e.g., bright lights, stress and irregular sleep patterns) that may exacerbate symptoms. Moreover, they may prescribe medications to alleviate symptoms or recommend specialized examinations, such as visual field testing or neuroimaging studies, to further evaluate the underlying cause of symptoms [67].

3.4. PFO and Impaired Eye Movement

Eye movements are coordinated motions of the eyes, which allow perception of the surrounding space, the tracking of objects and focusing on specific targets. These movements are controlled by a complex system, involving muscles, nerves and various brain regions. Oculomotor disfunctions are characterized by the weakness or paralysis of the muscles within or surrounding the eye, resulting in impaired ocular action or control (Figure 2A,B). These can be caused by different factors, including nerve damage, trauma, inflammation, underlying systemic disorders or ischemic strokes. Injuries at the level of brain visual-related areas can impair the oculomotor system, resulting in several alterations in coordination, visual acuity and visual field orientation [68].

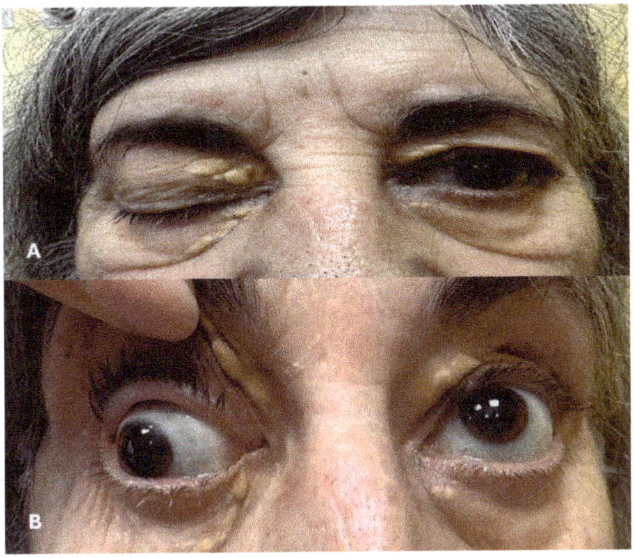

Figure 2. Impaired eye movement related to PFO: (**A**) Right eye third nerve palsy presenting a complete ptosis. (**B**) After eyelid elevation, the right eye appears to be positioned downward and outward, with inability to adduce, infraduce or overduce. The pupil is dilated with slow reaction.

The association between PFO and impaired eye movement is rare, and only few cases have been described [69–73] (Table 3). Cerebral lesions, involving the midbrain and other vision areas, were considered the consequence of paradoxical emboli resulting from the direct pass in the vascular system and in the cerebral circulation through the right–left shunt [69–73]. Internuclear ophthalmoplegia (IO)—a disorder characterized by a lesion of medial longitudinal fasciculus resulting in an ipsilesional adduction deficit with a nystagmus of the abducting eye—is often secondary to brain ischemia. A 39-year-old woman presented bilateral ptosis and IO associated with PFO diagnosed with TEE. After undergoing PFO closure and starting aspirin therapy for secondary prevention, the patient remained clinically stable over a one-year follow-up. [69]. A previously healthy 16-year-old girl experienced an IO secondary to a lesion of the left midbrain at the level of quadrigeminal lamina. Six months after aspirin therapy and PFO closure, her cerebral lesions and her eye movements were restored [70]. In addition, Zhuang and colleagues reported a case of a 55-year-old male who experienced a complete peripheral facial palsy and horizontal gaze palsy after Valsalva maneuver caused by paradoxical embolization from PFO. After 6 months and surgical closure, the symptoms improved [71]. Conversely, a 61-year-old man who had a severe embolic event involving the posterior cerebral artery territory, resulting in left hemiparesis, dysarthria, bilateral ptosis, and impaired eye movement on both sides, experienced only partial improvement after anticoagulant therapy. [72]. Khan described a case of an acute pupil-sparing complete third nerve palsy (complete ptosis, moderate hypotropia, large exotropia and no supraduction/infraduction/adduction) in a healthy young woman with PFO. After PFO closure, the neurological recovery was complete, except for diplopia and relatively comitant hypotropia, which responded well to conventional strabismus surgery [71]. Thus, despite only a few cases having been reported, PFO should be considered in cases of impaired eye movement secondary to embolic stroke in apparently healthy people [69–73].

Table 3. Summary of the articles showing correlation between impaired eye movement and PFO.

Author (Year)	Reference	Type of Study	Population	Outcomes
Xie et al. (2022)	[69]	Case report	1 case	A 39-year-old woman presented with sudden bilateral ptosis and diplopia exacerbated by leftward gaze, persisting for 3 days. Neurological examination and MRI confirmed acute midbrain infarction. The tests excluded other stroke causes but confirmed a large right-to-left shunt via PFO. She underwent PFO closure and received aspirin.
Mazurkiewicz-Bełdzińska et al. (2015)	[70]	Case report	1 case	A healthy 16-year-old girl had sudden diplopia and dizziness following a headache. MRI confirmed left midbrain ischemia with left internuclear ophthalmoplegia. PFO was discovered by TTE and TEE. Medical treatment led to full recovery of neurological deficits in two weeks. Six months after aspirin therapy and PFO closure, her cerebral lesions and her eye movements were restored.
Zhuang et al. (2021)	[71]	Case report	1 case	A 55-year-old man presented with sudden bilateral gaze palsy, upbeat nystagmus and facial paralysis. MRI revealed new pontine infarctions linked to PFO with significant shunt. He was treated with rivaroxaban and underwent PFO closure, resolving his symptoms. A follow-up MRI at 6 months showed no new lesions.
Takahashi et al. (2018)	[72]	Case report	1 case	A 61-year-old heavy smoker presented with sudden vision distortion and left leg weakness, revealing multiple brain infarctions correlated with PFO. Treatment included anticoagulants and antiplatelets, but severe residual deficits persisted after 12 weeks.
Khan (2012)	[73]	Case report	1 case	A healthy 23-year-old woman experienced sudden right third nerve palsy and facial weakness. MRI showed midbrain infarction linked to a large PFO. Surgical closure resolved the symptoms; strabismus surgery corrected residual right hypotropia, ensuring stable vision postoperatively.

3.5. PFO and Endogenous Eye Infections

Endophthalmitis refers to inflammation and infection of the fluids and tissues inside the eye and can result in devastating sight-threatening and systemic complications (Figure 3A–C). It can recognize an exogenous or endogenous origin. Most cases are of exogenous origin, typically arising from microbes entering the eye through an external source like penetrating trauma, intraocular surgery or corneal infection. Conversely, endogenous endophthalmitis results from the spread of bacterial or fungal infections from a distant site in the body, typically through the bloodstream [74]. In this type of endophthalmitis, the damage occurs mainly due to a septic embolus entering the posterior segment vasculature and acting as a trigger for the dissemination of micro-organisms into the surrounding tissues. After passing the blood–ocular barrier, the infection extends from the retina and choroid into the vitreous cavity, and subsequently, to the anterior chamber of the eye [75]. The common sources of infection leading to endogenous endophthalmitis include bacterial endocarditis, intravenous drug use and certain systemic infections like candidiasis or tuberculosis [74].

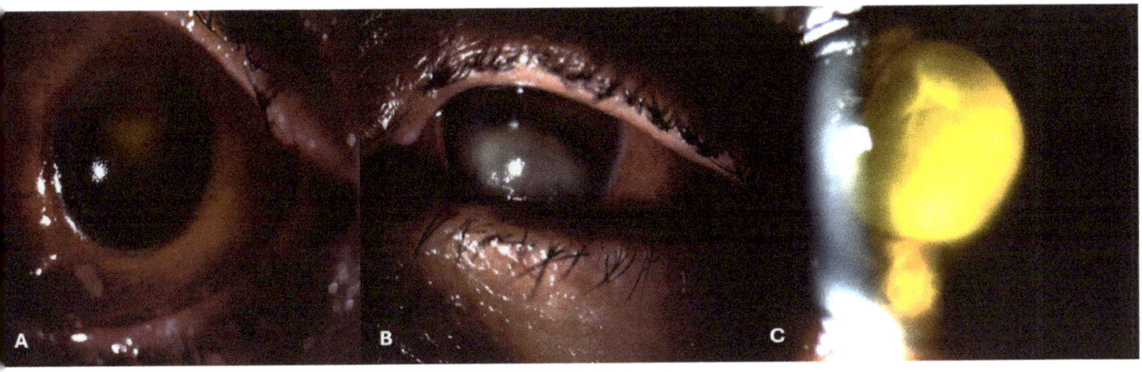

Figure 3. Endogenous eye infection related to PFO: (**A–C**) Slit lamp images of endophthalmitis showing conjunctival redness, purulent discharge, chemosis, hypopyon and fibrin in the pupillary field.

Rodrigues et al. described a case of endogenous endophthalmitis that developed as the first manifestation of right-sided endocarditis in a patient with an undiagnosed PFO [76]. A 66-year-old female with chronic renal failure presenting fever and eye endophthalmitis was treated with systemic antibiotics and enucleation. However, since a persistent systemic infection with positive blood cultures was observed, adjunctive analyses, including TEE, were performed, and a right endocarditis with a PFO was diagnosed [76]. Hence, even though paradoxical embolization through a PFO from right-sided endocarditis is rare [77], the presence of an interatrial defect caused ocular infection in this case. Therefore, an underlying cardiac defect should be taken into account in cases of endogenous endophthalmitis, where the source of primary infection is unidentified.

4. Discussion

The spectrum of clinical presentations associated with PFO encompasses a wide array of manifestations, including ophthalmological conditions like retinal artery occlusions, migraine with aura, impaired eye movements and endogenous infections (Figure 4).

The management of arterial occlusion remains a subject of ongoing debate. In the acute phase, the foremost goal for the ophthalmologist is to promptly restore retinal blood flow. Prolonged hypoxia has been demonstrated to lead to irreversible visual damage, underscoring the urgency of this intervention. Moving into the subacute phase, the ophthalmologist's focus shifts to assessing the patient in order to ascertain the underlying causative mechanism. This evaluation is crucial for preventing further ocular or systemic complications [34]. Despite the lack of clinical trials, the associations between PFO and acute retinal ischemic events have been described in multiple reports. According to retinal and ophthalmic artery occlusions guidelines provided by the American Academy of Ophthalmology, conditions like ophthalmic artery occlusion, CRAO and BRAO can potentially indicate life-threatening situations [78]. Therefore, particularly in cases where the initial examination does not reveal a causative mechanism for embolic disease, considering the significant risk of ischemic stroke associated with ocular arterial occlusions, ophthalmologists must refer patients to a stroke center for multidisciplinary medical evaluation, including echocardiography and other imaging analyses.

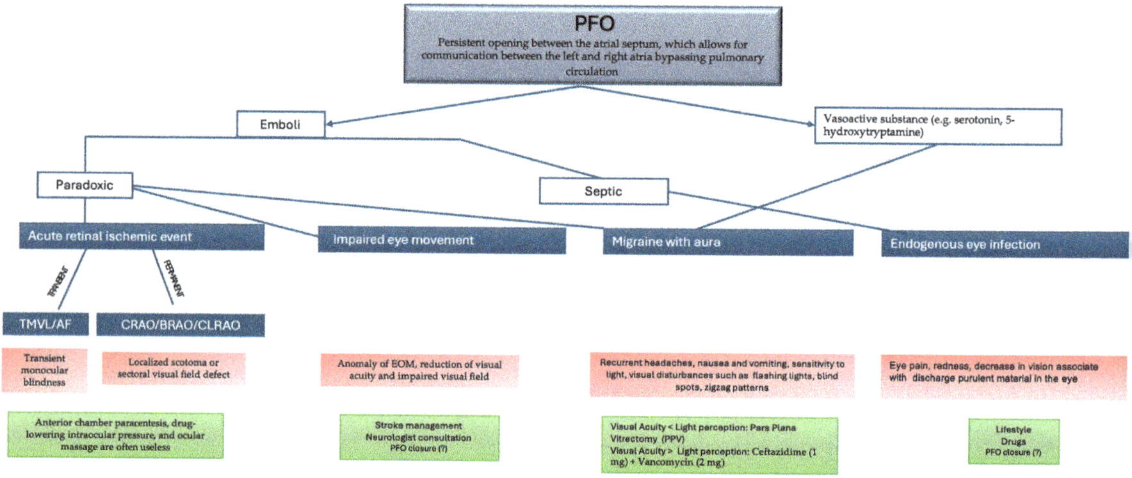

Figure 4. The diagram schematically illustrates the mechanism by which ophthalmic complications occur due to PFO. The symptoms of each condition are presented in the red squares, while the green squares show the possible management strategies.

Ophthalmologists frequently serve as the initial specialists to evaluate individuals experiencing visual symptoms related to migraines. The exact pathophysiological mechanisms linking PFO to migraine with aura remain uncertain. However, the higher prevalence of PFO among migraineurs with aura compared to the general population was shown in several studies, suggesting a relationship between these two entities. Although PFO closure has shown contrasting results in the management of migraine, considering the low complication rate of the procedure, surgical intervention, as secondary prevention, represents a valid option.

Managing ocular palsies typically involves several approaches, depending on the underlying cause, which need to be identified, and on the severity of the condition. Impaired eye movement in the presence of PFO is rarely reported. Nevertheless, in cases of cryptogenic embolic strokes affecting visual motility-related brain regions, the clinical suspicion of PFO should be raised, especially in young patients.

When suspecting endogenous endophthalmitis, an accurate diagnostic evaluation is crucial to identify a potential hematogenous spread of micro-organisms from a distant source in the body. It is worth noting that the presence of PFO may elevate the risk of paradoxical embolization. Indeed, particularly in patients with predisposing factors, such as bacterial endocarditis, endogenous ocular infection could be secondary to the presence of an undetected communication between the two atria. Despite ongoing debates, the consensus on the therapeutic approach to these conditions remains elusive. However, according to the guidelines from the European Society of Cataract and Refractive Surgery, pars plana vitrectomy appears to offer the most favorable visual outcomes in cases where visual acuity is limited to light perception. For patients with visual acuity exceeding light perception, the therapeutic strategies remain uncertain. Evidence suggests that combining the same antibiotics via both intravitreal and systemic routes is the most effective approach. Administering ceftazidime (1 mg) and vancomycin (2 mg) separately is considered the gold standard [79].

In summary, after diagnosing an ocular embolic event, ophthalmologists should ideally require further investigation, including a TTE or a TEE, by echocardiographic imaging specialists. Once a PFO is diagnosed, potential interventional therapies should be considered, including PFO closure and medical therapy. The meta-analysis by Vukadinović et al. indicated that percutaneous PFO closure significantly reduces the risk of ischemic recurrences compared to medical therapy, especially in cases of large or moderate shunts [80]. Similarly, Turc et al. stated that PFO closure is superior to antithrombotic therapy in preventing stroke recurrence after cryptogenic stroke despite an increased risk of atrial fibrillation after the surgical procedure [81]. Conversely, Liu and colleagues reported that, compared with drug therapy, PFO closure reduces the risk of recurrent stroke and the incidence of serious bleeding without increasing the risk of new-onset atrial fibrillation or atrial flutter [82].

Hence, while the direct involvement of ophthalmologists in diagnosing PFO itself may be limited, their expertise in assessing ocular health and recognizing subtle signs of systemic diseases is invaluable. The correlation between ocular signs and symptoms and systemic diseases has been well documented. Recently, the interest in identifying ocular risk factors or biomarkers for diagnosing or excluding systemic diseases has significantly increased, leading to the emergence of oculomics. By examining the eye's structure and function, oculomics aims to provide insights into a patient's overall health, identifying the potential risk factors for diseases beyond the eye [83]. In this context, the deep-learning algorithm RetiCAC, which uses retinal photographs to predict the presence of coronary artery calcium (CAC), has demonstrated improved cardiovascular risk stratification compared to traditional clinical parameters [84].

Nonetheless, collaboration with other specialists like cardiologists and neurologists still remains essential for ensuring timely diagnosis, comprehensive evaluation and appropriate treatment selection.

5. Conclusions

It should be noted that PFO is a highly common condition that can cause severe ocular complications. This review analyzed the diverse clinical scenarios in which PFO may be implicated, shedding light on the importance of early recognition and multidisciplinary management in optimizing patient care. Ophthalmologists, as the first healthcare professionals to encounter patients presenting with ocular symptoms and signs, upon identifying suspicious findings, should be aware of this possible subtle entity and promptly refer patients to appropriate specialists.

6. Future Directions

Given the limited number of reports on certain ocular disorders associated with PFO, future prospective studies and clinical trials are warranted to provide further insights into the preventive role and optimal therapeutic strategies for managing these conditions. Large-scale, multicenter studies with long-term follow-up periods would help elucidate the natural history of PFO-related ocular complications. Additionally, effective research comparing different treatment modalities and their impact on clinical outcomes would be valuable for guiding clinical decision making and optimizing patient care.

Author Contributions: F.L., L.F. and C.C. analyzed the literature and wrote the original draft; R.M. and G.G. conceived the article and reviewed the manuscript. All authors have read and agreed to the published version of the manuscript.

Funding: This research received no external funding.

Conflicts of Interest: The authors declare no conflicts of interest.

References

1. Homma, S.; Messé, S.R.; Rundek, T.; Sun, Y.-P.; Franke, J.; Davidson, K.; Sievert, H.; Sacco, R.L.; Di Tullio, M.R. Patent forame ovale. *Nat. Rev. Dis. Prim.* **2016**, *2*, 15086. [CrossRef] [PubMed]
2. Meissner, I.; Khandheria, B.K.; Heit, J.A.; Petty, G.W.; Sheps, S.G.; Schwartz, G.L.; Whisnant, J.P.; Wiebers, D.O.; Covalt, J.L Petterson, T.M.; et al. Patent foramen ovale: Innocent or guilty? Evidence from a prospective population-based study. *J. Am. Co Cardiol.* **2006**, *47*, 440–445. [CrossRef]
3. Koutroulou, I.; Tsivgoulis, G.; Tsalikakis, D.; Karacostas, D.; Grigoriadis, N.; Karapanayiotides, T. Epidemiology of Pater Foramen Ovale in General Population and in Stroke Patients: A Narrative Review. *Front. Neurol.* **2020**, *11*, 281. [CrossRe [PubMed] [PubMed Central]
4. Hagen, P.T.; Scholz, D.G.; Edwards, W.D. Incidence and size of patent foramen ovale during the first 10 decades of life: A autopsy study of 965 normal hearts. *Mayo Clin. Proc.* **1984**, *59*, 17–20. [CrossRef] [PubMed]
5. Homma, S.; Sacco, R.L. Patent foramen ovale and stroke. *Circulation* **2005**, *112*, 1063–1072. [CrossRef] [PubMed]
6. Serena, J.; Marti-Fàbregas, J.; Santamarina, E.; Rodríguez, J.J.; Perez-Ayuso, M.J.; Masjuan, J.; Segura, T.; Gállego, J.; Dávalos, A Recurrent stroke and massive right-to-left shunt: Results from the prospective Spanish multicenter (CODICIA) study. *Stroke* **200** *39*, 3131–3136. [CrossRef] [PubMed]
7. Alsheikh-Ali, A.A.; Thaler, D.E.; Kent, D.M. Patent foramen ovale in cryptogenic stroke: Incidental or pathogenic? *Stroke* **2009**, *4* 2349–2355. [CrossRef] [PubMed] [PubMed Central]
8. Katsanos, A.H.; Bhole, R.; Frogoudaki, A.; Giannopoulos, S.; Goyal, N.; Vrettou, A.R.; Ikonomidis, I.; Paraskevaidis, I.; Pappas, K Parissis, J.; et al. The value of transesophageal echocardiography for embolic strokes of undetermined source. *Neurology* **2016**, *8* 988–995. [CrossRef] [PubMed] [PubMed Central]
9. Dagra, A.; Lucke-Wold, B.; McGrath, K.; Mehkri, I.; Mehkri, Y.; Davidson, C.G.; Gilberstadt, N.; Douglas, B.W.; Hoh, B. Centra Retinal Artery Occlusion: A Review of Pathophysiological Features and Management. *Stroke Vasc. Interv. Neurol.* **2024**, *4*, e00097 [CrossRef]
10. Schwedt, T.J.; Demaerschalk, B.M.; Dodick, D.W. Patent foramen ovale and migraine: A quantitative systematic review. *Cephalalg* **2008**, *28*, 531–540. [CrossRef]
11. Collado, F.M.S.; Poulin, M.F.; Murphy, J.J.; Jneid, H.; Kavinsky, C.J. Patent Foramen Ovale Closure for Stroke Prevention an Other Disorders. *J. Am. Heart Assoc.* **2018**, *7*, e007146. [CrossRef] [PubMed]
12. Homma, S.; Di Tullio, M.R.; Sacco, R.L.; Mihalatos, D.; Li Mandri, G.; Mohr, J.P. Characteristics of patent foramen ovale associate with cryptogenic stroke. A biplane transesophageal echocardiographic study. *Stroke* **1994**, *25*, 582–586. [CrossRef] [PubMed]
13. Goel, S.S.; Tuzcu, E.M.; Shishehbor, M.H.; de Oliveira, E.I.; Borek, P.P.; Krasuski, R.A.; Rodriguez, L.L.; Kapadia, S.R. Morpholog of the patent foramen ovale in asymptomatic versus symptomatic (stroke or transient ischemic attack) patients. *Am. J. Cardio* **2009**, *103*, 124–129. [CrossRef] [PubMed]
14. Clarke, N.R.A.; Timperley, J.; Kelion, A.D.; Banning, A.P. Transthoracic echocardiography using second harmonic imaging wit Valsalva manoeuvre for the detection of right to left shunts. *Eur. J. Echocardiogr. J. Work. Gr. Echocardiogr. Eur. Soc. Cardiol.* **2004**, 176–181. [CrossRef] [PubMed]
15. Daniëls, C.; Weytjens, C.; Cosyns, B.; Schoors, D.; Desutter, J.; Paelinck, B.; Muyldermans, L.; Vancamp, G. Second harmoni transthoracic echocardiography: The new reference screening method for the detection of patent foramen ovale. *Eur. Echocardiogr. J. Work. Gr. Echocardiogr. Eur. Soc. Cardiol.* **2004**, *5*, 449–452. [CrossRef] [PubMed]
16. Takaya, Y.; Nakayama, R.; Akagi, T.; Yokohama, F.; Miki, T.; Nakagawa, K.; Toh, N.; Ito, H. Importance of saline contras transthoracic echocardiography for evaluating large right-to-left shunt in patent foramen ovale associated with cryptogeni stroke. *Int. J. Cardiovasc. Imaging* **2022**, *38*, 515–520. [CrossRef] [PubMed] [PubMed Central]
17. Schneider, B.; Zienkiewicz, T.; Jansen, V.; Hofmann, T.; Noltenius, H.; Meinertz, T. Diagnosis of patent foramen ovale by transesophageal echocardiography and correlation with autopsy findings. *Am. J. Cardiol.* **1996**, *77*, 1202–1209. [CrossRef [PubMed]
18. Zanette, E.M.; Mancini, G.; De Castro, S.; Solaro, M.; Cartoni, D.; Chiarotti, F. Patent foramen ovale and transcranial Doppler Comparison of different procedures. *Stroke* **1996**, *27*, 2251–2255. [CrossRef] [PubMed]
19. Job, F.P.; Ringelstein, E.; Grafen, Y.; Flachskampf, F.A.; Doherty, C.; Stockmanns, A.; Hanrath, P. Comparison of transcrania contrast Doppler sonography and transesophageal contrast echocardiography for the detection of patent foramen ovale in young stroke patients. *Am. J. Cardiol.* **1994**, *74*, 381–384. [CrossRef]
20. Klötzsch, C.; Janssen, G.; Berlit, P. Transesophageal echocardiography and contrast-TCD in the detection of a patent foramen ovale: Experiences with 111 patients. *Neurology* **1994**, *44*, 1603–1606. [CrossRef]
21. Mojadidi, M.K.; Roberts, S.C.; Winoker, J.S.; Romero, J.; Goodman-Meza, D.; Gevorgyan, R.; Tobis, J.M. Accuracy of transcrania Doppler for the diagnosis of intracardiac right-to-left shunt: A bivariate meta-analysis of prospective studies. *JACC Cardiovasc Imaging* **2014**, *7*, 236–250. [CrossRef] [PubMed]
22. Van, H.; Poommipanit, P.; Shalaby, M.; Gevorgyan, R.; Tseng, C.H.; Tobis, J. Sensitivity of transcranial Doppler versus intracardia echocardiography in the detection of right-to-left shunt. *JACC Cardiovasc. Imaging* **2010**, *3*, 343–348. [CrossRef]
23. Hayreh, S.S. Ocular vascular occlusive disorders: Natural history of visual outcome. *Prog. Retin. Eye Res.* **2014**, *41*, 1–25 [CrossRef] [PubMed]

24. Kvickström, P.; Lindblom, B.; Bergström, G.; Zetterberg, M. Amaurosis fugax: Risk factors and prevalence of significant carotid stenosis. *Clin. Ophthalmol.* **2016**, *10*, 2165–2170. [CrossRef] [PubMed]
25. Sverdlichenko, I.; Donaldson, L.; Margolin, E. Yield of Investigations in Young Patients Presenting With Transient Monocular Vision Loss: A Prospective Study. *Am. J. Ophthalmol.* **2024**, *257*, 137–142. [CrossRef] [PubMed]
26. Clifford, L.; Sievers, R.; Salmon, A.; Newsom, R.S.B. Central retinal artery occlusion: Association with patent foramen ovale. *Eye* **2006**, *20*, 736–738. [CrossRef] [PubMed]
27. Chang, Y.S.; Ho, C.H.; Chu, C.C.; Wang, J.J.; Tseng, S.H.; Jan, R.L. Risk of retinal artery occlusion in patients with diabetes mellitus: A retrospective large-scale cohort study. *PLoS ONE* **2018**, *13*, e0201627. [CrossRef] [PubMed]
28. Fekri, S.; Mahmoudimehr, P.; Jafari Fesharaki, M.; Hosseinjani, E.; Abtahi, S.H.; Nouri, H. Retinal arterial occlusion and patent foramen ovale: A case study-based review. *J. Fr. Ophtalmol.* **2024**, *47*, 104021. [CrossRef] [PubMed]
29. Schneider, M.; Molnar, A.; Angeli, O.; Szabo, D.; Bernath, F.; Hajdu, D.; Gombocz, E.; Mate, B.; Jiling, B.; Nagy, B.V.; et al. Prevalence of Cilioretinal Arteries: A systematic review and a prospective cross-sectional observational study. *Acta Ophthalmol.* **2021**, *99*, e310–e318. [CrossRef]
30. Draper, E.M.; Malloy, K.A. Case Report: Retinal Artery Occlusion Associated with Patent Foramen Ovale. *Clin. Insights Eyecare* **2023**, *1*, 1–9.
31. Jürgens, L.; Yaici, R.; Schnitzler, C.M.; Fleitmann, A.K.; Roth, M.; Schröder, K.; Guthoff, R. Retinal vascular occlusion in pregnancy: Three case reports and a review of the literature. *J. Med. Case Rep.* **2022**, *16*, 167. [CrossRef] [PubMed]
32. Wieder, M.S.; Blace, N.; Szlechter, M.M.; Shulman, E.; Thankenchen, J.; Mbekeani, J.N. Central retinal artery occlusion associated with patent foramen ovale: A case report and literature review. *Arq. Bras. Oftalmol.* **2021**, *84*, 494–498. [CrossRef]
33. Chatziralli, I.P.; Parikakis, E.A.; Mitropoulos, P.G. Undiagnosed patent foramen ovale as a rare cause for branch retinal artery occlusion. *Eur. J. Ophthalmol.* **2015**, *25*, e88–e90. [CrossRef]
34. Biousse, V.; Nahab, F.; Newman, N.J. Management of Acute Retinal Ischemia: Follow the Guidelines! *Ophthalmology* **2018**, *125*, 1597–1607. [CrossRef] [PubMed]
35. Sharma, S.; Sharma, S.M.; Cruess, A.F.; Brown, G.C. Transthoracic echocardiography in young patients with acute retinal arterial obstruction. RECO Study Group. Retinal Emboli of Cardiac Origin Group. *Can. J. Ophthalmol.* **1997**, *32*, 38–41.
36. Inatomi, Y.; Hino, H.; Hashimoto, Y.; Furuyoshi, N.; Misumi, I.; Uchino, M. Transesophageal echocardiography for detection of cardiac diseases in patients with retinal artery occlusion. *Intern. Med.* **2001**, *40*, 475–478. [CrossRef]
37. Tayyab, H.; Aamir, F.B.; Kirmani, S. Central retinal artery occlusion as a result of symptomatic patent foramen ovale. *Rom. J. Ophthalmol.* **2023**, *67*, 69–72. [CrossRef]
38. Ho, I.V.; Spaide, R. Central retinal artery occlusion associated with a patent foramen ovale. *Retina* **2007**, *27*, 259–260. [CrossRef] [PubMed]
39. Gabrielian, A.; Mieler, W.F.; Hariprasad, S.M. Retinal artery occlusion associated with a patent foramen ovale. *Eye* **2010**, *24*, 396–397. [CrossRef]
40. Nakagawa, T.; Hirata, A.; Inoue, N.; Hashimoto, Y.; Tanihara, H. A case of bilateral central retinal artery obstruction with patent foramen ovale. *Acta Ophthalmol. Scand.* **2004**, *82*, 111–112. [CrossRef]
41. Ascuitto, M.; Guertin, D.; Weaver, K. Acute unilateral vision loss from central retinal artery occlusion associated with an atrial septal aneurysm and a patent foramen ovale: A case report. *Fam. Pract.* **2021**, *38*, 834–836. [CrossRef] [PubMed]
42. Shoeibi, N.; Poorzand, H.; Abrishami, M. Branch retinal artery occlusion in a patient with patent foramen ovale. *J. Ophthalmic Vis. Res.* **2013**, *8*, 58–61. [PubMed]
43. Wisotsky, B.J.; Engel, H.M. Transesophageal echocardiography in the diagnosis of branch retinal artery obstruction. *Am. J. Ophthalmol.* **1993**, *115*, 653–656. [CrossRef] [PubMed]
44. Liu, X.; Calvert, P.A.; Arif, S.; Keane, P.A.; Denniston, A.K. Patent foramen ovale presenting as visual loss. *JRSM Open* **2016**, *8*, 2054270416669302. [CrossRef] [PubMed]
45. Grudzińska, E.; Nowacka, B.; Bania, B.; Lubiński, W.; Zaborski, D.; Modrzejewska, M. Patent foramen ovale as a cause of acute vision loss. *Int. J. Ophthalmol.* **2021**, *14*, 1125–1126. [CrossRef] [PubMed]
46. Sheth, H.G.; Laverde-Konig, T.; Raina, J. Undiagnosed patent foramen ovale presenting as retinal artery occlusion-an emerging association. *J. Ophthalmol.* **2009**, *2009*, 248269. [CrossRef] [PubMed]
47. Sabanis, N.; Zagkotsis, G.; Krikos, V.D.; Paschou, E.; Tapanlis, A. Central Retinal Artery Occlusion Secondary to Patent Foramen Ovale: The Unexpected Journey of a Paradoxical Embolus. *Cureus* **2020**, *12*, e9496. [CrossRef] [PubMed]
48. Kramer, M.; Goldenberg-Cohen, N.; Shapira, Y.; Axer-Siegel, R.; Shmuely, H.; Adler, Y.; Weinberger, D.; Sagie, A. Role of transesophageal echocardiography in the evaluation of patients with retinal artery occlusion. *Ophthalmology* **2001**, *108*, 1461–1464. [CrossRef]
49. Zhu, L.; Xu, N.; Li, Y. Monocular central retinal artery occlusion caused by bilateral internal carotid artery hypoplasia complicated with patent foramen ovale: A case report and review of literature. *Eur. J. Med. Res.* **2021**, *26*, 55. [CrossRef]
50. Si, M.; Wang, H. Retinal artery occlusion after facial filler injection in a patient with patent foramen ovale: A case report and literature review. *J. Int. Med. Res.* **2023**, *51*, 3000605231194514. [CrossRef]
51. Pipolo, G.R.; Neto, C.A.M.; Ishida, P.; Pereira, R.; Torres, R.; Barreto, G.; Moreira, C.A.M., Jr. OCT Angiography Use in Pregnancy: Branch Retinal Artery Occlusion Associated with Patent Foramen Ovale—A Case Report and Multimodal Analysis. *Case Rep. Ophthalmol.* **2023**, *14*, 29–33. [CrossRef] [PubMed]

52. Kapoor, K.M.; Kapoor, P.; Heydenrych, I.; Bertossi, D. Vision Loss Associated with Hyaluronic Acid Fillers: A Systematic Review of Literature. *Aesthetic Plast. Surg.* **2020**, *44*, 929–944. [CrossRef] [PubMed]
53. Kanwar, S.M.; Noheria, A.; DeSimone, C.V.; Rabinstein, A.A.; Asirvatham, S.J. Coincidental Impact of Transcatheter Patent Foramen Ovale Closure on Migraine with and without Aura—A Comprehensive Meta-Analysis. *Clin. trials Regul. Sci. Cardio* **2016**, *15*, 7–13. [CrossRef]
54. Lipton, R.B.; Stewart, W.F.; Diamond, S.; Diamond, M.L.; Reed, M. Prevalence and burden of migraine in the United States: Data from the American Migraine Study II. *Headache* **2001**, *41*, 646–657. [CrossRef] [PubMed]
55. Del Sette, M.; Dinia, L.; Bonzano, L.; Roccatagliata, L.; Finocchi, C.; Parodi, R.; Sivori, G.; Gandolfo, C. White matter lesions in migraine and right-to-left shunt: A conventional and diffusion MRI study. *Cephalalgia* **2008**, *28*, 376–382. [CrossRef] [PubMed]
56. Liu, K.; Wang, B.Z.; Hao, Y.; Song, S.; Pan, M. The Correlation Between Migraine and Patent Foramen Ovale. *Front. Neurol.* **2020**, *11*, 543485. [CrossRef] [PubMed]
57. Wilmshurst, P.T. Migraine with aura and persistent foramen ovale. *Eye* **2018**, *32*, 184–188. [CrossRef] [PubMed]
58. Dowson, A.; Mullen, M.J.; Peatfield, R.; Muir, K.; Khan, A.A.; Wells, C.; Lipscombe, S.L.; Rees, T.; De Giovanni, J.V.; Morrison, W.L et al. Migraine Intervention With STARFlex Technology (MIST) trial: A prospective, multicenter, double-blind, sham-controlled trial to evaluate the effectiveness of patent foramen ovale closure with STARFlex septal repair implant to resolve refractory migraine. *Circulation* **2008**, *117*, 1397–1404. [CrossRef]
59. Mattle, H.P.; Evers, S.; Hildick-Smith, D.; Becker, W.J.; Baumgartner, H.; Chataway, J.; Gawel, M.; Göbel, H.; Heinze, A.; Horlick E.; et al. Percutaneous closure of patent foramen ovale in migraine with aura, a randomized controlled trial. *Eur. Heart J.* **2016**, *37* 2029–2036. [CrossRef]
60. Tobis, J.M.; Charles, A.; Silberstein, S.D.; Sorensen, S.; Maini, B.; Horwitz, P.A.; Gurley, J.C. Percutaneous Closure of Patent Foramen Ovale in Patients With Migraine: The PREMIUM Trial. *J. Am. Coll. Cardiol.* **2017**, *70*, 2766–2774. [CrossRef]
61. Giardini, A.; Donti, A.; Formigari, R.; Salomone, L.; Palareti, G.; Guidetti, D.; Picchio, F.M. Long-term efficacy of transcatheter patent foramen ovale closure on migraine headache with aura and recurrent stroke. *Catheter. Cardiovasc. Interv. Off. J. Soc. Card. Angiogr. Interv.* **2006**, *67*, 625–629. [CrossRef]
62. Yan, S.; Wang, N.; Liu, H.; Wei, Y.; Liu, X.; Wang, L.; Huang, Y.; Lin, M. Patent Foramen Ovale Closure for Migraineurs with Massive Right-to-Left Shunt and White Matter Lesions: An Exploration on Curative Effects. *Altern. Ther. Health Med.* **2024** AT9388, *ahead of print*. [PubMed]
63. Elbadawi, A.; Barssoum, K.; Abuzaid, A.S.; Rezq, A.; Biniwale, N.; Alotaki, E.; Mohamed, A.H.; Vuyyala, S.; O Ogunbayo, G.; Saad, M. Meta-analysis of randomized trials on percutaneous patent foramen ovale closure for prevention of migraine. *Acta Cardiol.* **2019**, *74*, 124–129. [CrossRef] [PubMed]
64. Shi, Y.-J.; Lv, J.; Han, X.-T.; Luo, G.-G. Migraine and percutaneous patent foramen ovale closure: A systematic review and meta-analysis. *BMC Cardiovasc. Disord.* **2017**, *17*, 203. [CrossRef] [PubMed]
65. Zhang, Y.; Wang, H.; Liu, L. Patent Foramen Ovale Closure for Treating Migraine: A Meta-Analysis. *J. Interv. Cardiol.* **2022** *2022*, 6456272. [CrossRef]
66. Zhang, Q.-Q.; Lu, J.-J.; Yan, M.-Y.; Hu, X.-W.; Qin, Y.-R.; Wang, D.-P.; Jiang, J.-H.; Fang, Q.; Zhao, H.-R. The Efficacy of Percutaneous Patent Foramen Ovale Closure on Migraine: A Meta-Analysis of Randomized Controlled Trials and Observational Studies. *Biomed. Res. Int.* **2021**, *2021*, 6643266. [CrossRef]
67. Arunagiri, G.; Santhi, S. Migraine: An ophthalmologist's perspective. *Curr. Opin. Ophthalmol.* **2003**, *14*, 344–352. [CrossRef] [PubMed]
68. Ciuffreda, K.J.; Kapoor, N.; Rutner, D.; Suchoff, I.B.; Han, M.E.; Craig, S. Occurrence of oculomotor dysfunctions in acquired brain injury: A retrospective analysis. *Optometry* **2007**, *78*, 155–161. [CrossRef] [PubMed]
69. Xie, D.N.; Sun, Q. Bilateral ptosis caused by patent foramen ovale-associated stroke. *QJM An. Int. J. Med.* **2022**, *115*, 853–854. [CrossRef]
70. Mazurkiewicz-Bełdzińska, M.; Szmuda, M.; Zawadzka, M. Internuclear opthalmoplegia as a symptom of ischemic stroke in a girl with patent foramen ovale. *Pediatr. Neurol.* **2015**, *52*, 466–467. [CrossRef]
71. Zhuang, S.; Xie, W.; Mao, C. Bilateral facial colliculus syndrome caused by pontine tegmentum infarction: A case report. *BMC Neurol.* **2021**, *21*, 492. [CrossRef] [PubMed]
72. Takahashi, C. A Case of Progressive Stroke on Posterior Circulation with Transient Bilateral Oculomotor Palsy. *Case Rep. Neurol Med.* **2018**, *2018*, 1579426. [CrossRef] [PubMed]
73. Khan, A.O. Pupil-sparing complete third nerve palsy from cryptogenic midbrain stroke in an otherwise-healthy young adult with patent foramen ovale. *Middle East. Afr. J. Ophthalmol.* **2012**, *19*, 237–239. [CrossRef] [PubMed]
74. Durand, M.L. Endophthalmitis. *Clin. Microbiol. Infect. Off. Publ. Eur. Soc. Clin. Microbiol. Infect. Dis.* **2013**, *19*, 227–234. [CrossRef] [PubMed]
75. Sadiq, M.A.; Hassan, M.; Agarwal, A.; Sarwar, S.; Toufeeq, S.; Soliman, M.K.; Hanout, M.; Sepah, Y.J.; Do, D.V.; Nguyen, Q.D. Endogenous endophthalmitis: Diagnosis, management, and prognosis. *J. Ophthalmic Inflamm. Infect.* **2015**, *5*, 32. [CrossRef] [PubMed]
76. Rodrigues, A.C.; Ogawa, A.; Mota, J.; Carbone, A.; Arruda, A.L.; Furtado, M.; Pinheiro, J.; Andrade, J.L. Endophthalmitis as a first manifestation of right-sided endocarditis in a patient with patent foramen ovale. *J. Echocardiogr.* **2012**, *10*, 67–68. [CrossRef] [PubMed]

Nii, T.; Yoshikawa, H.; Okabe, T.; Tachibana, I. Septic pulmonary and systemic embolism in tricuspid endocarditis. *BMJ Case Rep.* **2014**, *2014*, 206569. [CrossRef] [PubMed]
Flaxel, C.J.; Adelman, R.A.; Bailey, S.T.; Fawzi, A.; Lim, J.I.; Vemulakonda, G.A.; Ying, G.-S. Retinal and Ophthalmic Artery Occlusions Preferred Practice Pattern®. *Ophthalmology* **2020**, *127*, P259–P287. [CrossRef] [PubMed]
Endophthalmitis Study Group, European Society of Cataract & Refractive Surgeons. Prophylaxis of postoperative endophthalmitis following cataract surgery: Results of the ESCRS multicenter study and identification of risk factors. *J. Cataract. Refract. Surg.* **2007**, *33*, 978–988. [CrossRef] [PubMed]
Vukadinović, D.; Schirmer, S.H.; Vukadinović, A.N.; Ukena, C.; Scheller, B.; Mahfoud, F.; Böhm, M. Interventional closure vs. medical therapy of patent foramen ovale for secondary prevention of stroke: Updated meta-analysis. *Clin. Res. Cardiol.* **2019**, *108*, 157–166. [CrossRef]
Turc, G.; Calvet, D.; Guérin, P.; Sroussi, M.; Chatellier, G.; Mas, J.L. Closure, Anticoagulation, or Antiplatelet Therapy for Cryptogenic Stroke With Patent Foramen Ovale: Systematic Review of Randomized Trials, Sequential Meta-Analysis, and New Insights from the CLOSE Study. *J. Am. Heart Assoc.* **2018**, *7*, e008356. [CrossRef] [PubMed]
Liu, Y.; Wu, Y.; Xiong, L. Surgical vs. drug therapy in patients with patent foramen ovale and cryptogenic stroke. *Herz* **2021**, *46*, 250–254. [CrossRef] [PubMed]
Rim, T.H.; Lee, C.J.; Tham, Y.C.; Cheung, N.; Yu, M.; Lee, G.; Kim, Y.; Ting, D.S.W.; Chong, C.C.Y.; Choi, Y.S.; et al. Deep-learning-based cardiovascular risk stratification using coronary artery calcium scores predicted from retinal photographs. *Lancet Digit. Health* **2021**, *3*, e306–e316. [CrossRef] [PubMed]
Wagner, S.K.; Fu, D.J.; Faes, L.; Liu, X.; Huemer, J.; Khalid, H.; Ferraz, D.; Korot, E.; Kelly, C.; Balaskas, K.; et al. Insights into Systemic Disease through Retinal Imaging-Based Oculomics. *Transl. Vis. Sci. Technol.* **2020**, *9*, 6. Erratum in *Transl. Vis. Sci. Technol.* **2021**, *10*, 13. https://doi.org/10.1167/tvst.10.8.13. [CrossRef] [PubMed]

Journal of *Personalized Medicine*

MDPI

Review

The Role of Oral Supplementation for the Management of Age-Related Macular Degeneration: A Narrative Review

Angela D'Angelo [1], Livio Vitiello [2], Vincenzo Gagliardi [2], Giulio Salerno [2], Ilaria De Pascale [2], Alessia Coppola [2], Giulia Abbinante [2], Alfonso Pellegrino [2] and Giuseppe Giannaccare [3,*]

[1] Department of Clinical Sciences and Community Health, University of Milan, 20133 Milan, MI, Italy; angela.dangelo@unimi.it

[2] Eye Unit, "Luigi Curto" Hospital, Azienda Sanitaria Locale Salerno, 84035 Polla, SA, Italy; gmed.vitiellol@aslsalerno.it (L.V.); v.gagliardi@aslsalerno.it (V.G.); gmed.salernog@aslsalerno.it (G.S.); i.depascale@aslsalerno.it (I.D.P.); ccc.coppolaa@aslsalerno.it (A.C.); ccc.abbinanteg@aslsalerno.it (G.A.); al.pellegrino@aslsalerno.it (A.P.)

[3] Eye Clinic, Department of Surgical Sciences, University of Cagliari, 09124 Cagliari, CA, Italy

* Correspondence: giuseppe.giannaccare@unica.it

Abstract: The majority of neurodegenerative eye disorders occur with aging and significantly impair quality of life. Age-related macular degeneration (AMD) is the third most common cause of visual impairment and blindness worldwide. One of the most important elements in the pathophysiology of neurodegenerative eye disease is certainly oxidative stress, with neuroinflammation and ocular ischemia which may also be significant factors. Antioxidants, either by food or oral supplementation, may be able to mitigate the deleterious effects of reactive oxygen species that build as a result of oxidative stress, ischemia, and inflammation. Over the past few decades, a number of research works examining the potential adjuvant impact of antioxidants in AMD have been published. In fact, there is not only more and more interest in already known molecules but also in new molecules that can help clinicians in the management of this complex multifactorial disease, such as astaxanthin and melatonin. However, while some studies showed encouraging outcomes, others were conflicting. In addition, more and more attention is also being paid to nutrition, considered a pivotal key point, especially to prevent AMD. For this reason, the purpose of this review is to analyze the main antioxidant molecules currently used as oral supplements for AMD treatment, as well as the role of diet and food intake in this ocular disease, to better understand how all these factors can improve the clinical management of AMD patients.

Keywords: age-related macular degeneration; AMD; diet; food intake; oral supplementation

1. Introduction

Age-related macular degeneration (AMD) is the third most common cause of severe irreversible vision loss worldwide and it is considered the leading cause of central blindness in industrialized countries, especially in people over 60 years of age [1]. In fact, prevalence data suggest that AMD affects around 200 million people today and it is expected to rise further to almost 300 million by 2040 [1].

AMD is a multifactorial disorder with multiple genetic and environmental risk factors, including genetic predisposition, older age, smoking, obesity, low dietary intake of several vitamins and minerals (A, C, E, and zinc), low dietary intake of lutein and omega-3 fatty acids, and unhealthy lifestyle related to cardiovascular risk factors [2,3].

In 2001, the Age-Related Eye Disease Study (AREDS) [4] first showed that patients with advanced AMD, or those with at least intermediate AMD (defined as bilateral large drusen with or without pigment changes) [5], could benefit from taking oral antioxidant vitamin and mineral supplements [4].

Indeed, one pivotal element in the pathophysiology of neurodegenerative eye disease such as AMD is certainly oxidative stress [6] (Figure 1).

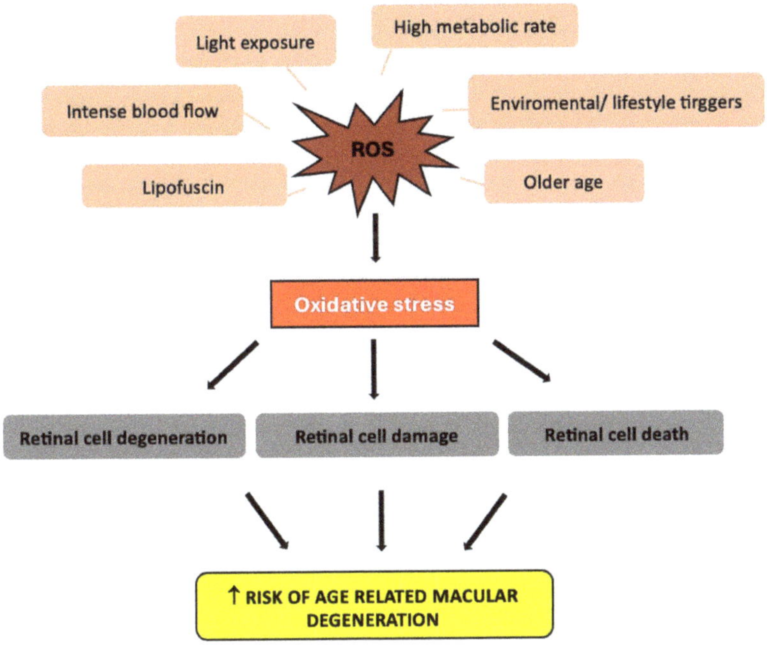

Figure 1. Factors predisposing the formation of reactive oxygen species (ROS), responsible for oxidative stress which can lead to an increased risk of age-related macular degeneration.

In response to oxidative stress, which can be induced by molecules like lipopolysaccharides, exosomes derived from retinal pigment epithelial cells (RPE) can induce inflammation in the retina and thus contribute to AMD pathogenesis. Among the key genes involved in oxidative stress, interleukin-1 beta (IL-1β), interleukin-6 (IL-6), Nuclear Factor Kappa B (NF-κB), and tumor necrosis factor alpha (TNF-α) are susceptible to upregulation [7], thus triggering an inflammatory cascade that contributes to disease progression [8].

Moreover, neuroinflammation and ocular ischemia also have a significant impact on the disease. Antioxidants, either by food or oral supplementation, may be able to mitigate the deleterious effects of reactive oxygen species (ROS) that build because of oxidative stress, ischemia, and inflammation by reducing the expression of the genes involved in retinal inflammation [6].

Over the past few decades, several studies examining the potential impact of antioxidants in AMD have been published [9,10], showing their potential use in AMD management and also as adjuvants to the therapeutic action of intravitreal anti-vascular endothelial growth factor (VEGF) drugs.

For this reason, the purpose of this narrative review was to explore a wide range of active substances, including not only vitamins and minerals as antioxidants, but also other substances such as saffron, curcumin, and melatonin, which are currently used as oral supplements for AMD. Our work differs from previous studies by including a broader range of these compounds [11]. Additionally, given the growing interest in understanding the impact of dietary factors on AMD progression, we aimed to integrate recent evidence on the role of diet and food intake in the management of this disease.

2. Main Oral Supplements for AMD Management

2.1. Lutein and Zeaxanthin

Lutein and zeaxanthin are pigments produced by plants and belong to the carotenoid family of xanthophylls. They are two fat-soluble antioxidants with very similar structures, differing in the location of one double bond in one of the hydroxyl groups. Lutein and zeaxanthin are only biosynthesized by plants, so these substances must be provided to the body through diet. Major sources of these carotenoids include broccoli, kale, spinach, corn, peas, and egg yolks. The recommended daily intake of lutein is about 10.0 mg, while for zeaxanthin, it is 2 mg [12–14]. Lutein and zeaxanthin are the only dietary carotenoids that accumulate in the retina, especially in the macula and in the lens of the human eye, and are called macular pigments, responsible for fine detail vision [12,15].

Given their accumulation in the retina, researchers have investigated the role of lutein and zeaxanthin in eye health. Their functions include enhancing visual function [16,17], acting as antioxidants to scavenge free radicals and protect the macula from oxidative damage [18,19], and filtering blue light [19,20]. Lutein and zeaxanthin are the most potent antioxidants for the prevention or risk reduction of AMD and various eye-related conditions [21]. Evidence suggests that these xanthophylls may protect the retina from damage and could potentially prevent or slow down the progression of AMD.

Numerous studies have explored the impact of lutein and zeaxanthin supplementation (both through whole foods and supplements) and their association with AMD. A multicenter case–control study conducted across five ophthalmological centers in the United States was the first epidemiological study to demonstrate a direct relationship between lutein intake and the risk of AMD [22]. Increasing the consumption of foods rich in specific carotenoids, particularly dark green, leafy vegetables, may help reduce the risk of developing advanced or exudative AMD [22].

The evidence supporting the protective effects of lutein and zeaxanthin intake against AMD development comes from the Age-Related Eye Disease Study 2 (AREDS2) published in 2013, an important clinical trial conducted in the United States [23]. The original Age-Related Eye Disease Study (AREDS1) was published in 2001 and was one of the first significant clinical trials to assess the association between nutrient intake and the progression of AMD [4]. In this original study, it was demonstrated that a combination of nutrient supplements (500 mg vitamin C, 400 IU vitamin E, 15 mg β-carotene, 80 mg zinc, and 2 mg cupric oxide) taken daily reduces the risk of developing advanced macular degeneration by 25% [4]. However, subsequent findings linking β-carotene to an increased risk of lung cancer among smokers led to revisions in the formulation [24]. Later, AREDS2 included lutein (10 mg) and zeaxanthin (2 mg) along with omega-3 long-chain polyunsaturated fatty acids, eliminating beta carotene and reducing zinc doses in the formulation [23]. While this modified formula did not further reduce the risk of late AMD progression compared to the previous one, the removal of β-carotene and the addition of lutein and zeaxanthin provided similar protective effects without introducing additional risks for smokers [23].

These studies have provided valuable clinical guidance on dietary supplementation for AMD patients [4,23]. Evidence also indicates that higher intake of lutein and zeaxanthin may offer significant protection against AMD, especially in individuals with a high genetic risk based on two major AMD genes [25]. A meta-analysis [21] involving seven controlled trials using lutein and zeaxanthin supplements [16,26–33] assessed the impact of this supplementation on visual performance in individuals with established AMD. The results of the meta-analysis suggest that lutein and zeaxanthin supplementation represents a safe and effective strategy for enhancing the visual performance and contrast sensitivity of AMD patients in a dose–response manner [26].

Determining effective doses of lutein and zeaxanthin is challenging due to a lack of long-term studies. However, current evidence suggests that higher dietary intake of these compounds may protect against AMD. A diverse diet rich in leafy greens and other foods can help achieve optimal levels of lutein and zeaxanthin, thus supporting eye health.

Further research is needed to improve our understanding of lutein and zeaxanthin and establish recommended targets for these eye-protective carotenoids.

2.2. Astaxanthin

Astaxanthin (3,3′-dihydroxy-β, β-carotene4,4′-dione), is a carotenoid that belongs to the family of oxygenated derivatives of carotenoids (xanthophylls) present in nature, mainly in marine environments, where it occurs as a red pigment, contributing to the red color of shrimp, lobsters, and shrimp pulp. Astaxanthin is biosynthesized by phytoplankton and microalgae, accumulating in various aquatic species that represent the main dietary sources of this carotenoid. It is a bioactive compound with promising structural and functional characteristics in the prevention of numerous human diseases as well as in maintaining good health [34,35].

Unlike most antioxidants, astaxanthin spans across the double layer of the membrane, providing protection against oxidative stress by neutralizing ROS and other free radicals both in the polar (hydrophilic) and nonpolar (hydrophobic) boundary zones of the cell membrane [36]. Astaxanthin has been shown to have antioxidant activity approximately ten times higher than that of zeaxanthin and lutein [37], as well as other carotenoids such as α-carotene, lycopene, and β-carotene [38]. Furthermore, it has been observed that astaxanthin can suppress the activation of NF-κB inflammatory gene expression induced by hydrogen peroxide by inhibiting the intracellular ROS accumulation [39]. Indeed, it has demonstrated multiple beneficial effects, including anti-inflammatory, antioxidant, anti-diabetic, and anti-cancer activities in addition to protective actions for the skin and the nervous and cardiovascular systems [36,37,40].

Several recent clinical trials emphasize the potential role of astaxanthin in enhancing eye health, as suggested by the significant improvement observed in the outcomes of various ocular conditions such as age-related macular degeneration, diabetic retinopathy, glaucoma, and cataracts [37].

In a randomized controlled trial, Parisi et al. evaluated the effects of short-term oral supplementation with carotenoids, including astaxanthin, on retinal function in non-advanced AMD patients [41]. Twenty-seven participants were randomly divided into two groups. One group received daily supplementation containing vitamin E (30 mg), vitamin C (180 mg), zinc (22.5 mg), copper (1 mg), lutein (10 mg), zeaxanthin (1 mg), and astaxanthin (4 mg) for 12 months, while the other group received no supplementation. The supplemented group showed improved central retinal function compared to the placebo group, highlighting the potential benefits of carotenoid supplementation in AMD management [41]. In another multicenter, prospective open-label randomized study, 145 patients were randomly divided into two treatment groups [27]. One group received a supplementation containing lutein (10 mg), zeaxanthin (1 mg), astaxanthin (4 mg), and antioxidants/vitamins, while the other group received no dietary supplementation for a duration of two years. Patients treated with lutein/zeaxanthin, astaxanthin, and other nutrients were more inclined to report clinically meaningful stabilization or improvements in visual acuity, contrast sensitivity, and vision-related functions over 24 months compared to untreated subjects [27].

Astaxanthin, due to its potent antioxidant activity, can influence choroidal neovascularization (CNV), another factor contributing to AMD. In fact, CNV is associated with oxidative stress and chronic inflammation in ocular tissues, caused by the overexpression of VEGF. Astaxanthin has demonstrated its ability to suppress CNV in murine experimental models, reducing the formation of abnormal new blood vessels in the retina [42]. These positive effects are supported by molecular mechanisms that regulate the production of inflammatory mediators such as ICAM-1, MCP-1, VEGF, IL-6, and VEGF receptors [42].

In conclusion, astaxanthin offers promising treatment prospects for combating ocular diseases and supporting eye health. However, to define optimal dosages and formulations, improving bioavailability and obtaining more data from clinical studies are essential, despite its broad safety profile and potential efficacy in various ocular conditions [37,43].

2.3. Vitamins and Minerals

High concentrations of certain antioxidant vitamins and minerals in the retina, coupled with the high levels of the carotenoids in the macula, suggest the hypothesis that micronutrient supplementation might protect against AMD. Vitamins A, C, and E are recognized as the most effective for reducing the risk of macular degeneration [4]. Vitamin A is essential for RPE cells of the human retina, while vitamins C and E are known to act as antioxidants. In addition to these vitamins, minerals such as zinc and selenium have also been associated with eye diseases.

AREDS is the first large multicenter randomized, placebo-controlled study initiated by the United States National Eye Institute, designed to investigate the effect of high-dose supplementation with vitamin C and E, beta-carotene, and zinc, either individually or in combination, on the progression of AMD and cataracts [4]. This study enrolled 3640 patients aged between 55 and 80 years diagnosed with AMD. The AREDS1 study showed a statistically significant benefit in consuming the AREDS formula, with a 25% reduced risk of AMD progression over 5 years; although vision loss continued, it occurred at a slower rate with a reduced risk of developing neovascularization [4]. However, the study has several limitations. Firstly, it is unclear to what extent and at what exact dosage vitamin C, vitamin E, and beta-carotene are beneficial for AMD patients because they were administered only in combination and at a single dosage. Additionally, concerns have been raised about the long-term safety of supplementation with dosages that clearly exceed the recommended daily intake [44]. To address some of the original AREDS limitations, the United States National Eye Institute sponsored a second large-scale randomized clinical trial. This study, known as AREDS2, aimed to investigate if additional nutritional supplements beyond AREDS1 supplements could further reduce the risk of progression to advanced AMD [23].

Although AREDS1 and AREDS2 are the most comprehensive studies on vitamin supplementation's impact on AMD progression, smaller-scale studies have also been carried out. However, research findings on the intake of these vitamins and minerals and their association with AMD risk remain conflicting.

2.3.1. β-Carotene and Vitamin A

Beta-carotene is a carotenoid and it is the precursor of vitamin A. Both compounds are liposoluble and excellent antioxidants, capable of counteracting the onset of free radicals [45].

In the AREDS1 study, the supplement formulation included beta-carotene at a dose of 15 mg, based on the structural similarities between the components of the macular pigment and beta-carotene [4]. Therefore, beta-carotene was long part of the recommendation for supplementation in AMD patients. However, it is now established that high doses of β-carotene (30 mg per day) increase the risk of lung cancer in smokers [24]. Although the mechanism behind this harmful effect has not been fully elucidated, side effects do not occur in non-smokers or when the carotenoid is administered at lower doses [46]. Based on these data, it was recommended to omit beta-carotene supplementation in smokers with AMD. Therefore, in the formulation of the AREDS2 study, beta-carotene was replaced with lutein/zeaxanthin [23].

The protective effect of vitamin A against AMD is demonstrated by epidemiological data from the National Health and Nutrition Examination Survey (NHANES I), which showed that those who consumed higher amounts of fruits and vegetables rich in vitamin A had a reduced risk of any stage of AMD [47]. A prospective population-based cohort study has demonstrated that the sustained consumption of fruits and vegetables containing provitamin A carotenoids can further decrease the risk of AMD [48].

However, other studies have not found a significant association between increased dietary vitamin A intake and reduced AMD risk [22,49]. This conflicting evidence highlights the need for additional studies to clarify the relationship between vitamin A and AMD.

2.3.2. Vitamin C

Vitamin C, chemically known as ascorbic acid, is synthesized by plants and certain mammals. However, humans have lost this ability over evolution making it necessary to obtain vitamin C from dietary sources. Therefore, vitamin C is an essential micronutrient for humans, with the recommended daily intake ranging from 75 mg for adult females to 90 mg for adult males per day [50]. Fruits and vegetables are the primary sources of vitamin C in the diet. Vitamin C plays a crucial role as a powerful antioxidant, contributing positively to redox oxidative pathways, inflammation, maintaining endothelial integrity, and regulating lipoprotein metabolism.

Vitamin C is plentiful in the retina, including in premature infants, and its potential protective role in age-related retinal diseases is supported by animal studies. Studies in the mid-1980s showed that ascorbic acid, specifically L-ascorbate, can reduce light-induced damage in rat retinas, likely due to its antioxidant properties [51]. Another study that supports the beneficial effect of Vitamin C is conducted by SanGiovanni et al. that found a reduced risk of neovascular AMD in individuals with a high intake of β-carotene, vitamin C, and vitamin E [52]. However, conflicting results were reported by Evans and Lawrenson, who did not find a significant association between vitamin C and the primary prevention of AMD [11]. This was consistent with other studies that also failed to show a clear link between dietary vitamin C intake and reduced AMD risk, as reported by Delcourt et al. [49] and Seddon et al. [22]. The Eye Diseases Control Study noted a significant correlation between an increased intake of green vegetables and a markedly reduced risk of AMD [53]. However, they found that total vitamin C consumption did not show a significant association with reduced AMD risk [22]. Additionally, the study observed that lower plasma levels of vitamin C were linked to a higher risk of AMD, whereas higher plasma concentrations did not offer protection [22]. Furthermore, a 10-year follow-up study did not find significant effects of vitamin C supplementation on AMD risk [54].

Overall, while some studies suggest a potential protective role for vitamin C against AMD, the evidence remains inconclusive and further research on a larger scale is necessary to clarify this relationship.

2.3.3. Vitamin E

Vitamin E is a fat-soluble vitamin and comprises four chemical compounds, among which α-tocopherol is considered the most biologically active and an effective scavenger of free radicals [55].

The recommended daily dose of 15 mg for adult males is based on α-tocopherol [50]. Photoreceptors and RPE cells, which have a high concentration of vitamin E, respond to increased oxidative stress by increasing their levels of this vitamin [56]. Some evidence supports the idea that vitamin E might offer benefits to those with AMD. Several studies have indicated a correlation between low serum levels of tocopherol and AMD [57,58], suggesting that elevated plasma carotenoid levels may offer protective effects [59].

An interventional study evaluated the effect of vitamin E on 1193 subjects, administering 500 IU of vitamin E (equivalent to 335 mg/day of α-tocopherol) or placebo [60]. After 4 years, no significant benefit was found in vitamin E supplementation for AMD prevention or risk reduction [60].

Most randomized prospective studies evaluating the effect of vitamin E on AMD have administered vitamin E in combination with other antioxidants, not allowing them to establish the actual role of vitamin E in protecting against AMD. In fact, while high blood levels of vitamin E may be considered protective, evidence regarding the influence of vitamin E alone on the incidence or progression of AMD is currently limited.

2.3.4. Zinc

Zinc is an essential trace element, and it is the second most abundant transition metal in the human body, following iron [61]. The human body contains approximately 2 g of this element, with high concentrations in bones, skeletal muscles, liver, and eyes. The eye exhibits a relatively high concentration of zinc compared to other organs and tissues, with the peak concentration reaching around 300 μg/g of dry tissue in the RPE [62]. Zinc is not stored in the human body; thus, daily diet is the only way for humans to acquire zinc. It occurs naturally in the form of sulfides or oxides and in food, it is most abundant in meat, saltwater fish, sunflower and pumpkin seeds, bran, wheat, egg yolks, onion, garlic, and tea [63]. The recommended daily intake of zinc for adults ranges from 12 to 15 mg/day [50]. Zinc is generally considered safe, particularly when taken orally, although long-term use, even at low doses, may lead to anemia. There is evidence suggesting that zinc can affect the utilization of other nutrients, particularly copper [64].

Zinc acts as a cofactor for hundreds of enzymes across all enzymatic classes and thus participates in a broad range of metabolic functions [65]. Zinc is recognized as important in the pathophysiology of several groups of diseases, including neurodegenerative diseases [62]. Growing evidence suggests that zinc, due to its antioxidant properties, protects cells from the damaging effects of oxidative stress, presumed to be a causative factor in the development of various age-related retinal disorders [66,67].

The first study assessing the effects of oral zinc administration in AMD patients was conducted in 1988 by Newsome et al. [68]. This was a randomized, 2-year, placebo-controlled clinical trial involving 151 subjects with drusen or macular degeneration, finding a statistically significant reduction in visual acuity loss in the group treated with zinc [68]. The study recommended a more definitive trial before making a general recommendation for zinc supplementation in individuals at risk of vision loss from advanced AMD [68]. Contrary to this finding, two epidemiological studies did not confirm this outcome, where zinc supplementation had no short-term effect on the progression of AMD [69] and was not associated with a reduced risk of AMD [70]. After these, the large randomized, placebo-controlled AREDS/AREDS2 studies were published [4,23]. These studies evaluated supplementation with relatively high doses of some vitamins with or without some minerals, including zinc administered as zinc oxide at 80 mg and copper at 2 mg per day. Copper was included in the AREDS formulations along with zinc to prevent copper deficiency anemia, which can occur due to metabolic competition with zinc during supplementation. These studies suggested that zinc supplementation in combination with the AREDS formula and other antioxidants could suppress retinal degeneration [71].

In conclusion, zinc supplementation has shown potential benefits for AMD patients in certain studies, with some indicating a slowdown in progression. However, there is no universal consensus on its efficacy, as other studies either found no effect or, in rare cases, even suggested an adverse effect [62].

2.3.5. Selenium

Selenium is an essential trace element in human body, with recommended daily levels set at 55 μg for both adult women and men [50]. Known for its antioxidant properties, recent studies have explored whether selenium can mitigate the risk of AMD, especially through its role in selenium-dependent glutathione peroxidase, which protects cellular lipids from oxidative damage [72]. However, current evidence is inconclusive and does not clearly confirm that selenium can effectively protect the macula from AMD [53]. The role of selenium in protecting against AMD is still unclear due to a lack of case–control studies. Further research is needed to determine if selenium can effectively prevent AMD and associated eye complications.

2.4. Omega-3 Fatty Acids

Omega-3 fatty acids are polyunsaturated fatty acids (PUFAs) defined as essential fats because humans lack the enzymatic mechanism necessary to synthesize them [73]. Their primary sources include fatty fish such as mackerel, salmon, trout, and tuna, which are particularly rich in omega-3 eicosapentaenoic acid (EPA) and docosahexaenoic acid (DHA) [74]. Omega-3 PUFA supplements, such as fish oil, are popular for their recognized anti-inflammatory properties [75]. EPA and DHA can modulate the immune response by reducing the production of pro-inflammatory cytokines (TNF-α, IL-1, IL-6, LTB4) and leukocyte activation, and by increasing anti-inflammatory derivatives like PGD2 [76,77]. Their anti-inflammatory mechanisms include altering the composition of phospholipid fatty acids in cell membranes, disrupting lipid rafts, and inhibiting the pro-inflammatory nuclear transcription factor κB activation, thereby reducing inflammatory gene expression and activating anti-inflammatory responses [78]. Although generally safe and well-tolerated, omega-3 fatty acid supplements may exacerbate bleeding and anticoagulation in individuals using anticoagulants [79].

In recent years, there has been growing interest in the potential protective role of omega-3 PUFAs against various retinal diseases linked to inflammation, ischemia, light exposure, oxidative stress, and aging [80]. DHA is a major structural component of the retina, and EPA may play a role as a precursor to signaling molecules with a potential role to influence retinal function [76]. PUFAs have also shown anti-inflammatory and antioxidant properties, anti-angiogenic, anti-vasoproliferative, and neuroprotective effects [76].

Studies on animal models of macular degeneration have also demonstrated encouraging outcomes with PUFA supplementation [77–82]. Moreover, they reduce pathological angiogenesis across cellular and animal models by influencing numerous angiogenic factors like platelet-derived growth factor (PDGF) and VEGF [80,83]. The AREDS2 trial included, in addition to lutein and zeaxanthin, omega-3 long-chain PUFAs (DHA 350 mg + EPA 650 mg) in the oral formulation for treating the progression to advanced AMD [23]. Overall, there was no additional benefit observed from the addition of these components to the formulation. Although the addition of omega-3 to the AREDS formulation did not prove to be beneficial, it is believed that higher doses of EPA and DHA may have a desirable effect [84]. Additionally, unsaturated fats aid in the absorption of lutein and zeaxanthin [12].

In an observational study conducted by Georgiou and Prokopiou, patients with dry AMD were supplemented with EPA and DHA for up to 6 months at doses ranging from 5 to 7.5 g per day, showing a significant improvement in vision, with patients experiencing a gain of at least 15 letters [85].

2.5. Curcumin

Curcumin (diferuloylmethane) is the main bioactive component of the popular Indian spice turmeric (*Curcuma longa*) and is a water-insoluble yellowish-orange colored polyphenol. It is isolated from the dried rhizome of *Curcuma longa* L. which belongs to the *Zingiberaceae* family [86,87]. Belonging to the group of phytochemicals, curcumin is considered a bioactive molecule with pleiotropic effects, demonstrating antioxidative, anti-inflammatory, antimicrobial, antimutagenic, and antiproliferative properties [88–90]. The mechanism by which curcumin induces its effects is still not fully understood, but it is considered as a nutraceutical substance for the treatment of some chronic diseases such as diabetes, neurodegenerative diseases, pulmonary infectious, rheumatism, and oncological diseases [91,92].

Curcumin exhibits promising therapeutic potential in treating various eye conditions, including diabetic retinopathy, chronic anterior uveitis, glaucoma, dry eye syndrome, and AMD [93]. Its mechanisms of action involve reducing apoptosis rates in RPE cells and decreasing overall inflammation by downregulating genes associated with inflammation in AMD [93,94]. Specifically, curcumin's biological, nutraceutical, and pharmaceutical properties has been linked to its ability to lower levels of TNF-α and proinflammatory interleukins (IL-1, IL-6, IL-8) [86]. Moreover, curcumin protects RPE against oxidative stress and inflammation by activating Nrf2/HO-1 signaling and modulating the ERK pathway, offering potential therapeutic benefits for diabetic retinopathy and AMD [86] (Figure 2).

These positive effects make curcumin a candidate for treating inflammatory and degenerative retinal eye conditions [86], but research studies on the efficacy of curcumin are mainly limited to in vitro and in vivo studies.

In an animal study, Mandal et al. observed significant retinal neuroprotection in rats fed diets supplemented with curcumin (0.2% in diet) for 2 weeks [95]. This effect was attributed to curcumin's ability to downregulate cellular inflammatory genes and inhibit NF-κB activation [95]. Another study found that curcumin reduced the expression of free radicals and gene expression of oxidative biomarkers such as superoxide dismutase (SOD), glutathione, and malondialdehyde [96]. In this study, AMD was modeled by inducing aging in RPE cells with pulsed H_2O_2, demonstrating that curcumin led to decreased apoptosis and thus higher cell viability [96]. In addition, a study demonstrated that curcumin has post-transcriptional regulatory effects and can induce gene silencing [97]. Curcumin was also observed to both up-regulate and down-regulate specific microRNAs (miRNAs) that could play a role in regulating the antioxidant system [97].

Curcumin, as a PPAR-γ agonist, may help slow AMD progression by reducing microglia's proinflammatory effects. Saberi et al. found that curcumin activates PPAR-γ, leading to lower production of matrix metalloproteinases (MMPs), particularly MMP-9, which is involved in AMD pathogenesis by promoting RPE cell migration and extracellular matrix degradation [98]. However, exploiting the biomedical potential of curcumin is difficult due to its limited solubility and poor oral bioavailability. The main factors contributing to the low levels of curcumin in plasma and tissues seem to be attributed to its poor absorption, rapid metabolism, and rapid systemic elimination [99]. For this reason, there has been a growing interest on nanoparticles and liposomes to enhance curcumin's bioavailability [100].

In conclusion, curcumin has good tolerance and does not exhibit dose-limiting toxicity and it could be considered safe even at high doses (6 g/day orally for 4–7 weeks) in humans [101].

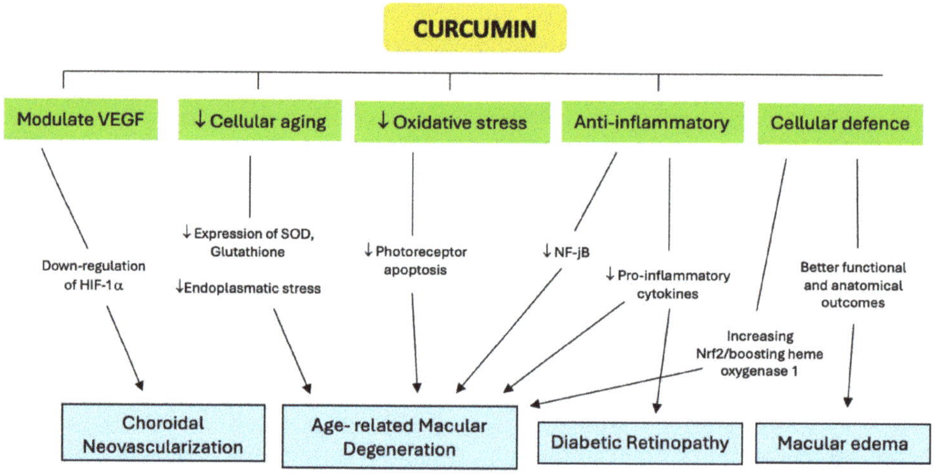

Figure 2. Beneficial mechanisms of action of curcumin on retinal diseases.

2.6. *Saffron*

Saffron is a spice obtained from *Crocus sativus* L., a plant of the Iridaceae family. Since ancient times, it has been used as an herbal medicine and as a coloring and flavoring spice. Saffron and its major constituents, such as crocetin, crocin, picrocin, and safranal, are natural carotenoids with antioxidant, anti-inflammatory, and neuroprotective effects [102]. These neuroprotective effects have been studied in neurodegenerative diseases such as Alzheimer's and Parkinson's [103] and in ocular diseases including AMD, glaucoma, and other retinal diseases. An increasing number of studies have explored the effects and mechanistic pathways of saffron and its compounds to assess their potential therapeutic use in ocular diseases. Most studies showed that saffron has a strong antioxidant activity, due to its carotenoids, especially crocin, protecting biomolecules from free radicals [104]. Additionally, saffron components exhibited anti-inflammatory and antiapoptotic effects possibly by inhibiting apoptosis mediated by caspase after retinal damage [105,106]. Moreover, crocin and crocetin are also known to enhance oxygen diffusion and improve ocular blood flow in the retina and choroid, which are crucial factors in AMD progression [107]. Considering AMD patients, six clinical studies assessed vision-related parameters after oral saffron supplementation [108–113]. All these studies showed significant improvement in visual acuity across different saffron dosages (ranging from 20 to 50 mg daily), even with short-term supplementation of around three months [108–113].

It is not possible to make a direct quantitative comparison because the above-mentioned studies had differences in formulation, dosage, intervention length, test methods, and outcome measures.

Longer-term data are available from only two non-randomized control trials, both showing improvements within three months of saffron supplementation (20 mg daily), with a stabilization over time [109,110].

2.7. Melatonin

Melatonin (N-acetyl-5-methoxytryptamine) is a neurohormone produced by the pineal gland in the human brain. Is a ubiquitous biomolecule in nature, also produced by other species of animals, plants, and microorganisms [114]. Additionally, this hormone is synthesized in human ocular tissues, including the retina and ciliary body, which have specific melatonin receptors [115]. Both melatonin and melanopsin, a regulator of melatonin synthesis in the eyes, are produced in the human lens [116]. Melatonin controls the circadian rhythm and sleep–wake regulation. Furthermore, it regulates various physiological functions including immune response, retinal physiology, sexual behavior, body temperature, and aging processes [117]. Melatonin acts as a scavenger for free radicals, playing a crucial role in detoxifying ROS. This protective action not only shields cells from damage caused by oxidative stress but also regulates the transcription of antioxidant genes through Nrf2 activation [118,119]. Additionally, melatonin influences several other molecular pathways including inflammation, apoptosis, angiogenesis, and autophagy [120]. Recent studies suggest that melatonin may decrease inflammation, oxidative stress, and apoptosis in the retina and increase viability of RPE cells as well as of photoreceptors, indicating its potential role in preventing and treating AMD [121,122]. One study reported that AMD patients have lower levels of nocturnal melatonin production compared to age-matched controls [123]. This could suggest that the decreased synthesis of melatonin may contribute to oxidative stress and the onset of AMD. Moreover, another study showed that the daily use of 3 mg of exogenous melatonin, for 3 months, in one hundred patients with AMD could protect the retina and delay AMD onset [124].

Phagocytic and autophagic processes in RPE cells are influenced by circadian rhythms [125], but the specific role of melatonin is not yet clear. Some studies indicated that melatonin may regulate photoreceptor phagocytosis [126], while others did not confirm this relationship. Retinal circadian clocks protect photoreceptors by reducing melatonin secretion during light exposure [127].

Melatonin also protects RPE cells from light-induced apoptosis through the aggregation of melanosomes and the absorption of light by melanin, which acts as an antioxidant [128]. Melatonin plays a crucial role in protecting the blood-retinal barrier in AMD-associated neovascularization, triggered by the accumulation of ROS [129]. This molecule may reduce the levels of VEGF and nitric oxide in the retina [129], thus preventing degradation of the blood–retinal barrier. Such action of melatonin suggests its potential effect in the treatment of AMD and suggests that its administration, especially in combination with antiangiogenic agents, could increase the efficacy of AMD therapy [119].

3. Role of Diet and Food Intake

In the last few years, in addition to all the aforesaid molecules (Table 1), there has been a high interest in the role of diet and food intake since they are considered as modifiable factors for preventing or slowing the progression of AMD [130,131].

Table 1. Overview of the main effects of the discussed oral supplement compounds for the management of age-related macular degeneration.

Active Compounds	Daily Therapeutic Dosage	Prescription Duration	Effects	Bioavailability	Adverse Effect and Contraindications	References	Clinical Trial Number
Lutein	1–20 mg	Weeks–months	Antioxidant activity Improvement of visual function	Moderate	No adverse effects demonstrated	[23,31–33]	NCT00345176 NCT00763659 NCT01042860 ISRCTN94557601
Zeaxanthin	2–10 mg	Weeks–months	Antioxidant activity Improvement of visual function	Moderate	May give the skin a golden-yellow color in people with fair complexions	[10,23,31,33]	NCT01527435 NCT00345176 NCT00763659 ISRCTN94557601
Astaxanthin	4–20 mg	Months	Antioxidant activity Anti-inflammatory effects	Low/Moderate	Minimal toxicity	[37,42]	
Vitamin A	700–900 mcg	Weeks	Antioxidant activity	Moderate/High	Hypervitaminosis, with possible permanent damage to the liver and spleen	[4]	NCT00000145
Vitamin C	100–500 mg	Months	Antioxidant activity	High	Digestive problems, vomiting, diarrhea, gastritis; may increase the risk of kidney stones in men	[23,33]	NCT00345176 ISRCTN94557601
Vitamin E	400–500 UI	Months	Antioxidant activity	High	Digestive problems, vomiting, nausea; may increase blood pression and reduce thyroid hormones	[23,33]	NCT00345176 ISRCTN94557601
Zinc	2–80 mg	Weeks–months	Antioxidant activity	High	Vomiting, nausea or diarrhea, irritability, drowsiness, anemia, dizziness; may cause copper deficiency anemia	[23,33]	NCT00345176 ISRCTN94557601
Selenium	50–200 µg	Weeks–months	Antioxidant activity	High	Digestive problems, vomiting, diarrhea, nausea	[50,72]	
Eicosapentaenoic acid Docosahexaenoic acid	350 mg–7.5 g	Weeks–months	Anti-inflammatory effects Antioxidant properties Anti-angiogenic and anti-vasoproliferative effects Neuroprotective effects	Moderate	May increase the risk of bleeding	[23,31]	NCT00345176 NCT00763659
Curcumin	500 mg–3 g	3–4 weeks	Possible prevention of retinal pigment epithelium cell death Anti-inflammatory effects Antioxidant activity	Very Low	Minimal toxicity, predominantly gastrointestinal upsets; may interfere with antibiotics, cardiovascular drugs, anticancer drugs, and antidepressants	[86]	
Saffron	20–30 mg	Weeks–months	Anti-inflammatory effects Antioxidant activity	Moderate	Mood disorders, lethal dose of approximately 20 g; May interfere with cardiovascular drugs	[9,111]	ACTRN12612000 729820 IRCT2012052198 20N1
Melatonin	3–20 mg	Weeks–months	Antioxidant activity Anti-inflammatory effect Possible increase in RPE cell viability	Moderate	Drowsiness; may enhance sedative effects of some drugs such as benzodiazepines	[119,124]	

Recent studies have highlighted the relationship between the Mediterranean diet and AMD [132–134]. The Mediterranean diet is characterized by a high intake of vegetables, fruits, legumes, grains, and nuts; moderate consumption of poultry, dairy and fish; limited consumption of red meat; and low to moderate amounts of red wine may be consumed.

Olive oil is used instead of butter as the main condiment fat. High adherence to this dietary pattern has been associated with a lower risk of developing AMD [133,134] and has also been shown to be beneficial for reducing the progression of late AMD [135]. This dietary approach could potentially mitigate oxidative stress and inflammation and provide a shield against AMD progression. The consumption of specific foods also appears to protect against the risk of AMD, such as vegetables rich in carotenoids, especially dark green leafy vegetables [22,135], and fatty fish containing omega-3 fatty acids [82,136]. Conversely, high consumption of foods like animal fats containing omega-6 fatty acids [137] and red and processed meat [138] should be minimized to reduce the risk of AMD progression (Figure 3).

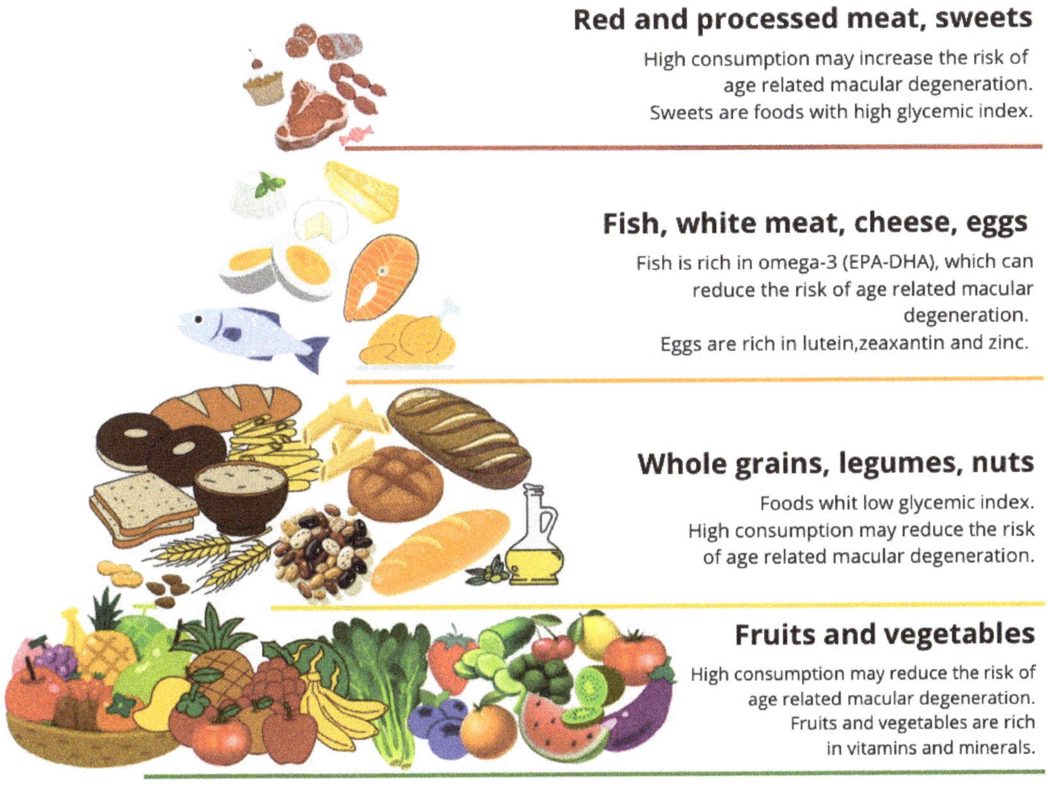

Figure 3. Simplified schematic representation of the food pyramid showing the possible role of food intake on age-related macular degeneration.

Table 2 provides a more in-depth overview of the potential role of diet and food intake in AMD.

Encouraging dietary improvements could help reduce AMD risk by focusing on nutrient-rich foods and avoiding those that cause oxidative damage. Providing nutritional guidance alongside standard treatments could be important for managing AMD effectively.

Table 2. Overview of the possible role of diet and food intake in age-related macular degeneration.

Dietary Factor	Possible Effects on AMD	General Considerations	References
Mediterranean diet	Lower risk of developing AMD Lower risk of AMD progression	High consumption of fruits, vegetables, legumes, whole grains and nuts; moderate consumption of fish, poultry and dairy; limited consumption of red meat; olive oil used as main fat; low to moderate amounts of red wine	[131–134]
Western diet	Increased AMD prevalence	Higher intake of red meat, processed meat, high-fat dairy products, fried potatoes, refined grains	[135]
High glycemic index diets	Increased risk of early AMD	Glycemic index is a measure that ranks carbohydrate-containing foods based on their impact on blood sugar levels over a 2 h period. Pure glucose is assigned the reference GI of 100. High consumption of foods with high GI (>70): white bread, potatoes, white rice, cereals, honey, and refined sugar Low consumption of foods with low GI (<55): whole fruit and vegetables, whole wheat bread, pasta, oats, bran, legumes, milk, and yoghurt	[139,140]
Vegetables and fruits	Lower risk of AMD	200 g per day of vegetables, in particular dark green leafy vegetables (broccoli, spinach…) and fruit two times per day	[22,48]
Fish and omega-3	Reduced risk of AMD	One or more servings of fish per week	[48,136,137]
Red and processed meat	Increased risk of developing AMD	High consumption especially of processed meat (salami or continental sausages)	[138]
Alcohol	Higher risk of development AMD	More than two drinks a day	[141,142]

AMD: Age-related macular degeneration; GI: glycemic index.

4. Discussion

This review focused on the preventive qualities and effects of several oral supplements as well as food intake for managing AMD. By shielding RPE cells from oxidative stress and preventing them from apoptosis, most of the oral supplements examined in this review provide therapeutic benefits through primarily antioxidant actions. While these supplements cannot replace traditional medical and surgical treatment, they can have a positive synergistic effect that boosts the efficacy of gold-standard therapies and aids in stabilizing the patient's general state of health.

In fact, the growing use of these oral supplements in clinical practice for the management of AMD has aroused considerable interest on the part of researchers to better understand their potential beneficial effects for the treatment of this ocular disease, adding them to conventional therapy characterized by intravitreal anti-VEGF drugs.

Considering oral supplements, all have shown substantially protective activities towards the retina in case of AMD, both in reducing the risk of development and progression of the disease. Furthermore, except for curcumin, all of these substances have moderate to high bioavailability when taken orally, with a good safety and tolerability profile. In fact, excluding curcumin and zinc, which showed a greater interaction with other drugs and a greater onset of undangerous gastrointestinal disorders, all molecules have demonstrated minimal toxicity in the clinical studies published in the literature.

While lutein and zeaxanthin are well recognized as retinal protective molecules, having already been included in the AREDS2 study [23], of particular interest are certainly astaxanthin, EPA, and DHA, which have shown very promising effects thanks to their anti-inflammatory, anti-angiogenic, anti-vasoproliferative and neuroprotective properties. In particular, all these molecules can exert their beneficial effects by modulating the immune response, thus reducing the production of pro-inflammatory cytokines and leukocyte activation, together with the increase of anti-inflammatory derivatives [76,77].

In addition to oral supplements, diet and food intake have also recently attracted increasing interest in the ophthalmology field, in particular in the clinical management of degenerative diseases such as AMD. In fact, several studies in the literature have demonstrated the protective effects of some foods, such as fish, fruit, and vegetables, and the harmful effects of others, such as red and processed meat, alcohol, and all foods with a high glycemic index. However, more scientific evidence is needed to better establish the relationship between AMD and diet, and to better understand the potential benefits of healthy food for the management and the prevention of this ocular disease.

The narrative and non-systematic nature of this review, together with the fact that it was composed using only one scientific database (PubMed), could be considered limitations of this study. Furthermore, only some of the main oral supplements that are currently used in clinical practice to control AMD have been reviewed in this study.

5. Conclusions

The integrative use of antioxidants, vitamins, organic compounds, and micronutrients, along with a balanced and healthy diet, may be beneficial for the treatment of AMD, as well as glaucoma and other ocular disorders [143–145].

However, effective oral supplementation strategies are challenging to design due to a number of limiting factors, including the complexity of the anatomy and tissues of the visual system, the timing of patient enrollment in clinical trials, the lack of valid endpoints, and our incomplete understanding of the underlying molecular causes of neurodegenerative diseases, including AMD.

For this reason, more investigations and even large-scale multicenter clinical trials are continuously required to confirm the efficacy of these oral supplements and to gain a deeper understanding of their mechanisms of action to fully utilize their therapeutical properties as adjuvant therapeutic alternatives in treatment regimens for AMD, in addition to the promotion of a healthy diet, given the potential benefits it can bring to AMD patients.

Author Contributions: A.D., L.V., V.G., G.S., I.D.P., A.C. and G.A. analyzed the literature and wrote the original draft. A.P. and G.G. conceived the article and reviewed the manuscript. All authors have read and agreed to the published version of the manuscript.

Funding: This research received no external funding.

Institutional Review Board Statement: Not applicable.

Informed Consent Statement: Not applicable.

Data Availability Statement: The data can be shared upon request.

Conflicts of Interest: The authors declare no conflicts of interest.

eferences

Carnevali, A.; Mastropasqua, R.; Gatti, V.; Vaccaro, S.; Mancini, A.; D'aloisio, R.; Lupidi, M.; Cerquaglia, A.; Sacconi, R.; Borrelli, E.; et al. Optical Coherence Tomography Angiography in Intermediate and Late Age-Related Macular Degeneration: Review of Current Technical Aspects and Applications. *Appl. Sci.* **2020**, *10*, 8865. [CrossRef]

Fleckenstein, M.; Schmitz-Valckenberg, S.; Chakravarthy, U. Age-Related Macular Degeneration: A Review. *JAMA* **2024**, *331*, 147–157. [CrossRef] [PubMed]

Lim, L.S.; Mitchell, P.; Seddon, J.M.; Holz, F.G.; Wong, T.Y. Age-related macular degeneration. *Lancet* **2012**, *379*, 1728–1738. [CrossRef] [PubMed]

Age-Related Eye Disease Study Research Group. A randomized, placebo-controlled, clinical trial of high-dose supplementation with vitamins C and E, beta carotene, and zinc for age-related macular degeneration and vision loss: AREDS report no. 8. *Arch. Ophthalmol.* **2001**, *119*, 1417–1436. [CrossRef] [PubMed]

Klein, R.; Klein, B.E.; Linton, K.L. Prevalence of age-related maculopathy: The Beaver Dam Eye Study. *Ophthalmology* **1992**, *99*, 933–943. [CrossRef] [PubMed]

Semenova, Y.; Bjørklund, G. Antioxidants and neurodegenerative eye disease. *Crit. Rev. Food Sci. Nutr.* **2023**, 1–19. [CrossRef] [PubMed]

7. Zhang, Z.; Gu, Q.; Chen, L.; Yuan, D.; Gu, X.; Qian, H.; Xie, P.; Liu, Q.; Hu, Z. Selective microRNA expression of exosomes fror retinal pigment epithelial cells by oxidative stress. *Vis. Res.* **2024**, *220*, 108388. [CrossRef] [PubMed]
8. Tan, W.; Zou, J.; Yoshida, S.; Jiang, B.; Zhou, Y. The Role of Inflammation in Age-Related Macular Degeneration. *Int. J. Biol. Sc* **2020**, *16*, 2989–3001. [CrossRef] [PubMed]
9. Broadhead, G.K.; Grigg, J.; McCluskey, P.J.; Hong, T.; Schlub, T.E.; Chu, E.; Chang, A.A. Saffron therapy for the ongoing treatmer of age-related macular degeneration. *BMJ Open Ophthalmol.* **2024**, *9*, e001399. [CrossRef]
10. Brown, G.C.; Brown, M.M.; Gierhart, D.; Olk, R.J. Prevention Surpasses Treatment: 5-year Follow-Up, Cost-Utility, and Cos Benefit of Zeaxanthin Therapy for Neovascular Age-Related Macular Degeneration. *Ophthalmol. Ther.* **2023**, *12*, 2583–260 [CrossRef]
11. Evans, J.R.; Lawrenson, J.G. Antioxidant vitamin and mineral supplements for preventing age-related macular degeneratio *Cochrane Database Syst. Rev.* **2017**, *7*, CD000253. [CrossRef] [PubMed]
12. Mrowicka, M.; Mrowicki, J.; Kucharska, E.; Majsterek, I. Lutein and Zeaxanthin and Their Roles in Age-Related Macula Degeneration—Neurodegenerative Disease. *Nutrients* **2022**, *14*, 827. [CrossRef] [PubMed]
13. Li, L.H.; Lee, J.C.-Y.; Leung, H.H.; Lam, W.C.; Fu, Z.; Lo, A.C.Y. Lutein Supplementation for Eye Diseases. *Nutrients* **2020**, *12*, 172 [CrossRef] [PubMed]
14. Eisenhauer, B.; Natoli, S.; Liew, G.; Flood, V.M. Lutein and Zeaxanthin-Food Sources, Bioavailability and Dietary Variety i Age-Related Macular Degeneration Protection. *Nutrients* **2017**, *9*, 120. [CrossRef] [PubMed]
15. Carpentier, S.; Knaus, M.; Suh, M. Associations between lutein, zeaxanthin, and age-related macular degeneration: An overviev *Crit. Rev. Food Sci. Nutr.* **2009**, *49*, 313–326. [CrossRef] [PubMed]
16. Richer, S.; Stiles, W.; Statkute, L.; Pulido, J.; Frankowski, J.; Rudy, D.; Pei, K.; Tsipursky, M.; Nyland, J. Double-masked, placebc controlled, randomized trial of lutein and antioxidant supplementation in the intervention of atrophic age-related macula degeneration: The Veterans LAST study (Lutein Antioxidant Supplementation Trial). *Optometry* **2004**, *75*, 216–230. [CrossRef [PubMed]
17. Falsini, B.; Piccardi, M.; Iarossi, G.; Fadda, A.; Merendino, E.; Valentini, P. Influence of short-term antioxidant supplementation o macular function in age-related maculopathy. A pilot study including electrophysiologic assessment. *Ophthalmology* **2003**, *11* 51–60, discussion 61. [CrossRef] [PubMed]
18. Sujak, A.; Gabrielska, J.; Grudziński, W.; Borc, R.; Mazurek, P.; Gruszecki, W.I. Lutein and zeaxanthin as protectors of lipi membranes against oxidative damage: The structural aspects. *Arch. Biochem. Biophys.* **1999**, *371*, 301–307. [CrossRef] [PubMed]
19. Bone, R.A.; Ruiz, C.A.; Landrum, J.T.; Guerra, L.H. Lutein and zeaxanthin dietary supplements raise macular pigment densit and serum concentrations of these carotenoids in humans. *J. Nutr.* **2003**, *133*, 992–998. [CrossRef]
20. Junghans, A.; Sies, H.; Stahl, W. Macular pigments lutein and zeaxanthin as blue light filters studied in liposomes. *Arch. Biochem Biophys.* **2001**, *391*, 160–164. [CrossRef]
21. Krinsky, N.I.; Landrum, J.T.; Bone, R.A. Biologic mechanisms of the protective role of lutein and zeaxanthin in the eye. *Annu. Re Nutr.* **2003**, *23*, 171–201. [CrossRef] [PubMed]
22. Seddon, J.M.; Ajani, U.A.; Sperduto, R.D.; Hiller, R.; Blair, N.; Burton, T.C.; Farber, M.D.; Gragoudas, E.S.; Haller, J.; Miller, D.T et al. Dietary carotenoids, vitamins A, C, and E, and advanced age-related macular degeneration. *JAMA* **1994**, *272*, 1413–142 [CrossRef] [PubMed]
23. Age-Related Eye Disease Study 2 Research Group. Lutein + zeaxanthin and omega-3 fatty acids for age-related macula degeneration: The Age-Related Eye Disease Study 2 (AREDS2) randomized clinical trial. *JAMA* **2013**, *309*, 2005–2015. [CrossRef [PubMed]
24. Tanvetyanon, T.; Bepler, G. Beta-carotene in multivitamins and the possible risk of lung cancer among smokers versus forme smokers: A meta-analysis and evaluation of national brands. *Cancer* **2008**, *113*, 150–157. [CrossRef] [PubMed]
25. Wang, J.J.; Buitendijk, G.H.; Rochtchina, E.; Lee, K.E.; Klein, B.E.; van Duijn, C.M.; Flood, V.M.; Meuer, S.M.; Attia, J.; Myers, C et al. Genetic susceptibility, dietary antioxidants, and long-term incidence of age-related macular degeneration in two population *Ophthalmology* **2013**, *121*, 667–675. [CrossRef] [PubMed]
26. Liu, R.; Wang, T.; Zhang, B.; Qin, L.; Wu, C.; Li, Q.; Ma, L. Lutein and zeaxanthin supplementation and association with visua function in age-related macular degeneration. *Investig. Ophthalmol. Vis. Sci.* **2014**, *56*, 252–258. [CrossRef] [PubMed]
27. The Carmis Study Group; Piermarocchi, S.; Saviano, S.; Parisi, V.; Tedeschi, M.; Panozzo, G.; Scarpa, G.; Boschi, G.; Giudice, G.L Sartore, M.; et al. Carotenoids in Age-related Maculopathy Italian Study (CARMIS): Two-year results of a randomized study. *Eu J. Ophthalmol.* **2012**, *22*, 216–225. [CrossRef]
28. Bartlett, H.E.; Eperjesi, F. Effect of lutein and antioxidant dietary supplementation on contrast sensitivity in age-related macula disease: A randomized controlled trial. *Eur. J. Clin. Nutr.* **2007**, *61*, 1121–1127. [CrossRef] [PubMed]
29. Ma, L.; Yan, S.-F.; Huang, Y.-M.; Lu, X.-R.; Qian, F.; Pang, H.-L.; Xu, X.-R.; Zou, Z.-Y.; Dong, P.-C.; Xiao, X.; et al. Effect of lutein and zeaxanthin on macular pigment and visual function in patients with early age-related macular degeneration. *Ophthalmology* **2012**, *119*, 2290–2297. [CrossRef] [PubMed]
30. Weigert, G.; Kaya, S.; Pemp, B.; Sacu, S.; Lasta, M.; Werkmeister, R.M.; Dragostinoff, N.; Simader, C.; Garhöfer, G.; Schmidt-Erfurth U.; et al. Effects of lutein supplementation on macular pigment optical density and visual acuity in patients with age-related macular degeneration. *Investig. Opthalmol. Vis. Sci.* **2011**, *52*, 8174–8178. [CrossRef]

Dawczynski, J.; Jentsch, S.; Schweitzer, D.; Hammer, M.; Lang, G.E.; Strobel, J. Long term effects of lutein, zeaxanthin and omega-3-LCPUFAs supplementation on optical density of macular pigment in AMD patients: The LUTEGA study. *Graefe's Arch. Clin. Exp. Ophthalmol.* **2013**, *251*, 2711–2723. [CrossRef] [PubMed]
Murray, I.J.; Makridaki, M.; van der Veen, R.L.P.; Carden, D.; Parry, N.R.A.; Berendschot, T.T.J.M. Lutein supplementation over a one-year period in early AMD might have a mild beneficial effect on visual acuity: The CLEAR Study. *Investig. Opthalmol. Vis. Sci.* **2013**, *54*, 1781–1788. [CrossRef] [PubMed]
Beatty, S.; Chakravarthy, U.; Nolan, J.M.; Muldrew, K.A.; Woodside, J.V.; Denny, F.; Stevenson, M.R. Secondary outcomes in a clinical trial of carotenoids with coantioxidants versus placebo in early age-related macular degeneration. *Ophthalmology* **2013**, *120*, 600–606. [CrossRef] [PubMed]
Ambati, R.R.; Phang, S.M.; Ravi, S.; Aswathanarayana, R.G. Astaxanthin: Sources, extraction, stability, biological activities and its commercial applications-a review. *Mar. Drugs* **2014**, *12*, 128–152. [CrossRef] [PubMed]
Yuan, J.; Peng, J.; Yin, K.; Wang, J. Potential health-promoting effects of astaxanthin: A high-value carotenoid mostly from microalgae. *Mol. Nutr. Food Res.* **2010**, *55*, 150–165. [CrossRef] [PubMed]
Fakhri, S.; Abbaszadeh, F.; Dargahi, L.; Jorjani, M. Astaxanthin: A mechanistic review on its biological activities and health benefits. *Pharmacol. Res.* **2018**, *136*, 1–20. [CrossRef] [PubMed]
Giannaccare, G.; Pellegrini, M.; Senni, C.; Bernabei, F.; Scorcia, V.; Cicero, A.F.G. Clinical Applications of Astaxanthin in the Treatment of Ocular Diseases: Emerging Insights. *Mar. Drugs* **2020**, *18*, 239. [CrossRef] [PubMed]
Naguib, Y.M.A. Antioxidant Activities of Astaxanthin and related carotenoids. *J. Agric. Food Chem.* **2000**, *48*, 1150–1154. [CrossRef]
Lee, S.J.; Bai, S.K.; Lee, K.S.; Namkoong, S.; Na, H.J.; Ha, K.S.; Han, J.A.; Yim, S.V.; Chang, K.; Kwon, Y.G.; et al. Astaxanthin inhibits nitric oxide production and inflammatory gene expression by suppressing I(kappa)B kinase-dependent NF-kappaB activation. *Mol. Cells* **2003**, *16*, 97–105. [CrossRef]
Kidd, P. Astaxanthin, cell membrane nutrient with diverse clinical benefits and anti-aging potential. *Altern. Med. Rev.* **2011**, *16*, 355–364.
Parisi, V.; Tedeschi, M.; Gallinaro, G.; Varano, M.; Saviano, S.; Piermarocchi, S.; CARMIS Study Group. Carotenoids and antioxidants in age-related maculopathy italian study: Multifocal electroretinogram modifications after 1 year. *Ophthalmology* **2008**, *115*, 324–333.e2. [CrossRef] [PubMed]
Izumi-Nagai, K.; Nagai, N.; Ohgami, K.; Satofuka, S.; Ozawa, Y.; Tsubota, K.; Ohno, S.; Oike, Y.; Ishida, S. Inhibition of choroidal neovascularization with an anti-inflammatory carotenoid astaxanthin. *Investig. Ophthalmol. Vis. Sci.* **2008**, *49*, 1679–1685. [CrossRef] [PubMed]
Cicero, A.F.; Colletti, A. Effects of Carotenoids on Health: Are All the Same? Results from Clinical Trials. *Curr. Pharm. Des.* **2017**, *23*, 2422–2427. [CrossRef] [PubMed]
Gaynes, B.I. AREDS misses on safety. *Arch. Ophthalmol.* **2003**, *121*, 416–417. [CrossRef]
Bates, C.J. Vitamin A. *Lancet* **1995**, *345*, 31–35. [CrossRef]
Schmidl, D.; Garhöfer, G.; Schmetterer, L. Nutritional supplements in age-related macular degeneration. *Acta Ophthalmol.* **2015**, *93*, 105–121. [CrossRef] [PubMed]
Goldberg, J.; Flowerdew, G.; Smith, E.; Brody, J.A.; Tso, M.O. Factors associated with age-related macular degeneration. An analysis of data from the first National Health and Nutrition Examination Survey. *Am. J. Epidemiol.* **1988**, *128*, 700–710. [CrossRef]
de Koning-Backus, A.P.; Buitendijk, G.H.; Kiefte-de Jong, J.C.; Colijn, J.M.; Hofman, A.; Vingerling, J.R.; Haverkort, E.B.; Franco, O.H.; Klaver, C.C. Intake of Vegetables, Fruit, and Fish is Beneficial for Age-Related Macular Degeneration. *Am. J. Ophthalmol.* **2019**, *198*, 70–79. [CrossRef] [PubMed]
Delcourt, C.; Cristol, J.-P.; Tessier, F.; Léger, C.L.; Descomps, B.; Papoz, L. Age-related macular degeneration and antioxidant status in the POLA study. *Arch. Ophthalmol.* **1999**, *117*, 1384–1390. [CrossRef]
Monsen, E.R. Dietary reference intakes for the antioxidant nutrients: Vitamin C, vitamin E, selenium, and carotenoids. *J. Am. Diet. Assoc.* **2000**, *100*, 637–640. [CrossRef]
Organisciak, D.; Jiang, Y.; Wang, H.; Bicknell, I. The protective effect of ascorbic-acid in retinal light damage of rats exposed to intermittent light. *Investig. Ophthalmol. Vis. Sci.* **1990**, *31*, 1195–1202.
SanGiovanni, J.P.; Chew, E.Y.; Clemons, T.E.; Ferris, F.L., 3rd; Gensler, G.; Lindblad, A.S.; Milton, R.C.; Seddon, J.M.; Sperduto, R.D. The relationship of dietary carotenoid and vitamin A, E, and C intake with age-related macular degeneration in a case-control study: AREDS Report No. 22. *Arch. Ophthalmol.* **2007**, *125*, 1225–1232.
Eye Disease Case-Control Study Group. Antioxidant status and neovascular age-related macular degeneration. *Arch. Ophthalmol.* **1993**, *111*, 104–109. [CrossRef] [PubMed]
Olmedilla, B.; Granado, F.; Blanco, I.; Vaquero, M. Lutein, but not α-tocopherol, supplementation improves visual function in patients with age-related cataracts: A 2-y double-blind, placebo-controlled pilot study. *Nutrition* **2003**, *19*, 21–24. [CrossRef]
Alvarez, R.A.; Liou, G.I.; Fong, S.L.; Bridges, C.D. Levels of alpha- and gamma-tocopherol in human eyes: Evaluation of the possible role of IRBP in intraocular alpha-tocopherol transport. *Am. J. Clin. Nutr.* **1987**, *46*, 481–487. [CrossRef] [PubMed]
Stephens, R.; Negi, D.; Short, S.; van Kuijk, F.; Dratz, E.; Thomas, D. Vitamin E distribution in ocular tissues following long-term dietary depletion and supplementation as determined by microdissection and gas chromatography-mass spectrometry. *Exp. Eye Res.* **1988**, *47*, 237–245. [CrossRef]

57. West, S.; Vitale, S.; Hallfrisch, J.; Muñoz, B.; Muller, D.; Bressler, S.; Bressler, N.M. Are antioxidants or supplements protective f age-related macular degeneration? *Arch. Ophthalmol.* **1994**, *112*, 222–227. [CrossRef]
58. Mares-Perlman, J.A.; Brady, W.E.; Klein, R.; Klein, B.E.K.; Bowen, P.; Stacewicz-Sapuntzakis, M.; Palta, M. Serum antioxidants an age-related macular degeneration in a population-based case-control study. *Arch. Ophthalmol.* **1995**, *113*, 1518–1523. [CrossRef
59. Thurnham, D.I. Macular zeaxanthins and lutein—A review of dietary sources and bioavailability and some relationships wi macular pigment optical density and age-related macular disease. *Nutr. Res. Rev.* **2007**, *20*, 163–179. [CrossRef]
60. Taylor, H.R.; Tikellis, G.; Robman, L.D.; McCarty, C.A.; McNeil, J.J. Vitamin E supplementation and macular degeneratio Randomised controlled trial. *BMJ* **2002**, *325*, 11. [CrossRef]
61. King, J.C.; Shames, D.M.; Woodhouse, L.R. Zinc homeostasis in humans. *J. Nutr.* **2000**, *130* (Suppl. 5S), 1360S–1366S. [CrossRe [PubMed]
62. Blasiak, J.; Pawlowska, E.; Chojnacki, J.; Szczepanska, J.; Chojnacki, C.; Kaarniranta, K. Zinc and Autophagy in Age-Relate Macular Degeneration. *Int. J. Mol. Sci.* **2020**, *21*, 4994. [CrossRef] [PubMed]
63. Duan, M.; Li, T.; Liu, B.; Yin, S.; Zang, J.; Lv, C.; Zhao, G.; Zhang, T. Zinc nutrition and dietary zinc supplements. *Crit. Rev. Foc Sci. Nutr.* **2021**, *63*, 1277–1292. [CrossRef] [PubMed]
64. Fosmire, G.J. Zinc toxicity. *Am. J. Clin. Nutr.* **1990**, *51*, 225–227. [CrossRef] [PubMed]
65. McCall, K.A.; Huang, C.-C.; Fierke, C.A. Function and mechanism of zinc metalloenzymes. *J. Nutr.* **2000**, *130* (Suppl. 5S 1437S–1446S. [CrossRef] [PubMed]
66. Ripps, H.; Chappell, R.L. Zinc's functional significance in the vertebrate retina. *Mol. Vis.* **2014**, *20*, 1067–1074. [PubMed]
67. Leung, E.; Landa, G. Update on current and future novel therapies for dry age-related macular degeneration. *Expert Rev. Cli Pharmacol.* **2013**, *6*, 565–579. [CrossRef]
68. Newsome, D.A.; Swartz, M.; Leone, N.C.; Elston, R.C.; Miller, E. Oral zinc in macular degeneration. *Arch. Ophthalmol.* **1988**, *10* 192–198. [CrossRef]
69. Tittl, M.; Reitner, A.; Meisinger, V.; Stur, M. Oral zinc and the second eye in age-related macular degeneration. *Investig. Ophthalmc Vis. Sci.* **1996**, *37*, 1225–1235. [CrossRef]
70. Cho, E.; Stampfer, M.J.; Seddon, J.M.; Hung, S.; Spiegelman, D.; Rimm, E.B.; Willett, W.C.; Hankinson, S.E. Prospective study c zinc intake and the risk of age-related macular degeneration. *Ann. Epidemiol.* **2001**, *11*, 328–336. [CrossRef]
71. Wong, P.; Markey, M.; Rapp, C.M.; Darrow, R.M.; Ziesel, A.; Organisciak, D. Enhancing the efficacy of AREDS antioxidants i light-induced retinal degeneration. *Mol. Vis.* **2017**, *23*, 718–739. [PubMed]
72. Ursini, F.; Bindoli, A. The role of selenium peroxidases in the protection against oxidative damage of membranes. *Chem. Phy Lipids* **1987**, *44*, 255–276. [CrossRef] [PubMed]
73. Surette, M.E. The science behind dietary omega-3 fatty acids. *CMAJ* **2008**, *178*, 177–180. [CrossRef] [PubMed]
74. Cholewski, M.; Tomczykowa, M.; Tomczyk, M. A Comprehensive Review of Chemistry, Sources and Bioavailability of Omega- Fatty Acids. *Nutrients* **2018**, *10*, 1662. [CrossRef] [PubMed]
75. Calder, P.C.; Grimble, R.F. Polyunsaturated fatty acids, inflammation and immunity. *Eur. J. Clin. Nutr.* **2002**, *56* (Suppl. 3), S14–S1 [CrossRef] [PubMed]
76. SanGiovanni, J.P.; Chew, E.Y. The role of omega-3 long-chain polyunsaturated fatty acids in health and disease of the retina. *Pro Retin. Eye Res.* **2004**, *24*, 87–138. [CrossRef] [PubMed]
77. Tuo, J.; Ross, R.J.; Herzlich, A.A.; Shen, D.; Ding, X.; Zhou, M.; Coon, S.L.; Hussein, N.; Salem, N., Jr.; Chan, C.-C. A High omega- fatty acid diet reduces retinal lesions in a murine model of macular degeneration. *Am. J. Pathol.* **2009**, *175*, 799–807. [CrossRe [PubMed]
78. Calder, P.C. Omega-3 fatty acids and inflammatory processes: From molecules to man. *Biochem. Soc. Trans.* **2017**, *45*, 1105–111 [CrossRef] [PubMed]
79. Gross, B.W.; Gillio, M.; Rinehart, C.D.; Lynch, C.A.; Rogers, F.B. Omega-3 Fatty Acid Supplementation and Warfarin: A Letha Combination in Traumatic Brain Injury. *J. Trauma Nurs.* **2017**, *24*, 15–18. [CrossRef] [PubMed]
80. Prokopiou, E.; Kolovos, P.; Kalogerou, M.; Neokleous, A.; Papagregoriou, G.; Deltas, C.; Malas, S.; Georgiou, T. Therapeuti potential of omega-3 fatty acids supplementation in a mouse model of dry macular degeneration. *BMJ Open Ophthalmol.* **201** *1*, e000056. [CrossRef]
81. Dornstauder, B.; Suh, M.; Kuny, S.; Gaillard, F.; MacDonald, I.M.; Clandinin, M.T.; Sauvé, Y. Dietary docosahexaenoic aci supplementation prevents age-related functional losses and A2E accumulation in the retina. *Investig. Opthalmol. Vis. Sci.* **2012**, *5* 2256–2265. [CrossRef] [PubMed]
82. Ramkumar, H.L.; Tuo, J.; Shen, D.F.; Zhang, J.; Cao, X.; Chew, E.Y.; Chan, C.C. Nutrient supplementation with n3 polyunsaturate fatty acids, lutein, and zeaxanthin decrease A2E accumulation and VEGF expression in the retinas of Ccl2/Cx3cr1-deficient mic on Crb1rd8 background. *J. Nutr.* **2013**, *143*, 1129–1135. [CrossRef] [PubMed]
83. Qiu, S.; Wei, Y.; Zhou, X.; Jiang, Z.; Zhang, T.; Jiang, X.; Zhang, S. Intravitreal injection of docosahexaenoic acid attenuate photoreceptor cell injury in a NaIO 3 -induced age-related macular degeneration rat model. *Neurosci. Lett.* **2017**, *657*, 53–6 [CrossRef] [PubMed]
84. Chew, E.Y.; Clemons, T.; SanGiovanni, J.P.; Danis, R.; Domalpally, A.; McBee, W.; Sperduto, R.; Ferris, F.L.; AREDS2 Researc Group. The Age-Related Eye Disease Study 2 (AREDS2): Study design and baseline characteristics (AREDS2 report number 1 *Ophthalmology* **2012**, *119*, 2282–2289. [CrossRef] [PubMed]

85. Georgiou, T.; Prokopiou, E. The New Era of Omega-3 Fatty Acids Supplementation: Therapeutic Effects on Dry Age-Related Macular Degeneration. *J. Stem Cells* **2015**, *10*, 205–215. [PubMed]
86. Franzone, F.; Nebbioso, M.; Pergolizzi, T.; Attanasio, G.; Musacchio, A.; Greco, A.; Limoli, P.G.; Artico, M.; Spandidos, D.A.; Taurone, S.; et al. Anti-inflammatory role of curcumin in retinal disorders (Review). *Exp. Ther. Med.* **2021**, *22*, 790. [CrossRef]
87. Martínez-Solís, I.; Bosch-Morell, F.; Villagrasa, V.; Ortega, T.; Acero, N.; Muñoz-Mingarro, D.; González-Rosende, M.E.; Castillo, E.; Sanahuja, M.A.; Soriano, P. Medicinal plants and natural products as neuroprotective agents in age-related macular degeneration. *Neural Regen. Res.* **2020**, *15*, 2207–2216. [CrossRef] [PubMed]
88. Jurenka, J.S. Anti-inflammatory properties of curcumin, a major constituent of Curcuma longa: A review of preclinical and clinical research. *Altern. Med. Rev.* **2009**, *14*, 141–153. [PubMed]
89. Aggarwal, B.B.; Harikumar, K.B. Potential therapeutic effects of curcumin, the anti-inflammatory agent, against neurodegenerative, cardiovascular, pulmonary, metabolic, autoimmune and neoplastic diseases. *Int. J. Biochem. Cell Biol.* **2008**, *41*, 40–59. [CrossRef]
90. Schaffer, M.; Schaffer, P.M.; Zidan, J.; Sela, G.B. Curcuma as a functional food in the control of cancer and inflammation. *Curr. Opin. Clin. Nutr. Metab. Care* **2011**, *14*, 588–597. [CrossRef]
91. Hewlings, S.J.; Kalman, D.S. Curcumin: A Review of Its Effects on Human Health. *Foods* **2017**, *6*, 92. [CrossRef] [PubMed]
92. Allegra, A.; Innao, V.; Russo, S.; Gerace, D.; Alonci, A.; Musolino, C. Anticancer Activity of Curcumin and Its Analogues: Preclinical and Clinical Studies. *Cancer Investig.* **2017**, *35*, 1–22. [CrossRef] [PubMed]
93. Radomska-Leśniewska, D.M.; Osiecka-Iwan, A.; Hyc, A.; Góźdź, A.; Dąbrowska, A.M.; Skopiński, P. Therapeutic potential of curcumin in eye diseases. *Cent. Eur. J. Immunol.* **2019**, *44*, 181–189. [CrossRef] [PubMed]
94. Peddada, K.V.; Brown, A.; Verma, V.; Nebbioso, M. Therapeutic potential of curcumin in major retinal pathologies. *Int. Ophthalmol.* **2018**, *39*, 725–734. [CrossRef] [PubMed]
95. Mandal, N.A.; Patlolla, J.M.; Zheng, L.; Agbaga, M.-P.; Tran, J.-T.A.; Wicker, L.; Kasus-Jacobi, A.; Elliott, M.H.; Rao, C.V.; Anderson, R.E. Curcumin protects retinal cells from light-and oxidant stress-induced cell death. *Free Radic. Biol. Med.* **2009**, *46*, 672–679. [CrossRef] [PubMed]
96. Lu, J.; Zhu, W.; Wu, Y.; Meng, Y.-F.; Wang, J.-Y.; Xu, M.; Tao, J.-J. Effect of curcumin on aging retinal pigment epithelial cells. *Drug Des. Dev. Ther.* **2015**, *9*, 5337–5344. [CrossRef] [PubMed]
97. Howell, J.C.; Chun, E.; Farrell, A.N.; Hur, E.Y.; Caroti, C.M.; Iuvone, P.M.; Haque, R. Global microRNA expression profiling: Curcumin (diferuloylmethane) alters oxidative stress-responsive microRNAs in human ARPE-19 cells. *Mol. Vis.* **2013**, *19*, 544–560. [PubMed]
98. Saberi-Karimian, M.; Katsiki, N.; Caraglia, M.; Boccellino, M.; Majeed, M.; Sahebkar, A. Vascular endothelial growth factor: An important molecular target of curcumin. *Crit. Rev. Food Sci. Nutr.* **2019**, *59*, 299–312. [CrossRef] [PubMed]
99. Anand, P.; Kunnumakkara, A.B.; Newman, R.A.; Aggarwal, B.B. Bioavailability of curcumin: Problems and promises. *Mol. Pharm.* **2007**, *4*, 807–818. [CrossRef]
100. Pescosolido, N.; Giannotti, R.; Plateroti, A.M.; Pascarella, A.; Nebbioso, M. Curcumin: Therapeutical potential in ophthalmology. *Planta Medica* **2013**, *80*, 249–254. [CrossRef]
101. Soleimani, V.; Sahebkar, A.; Hosseinzadeh, H. Turmeric (Curcuma longa) and its major constituent (curcumin) as nontoxic and safe substances: Review. *Phyther. Res.* **2018**, *32*, 985–995. [CrossRef] [PubMed]
102. Heitmar, R.; Brown, J.; Kyrou, I. Saffron (*Crocus sativus* L.) in Ocular Diseases: A Narrative Review of the Existing Evidence from Clinical Studies. *Nutrients* **2019**, *11*, 649. [CrossRef] [PubMed]
103. Hatziagapiou, K.; Kakouri, E.; Lambrou, G.I.; Bethanis, K.; Tarantilis, P.A. Antioxidant Properties of *Crocus sativus* L. and Its Constituents and Relevance to Neurodegenerative Diseases; Focus on Alzheimer's and Parkinson's Disease. *Curr. Neuropharmacol.* **2019**, *17*, 377–402. [CrossRef] [PubMed]
104. Di Marco, S.; Carnicelli, V.; Franceschini, N.; Di Paolo, M.; Piccardi, M.; Bisti, S.; Falsini, B. Saffron: A Multitask Neuroprotective Agent for Retinal Degenerative Diseases. *Antioxidants* **2019**, *8*, 224. [CrossRef] [PubMed]
105. Nam, K.N.; Park, Y.-M.; Jung, H.-J.; Lee, J.Y.; Min, B.D.; Park, S.-U.; Jung, W.-S.; Cho, K.-H.; Park, J.-H.; Kang, I.; et al. Anti-inflammatory effects of crocin and crocetin in rat brain microglial cells. *Eur. J. Pharmacol.* **2010**, *648*, 110–116. [CrossRef] [PubMed]
106. Ohno, Y.; Nakanishi, T.; Umigai, N.; Tsuruma, K.; Shimazawa, M.; Hara, H. Oral administration of crocetin prevents inner retinal damage induced by N-methyl-d-aspartate in mice. *Eur. J. Pharmacol.* **2012**, *690*, 84–89. [CrossRef]
107. Xuan, B.; Zhou, Y.-H.; Li, N.; Min, Z.-D.; Chiou, G.C. Effects of crocin analogs on ocular blood flow and retinal function. *J. Ocul. Pharmacol. Ther.* **1999**, *15*, 143–152. [CrossRef] [PubMed]
108. Falsini, B.; Piccardi, M.; Minnella, A.; Savastano, C.; Capoluongo, E.; Fadda, A.; Balestrazzi, E.; Maccarone, R.; Bisti, S. Influence of saffron supplementation on retinal flicker sensitivity in early age-related macular degeneration. *Investig. Ophthalmol. Vis. Sci.* **2010**, *51*, 6118–6124. [CrossRef]
109. Piccardi, M.; Marangoni, D.; Minnella, A.M.; Savastano, M.C.; Valentini, P.; Ambrosio, L.; Capoluongo, E.; Maccarone, R.; Bisti, S.; Falsini, B. A Longitudinal follow-up study of saffron supplementation in early age-related macular degeneration: Sustained benefits to central retinal function. *Evid.-Based Complement. Altern. Med.* **2012**, *2012*, 429124. [CrossRef]

110. Marangoni, D.; Falsini, B.; Piccardi, M.; Ambrosio, L.; Minnella, A.M.; Savastano, M.C.; Bisti, S.; Maccarone, R.; Fadda, A. Mello, E.; et al. Functional effect of Saffron supplementation and risk genotypes in early age-related macular degeneration: A preliminary report. *J. Transl. Med.* **2013**, *11*, 228. [CrossRef]
111. Lashay, A.; Sadough, G.; Ashrafi, E.; Lashay, M.; Movassat, M.; Akhondzadeh, S. Short-term Outcomes of Saffron Supplementatio in Patients with Age-related Macular Degeneration: A Double-blind, Placebo-controlled, Randomized Trial. *Med. Hypothesi Discov. Innov. Ophthalmol.* **2016**, *5*, 32–38.
112. Riazi, A.; Panahi, Y.; Alishiri, A.A.; Hosseini, M.A.; Karimi Zarchi, A.A.; Sahebkar, A. The impact of saffron (*Crocus sativus* supplementation on visual function in patients with dry age-related macular degeneration. *Ital. J. Med.* **2016**, *10*, 196–201 [CrossRef]
113. Broadhead, G.K.; Grigg, J.R.; McCluskey, P.; Hong, T.; Schlub, T.E.; Chang, A.A. Saffron therapy for the treatment o mild/moderate age-related macular degeneration: A randomised clinical trial. *Graefes Arch. Clin. Exp. Ophthalmol.* **2019**, *257* 31–40. [CrossRef]
114. Amaral, F.G.D.; Cipolla-Neto, J. A brief review about melatonin, a pineal hormone. *Arq. Bras. de Endocrinol. Metabol.* **2018**, *62* 472–479. [CrossRef] [PubMed]
115. Alarma-Estrany, P.; Pintor, J. Melatonin receptors in the eye: Location, second messengers and role in ocular physiology. *Pharmaco Ther.* **2006**, *113*, 507–522. [CrossRef]
116. Alkozi, H.A.; Wang, X.; de Lara, M.J.P.; Pintor, J. Presence of melanopsin in human crystalline lens epithelial cells and its role ir melatonin synthesis. *Exp. Eye Res.* **2017**, *154*, 168–176. [CrossRef]
117. Reiter, R.J.; Tan, D.X.; Fuentes-Broto, L. Melatonin: A multitasking molecule. *Prog Brain Res.* **2010**, *181*, 127–151.
118. Poeggeler, B.; Reiter, R.J.; Tan, D.X.; Chen, L.D.; Manchester, L.C. Melatonin, hydroxyl radical-mediated oxidative damage, and aging: A hypothesis. *J. Pineal Res.* **1993**, *14*, 151–168. [CrossRef]
119. Crooke, A.; Huete-Toral, F.; Colligris, B.; Pintor, J. The role and therapeutic potential of melatonin in age-related ocular diseases. *J Pineal Res.* **2017**, *63*, e12430. [CrossRef] [PubMed]
120. Dehdashtian, E.; Mehrzadi, S.; Yousefi, B.; Hosseinzadeh, A.; Reiter, R.J.; Safa, M.; Ghaznavi, H.; Naseripour, M. Diabetic retinopathy pathogenesis and the ameliorating effects of melatonin; involvement of autophagy, inflammation and oxidative stress. *Life Sci.* **2018**, *193*, 20–33. [CrossRef]
121. Mehrzadi, S.; Hemati, K.; Reiter, R.J.; Hosseinzadeh, A. Mitochondrial dysfunction in age-related macular degeneration: Melatonir as a potential treatment. *Expert Opin. Ther. Targets* **2020**, *24*, 359–378. [CrossRef] [PubMed]
122. Fu, Y.; Tang, M.; Fan, Y.; Zou, H.; Sun, X.; Xu, X. Anti-apoptotic effects of melatonin in retinal pigment epithelial cells. *Front Biosci.* **2012**, *17*, 1461–1468. [CrossRef] [PubMed]
123. Rosen, R.; Hu, D.-N.; Perez, V.; Tai, K.; Yu, G.-P.; Chen, M.; Tone, P.; McCormick, S.A.; Walsh, J. Urinary 6-sulfatoxymelatonin level in age-related macular degeneration patients. *Mol. Vis.* **2009**, *15*, 1673–1679. [PubMed]
124. Yi, C.; Pan, X.; Yan, H.; Guo, M.; Pierpaoli, W. Effects of melatonin in age-related macular degeneration. *Ann. N. Y. Acad. Sci.* **2005** *1057*, 384–392. [CrossRef] [PubMed]
125. Yao, J.; Jia, L.; Shelby, S.J.; Ganios, A.M.; Feathers, K.; Thompson, D.A.; Zacks, D.N. Circadian and noncircadian modulation of autophagy in photoreceptors and retinal pigment epithelium. *Investig. Opthalmol. Vis. Sci.* **2014**, *55*, 3237–3246. [CrossRef] [PubMed]
126. Grace, M.S.; Chiba, A.; Menaker, M. Circadian control of photoreceptor outer segment membrane turnover in mice genetically incapable of melatonin synthesis. *Vis. Neurosci.* **1999**, *16*, 909–918. [CrossRef] [PubMed]
127. Organisciak, D.T.; Darrow, R.M.; Barsalou, L.; Kutty, R.K.; Wiggert, B. Circadian-dependent retinal light damage in rats. *Investig Ophthalmol. Vis. Sci.* **2000**, *41*, 3694–3701.
128. Seagle, B.-L.L.; Rezai, K.A.; Kobori, Y.; Gasyna, E.M.; Rezaei, K.A.; Norris, J.R. Melanin photoprotection in the human retinal pigment epithelium and its correlation with light-induced cell apoptosis. *Proc. Natl. Acad. Sci. USA* **2005**, *102*, 8978–8983 [CrossRef] [PubMed]
129. Kaur, C.; Sivakumar, V.; Yong, Z.; Lu, J.; Foulds, W.; Ling, E. Blood–retinal barrier disruption and ultrastructural changes in the hypoxic retina in adult rats: The beneficial effect of melatonin administration. *J. Pathol.* **2007**, *212*, 429–439. [CrossRef]
130. Ambati, J.; Ambati, B.K.; Yoo, S.H.; Ianchulev, S.; Adamis, A.P. Age-related macular degeneration: Etiology, pathogenesis, and therapeutic strategies. *Surv. Ophthalmol.* **2003**, *48*, 257–293. [CrossRef]
131. Pameijer, E.M.; Heus, P.; Damen, J.A.A.; Spijker, R.; Hooft, L.; Ringens, P.J.; Imhof, S.M.; van Leeuwen, R. What did we learn in 35 years of research on nutrition and supplements for age-related macular degeneration: A systematic review. *Acta Ophthalmol.* **2022** *100*, E1541–E1552. [CrossRef] [PubMed]
132. Wu, Y.; Xie, Y.; Yuan, Y.; Xiong, R.; Hu, Y.; Ning, K.; Ha, J.; Wang, W.; Han, X.; He, M. The Mediterranean Diet and Age-Related Eye Diseases: A Systematic Review. *Nutrients* **2023**, *15*, 2043. [CrossRef] [PubMed]
133. Merle, B.M.; Silver, R.E.; Rosner, B.; Seddon, J.M. Adherence to a Mediterranean diet, genetic susceptibility, and progression to advanced macular degeneration: A prospective cohort study. *Am. J. Clin. Nutr.* **2015**, *102*, 1196–1206. [CrossRef]
134. Merle, B.M.; Colijn, J.M.; Cougnard-Grégoire, A.; de Koning-Backus, A.P.; Delyfer, M.N.; Kiefte-de Jong, J.C.; Meester-Smoor, M. Féart, C.; Verzijden, T.; Samieri, C.; et al. Mediterranean Diet and Incidence of Advanced Age-Related Macular Degeneration: The EYE-RISK Consortium. *Ophthalmology* **2019**, *126*, 381–390. [CrossRef] [PubMed]

5. Chapman, N.A.; Jacobs, R.J.; Braakhuis, A.J. Role of diet and food intake in age-related macular degeneration: A systematic review. *Clin. Exp. Ophthalmol.* **2018**, *47*, 106–127. [CrossRef] [PubMed]
6. Chong, E.W.; Kreis, A.J.; Wong, T.Y.; Simpson, J.A.; Guymer, R.H. Dietary omega-3 fatty acid and fish intake in the primary prevention of age-related macular degeneration: A systematic review and meta-analysis. *Arch. Ophthalmol.* **2008**, *126*, 826–833. [CrossRef] [PubMed]
7. Christen, W.G.; Schaumberg, D.A.; Glynn, R.J.; Buring, J.E. Dietary omega-3 fatty acid and fish intake and incident age-related macular degeneration in women. *Arch. Ophthalmol.* **2011**, *129*, 921–929. [CrossRef] [PubMed]
8. Chong, E.W.-T.; Simpson, J.A.; Robman, L.D.; Hodge, A.M.; Aung, K.Z.; English, D.R.; Giles, G.G.; Guymer, R.H. Red meat and chicken consumption and its association with age-related macular degeneration. *Am. J. Epidemiol.* **2009**, *169*, 867–876. [CrossRef] [PubMed]
9. Kaushik, S.; Wang, J.J.; Flood, V.; Tan, J.S.L.; Barclay, A.W.; Wong, T.Y.; Brand-Miller, J.; Mitchell, P. Dietary glycemic index and the risk of age-related macular degeneration. *Am. J. Clin. Nutr.* **2008**, *88*, 1104–1110. [CrossRef]
0. Chiu, C.-J.; Milton, R.C.; Klein, R.; Gensler, G.; Taylor, A. Dietary carbohydrate and the progression of age-related macular degeneration: A prospective study from the Age-Related Eye Disease Study. *Am. J. Clin. Nutr.* **2007**, *86*, 1210–1218. [CrossRef]
1. Dinu, M.; Pagliai, G.; Casini, A.; Sofi, F. Food groups and risk of age-related macular degeneration: A systematic review with meta-analysis. *Eur. J. Nutr.* **2019**, *58*, 2123–2143. [CrossRef] [PubMed]
2. Kuan, V.; Warwick, A.; Hingorani, A.; Tufail, A.; Cipriani, V.; Burgess, S.; Sofat, R.; Fritsche, L.G.; Igl, W.; Bailey, J.N.; et al. Association of Smoking, Alcohol Consumption, Blood Pressure, Body Mass Index, and Glycemic Risk Factors With Age-Related Macular Degeneration: A Mendelian Randomization Study. *JAMA Ophthalmol.* **2021**, *139*, 1299–1306. [CrossRef] [PubMed]
3. Lixi, F.; Vitiello, L.; Giannaccare, G. Marine Natural Products Rescuing the Eye: A Narrative Review. *Mar. Drugs* **2024**, *22*, 155. [CrossRef] [PubMed]
4. Vitiello, L.; Capasso, L.; Cembalo, G.; De Pascale, I.; Imparato, R.; De Bernardo, M. Herbal and Natural Treatments for the Management of the Glaucoma: An Update. *BioMed Res. Int.* **2023**, *2023*, 3105251. [CrossRef]
5. D'angelo, A.; Vitiello, L.; Lixi, F.; Abbinante, G.; Coppola, A.; Gagliardi, V.; Pellegrino, A.; Giannaccare, G. Optic Nerve Neuroprotection in Glaucoma: A Narrative Review. *J. Clin. Med.* **2024**, *13*, 2214. [CrossRef]